THE ROUTLEDGE INTERNATIONAL HANDBOOK OF PSYCHOLINGUISTIC AND COGNITIVE PROCESSES

This handbook provides a comprehensive overview of the theories of cognition and language processing relevant to the field of communication disorders. Thoroughly updated in its second edition, the book explores a range of topics and issues that illustrate the relevance of a dynamic interaction between both theoretical and applied clinical work.

Beginning with the origins of language evolution, the authors explore a range of both developmental and acquired communication disorders, reflecting the variety and complexity of psycholinguistics and its role in extending our knowledge of communication disorders. The first section outlines some of the major theoretical approaches from psycholinguistics and cognitive neuroscience that have been influential in research focusing on clinical populations, while Section II features examples from researchers who have applied this body of knowledge to developmental disorders of communication. Section III features examples focusing on acquired language disorders, and finally, Section IV considers psycholinguistic approaches to gesture, sign language, and alternative and augmentative communication (AAC). The new edition features new chapters offering fresh perspectives, further reading recommendations, and a new epilogue from Jackie Guendouzi.

This valuable text serves as a single interdisciplinary resource for graduate and upper-level undergraduate students in cognitive neurosciences, psychology, communication sciences and disorders, as well as researchers new to the field of communication disorders or to psycholinguistic theory.

Jackie Guendouzi, Ph.D., is a Professor and department head of Health and Human Sciences at Southeastern Louisiana University, United States.

Filip Loncke, Ph.D., is a Professor at the University of Virginia's School of Education and Human Development, United States.

Mandy J. Williams, Ph.D., CCC-SLP, is an Associate Professor of Communication Sciences and Disorders at the University of South Dakota, United States.

THE ROUTLEDGE INTERNATIONAL HANDBOOK OF PSYCHOLINGUISTIC AND COGNITIVE PROCESSES

Second Edition

Edited by Jackie Guendouzi, Filip Loncke and Mandy J. Williams

Routledge
Taylor & Francis Group
NEW YORK AND LONDON

Designed cover image: © Getty Images

Second edition published 2023
by Routledge
605 Third Avenue, New York, NY 10158

and by Routledge
4 Park Square, Milton Park, Abingdon, Oxon, OX14 4RN

Routledge is an imprint of the Taylor & Francis Group, an informa business

First edition published by Psychology Press 2010

Library of Congress Cataloging-in-Publication Data
A catalog record has been requested for this book

ISBN: 978-1-032-06866-4 (hbk)
ISBN: 978-1-032-06864-0 (pbk)
ISBN: 978-1-003-20421-3 (ebk)

DOI: 10.4324/9781003204213

Typeset in Bembo
by Deanta Global Publishing Services, Chennai, India

CONTENTS

EDITORS

Jackie Guendouzi, Ph.D., is a Professor and Department Head of Health and Human Sciences at Southeastern Louisiana University, USA. She obtained both her undergraduate and graduate degrees in Linguistics and Communication at Cardiff University in Wales, UK. Her main area of clinical research has been investigating communication in the context of dementia.

Filip Loncke, Ph.D., is a Professor of Education at the University ofVirginia School of Education and Human Development, USA. He teaches courses in Psycholinguistics, Speech Science, and Augmentative and Alternative Communication. His interest is in commonalities and distinctions between natural speech generation and processing and the generation and processing of messages in non-speech modalities. isHis

Mandy J. Williams, Ph.D., CCC-SLP, is an Associate Professor in the Department of Communication Sciences & Disorders at the University of South Dakota, USA. She is a licensed Speech Language Pathologist. She obtained her master's and graduate degrees at the University of Nevada, USA. Her research focuses on children and adults with fluency disorders. She teaches graduate courses in acquired disorders of language and cognition, fluency disorders, craniofacial anomalies, and voice disorders.

CONTRIBUTORS

Lise Abrams is the Peter W. Stanley Chair of Linguistics and Cognitive Science at Pomona College, USA. She double-majored in psychology and mathematics at Pomona, then earned her graduate degree in Cognitive Psychology from the University of California, USA. After 20 years as a faculty member in the Department of Psychology at the University of Florida, USA, she returned to Pomona as a faculty member in 2018 and established the Psycholinguistic Research in Memory (PRIME) Laboratory. Her research investigates the causes underlying real-world retrieval problems, including tip-of-the-tongue states, difficulties retrieving proper names, and interference from emotional words during speech production. She is also an Associate Editor for the journal *Psychology and Aging*.

Hermann Ackermann has a master's degree in Philosophy and Psychology, and a medical degree in Neurology. He is a Professor for Neurological Rehabilitation at the Medical School, University of Tübingen, Germany, and head of the Research Group Neurophonetics at the HERTIE-Institute for Clinical Neurosciences, University ofTübingen. He is also head of the Department of Neurological Rehabilitation at the Rehabiliation Center Hohenurach, Bad Urach.

Roa'a Alsulaiman was awarded her graduate degree in 2022 by the University College London (UCL), UK, for work conducted in the division of Psychology and Language sciences. She trained in the Speech and Intervention lab and worked primarily on assessment of stuttering in preschool children, with a focus on Arabic children with English as an additional language. She continues to work on research projects related to speech disfluencies and early intervention in Saudi Arabia and in collaboration with UCL. She is currently an assistant professor in the college of Education at King Saud University.

Sharon Armon-Lotem finished her graduate degree in Linguistics (syntax and language acquisition) at Tel-Aviv University, Israel, in 1997. She is a Professor of Linguistics at Bar-Ilan University, Israel. She studies language acquisition in typically developing bilingual preschool children and bilingual children with specific language impairments (SLI) focusing on syntax and morphosyntax.

Dana Arthur is an Assistant Professor in the Department of Communication Sciences at the State University of New York, USA. Her research interests include the language literacy connection in language-disordered populations, particularly in children with SLI.

Hadeel Ayyad is an Assistant Professor in the Department of Communication Disorders and Sciences (Life Sciences) at Kuwait University. Her area of interest is phonological development and disorders of Kuwaiti children from a nonlinear phonological perspective, including for children with Down Syndrome. She is a collaborator on the cross-linguistic project of Drs Bernhardt and Stemberger on phonological acquisition, and also on a project in speech development in children with cleft lip and palate.

Martin J. Ball is an Honorary Professor of Linguistics at Bangor University and Visiting Professor in Speech-Language Pathology at Wrexham Glyndŵr University, both in Wales, UK. He previously held positions in Wales, Ireland, the US, and Sweden. He co-edits two academic journals and two book series. He has published widely in communication disorders, phonetics, sociolinguistics, bilingualism, and Welsh linguistics. He recently edited the *Manual of Clinical Phonetics* for Routledge publishers (2021). He is an honorary fellow of the Royal College of Speech and Language Therapists, and a fellow of the Learned Society of Wales. He currently lives in the Republic of Ireland.

Ursula Bellugi passed away on April 17, 2022. She was a pioneer in the study of the biological foundation of language. She is regarded as the founder of the neurobiology of American Sign Language because her work was the first to show it is a true language, complete with grammar and syntax, and is processed by many of the same parts of the brain that process spoken language. Her work has led to the discovery that the left hemisphere of the human brain becomes specialized for languages, whether spoken or signed, a striking demonstration of neuronal plasticity. She studied cognitive neuroscience with emphasis on American Sign Language and Williams Syndrome.

Barbara M. Bernhardt is a Professor Emerita (since 2017) and was also a speech-language pathologist (to 2019). Her primary focus is children's phonological acquisition, assessment, and intervention, (including visual feedback in speech habilitation); she has been involved in a cross-linguistic project since 2006 with Dr Joseph Stemberger, and international colleagues.

Martha S. Burns is employed in the neuroscience education industry and serves on the Faculty of Northwestern University, USA, in the area of cognitive and communication neuroscience. She is a Fellow of the American Speech-Language-Hearing Association and has received honors from Northwestern University, other universities, hospitals, and professional organizations. She has authored five books and over 100 book chapters and articles.

Hiram Brownell is a Professor in the Department of Psychology and Neuroscience at Boston College, UAS. His areas of interest include cognitive-linguistic disorders in adults with acquired brain injury and methodology.

José G. Centeno is a Professor in the Department of Rehabilitation and Movement Sciences at Rutgers University, USA. His teaching and research focus on stroke-related impairments and aspects of service delivery in monolingual Spanish/bilingual Spanish–English adults.

Beverly Collisson is a Research Associate Professor at the University of Calgary. She is affiliated with the Department of Pediatrics, Cumming School of Medicine, the Owerko Centre at the Alberta Children's Hospital Research Institute, University of Calgary, Canada. Her clinical and research interests lie in the area of semantic development in typical and atypical language learners.

Nelson Cowan obtained his graduate degree in 1980, from the University of Wisconsin, USA. He is a Curators' Professor of Psychological Sciences at the University of Missouri, UAS. His research on working memory, its relation to attention, and its childhood development has recently demonstrated a capacity limit in adults of only three to five items, unless the items can be rehearsed or grouped together. His books include *Working Memory the State of the Science, Attention and Memory: An Integrated Framework*, and *Working Memory Capacity*.

Clothilde Degroot is Managing Director of the Neuro Genomics Partnership at the Neuro (Montreal Neurological Institute-Hospital) – McGill University, Canada. She has published widely in the area of neurodegenerative diseases.

Devin Dickinson received their undergraduate degree in Psychology at the University of South Alabama, USA. They are currently a master's student enrolled in the University of South Alabama's Behavioral and Brain Sciences program. Their recent research interest focuses on semantic processing in visual word recognition with verbs and how this interacts with individual differences in participants.

Susan Duncan is a psycholinguist and has published widely on the topic of gesture.

Manuela Friedrich obtained a graduate degree from the Institute for Psychology, Humboldt-University, Berlin, and also a diploma in mathematics from the University of Rostock, Germany. She has worked at the Institute for Psychology, Humboldt-University, Berlin; the Centre for General Linguistics (ZAS), Berlin; the MPI for Human Cognitive and Brain Sciences, Leipzig; the Department of Neuropsychology at the Max Planck Institute for Human Cognitive and Brain Sciences, Berlin; and is currently involved with the research program *The Origins of Episodic Memory Formation* at Humboldt-University, Berlin.

Bernard Grela is an Associate Professor in the Department of Communication Sciences at the University of Connecticut, USA, whose area of expertise is children with specific language impairment. His research focuses on the impact of linguistic complexity on grammatical errors in this population of children.

Gregory Hickok is a Professor of Cognitive Sciences and Director of the Center for Cognitive Neuroscience at the University of California, USA. Hickok's research centers on the neural basis of both signed and spoken language as well as human auditory perception.

Peter Howell is a Professor of Experimental Psychology at the University College London, UK. His long-term interests are on the relationship between speech perception and speech production. This motivated his interest in stuttering.

William Hula is a research speech pathologist at the VA Pittsburgh Healthcare System. His research interests include measurement of language performance and health outcomes in aphasia and the use of dual-task methods and theories to help identify specific points of breakdown in word production and comprehension in aphasia.

Yves Joanette is a Professor at the Faculty of Medicine of the Université de Montréal and Lab Director at the Centre de Recherche of the Institut Universitaire de Gériatrie de Montréal, Canada. His work has focused on the relative contribution of each cerebral hemisphere to language and communication, as well as on the neuro-biological determinants of successful aging for communication abilities. He was honored by a Doctorat Honoris Causa by the Université Lyon 2.

Karima Kahlaoui holds a doctoral degree in Psychology from the University of Nice, France. She was a Postdoctoral Fellow at the Université de Montréal, Canada. Her research includes studies of the semantic processing of words across the hemispheres, semantic memory, and aging. In order to investigate these topics, she has made use of behavioral methods, event-related potentials (ERPs), and near infrared spectroscopy (NIRS). She is also a clinical neuropsychologist.

Juliane Kappes is a trained speech-language pathologist with a diploma in Patholinguistics from the University of Potsdam, Germany. She worked with the Clinical Neuropsychology Research Group (*From Dynamic Sensorimotor Interaction to conceptual Representation: Deconstructing Apraxia*) a grant funded project by the German Fed. Ministry of Research and Education.

Michael Kiang is an Associate Professor in the Department of Psychiatry at the University of Toronto, Canada, and a Clinician-Scientist at the Centre for Addiction and Mental Health in Toronto, Canada.

Marta Kutas is the Director of the Center for Research in Language, University of California, USA, and a Distinguished Professor in the Departments of Cognitive Science and Neurosciences, University of California.

Eeva Leinonen is a Professor of Psycholinguistics and President of Maynooth University, Ireland. She achieved private docent in clinical linguistics at the University of Oulu, Finland. Her research focus is on clinical pragmatics and pragmatic language comprehension difficulties in children.

John Locke is interested in the biology of human communication. He is currently working on a selection-based account of various aspects of language and speech.

Catherine Longworth obtained her graduate degree in Cognitive Neuroscience at the Centre for Speech and Language in the Department of Experimental Psychology at Cambridge University, UK, where she then went on to hold the Pinsent Darwin Research Fellowship in Mental Pathology before obtaining a doctorate in clinical psychology. Her clinical and research interests include the cognitive and neural basis of morphological impairments in aphasia and psychological adjustment to acquired language disorders.

Kristine Lundgren is a Professor and Chair in the Department of Communication Sciences and Disorders at the University of North Carolina Greensboro, USA. Her areas of interest include cognitive-linguistic disorders in adults with acquired brain injury and the use of complementary and integrative approaches to treating communication disorders.

Brian MacWhinney is the Teresa Heina Professor of Cognitive Psychology whose research spans language acquisition and psycholinguistics. His most well-known contributions to the field include work on emergentist theory and the Competition Model of language processing (MacWhinney, 2015). He also manages the NIH and NSF-funded CHILDES and TalkBank (including SLABank) corpora.

William Marslen-Wilson is the Director of the MRC Cognition and Brain Sciences Unit in Cambridge, UK, and Honorary Professor of Language and Cognition at the University of Cambridge, UK. He is an influential and prominent figure in the cognitive science and neuroscience of language, studying the comprehension of spoken language in the mind and the brain. His work is interdisciplinary and cross-linguistic, aimed at identifying the neural processing streams that support the immediate interpretation of spoken utterances.

Chloë Marshall is a Professor in Psychology, Language, and Education at the UCL Institute of Education, University College London, UK. Her research interests include language and literacy development; developmental disorders of language, speech, and literacy (SLI, dyslexia, stuttering); phonology and its developmental relationship to morphology, syntax, and the lexicon; the cognitive skills underlying typical and atypical language/literacy acquisition in hearing and deaf children; and the phonology of English and British Sign Language.

Malcolm McNeil is a Distinguished Professor Emeritus of the Department of Communication Science and Disorders at the University of Pittsburgh, USA. His research interests included the cognitive mechanisms underlying the language behaviors in aphasia, aphasia test development, and in the mechanisms and treatment for apraxia of speech.

David McNeill is a Professor Emeritus in the Department of Psychology and Linguistics at the University of Chicago, USA. For 20 years, he led the McNeill Lab: Center for Gesture and Speech

Research. He has published several books on gesture, thought, and language. His 1992 book, *Hand and Mind*, received the Laing Prize in 1994 from the University of Chicago Press.

Elise Money-Nolan is pursuing her graduate degree in Communication Sciences and Disorders and her clinical Doctorate in Audiology from the University of South Alabama, USA. Her research interests include vestibular assessment and balance rehabilitation, auditory evoked potentials, and using event-related potentials to index semantic processing.

Gareth Morgan was a Postdoctoral Fellow at The University of Texas, Austin, USA. His research interests included: Bilingual child language development and disorders, issues in assessment and treatment of bilingual children with language disorders, language proficiency, Test and Scale Development, language assessment and screening measures, use of Classical Test Theory, and Item Response Theory as they pertain to measurement in education and the inclusion of cognitive models in test and scale development. Currently, he is the Vice President of Morgan Scientific, Inc.

Katherine Morton studied biopsychology at the University of Chicago, UAS, and linguistic phonetics at the University of California, USA. Her current research is in modeling how speaking and understanding speech might be mediated by biological and cognitive systems.

Maria Adelaida Restrepo is a Professor and Chairperson in the Department of Communication Sciences & Disorders at the University of South Florida, USA. She is a bilingual speech–language pathologist and obtained her graduate degree from the University of Arizona, USA. Restrepo's research deals with differentiating language differences from language disorders, assessment in culturally diverse children, especially those from Spanish-speaking homes; further, she studies language maintenance, loss, and intervention in children developing language typically and those with language disorders. She has published in a range of national and international journals in Spanish and English and collaborates with international investigators on matters relating to language disorders and children with attention deficit and hyperactivity disorders.

Ardi Roelofs is a Full Professor in the Donders Institute for Brain, Cognition and Behaviour at Radboud University, the Netherlands. His research is on attention and language performance, which he investigates in healthy individuals and patients using a multi-method approach including measurement of response time and accuracy, eye tracking, electrophysiological and hemodynamic neuroimaging, brain stimulation, tractography, imaging genetics, and computational modeling.

Ben Rutter is a Lecturer in Clinical Linguistics in the Division of Human Communication Sciences, Health Sciences School at the University of Sheffield, UK. He holds undergraduate dgree in Linguistics from the University ofYork, USA, and a graduate degree in Clinical Linguistics from the University of Louisiana at Lafayette, USA. His research interests are in the application of phonetics and linguistics to the study of communication disorders with a particular focus on motor speech.

Nuala Ryder is currently in the Department of Psychology at the University of Hertfordshire. Her research focuses on children's language development and executive function development (including prospective memory) and understanding the role of inhibition in the language development of children with DLD (monolingual and bilingual) and prospective memory in typical and atypical populations. Her interests extend to qualitative analysis from a clinical perspective (language assessment, understanding experiences of parents with children with autism) and health (adherence to medication).

John (Jack) Shelley-Tremblay is a Professor and Chair of Psychology at the University of South Alabama, USA. His graduate degree is from the City University of New York Graduate Center in Experimental Psychology/Psycholinguistics, USA. He uses psychophysiological methods to study attention, semantics, and broad topics in applied health psychology.

Diana Sidtis is a Professor Emeritus at New York University, UAS, and Research Scientist at the Nathan Kline Institute. She has published widely on a variety of research topics in linguistics, voice, and communicative sciences and disorders. Her book, *Foundations of Voice Studies*, published by Wiley-Blackwell with co-author Jody Kreiman, received the 2011 Prose Award from the Association of American Publishers and is still widely cited. Her second book, *Foundations of Familiar Language*, appeared in 2021.

Bernadette Ska obtained a doctoral degree is Cognitive Psychology from the Université catholique de Louvain, Belgium, and a specialization in neuropsychology at the centre de recherche de l'institut universitaire de gériatrie de Montréal, Canada. She is now a professor at the faculty of medicine (department of speech and language pathology), université de Montréal. Her research interest focuses on the effects of aging on cognition and neuropsychology in dementia. She also is interested in the effects of cerebral lesions on semantic and pragmatic aspects of verbal and non-verbal communication.

Ekaterina Smyk is currently an Adjunct Faculty Member at Portland State University, USA, as well as a speech-language pathologist in the Hillsboro School District in Portland. Her research has focused on the areas of typical and atypical language acquisition in bilingual children and identification of language impairment in bilingual populations. Her dissertation project investigated the effects of language impairment on English language acquisition in bilingual children and differentiation between bilingual children with and without language impairment at different levels of English language proficiency. She has also worked on several research projects that investigated the language skills of bilingual children with and without language disorders and the effects of bilingual and English-only intervention on the development of two languages. In addition, she worked on the development and validation of a criterion-based measure of oral language proficiency for bilingual children.

Clarissa Sorger completed her graduate degree in Developmental Neurosciences at University College London, UK. Her previous undergraduate degree in Psychology and Language Sciences, and her master's degree in Research in Speech, Language, and Cognition, for which she has received a Student Excellence Award for outstanding academic achievement, focused on identifying speech production difficulties in primary school children from diverse language backgrounds.

Joseph P. Stemberger is a Professor Emeritus (since 2018). He specializes in adult psycholinguistics (especially phonology and morphology in language production, and the interactions between them) and first language acquisition, most recently the phonological acquisition ofValley Zapotec in Mexico and a crosslinguistic project with Dr Bernhardt and international colleagues.

Holly Storkel is a program officer for the language program at the National Institute on Deafness and Other Communication Disorders (NIDCD). Her research has focused on sound and word learning by typically developing children and children with phonological or language impairments.

Jee Eun Sung gained her graduate degree from the University of Pittsburgh, USA, and is currently at Ewha Women's University, Korea. Her research interest is sentence processing and its underlying cognitive mechanism in normal elderly adults and persons with aphasia.

Mark Tatham has worked at the University of Essex, UK (where he is an Emeritus Professor), Ohio State University, USA, and the University of California, USA. His current research is in building computationally adequate models of speech production and perception.

Heather van der Lely passed away in 2014. She pioneered the study of Grammatical-Specific Language Impairment. She was a Professor and Director of the Centre for Developmental Language Disorders and Cognitive Neuroscience, at University College London, UK.

Mieke Van Herreweghe is a Senior Full Professor and current Vice-Rector at Ghent University, UK. She has published widely on grammatical, lexicographical and sociolinguistic aspects of Flemish Sign Language (VGT). Mieke is also a certified sign language interpreter, co-founder and former chair of the Flemish Sign Language Centre, recognised by the Flemish Government as a "knowledge and coordination centre for Flemish Sign Language" and the first chair of the Advisory Committee on Flemish Sign Language, installed by the Flemish government in 2008.

Rosemary Varley is a Professor in Language and Cognition at University College London, UK. She works primarily in the field of neurodisability, exploring speech and language capacities in aphasia and dementia, as well as residual cognition in severe aphasia. Her current psycholinguistic work applies usage-based perspectives to speech and language in aphasia, including designing and testing digital interventions for these impairments.

Myriam Vermeerbergen is a Professor at KU Leuven, Belgium, where she teaches general linguistics, general sign language linguistics, and several courses on (socio)linguistic aspects of Flemish Sign Language (VGT). She is also a Professor Extraordinary at the Department of Dutch and Afrikaans at the University of Stellenbosch, South Africa. In the early 1990s, Myriam pioneered research on VGT and the Flemish Deaf community. Her current research interests include the linguistics of Flemish Sign Language, the gesture/sign interface, and (Flemish) Sign Language interpreting. Myriam is co-founder and former chair of the Flemish Sign Language Centre, recognized by the Flemish Government as a "knowledge and coordination centre for Flemish Sign Language" (www.vgtc.be) and the current Vice-Chair of the Advisory Committee on Flemish Sign Language.

Grant M. Walker is an Assistant Project Scientist in the Auditory and Language Neuroscience Lab at the University of California, USA, and is a Co-Investigator at the Center for the Study of Aphasia Recovery (C-STAR), a multi-site collaboration funded by the National Institutes of Health. He received an undergraduate degree in Cognitive Science and Communications from the University of Pennsylvania, USA, in 2006, a master's degree in Cognitive Neuroscience from the University of California, USA, in 2014, and a graduate degree in Psychology in 2016, also from the University of California. His research is focused on understanding the mechanisms that support speech and language functions, how these mechanisms are impaired by brain injury, and how best to repair them. The methods typically involve the development of computational models to extract meaningful measures of latent cognitive abilities from behavioral tests and neuroimaging data.

Joel Walters is the Chair of the M.Ed. Program in English as an International Language at Talpiot Academic College of Education, Israel. He trained in applied psycholinguistics at Boston University, where he worked on pragmatics in bilingual children. His book *Bilingualism: The Sociopragmatic and Psycholinguistic Interface* was published in 2005. His current work focuses on language impairment in bilinguals and implications for social integration and language policy.

Katherine White is a Professor of Psychology at Rhodes College, USA. She received her graduate degree in Cognitive and Sensory Processes, with a Certificate in Gerontology, from the University of Florida, USA, in 2002. Her research aims to better understand how humans produce language, with specific emphasis on factors that influence spoken and written word retrieval in younger and older adults. She is also interested in how language production is supported by other cognitive processes such as memory and attention, and how engagement with emotion influences language fluency. She employs diverse research methods to study language production, including experiments where participants produce language under certain constraints (e.g., when distractors are present) and more naturalistic communicative settings (e.g., where participants share narratives about events in their lives).

Emma Willis was, at the time the manuscript of the AAC chapter was written, finalizing her master's degree in Speech Language Pathology at the University ofVirginia, USA. She has coordinated several research projects examining psycholinguistic and cognitive processes in using augmentative and alternative communication. After graduation, she intends to remain involved in AAC research.

Mark Yates obtained his graduate degree from the University of Kansas, USA. Currently, he is an Associate Professor at the University of South Alabama, USA. His research has focused on phonological and semantic processing during visual word recognition and how these are influenced by reader individual differences.

Zhixing Yang attained her undergraduate degree in Psychology at University College London (UCL), UK, and is currently undertaking a master's degree in Clinical Mental Health Sciences at UCL. She has interests in clinical psychology and developmental psychology, especially in children's language and mental development. She has participated in internship programmes in the children's psychology department at several mental health hospitals. She has special concerns about helping kids and adolescents in underdeveloped socioeconomic situations.

Jing Zhao practiced as a developmental pediatrician for seven years before she came to Canada from Shanghai in 2003. She received a master's degree in Speech-Language Pathology from the School of Audiology and Speech Sciences, University of British Columbia, Canada, in 2007 and is a practicing speech-language pathologist. Her research focuses on speech-language development in Mandarin-speaking and bilingual children, and she is a collaborator on the cross-linguistic project of Drs Bernhardt and Stemberger.

Wolfram Ziegler has a diploma and doctoral degree in mathematics. He worked as a research assistant at the Max-Planck-Institute for Psychiatry and is now head of the Clinical Neuropsychology Research Group (EKN), City Hospital Munich, and a lecturer of phonetics and neurophonetics at the Phonetics Department and at the Speech Pathology School, University of Munich.

PSYCHOLINGUISTICS

Some basic considerations

Jackie Guendouzi and Filip Loncke

Introduction

As noted in the first edition we did not intend this collection to be an extensive survey of the field of psycholinguistics. Rather, the aim of the book was to provide a tutorial resource that combines research from psycholinguistics and cognitive sciences with the field of communication disorders. The information presented here does not require prior knowledge but it does assume some basic knowledge in the area of linguistics or cognitive sciences. The second edition includes 18 updated or revised chapters that include new authors. However, several of the original chapters remain because they reflect seminal areas of knowledge in the fields of psycholinguistics and communication disorders. Sadly, since the first edition, Heather van der Lely and Ursula Bellugi both passed away. Van der Lely's research (see Chapter 20) was influential in generating debate in the area of Specific Language Impairment (SLI) while Bellugi's phenomenal career pioneered work that aligned cognitive science with the study of sign language (see Chapter 32). In both cases, their contributions to this book reflect their influence within their respective areas of research and make for compelling reading.

The field of psycholinguistics has yielded many diverse and competing theories over the years; some more than others have dominated language research. As seen in this text, there are multiple approaches to the question of how we process language. Readers should draw their own conclusions as to the robustness of specific models or theories; exploring theoretical questions is an ongoing process that rarely arrives at a definitive answer, there is always more to discover. As with the first edition, we feel it is helpful to start the introduction by providing some historical context to the field of psycholinguistics and its relationship with communication disorders.

Psycholinguistics: A historical perspective

Psycholinguistics has always involved the art of finding models to help us understand why and how people speak, listen, read, and write. In some of the earliest reflections on language and speech, it raises questions that still spark the interest of scholars to this day. Plato's *Cratylus* (Sedley, 2003) discusses the relationship between words and their referents, an issue that has remained central both in developmental accounts of language (Piaget, 1929/1997) and its disorders and in the field of cognitive semantics (Evan & Green, 2006).

A general fascination with language, where it came from, its potential synaptic plasticity, and its disorders is reflected in discussions from the time of the Enlightenment on. Twentieth-century

DOI: 10.4324/9781003204213-1

linguists explicitly trace back their line of thinking to Descartes's reasoning on the nature of ideas and mental functioning (Chomsky, 1966).

The 19th century was the time of the precursors of our understanding of the neurolinguistic underpinnings of language, starting with Gall's speculation of the brain's mental areas to Broca's and Wernicke's description of types of aphasia. Theories about localization led to a rudimentary psycholinguistic theory, most notably reflected in the Wernicke/Lichtheim model (Caplan, 1987). This model assumed the existence of an (anatomically based) system of connections between brain centers; problems in processing language were described as a breakdown, a deletion, or a distortion in the communication system. The Wernicke/Lichtheim classification may be considered the earliest model of internal linguistic processing, combining a brain localization approach with an information processing approach. The study of aphasia also led to the first classifications and distinctions between subcomponents of language and language processing. The terms motor aphasia, conduction aphasia, receptive aphasia, and transcortical aphasia reflect an attempt to grasp both the internal organization of language and its interaction with the brain. For a century and a half, these distinctions have been a basis on which intervention rationales have been built. At the same time, already in the early 20th century, the accuracy of these approaches was challenged and criticized. These early neurolinguistics models served as a framework to understand language disorders in children: Until the 1970s childhood language problems were often referred to as developmental dysphasia (Wyke, 1978), a clear reference for a purported neuropsychological explanation of the phenomenon. These approaches initially have helped to conceptualize the relationship between language and brain.

Language as a system was the object of study of De Saussure's *Cours de Linguistique Générale*, published in 1916, This influential work marks the beginning of a strong structuralist view in language theory. Although De Saussure described language as rooted in historical "diachronic" development, he also thought that a "panchronic" (p. 134) approach would be possible. This latter concept corresponds with today's "universal" view on language, a view that implies that explanatory models of language, language disorders, and language intervention should be valid and applicable across languages.

Today's schools of thought on language acquisition are often categorized in empiricism, rationalism, and pragmaticism (Russell, 2004). The influence of the empiricists in speech–language intervention was the most obvious in the 1950s and 1960s but remains powerful and obvious to this day. The empiricist approach apparently offers a framework that easily lends itself into concepts of trainability and modifiability, which are central for interventions. Rationalism tends to consider language as a semiautonomous self-developing system. An underlying hypothesis is that understanding the rules of languages helps with the grasp of language functioning and will lead to most effective interventions. In the period of linguistic structuralism, we find an interest in patterns that learners would use as reference frames to build language structures. One example here is the Fitzgerald key (1954), meant to make syntactic structures transparent and to help the student to "build" sentences according to visually laid out patterns.

In the past 20 years, the influence of linguistics on language intervention has waned. Its place is taken by a more cognitivist, emergentist, and information-processing oriented focus, as is the case for much of the entire field of psycholinguistics (Harley, 2008).

Interestingly, for a long time, the pragmaticists did not become a dominant factor in the theory of speech, language, and their disorders until the 1970s, a time when interest in research areas such as early development, social interaction, and sociolinguistics started to rise. It changed the field of speech–language pathology, with a stronger emphasis on early and functional intervention, and especially the involvement of communication partners.

The developments in the first decade of the 21st century maintain some of the old debates. However, many of the therapeutic approaches integrate and motivate multiple approaches. For example, Nelson (2000) proposes the "tricky mix approach," which strives to create multiple conditions that converge to increase learning. Nelson suggests that attention, motivation, and the right contrastive examples work together to make learning possible in typically developing children. Knowing this, the clinician's task is to recreate similar favorable conditions. Throughout history, psycholinguistic theory and intervention have always benefited from clinical research, starting with Broca, to today's genetic studies, syndrome studies, and neuroimaging studies.

Roots of the language debate

Historically, two theories had a major influence on language research in the 1950s, Skinner's behaviorist model emphasizing the effects of reinforcement and environmental input (1957), and Chomsky's nativist (cognitive) approach (1957). Chomsky's work stimulated research that hypothesized the mind of the ideal speaker when forming a sentence. Thus, the emphasis of research in linguistics shifted toward the study of a speaker's competence (rather than their performance) and the pursuit of uncovering the underlying cognitive mechanisms of language. Chomsky's work also stimulated interest in the role of biological factors by suggesting a language acquisition device (LAD) innate to humans. Chomsky's subsequent critique of Skinner's Verbal Behaviors (1959) led to nativist approaches becoming the agenda of most linguistic programs during that period.

However, despite the primacy of Chomsky's work during the 1970s and 1980s, work in language acquisition has continued to explore both physiological factors and environmental influences. Current research is more likely to draw on the interaction between physiological factors and socio-environmental factors. Furthermore, advances in artificial intelligence, neurosciences, and computational modeling have resulted in a research agenda focusing on the notion of language as an emergent property of competing systems.

The structure of language

For the purposes of teaching, language is typically broken up into its component parts; however, it is important to note that these parts are to some extent artificial constructs. That is, the degree to which any language system (e.g., phonology or morphology) is independent of other systems is debatable. Perhaps a good analogy is that of driving a car; in order for the car to move, all the component parts and systems of the car need to be operating. In addition, a driver is required to coordinate the exercise; thus, one event "driving down the road" is the sum of many interrelating and synchronized systems. However, if the car stops moving in order to repair the damage, we need to establish which system, or mechanical part, failed. A global failure of the car may be due to a minor disruption in the electrical system rather than major engine damage.

A similar situation occurs with language. When hearing an acoustic stimulus (e.g., a request for coffee) our language processing system (LPS) must carry out several processing tasks; first we have to focus on the speaker (attention), retain the auditory information (working memory), interpret the acoustic signal (auditory discrimination system), parse the utterance (morpho-syntactic system), and then interpret the message (semantic and conceptual systems). In addition, we need integrate any visual stimuli such as gesture and facial expressions that may affect the speaker's intended meaning. Yet this simple action takes place in a split second of time as a holistic event and listeners are not aware of the separate systems operating to process the utterance; one is only aware that someone requested a cup of coffee. Thus, using language is similar to driving a car; in order to process what we hear or see, all the interconnected systems need to be functional. If there is a central theme in this book, it is the notion of language as an emergent property of dynamic interacting systems.

Models and theories drive research, yet it is not always easy to see the connection between theory and practice. As early as 1997, Stackhouse and Wells noted that although traditional linguistic approaches offer very detailed descriptions, they do not always offer adequate explanations for the development of linguistic systems in individuals with disorders. Baker, Croot, McLeod, and Paul

(2001) suggested that a psycholinguistic approach to communication disorders would ultimately help identify treatments that are more effective. It is also encouraging to note that, more recently, there has been greater interest in applying psycholinguistic approaches to translatable, clinical contexts. For example, Terbrand, Maassen, and Maas (2019) suggested a psycholinguistic framework that may help when diagnosing and treating developmental speech disorders.

We hope this new edition of the book will continue to generate interest in the application of psycholinguistics to the field of communication disorders. More importantly, we hope it will stimulate further debate and encourage continued research into this area. Many of the chapters in this book have overlapping interests, but in some cases, the content may reflect theoretical differences. This is a natural part of the research process, and we encourage readers to consider all approaches when seeking to find answers to difficult questions about the ways in which we process language. This edition of the text retains the original four sections. Section I focuses on theories of language processing, Section II on work that expands theory in the area of developmental disorders, Section III considers language processing in the context of acquired disorders, and Section IV contains work that considers other modalities such as gesture, sign language, and Augmentative and Alternative Communication (AAC).

Section I: Theories of language processing

Locke's examination of the evolution of language (Chapter 1) suggests that it may be hard to disentangle the two driving forces of biological and social need. His discussion of the development of human language explains gender and cultural differences within, and across, language use. Interactionist approaches such as Locke's consider both the biological and genetic bases of language, and the role the child's environment plays in sculpting the brain for language. MacWhinney (Chapter 2) has updated his chapter considerably to discuss how "emergentism" and "competition" might offer explanations that account for language disorders in the context of SLI and aphasia. MacWhinney suggests 16 mechanisms involved in language processing, that when considered in conjunction with the impact of specific genetic variations, may help us better understand language disorders such as stuttering and Specific Language Impairment (SLI).

Abrams and White have revised Chapter 3 to focus on the issue of fluency in healthy aging. Drawing on recent research, they consider the interaction between cognition, fluency, and gesture and note that this area of research has been unexplored, particularly with respect to aging and bilingualism. Cowan (Chapter 4) contrasts his model of working memory (WM) with that of Baddeley (1986) to discuss how attention and working memory interact, both with each other, and with other areas of the language processing system (LPS). His seminal work in the area of working memory (WM) also raises questions relating to research that might be considered as deriving from a Chomskyan paradigm (Caplan, Waters, & DeDe, 2007) by linking WM specifically to syntax. Cowan and colleagues have been actively researching memory and cognition over the past decade; a list of his more recent work for further reading can be found at the conclusion of his chapter; in particular we recommend Cowan's review of 50 years of research investigating the topic of working memory (Cowan, 2022).

Advances in brain imaging techniques have led to greater understanding of the neurobiological aspects of language processing. In Chapter 5, Kahlaoui, Ska, Degroot, and Joanette review imaging methods, then consider what each method can tell us about the neurobiological bases of semantic processing. Kutas and Kiang (Chapter 6) note that, when compared to other neuroimaging methods, electrophysiological studies are not only economical but they can also provide a potential "window" on the brain's language related processing operations. Their updated chapter includes work that is more recent to consider what such paradigms reveal about normal and abnormal language processing. In Chapter 7, Friedrich compares mathematical models and artificial neural networks (connectionist models) to brain imaging techniques. In particular, she reflects on what ERP studies can contribute to our knowledge of early word learning. As with several other chapters in this section, Friedrich's original chapter is a valuable starting point to this area of study.

Research based on connectionist approaches has been very influential in the field of communication disorders, particularly when considering acquired disorders of language and cognition such as aphasia. In Chapter 8, Walker has extended the work of Dell and Kittredge (2013) to provide an updated overview of connectionist approaches to the context of aphasia and other communication impairments. He suggests a cooperative view of language that argues for models based on interaction between processing parts. Roelofs (Chapter 9) considers vocal utterance production from the standpoint of Wernicke's classical model to the current version of the WEAVER++ model. Roelofs stresses it is important that future research draws on such models to develop intervention methods. In Chapter 10, Money-Nolan and Shelley-Tremblay review some of the more influential and widely researched theories of semantic representation. They focus on models of semantic memory, word identification, and semantic priming to assess the efficacy of local theories, feature-based theories, and distributed models.

The work of Marslen-Wilson has been highly influential in the field of psycholinguistics and cognitive sciences, and for that reason we chose to include the original chapter (Chapter11) that he and Longworth contributed to the first edition. They examine language comprehension from the perspective of what occurs within the milliseconds that it takes the brain to recognize individual words. Exploring this aspect of connectivity and language processing through a clinical example, they go on to suggest a neurocognitive model that contrasts with the classic model of a single processing pathway. Their model formed part of the "Words and Rules" debate in cognitive science and is an important contribution to the field.

Sidtis (Chapter 12) has introduced the use of an umbrella term "familiar language" to extend her discussion of formulaic language. Her new chapter summarizes over 20 years of work in this area of language processing and is essential reading for anyone who is interested in researching this often-neglected area of language. Ryder and Leinonen (Chapter 13) draw on Relevance Theory (Sperber & Wilson, 1995; Novek & Sperber, 2004) to discuss both acquired and developmental language processing disorders. As will be shown in the Epilogue (Chapter 35), Relevance Theory also helps provide explanations for some of the communication patterns that emerge in dementia.

In Chapter 14, Yates and Dickinson note that single word recognition and similarity in phonological and orthographic forms are issues of cognitive psychology that have been widely studied. This area of language processing is highly relevant when we consider the issue of literacy and language processing. Yates and Dickinson consider models of Interactive Activation and Competition (IAC) that have been influential in examining the effects of inhibition by words that have orthographic or phonological competitors.

Phonology has been an area of psycholinguistics that has been in the foreground of research in communication disorders for some time. The move away from linear phonetics and phonology to nonlinear approaches (e.g., autosegmental, feature geometry, and optimality theory) led to a great deal of research in constraint-based phonology. However, this area of psycholinguistics has been highly debated in the research arena, particularly in relation to the issue of phonological representation. Tatham and Morton's chapter (Chapter 15) although not updated is essential reading for students and researchers new to the area. In their work, they compare classical phonetic approaches to speech production to a cognitive approach, examining theories that posit speech as a continuous dynamic process. Rutter and Ball's work (Chapter 16) adds to this discussion through an overview of phonological theories. In particular, theories that have moved away from the notion that children store a representation of their ambient language's system of sounds. Such theories suggest that we have exemplars of each sound that enable us to process speech sounds online. In contrast, Ziegler, Ackermann, and Kappes' original chapter (Chapter 17) draws on neuro-phonetics and brain imaging to examine what happens in the processing chain, from initial abstract phonological representations to the intended motor acts of articulation. As Ziegler and colleagues note, there has been considerable disagreement about the separation of phonological and phonetic encoding; they argue there is a need for further research that incorporates a neurological approach.

Section II: Developmental disorders

In this section, the chapters focus on how the use of theoretical constructs helps us better understand particular disorders and provides the basis of evidence-based practice. Burns (Chapter 18) discusses the temporal processing hypothesis in children with language disorders. She draws on the seminal work of Tallal and colleagues (1981) to explore the notion of bottom-up and top-down processing and their role in language interventions. Her recent book (2021) is an excellent resource that highlights this topic over the past decade.

In Chapter 19, Grela, Collisson, and Arthur provide a comprehensive review of theories that attempt to explain Specific Language Impairment (SLI). They suggest the original classification of SLI was intended to differentiate between children with language related conditions accompanied by other cognitive impairments (e.g., low IQ) and children who did not manifest noticeable cognitive impairment but presented with language specific deficits. Grela and colleagues suggest that children with SLI are a heterogeneous population with different underlying causes to their language deficit. In contrast, Marshall and van der Lely (Chapter 20) make the case for a subgroup of children with specific problems in the morphosyntactic and phonological systems. Van der Lely labeled this group Grammatical Specific Language Impairment (G-SLI), and suggests this group manifests domain specific deficits and domain general deficits. They suggest that the Computational Grammatical Complexity (CGC) hypothesis can provide a framework for the G-SLI subgroup. Storkel (Chapter 21) extends the discussion of SLI by examining a subset of properties in lexical items typically incorporated within both adult and child models of spoken language processing. She considers several models of the lexicon in relation to normal development before applying these theories to the case of SLI.

Howell and his new co-authors (Chapter 22) draw on activation theories (Dell & Kittredge, 2013) to elaborate on EXPLAN, a theory they contrast with the covert repair hypothesis (Kolk & Postma, 1997) and the vicious cycle theory (Bernstein Ratner & Wijnen, 2007); both draw on Levelt's model of speech production (1983, 1989). In this revised chapter, Howell et al. report data collected from school age Arabic speakers ($n=63$) to consider assessment of people who stutter in the context of schools where there are multi-lingual populations.

The final three chapters in this section of the book apply theories of language processing to bilingual contexts. Armon-Lotem and Walters (Chapter 23) draw on models of lexical representation relating to inhibition and control to consider the notion that there is parallel activation in two languages even when a bilingual person is speaking in a single language. They highlight the work of Kroll and Green, including his more recent Control Process Model. Armon-Lotem and Walters then present Walters' model of bilingual production that uses a single framework to account for both psycholinguistic and socio-pragmatic information. They conclude with a discussion of how bilingual processing models apply to bilingual populations diagnosed with SLI and schizophrenia.

Bernhardt and colleagues (Chapter 24) discuss how constraints-based nonlinear phonological theories have influenced phonological descriptions since the 1970s. Nonlinear phonological theories describe the hierarchical representation of phonological form from the prosodic phrase to the individual feature. Constraints-based theories contrast possibilities and limitations for output (e.g., production of the feature [Labial] as possible or impossible) when a speaker attempts to produce a word. In the approach taken here, constraints are grounded in the processing of words and the access of phonological elements during the learning process. The chapter outlines constraints-based nonlinear phonological theories and describes their application to phonological assessment and/or intervention for English, Kuwaiti Arabic, and Mandarin. Key phonological characteristics of each language are described in turn, followed by a brief overview of phonological development for that language, and a summary of clinical applications, whether intervention (as in English) or assessment.

There is a growing need for cognitive researchers to turn their attention to dual and multi-language speakers when considering the role of the LPS in communication disorders. In Chapter 25, Restrepo, Morgan, and Smyk consider how SLI and bilingualism are at the crossroads of linguistic and psycholinguistic accounts of language. They suggest bilingualism interfaces with SLI from the theoretical position of Dynamic Systems Theory; their chapter provides a review of research evidence supporting the notion of SLI in bilingual populations. Although this chapter remains in its original form, it raises important questions for those interested in studying the effects of a multi-language processing system in the context of language disorders, an area where there is still a great need for further research.

Section III: Acquired disorders

Chapters in this section focus on acquired disorders of language. Varley (Chapter 26) notes the historical divide between generative approaches and more diverse work in cognitive and neurobiological approaches to language disorders. She explores conceptualizations of the processes involved in speech programming; in particular, a dual mechanism model and its implications for acquired apraxia of speech.

McNeil, Hula, and Sung's chapter (Chapter 27) discusses the traditional paradigm of aphasia research based on anatomical centers and pathways. This model, although influential, is untenable with many attributes of aphasia. McNeil et al. discuss the role of working memory suggesting the executive attentional component of working memory may be the source of the language impairments in persons with aphasia; constructs that are consistent with general attributes of aphasia supported by the research directed toward these alternative cognitive mechanisms. Evidence from their more recent work (2015) provides Lundgren and Brownell with strong statistical support for the suggestion that theory of mind (ToM) training can have benefits for clinical practice with clients who have a traumatic brain injury (TBI). In their updated chapter (Chapter 28) this additional support suggests ToM performance can be differentiated from performance in other cognitive domains.

In Chapter 29, Shelley-Tremblay draws on his previous chapter (Chapter 10) outlining theories of semantic processing to provide further support for the hypothesis that many of the problems noted in dementia and aphasia are related to both the representation of semantic information and the allocation of attention resources. He reviews ERP studies of dementia and relates their findings to the Center Surround Model (CSM), suggesting that it is necessary to identify in what format the information is stored in the brain.

Finally, in Chapter 30 of this section, Centeno notes that the rise of age related cardio-vascular and neurogenic language disorders in a rapidly aging world population is being affected by growth in migration driven, multi-ethnic populations. Centeno discusses the strengths, limitations, and current trends in research examining the interaction of language and cognition in the case of the multilingual brain, in particular the case of aphasia in bilingual individuals. In this updated version of the chapter, the content draws on recent research to interpret the aphasia profiles exhibited by bi-/multilingual adults after a stroke. Centeno considers important information on bi-/multilingualism relevant to the understanding of the studies and theoretical constructs. The chapter provides a valuable review of research that references cerebral language organization and processing in multiple language users. Centeno ends with a discussion on future directions and implications in this area of research.

Section IV: Other modalities

Although this is a much smaller section, it remains a very important part of this collection. Nonverbal aspects of communication processing are an area of research that may not always receive as much attention as other areas of psycholinguistics. However, as McNeil and Duncan argue in Chapter 31, gesture is an integral part of the language system: indeed, gesture was likely the primary system of human communication with verbal forms being a later addition. Sign language is another area of language processing that should be included in any book relating to communication disorders. In Chapter 32, Hickok and Bellugi examine evidence from sign language to theorize on the neural organization of language. As noted above, Ursula Bellugi passed away in April 2022; however, her collaboration with Hickok published in the original edition remains seminal reading for new researchers and students. Vermeerbergen and Van Herreweghe have updated their chapter (Chapter 33) reviewing research in the area of sign language; as they note there have been important developments over the past decade; however, sign languages themselves have not undergone any real change. Their discussion of the structure of sign language and its role in the field of linguistics is an excellent starting point for researchers and students who are not familiar with this domain of study.

Loncke and Willis (Chapter 34) explore an area often overlooked in texts covering language processing, the psycholinguistics of Augmentative and Alternative Communiction (AAC). Loncke and Willis's chapter raises several questions, how for instance do AAC users incorporate the LPS when using alternate modalities of communication? AAC relies heavily on iconicity i.e., the symbol bears a physical resemblance to its referent and, as Loncke and Willis note, the age of the intended user of AAC is not always considered when creating iconicity of symbols. They suggest that children rely heavily on episodic memory to gain meaning, whereas, typically, adults draw more on their semantic memory. An additional consideration is the target user's disorder type, as Loncke and Willis note these factors should be given greater attention when designing AAC assistance for those with communication disorders.

The final chapter (Chapter 35) in Section IV takes the place of the traditional epilogue; rather than summarize such an extensive body of work, this chapter attempts to illustrate why it is important for the clinician to be aware of research in the area of psycholinguistics. Guendouzi provides examples of conversational data to illustrate how psycholinguistic theories can explain some of the divergent patterns of communication noted in the context of dementia.

References

Baddeley, A. D. (1986). *Working memory*. Oxford: Clarendon Press.

Baker, E., Croot, K., McLeod, S., & Paul, R. (2001). Pyscholinguistic models of speech development and their practice in clinical practice. *Journal of Speech, Language, and Hearing Research*, *44*(3), 685–702.

Bernstein Ratner, N., & Wijnen, F. (2007). The vicious cycle: Linguistic encoding, self monitoring and stuttering. In J. Au-Yeung & M. M. Leahy (Eds.), *Research, treatment and self help in fluency disorders: New horizons* (pp. 84–90). Proceedings of the Fifth World Congress on Fluency Disorders Dublin: The International Fluency Association.

Burns, M. S. (2021). *Cognitive & communication interventions: Neuroscience applications for speech-language pathologists*. San Diego, CA: Plural Publishers.

Caplan, D. (1987). *Neurolinguistics and linguistic aphasiology*. New York: Cambridge University Press.

Caplan, D., Waters, G., & Dede, G. (2007). Specialized verbal working memory for language comprehension. In A. R. Conway, C. Jerrold, M. J. Kane, A. Miyake, & J. N. Towse (Eds.), *Variation in working memory*. New York: Oxford University Press.

Chomsky, N. (1957). *Syntactic structures*. The Hague: Mouton.

Chomsky, N. (1966). *Cartesian linguistics*. New York: Harper and Row.

Chomsky, N., & Skinner, B. F. (1959). Review of Skinner's verbal behavior. *Language*, *35*(1), 26–58.

Cowan, N. (2022). Working memory development: A 50-year assessment of research and underlying theories. *Cognition*, *224*, 1–18.

Dell, G., & Kittredge, A. (2013). Connectionist models of aphasia and other language impairments. In J. Guendouzi, F. Loncke, & M. Williams (Eds.), *Handbook of psycholinguistics & cognitive processes: Perspectives in communication disorders*. New York: Taylor & Francis.

de Saussure, F. (1916). *Cours de linguistique générale*. Paris: Payot.

Evan, V., & Green, M. (2006). *Cognitive linguistics: An introduction*. Mahwah, NJ: Lawrence Erlbaum Associates.

Fitzgerald, E. (1954). *Straight language for the deaf: A system of instruction for deaf children*. Washington, DC: Volta.
Harley, T. A. (2008). *The psychology of language: From data to theory* (3rd ed.). New York: Psychology Press.
Kolk, H., & Postma, A. (1997). Stuttering as a covert repair phenomenon. In R. F. Curlee & G. M. Siegel (Eds.), *Nature and treatments of stuttering: New directions* (pp. 182–203). Needham Heights, MA: Allyn & Bacon.
Levelt, W. (1983). Monitoring and self-repair in speech. *Cognition, 14*(1), 41–104.
Levelt, W. (1989). *Speaking: From intention to articulation*. Cambridge, MA: Bradford Books.
Lundgren, K., & Brownell, H. (2015). Selective training in theory of mind in traumatic brain injury: A series of single subject treatment studies. *Open Behavioral Science Journal, 9*, 1–11.
Nelson, K. (2000). Methods for stimulating and measuring lexical and syntactic advances. Why fiffins and lobsters can tag along with other recast friends. In L. Menn & N. Bernstein Ratner (Eds.), *Methods for studying language production* (pp. 115–148). Mahwah, NJ: Lawrence Erlbaum Associates.
Novek, I. A., & Sperber, D. (2004). *Experimental pragmatics*. Hampshire: Palgrave Macmillan.
Piaget, J. (1997). *The child's conception of the world: Jean Piaget: Selected works* (A. Tomlinson & J. Tomlinson, Trans.). London: Routledge. (Original work published 1929).
Russell, J. (2004). *What is language development? Rationalist, empiricist, and pragmaticist approaches to the acquisition of syntax*. Oxford: Oxford University Press.
Sedley, D. N. (2003). *Plato's Cratylus*. New York: Cambridge University Press.
Skinner, B. F. (1957). *Verbal behavior*. New York: Appleton, Century & Croft.
Sperber, D., & Wilson, D. (1995). *Relevance: Communication & cognition*. Oxford: Oxford University Press.
Stackhouse, J., & Wells, B. (1997). *Children's speech and literacy difficulties: A psycholinguistic framework*. London: Whurr.
Tallal, P., & Stark, R. E. (1981). Speech acoustic-cue discrimination abilities of normally developing and language-impaired children. *Journal of the Acoustic Society of America, 69*(2), 568–574.
Terband, H., Maassen, B., & Maas, E. (2019). A psycholinguistic framework for diagnosis and treatment planning of developmental speech disorders. *Folia Phoniatrica et Logopaedica, 71*(5–6), 216–227. https://doi.org/10.1159/000499426.
Wyke, M. (1978). *Developmental dysphasia*. London: Academic Press.

SECTION I

Language processing

1

THE DEVELOPMENT OF LINGUISTIC SYSTEMS

Insights from evolution

John Locke

Introduction

Some years ago, I encountered a statement that, on the surface, appeared to be eminently reasonable. It expressed the idea that linguistics may be able to grapple with evolutionary questions – a matter that has drawn new scholars at an exponential rate over the last 30 years – but not until linguists have come to a decision about what language is. One might suppose that similar thinking applies with equal force to development. How, according to the logic, can we possibly understand the development of language until we find out precisely what it is that develops?

There are at least two problems with this. The first is that it ignores the considerable merits of "reverse engineering." According to the methodology, we improve our understanding of language, and any other complex behavior, when we take it apart. Since language is a biological trait, this means, among other things, seeing how it was put together in evolution and comes together in development.

Reverse engineering contrasts sharply with the traditional approach. From the dawn of research on language development, the leitmotif has been to document the appearance of behaviors that seemed relevant to language or were actually linguistic. It was never clear that we might gain from knowing what these behaviors do for infants at the time of their appearance, if anything, nor was there an obvious way to find out. As a consequence, development was seen, by default, as something that "happens" to infants, not as an unfolding of new functions that contemporaneously benefit the infant and might, to some extent, be under the infant's own control.

There is, as mentioned, a second problem with the primacy of formal definition. It is a classic confrontation between internal evidence and external evidence. What if language met a series of discipline-internal tests but was later found to resist all attempts to characterize its emergence in the species and the child? Would we reject the principles of evolutionary and developmental change that have worked, with some success, for other traits, purely on the basis of the language experience; or would we argue that language is so unlike other complex traits that it emerged according to entirely different principles – ones unknown to biologists? Where evolution is concerned, one could argue that, to some extent, this has been happening for some time and is still taking place (e.g., Chomsky, 2002).

If we are more likely to understand language by looking at its evolution and development, I think we will be unusually advantaged if we look at the interactions that have occurred, and that still occur, between those processes (Locke, 2009). Evolution and development are collaborative.

DOI: 10.4324/9781003204213-3

They feed each other. If we treat them independently, the result can only be distortion of each process and of the faculty of language itself.

I will begin here with a brief summary of evidence that, in its totality, indicates that language is a biological trait, as Pinker (1994) famously declared, not a cultural trait or the product of some form of instruction. The emergence of "language" in the infant will be seen as the development of adaptive mechanisms that take in socially and linguistically relevant behaviors – among other "duties" that they might have – store this material long enough to extract organizing principles, and use the principles to generate novel utterances. This much relates to the code of language, but development also includes the activation of rather different mechanisms that oversee the application of linguistic knowledge by, and for the benefit of, the speaker in a variety of biosocial contexts. In the next section, I will examine a view of language that is widely shared in the linguistic community, one that has been unhelpfully influenced, paradoxically, by a factor that plays no role in its development – formal instruction – and by the cultural variables responsible for instructional institutions. In the succeeding section, I will ask what actually evolved, or could have evolved, according to a selection-based account in which observable behaviors enhanced fitness. The emergence of these evolved traits, I will submit, requires a new theoretical framework, one that provides a biological context for the development of neurological, cognitive, and social functions, as well as linguistic ones. Life history provides such a framework, partly because it enables one to trace critical effects of evolution on development, and partly because it is receptive, in principle, to reciprocal effects of development on evolution. In the end, what is needed is a strict evolutionary ↔ developmental ("evo-devo") approach or, better, evo-devo-evo-devo …

Language is biological trait

Language evolved in humans uniquely and develops in the young universally. A strong biological endowment was suspected over a half-century ago when it was noted that infants acquire linguistic material rapidly in view of the seeming inadequacy of ambient models and the rarity of teaching or corrective feedback (Chomsky, 1959, 1980). Later, it was observed that infants appear to invent aspects of linguistic structure, as when pidgins are transformed into creoles (Bickerton, 1984) and deaf children reconstruct sign languages that have been awkwardly modeled by their nonnatively signing parents (Senghas & Coppola, 2001; Senghas, Kita, & Ozyurek, 2004). If only a portion of the language known to these individuals originated outside of their heads, then the rest, it has been assumed, must have come from the inside.

One consequence of the strong role played by internal factors is a course of development that appears relatively uneventful to observers, who tend to think that language, given its size and complexity, should require more effort than is actually witnessed. In some societies, of course, parents do direct a great deal of talk to their infants, and speak more slowly, or with exaggerated prosody; and they usually supply the names of particularly salient objects, actions, and concepts. These practices, or the disposition to engage in them, may not facilitate language learning (Hart & Risley, 1995; Nelson, Carskaddon, & Bonvillian, 1973), and may be no more helpful than merely modeling speech (Akhtar, 2005). But they cannot be essential, since infant-directed speech is rare in some societies (Ochs, 1982), and it is unusual – in any culture – for caregivers to do much that is specifically tutorial. Chomsky saw this disparity between knowledge and experience as "the most striking fact about human language." Accounting for it, he wrote, "is the central problem of linguistic theory" (Chomsky, 1967, p. 438).

For Chomsky, "knowledge" is linguistic grammar, the primary function of which is cognitive (2002). But "speech," as de Laguna advised, "must be envisaged … as performing some objective and observable function, before one can hope to discern the factors which have led to its development" (1927, p. 10). Whether she meant to exclude "language" is unclear, but the distinction is salient, for speech does things that language does not do, and cannot do. These observable functions, we may assume, relate to the ways that people use language.

Some might consider questions of use to be outside the purview of language scientists. Others would surely rebut this contention, claiming that pragmatics, conversation rules, and other principles of usage are among the critical components of language. This division between lexical and grammatical knowledge on the one hand, and the social and communicative applications of language on the other, is one of the issues about which evolution and development have something important to say. But there is another issue here. Since we are dealing with an evolved trait, we must assume that the function of language determined its form in evolution, and to some extent continues to do so in development (Studdert-Kennedy, 1991). Since language evolved, it should be possible to locate cases where function was responsible for something about the physical nature of speech or ways of speaking.

Language is what linguists say it is

Speaking is one of the more dynamic forms of human action that one can imagine, one so dynamic that critical elements fade as rapidly as they appear (Hockett, 1960). Linguistics, however, has encouraged its followers to regard language as an object, a stable cache of knowledge about grammar that is stored in the brains of all normal individuals who are socially reared. Although Chomsky (2002) has been a strong proponent of this view, one can hardly blame him for the objectification of language. He was born four years after Jespersen complained that language was being viewed as a collection of "things or natural objects with an existence of their own" (Jespersen, 1924/1963, p.17). Later, objectification troubled Lakoff and Johnson (1980), who commented that words and sentences were being seen as "objects that have properties in and of themselves and stand in fixed relationships to one another, independently of any person who speaks them or understands them" (p. 204). This depersonalized view of language also concerned Linell (2005), who commented that when linguists consult their intuitions on matters of linguistic practice, they encounter "an inventory of forms, and rules for generating forms" (p. 4). Finally, Hermann (2008) called the language-as-thing metaphor a "systematically misleading expression." He suggested that it is time for a better metaphor, one that captures the fleeting and subjective nature of speech.

How did language come to be seen as an object? Most scholars blame literacy training (Goody, 1977; Jespersen, 1924/1963; Lakoff & Johnson, 1980; Linell, 2005; Olson, 1994). When people learn to read, they experience a cross-modal phenomenon that is on a par with hearing a taste or touching an odor. They see words. They also see spaces between the words in a sentence. If the language is alphabetic, they are conditioned to notice the sound symbols – hence the sounds – that make up words, and they additionally discover the spaces between these symbols. From capitalization and punctuation, their attention is further drawn to sentences and phrases.

It is instructive, I think, to consider the things that readers do not encounter on the printed page. They see no prosody, no voice quality, no tone of voice, no rate of speaking, no loudness, no vocal pitch, and no formant structure. As a consequence, they get little or no reliable information about the sender's identity, temperament, emotionality, attitude, social class, place of birth, height, age, sex, physical status, or hormonal status (Locke, 2021). These personal factors relate to important fitness variables such as social dominance and reproductive status, and therefore provide the raw material for evolutionary accounts of vocal communication and spoken language.

With speech literally off the page, it is not surprising that language would come to be conceptualized as whatever is left behind. But there is more, for literacy training is usually followed by five or six years of language arts instruction. Students learn the parts of speech. They are taught to recognize and correct sentences that are ungrammatical. They learn about topic sentences and paragraph structure and the importance of making sense. They become conscious of rules that they inferred in infancy and memorize others. It is a festival of linguistic prescription.

Predictably, literacy training affects the way individuals process linguistic material. In a study carried out in Portugal, subjects who were literate or culturally illiterate were enrolled in a lexical decision task. Concurrent brain scans revealed unequal activation of the right front opercular-anterior insular region, left anterior cingulate, left lentiform nucleus, and anterior thalamus and hypothalamus in the two groups. In a separate repetition task, the illiterate subjects substituted real words for nonsense constructions 25 times more often than the literate subjects (Castro-Caldas, Petersson, Reis, Stone-Elander, & Ingvar, 1998; also see Ostrosky-Solis, Ramirez, & Ardila, 2004).

This work relates to the ways people think about and process language, but there are also huge measurement issues. Language is learned in one modality and tested in another. The result is a personal problem for good speakers who are poor readers, and a theoretical problem for scholars who wish to find out what the evolved trait of language actually entails (Locke, 2008a).

But it is not just a matter of conflicting modalities. Most standard measures of language are, in fact, evaluations of the ability to use linguistic knowledge to solve cognitive problems (e.g., anagrams). The relevant skills are usually classified as "metalinguistic." Individuals with metalinguistic ability are able "to deliberately reflect on and manipulate the structural features of spoken language" (Tunmer & Cole, 1991, p. 387). This ability does not naturally emerge from the biological trait of language. If untrained in literacy, normally speaking adults tend to perform poorly on metalinguistic tests (Morais, 2001; Navas, 2004; see Locke, 2008a for other references).

It is serious enough that academic training affects the way people process and use language and that scientists measure it, but instructed material forms a significant portion of the language that is tested. Some years ago, I analyzed some data collected on an unusual population – the canal boat children of early 20th century England (Locke, 2008a). These children lived on boats, in constant interaction with their parents and siblings, but rarely went ashore or set foot in a classroom. Governmental concern brought about the evaluation of a number of the canal boat children using a standardized intelligence test. This instrument revealed that at six years, when all tests were necessarily oral, the canal boat children scored in the normal range on language measures. However, as the years went by, they sank further and further below the norms on four oral subtests – language comprehension, vocabulary knowledge, sentence construction, and verbal fluency – while displaying age-appropriate abilities on nonverbal subtests. The children were not forgetting what they had learned about language, they were simply not improving at the same rate as their academic peers in the areas affected by instruction. At 12, their scores on the oral subtests approached zero. The results thus dramatized the fact that language, as tested, is heavily influenced by what children learn in schools.

All of these assessments, neuropsychological and linguistic problems are significant, but they converge upon a hugely important biological issue. For it appears that formal training transforms language from a trait that was selected to a talent that is instructed (Locke, 2008a). A talent, according to Simonton (1999), is "any innate capacity that enables an individual to display exceptionally high performance in a domain that requires special skills and training" (p. 436). Competitive chess is considered a talent. No language scientist would assert that the faculty of human language requires instruction – we have already seen that it does not – but my claim here is that language, as it has come to be defined, reflects it. Formal instruction makes a talent out of a trait.

Having said all of this, I would not be particularly worried about these issues if my focus were the development of language in preschool children, as it once was (Locke, 1993a). But why stop studying the development of language (or anything else) just because the child starts school? Of course we know the answer – at this age, they know enough language and are cognitively mature enough to learn to read and take classroom instruction. But an evolutionary approach is necessarily blind to cultural inventions. We will see below and in the section on life history that the trait of language continues to develop well into adolescence.

Language is what evolved

There are some 6,912 natural languages in the world (Gordon, 2005). All of them are spoken. If just one of these languages was produced in a different modality, the incidence of nonvocal languages would be about 0.0001%, but the true incidence is zero. We do not know why the vocal modality is so robust, possibly because few scholars have taken the question seriously, or even recognized that this is a question that needs to be answered (Locke, 1998a). But it is possible that when we know what caused our ancestors to "go vocal" we will be a step closer to an explanation for language itself.

In the past, the higher primates have seemed to give us very little to work with. For some time, it appeared that apes were more gestural than vocal (Locke, 2001a). Even in recent years, linguists have looked at the ape literature and found little more than "a few calls and grunts" (Newmeyer, 2003). How, under the circumstances, could language-as-mental-code have entered the heads of their successors? If we are tacitly discouraged from addressing the modality of language, the medium that contains all of the physical cues, how do we get to the object? Framed in this way, the problem seems insoluble.

Fortunately, we have about six million years to work with – the time elapsed since the Homo line diverged from that of the apes. In that period, there were significant environmental changes that brought about a number of different adaptations. As we will see, two that were heavily deterministic were the shift to bipedalism and increased social complexity. It is also the case that the cognitive and communicative abilities of our last common ancestors were closer to those of humans than has generally been thought. For one thing, the functional value of ape vocalization has been greatly underestimated. While linguists were busily noting the vocal poverty of the apes, animal behaviorists were conducting field studies that revealed unsuspected vocal riches. It is now clear that apes' calls and grunts carry a great deal of information about the age, size, and sex of individuals, as well as their location. They also carry information about the motivational state of the individual, and his intentions with respect to aggression and sex (Seyfarth & Cheney, 2003; see review in Locke, 2009, 2021). In its totality, this literature makes it less strange to ask where the human affection for vocal communication came from, even if we are left wondering how our species, and not the apes, evolved the capacity to control and process particularized vocalization (Oller, 2004; Studdert-Kennedy, 2005).

At the other end of the evolutionary spectrum – the theoretical endpoint – it is not psychologists' and linguists' ability to use and think about language that needs to be explained, but the ability of traditionally living individuals. For them, speaking seems to be more important than speech, the ability to joke, riddle, and tell stories more highly appraised than phonological (and grammatical) knowledge. The task, then, is to find links between the "more vocal than previously suspected" apes and the verbally artful members of traditional societies, and to ask how environmental changes produced fitness-enhancing behaviors that edged our evolutionary ancestors closer to spoken language.

In preliterate societies, language is heavily situational. This allows individuals to speak in a relatively inexplicit way (Linell, 2005). Some have difficulty thinking about the concept of "word" (Goody, 1977). Others act puzzled when asked what a word "means," possibly because words take their meaning from the context in which they are used (Malinowski, 1923). In some societies, words are thought to possess a "magical" quality (Tambiah, 1983). In none of these preliterate societies can a word's meaning be "looked up," nor can one know a word but wonder how it is pronounced.

In these societies, there are few if any schools, and no standardized language tests. Thus, what we know is what anthropologists have mentioned in their accounts. These descriptions make it clear that the communicative practices of traditionally living individuals appear neither as language nor speech. They appear as speaking. In these societies as with the apes, there is a special relationship between speaking and status. In a range of human societies anthropologists have noted unusual linguistic knowledge and rhetorical skill in individuals, invariably men, who have risen to positions of authority and power (Burling, 1986; Locke, 2001a; Locke & Bogin, 2006). I have speculated elsewhere that selection for vocal extravagance expanded the capacity to coordinate and control longer sequences of phonetic material, and that listeners who were able to evaluate these sequences received fitness information that others did not (Locke, 2008a,b, 2009).

There are links between speaking and sex, too. Miller's (2000) claim is that sexual selection shaped human language directly, through mate choice, and indirectly, through its effects on social status.

Verbal courtship can be viewed narrowly as face-to-face flirtation, or broadly as anything we say in public that might increase our social status or personal attractiveness in the eyes of potential mates. Sexual flirtation during early courtship accounts for only a small percentage of language use, but it is the percentage with the most important evolutionary effects. This is the time when the most important reproductive decisions are made, when individuals are accepted or rejected as sexual partners on the basis of what they say (Miller, 2000, pp. 356–357).

Spoken language may also have played a role in sexual selection outside of courtship by advertising various male qualities. It was through public speaking and debate that individuals were able to advertise their knowledge, clear thinking, social tact, good judgment, wit, experience, morality, imagination, and self-confidence. Under Pleistocene conditions, the sexual incentives for advertising such qualities would have persisted throughout adult life, in almost every social situation. Language put minds on public display, where sexual choice could see them clearly for the first time in evolutionary history (Miller, 2000, p. 357).

I agree that language helped to exhibit these qualities, but it could only do so when people spoke. Then, I propose, the variables facilitative of status and sex had less to do with grammar than various aspects of speaking, including prosody, fluency, rhythm, tone of voice, rate, loudness, and humor (Locke, 2001a). But these elements would have exerted no effect had they not enjoyed some relationship to fitness variables such as dominance and attractiveness for mating.

Below, in the section on life history, I will offer proposals as to how our ancestors evolved the capacity for controlled vocalization and speech at a level of complexity that prepared them for modern language, and suggest some functions of various events or milestones in the development of language.

Language is what develops

Purely by cataloguing the world's languages, we find out about the range of linguistic elements that can be handled by the nervous system of young humans. But what is language from the infant's point of view? Over 40 years ago, Miller made a simple but provocative statement. The child, he wrote, "learns the language because he is shaped by nature to pay attention to it, to notice and remember and use significant aspects of it" (1965, p. 20). When I first thought about this I wondered what "it" was from the infant's perspective (Locke, 1993a). My reaction was that "it" must refer to the things people do while talking. This vocal, facial, and gestural activity, and associated situational cues, comprise the totality of linguistically relevant stimulation (Locke, 1993b, 1994).

The process gets off to an early start. Because fetuses eavesdrop on their mother's voice, infants are born with a preference not only for maternal vocalization, but for the language she spoke during this period, even when the speaker is someone else (DeCasper & Fifer, 1980; Moon, Cooper, & Fifer, 1993). But in an astonishingly short time, the mother's tongue lays the physical groundwork for what will become the infant's mother tongue. The most obvious function at this point is indexical learning – learning about people – but it incidentally produces linguistic learning.

So does what I have called "vocal communion," a continuous state or feeling of connectedness that is maintained largely by the vocalizations of infants and caregivers (Locke, 2001b). As we will see, infants place certain kinds of vocal behaviors in this channel, and are rewarded with physical approach, handling, and other forms of care. Several of the social behaviors that predict lexical learning, including joint attention and vocal imitation, may also be associated with maternal attachment. Since quality of attachment predicts language development (van Ijzendoorn, Kijkstra, & Bus,

1995), research is needed to determine those behaviors that are functionally related to language learning and that are only symptomatic of a relationship that is independently influential.

But of course infants do not merely listen. There is a call-response aspect to vocal signaling. When mothers vocalize, infants tend to respond and vice versa. This sort of communications link resembles what Schleidt (1973) called tonic communication. When they respond, there is a tendency on the part of caregivers and infants to do so "in kind"; that is, to produce like behaviors (Locke, 1993a). One might suppose that infants are "attempting" to learn to speak. But if that is the purpose, how do we explain mothers' frequent imitations of their infants (Pawlby, 1977; Veneziano, 1988)?

It is beginning to appear that vocal imitation may be an important way of demonstrating pacifistic intent and willingness to relate, possibly even to establish the identity of the other. Several years ago, Meltzoff and Moore (1994) published a relevant paper on a six-week-old infant's imitation of an adult's facial gestures. Each of several assistants came into the lab at various times and made a distinctive gesture, then left. When they returned to the lab the next day, the same assistants entered the room. Infants responded by reproducing the gesture that the assistants had made the day before, even if they merely saw the person on the second occasion. The results thus suggested that the infants were attempting to relate to, and possibly identify, individuals on the basis of characteristic behaviors.

These results make it possible to see the function of a particular behavior – imitation – that would otherwise merely pass as something that infants do at certain ages. If the adult were to speak instead of gesture, there is nothing here to suggest that the infant would not reproduce aspects of his speaking voice as a means of relating to or identifying him. This would make it appear that the infant was learning language, and might suggest to some observers that the infant was aware of the existence of language, and was attempting to learn it.

Infants who traffic in speech are likely to be credited with progress in the acquisition of language. Nevertheless, perhaps this is not altogether inappropriate. In a prospective study of normally developing children, Nelson et al. (1973) found a relationship between the sheer number of utterances recorded in a session held at 20 months and the age at which a 50-word expressive vocabulary was attained. The number of utterances also was correlated with the age of children at their tenth phrase, and with their rate of lexical acquisition and mean length of utterances. Other work indicates that lexically delayed infants exhibit fewer vocally communicative intentions per minute than normally developing children (Paul & Shiffer, 1991), and produce far fewer utterances, independent of their quality (Paul & Jennings, 1992). Similar findings have been reported by others (Rescorla & Ratner, 1996; Thal, Oroz, & McCaw, 1995).

This is consistent with a paradox about language development. Infants rarely vocalize at normal levels of frequency and complexity during the babbling stage, imitate aspects of their mother's speech, and produce isolated words – behaviors that ostensibly require no grammatical ability at all – later stumble as they enter the domains of morphology and syntax (Locke, 1998b). Whatever problems arise at the grammatical level of language are typically forecast by deficiencies in early lexical development (Bates & Goodman, 1997), just as the rate of word learning is predicted, to some degree, by the level of vocal sophistication and control revealed in the babbling stage (Oller, Eilers, Neal, & Schwartz, 1999).

But it gets better. Grammatical development is also linked to personality factors. Slomkowski, Nelson, Dunn, and Plomin (1992) found that a measure of introversion and extroversion at the age of two years was highly predictive of scores on eight different standardized language measures at the age of seven. Infants who were extraverted learned language with unusual speed. Thus, it appears that sociability and volubility – measures that are neither linguistic nor cognitive – predict the development of language even when it is defined as code.

How do we make sense of these links between volubility and the lexicon, and between personality and grammar? Earlier I referred to species-specific linguistic mechanisms. Language development involves the activation of these mechanisms, but there is no evidence that the mechanisms are turned on solely by maturation or exposure to people who talk. It makes more sense to suppose that they, like other neural systems, are pressured to turn on. I have suggested elsewhere that the precipitating event is a storage problem, created by the accumulation of utterances that are appropriately analyzed prosodically, but underanalyzed phonetically (Locke, 1997). It has been suggested that children must have a "critical mass" of words in their expressive lexicon – perhaps as many as 70 verbs, and 400 words overall – before they discover and begin to apply the rules of linguistic morphology (Bates, Dale, & Thal, 1994; Marchman & Bates, 1994; Plunkett & Marchman, 1993).

With language presupposing the operation of mechanisms that do various things, there is naturally a question about what the language faculty can be said to include. Hauser, Chomsky, and Fitch (2002) solved this problem, to their satisfaction, by positing a broad and a narrow faculty, the former including social and cognitive mechanisms, the latter excluding them. This is a reasonable way of thinking about linguistic systems, in a logical sense, but when it comes to development a different kind of "sense" creeps in. If social factors are critical to language, then they are critical components in the developmental system that is responsible for language. Here we begin to see the problem - the difference between a developmentally and a theoretically based definition of language.

We have seen that evolution plays a role in development. It supplied the mechanisms that, with appropriate experience, carry out linguistic operations. But it has been overlooked until recently that evolution also supplied the developmental stages in which language develops, so that when evolution produced new and modified developmental stages, they fed back new candidate behaviors for selection.

The evolution of development

To evolve, genetically supported traits must offer a selective advantage. Pinker and Bloom (1990) argued that natural selection is the only way to explain the origin of language and other complex abilities. In doing so, they said little about any role that selection might have played in development. But as Hogan (1988) has pointed out, natural selection "should operate at all stages of development, and not only on the adult outcome, since any developmental process that reduces the probability of reaching adulthood will be very strongly selected against" (p. 97). Thus, in this section I offer several new proposals relating to vocal and verbal selection as it may have operated in infancy and childhood.

There are lots of theories (or pseudotheories) of evolution in which language, like a deus ex machina, enters the hominin scene in the nick of time, supplying our ancestors with just the communicative tool they need to solve some pressing environmental problem. But evolution is a tinker who works from available parts. No species can manufacture a new part just because having it would become in handy.

Nor can an adult member of any species do this. No trait can evolve unless precursory forms appear during a stage of development, and this is the only time when he suggested that new species emerged from "affections of their generative system" (1871, p.267). A half-century later, Garstang wrote that ontogeny "creates" phylogeny. It is "absurd," he said, to think that a new trait could evolve in adults (Garstang, 1922).

In the interim, a number of respected biologists have embraced and elaborated upon Garstang's claim (Gottlieb, 2002; Gould, 1977; Northcutt. 1990; West-Eberhard, 2003; see other references in Locke, 2009). It is now understood that evolution is a two-step process (West-Eberhard, 2003). In the first step, a plastic phenotype responds to environmental variation – in development – producing novel forms that vary genetically. In the second step, selection acts on the variants. A selection-based account of language cannot be complete unless it identifies the linguistically favorable genetic variations that arise in ontogeny and the processes of selection that reinforced and expanded those variations.

If development occurs in stages, then behaviors that develop owe their existence to some feature of those stages. This implores us to look beyond the development of mechanisms that evolved and explore the evolution of development. I believe the case can be made that in evolution, some type of selection occurred for language – or what was to become language – at every stage of development from infancy to sexual maturity – and that each new behavior that develops serves a distinct function. I have suggested elsewhere that selection in infancy helped produce the vocal complexity and social functionality that were later reselected in the rather different biological contexts supplied by childhood, juvenility, and adolescence (Locke, 2006). But even if selection had initially applied in adolescence, the behaviors reinforced at that stage would already have to have "been there" in some form, even if they had never functioned in the new way.

To be prepared for a socially complex adulthood, there must be appropriately structured intervals for development and learning. Humans have four such stages – two more than the other primates. We also have two stages that were remodeled (Bogin, 1999a). I propose that all four of these new and remodeled stages were needed for language to evolve, and that all four are needed for the young to acquire knowledge of language and to become fully proficient in its use (Locke, 2009; Locke & Bogin, 2006).

The approach to human life history that will be used here was developed by Bogin (1988; 1999a). Much of what will be said about the individual stages is adapted from a paper coauthored with Bogin several years ago (see Locke & Bogin, 2006, 2021, for details and references).

Infancy

Infancy begins at or before birth and ends at about 30 to 36 months when, in traditional societies, weaning takes place. This stage is characterized by rapid physical growth, provision of nourishment by maternal lactation, and eruption of deciduous dentition. Human infants are more helpless than ape and monkey infants, a "deficiency" that requires a long period of continuous care.

It is thought that the initial change that produced greater helplessness was bipedal locomotion, which realigned the spine and narrowed the pelvis. This produced problems at birth for the mother and her large-headed fetus. There being a range of variation among infants, some had smaller heads at the time of birth, and these infants – and their mothers – were more likely to survive the delivery. Over time, differential rates of survival caused a shift in skull and brain development from the prenatal to the postnatal period. This increased infant dependency and need of care.

These changes remodeled the premodern human infancy. In doing so, they positioned it for language and other complex behaviors. For, in a number of important respects, the conditions above – in danger of being seen as design flaws – offered more and better opportunities for social, vocal, lexical, and symbolic learning (Bjorklund, 1997; Locke, 1993a, 1999).

This tendency to view helplessness and heightened care as socially and cognitively beneficial is supported by anthropological accounts, which indicate that most hunter-gatherer mothers rarely put their babies down, and then do so for no more than a few seconds. Separation cries usually evoke pick up and breast feeding. When infants cannot be carried, they are often left in the care of others (Hardy, 2006).

Beginning prenatally, infants learn aspects of the prosodic and segmental characteristics of the ambient language. By six months, most infants have heard enough speech to recognize a few words and stereotyped phrases, and to experience some perceptual reorganization, a process that continues in succeeding months.

From a variety of developments in the first year or life, parents and language scientists alike conclude that infants are learning speech or acquiring language. Undoubtedly they are, but in some sense, these advances are unintended consequences. There are many reasons why helpless individuals might benefit by attending to, storing, and reproducing caregiver speech, most of which have a great deal to do with the negotiation of their own care (Locke, 1996).

In our species, weaning comes earlier than it does in the apes. It is generally held that earlier weaning would have shortened the interbirth interval, enabling women to have more infants in their reproductive lifetime. I have proposed that this produced an increase in the number of siblings – competitors for care. This heightened competition, combined with unprecedented levels of helplessness, forced infants to explore clever new ways of using the voice to secure and maintain maternal proximity, and to monitor and "read" maternal feedback; and that, therefore, some of the vocal ability presupposed by spoken language was asserted initially by hominin infants and reinforced by successful interactions with their parents.

According to the proposal, infants who issued more effective care-elicitation signals received more care, and were marginally more likely to live on to reproductive age (Locke, 2006). The parental selection hypothesis proposes that some of the vocal ability presupposed by spoken languages emerged from infancy, having been asserted initially by hominin infants and supported by interactions with their parents. This hypothesis holds that infants who issued more effective care-elicitation signals (e.g., measured or strategic levels of cry) were better positioned to receive care than infants who issued stress vocalizations noxiously or incosably – behaviors that invite neglect and abuse in primates generally, and forecast language-learning problems in humans. The hypothesis also envisions that infants who cooed and babbled at appropriate intervals were more likely to engage with adults, to be liked by them, to receive more sophisticated forms of care as infancy progressed, and to generate and learn complex phonetic patterns. Infants who were able to monitor adult reactions to their behaviors would have been able to discover those vocalizations that had the most beneficial effects, and thus could use structured vocalization to maximum effect.

It is also possible that syllabic and articulatory activity played a "decoupling" role (Oller, 2004), making available for recombination the discrete movements, hence the phonetic segments that make phonological systems possible (Studdert-Kennedy, 1998, 2005; Studdert-Kennedy & Goldstein, 2003). I propose that further elaboration of vocal repertoires would have occurred later in development under different pressures, potentially enhancing fitness in one or more of these stages, particularly adolescence. The result is a system flexible enough to be used for speech, and there is evidence that vocal abilities presupposed by variegated babbling are in fact adequate for infants' initial words (Vihman, Macken, Miller, Simmons, & Miller, 1985).

It is generally recognized that development is continuous, but continuity would also have played a role in evolution. I have proposed that new levels of vocal complexity, flexibility, and control that emerged from infancy were carried into later ontogenetic stages where – development being continuous and cumulative – they were reinforced and elaborated (Locke & Bogin, 2006). In the new childhood that evolved (see below), these signaling capabilities would surely have proved beneficial, for if children are to avoid hazardous aspects of their environment, they must be warned if not "instructed."

It is at this point that we begin to see the first of several sets of discontinuities. In the typical case, the close of intimacy is co-timed with evidence that the mechanisms responsible for each of the recognized components of language-as-code – the lexicon, phonology, morphology, and syntax – are operating at some level of efficiency.

Childhood

Childhood is a uniquely human stage that is thought to have entered the Homo line about two million years ago (Bogin, 2001, 2003). Since chimpanzees wean at about five years, it is assumed that earlier weaning liberated about two years from infancy. This is what created childhood (Bogin, 1990). It has been suggested that the extension of childhood to its present length – which extends from about three to nearly seven years – was due, at least in part, to the increasing functionality of communicative behaviors in this stage (Locke & Bogin, 2006).

The childhood stage is peculiar to humans, having been evolutionarily inserted between the infant and juvenile stages that characterize social mammals. Childhood, according to Bogin, is defined by several developmental characteristics, including a deceleration and stabilization of the rate of growth, immature dentition, dependence on older people for food, and immature motor control. The evolutionary value of childhood is associated with the mother's freedom to stop breast-feeding her three-year-old, enabling her to become pregnant again. This enhanced reproductive output without increasing the risk of mortality for the mother or her infant or older children, for in cooperatively breeding societies, others were available to help care for the young.

Childhood is largely defined by the long period, extending from three to seven years, in which food must be provided. By seven, dentition is becoming adult-like, and with parallel increases in jaw control, it becomes possible for children to eat adult foods. Socially, childhood produces new friendships outside of the home as well as increased disenchantment with siblings. In some modern societies, five-year-olds have social hierarchies. In these hierarchies, low-status children behave positively toward their higher status peers, without reciprocity. Children with good communication skills are likely to be popular (Asher & Renshaw, 1981; Putallaz & Gottman, 1981), whereas children with speech and language disorders are typically unpopular, and may even be victimized (Conti-Ramsden & Botting, 2004). Children with pragmatic or higher-level language processing disorders are likely to experience serious peer interaction problems (Botting & Conti-Ramsden, 2000). Delayed language predicts poor quality of friendship in adolescence; it may independently impair friendship or do so in conjunction with poor social cognition (Botting & Conti-Ramsden, 2008; Durkin & Conti-Ramsden, 2007).

As childhood draws to an end, a second set of discontinuities in native language learning occurs. One relates to the fact that languages acquired after large epidemiological samples of midwestern American children, six years of age was also treated as the approximate age of native language mastery, based on standardized tests that are oriented to school performance (Shriberg, Tomblin, & McSweeny, 1999; Tomblin et al., 1997). Thus, in one modern society, and undoubtedly far more, much of the childhood period is needed to master the basic structure and elementary vocabulary of a knowledge-based linguistic system.

But there is more to be accomplished in childhood. One advance involves verbal fluency, which continues to improve throughout this stage (Starkweather, 1987). Other developments relate to automaticity and rate of speaking (Smith, 2006). If something goes wrong with the sensory system that guides ambient learning during childhood, there is likely to be significant deterioration of speech. Clinical studies indicate that all of childhood is needed to achieve a speaking ability that can tolerate the discontinued stimulation entailed by acquired deafness (Waldstein, 1990; also see Locke & Bogin, 2006).

Some of the communicative skills arising in childhood do so in tandem with certain cognitive advances. One such development is the "theory of other minds," which typically emerges between two and four years of age (Baron-Cohen, Tager-Flusberg, & Cohen, 1993), enabling children to take the perspective of others. There is also an improvement in autobiographical memory, which usually occurs between three and eight years of age (Nelson, 1996), enabling children to describe sequential events and to share memories of their own experience. This comports with the fact that childhood also sees improvement in discourse and narration (Girolametto, Wiigs, Smyth, Weitzman, & Pearce, 2001).

In recent years, there has been increased attention to pragmatics, but there are few if any accounts of language development that seriously address verbal performance. Some of the developments that occur in childhood relate to verbal competition and performance. These include joking (McGhee, 1979; Shultz & Horibe, 1974) and the use of "off the shelf" verbal routines (Gleason & Weintraub, 1976). In many cultures, jokes and riddles mark the beginning of various sorts of verbal competition (Gossen, 1976a,b; Sanches & Kirshenblatt-Gimblett, 1976).

During childhood, males tend to speak assertively to get and maintain attention and to make evident their desires, and girls tend to speak softly in order to promote interpersonal closeness and harmony (see review in Locke & Bogin, 2006). The linguistic acquisitions of infancy are thus joined, in childhood and succeeding stages, by other factors that elevate the quality of verbal expression and facilitate development of communicative skills (e.g., Sherzer, 2002).

Since it begins with weaning, childhood liberated the young from continuous maternal restraint. Naïve children's exploration of their physical environment presumably increased the need for parents to warn and instruct, giving them and other kin self-serving reasons to send honest signals. But childhood also positioned the young to know about, thus to convey information about, events occurring in the absence of others. I would suggest that childhood handed the young and their families a key ingredient of human language – displacement – in the form of new opportunities and needs to talk about things not physically present (Fitch, 2004; Hockett, 1960). It is possible that the swing period in development of native-like language abilities – six to eight years of age – is related to changing pressures associated with the transition to a more independent and autonomous stage of development.

In development, childhood would have given the young opportunities to integrate and automate linguistic operations, to introspect on language and to analyze it, and to develop an appreciation of rhyme, alliteration, fluency – all of which would be needed in juvenility.

Juvenility

Juvenility is the next stage of human development. In mammals generally and primates more specifically, juveniles are sexually immature but independent of others for survival. It is not unusual in traditional human societies for juveniles to find much of their own food, avoid predators, and compete with adults for food and space (see Locke & Bogin, 2006).

Juvenility begins at seven years, with the onset of adrenarche and associate cognitive and social advances. This stage ends at ten and 12 years in females and males, respectively. Juveniles are sexually immature but more independent of older individuals than children. Since it comes after a remodeled infancy and new childhood, the juvenile stage of our evolutionary ancestors could hardly have remained unchanged. In various species of mammals, juvenility provides additional time for the brain growth and learning that is required for reproductive success (Janson & van Schaik, 1993; Joffe, 1997). In complex human societies, it takes all of juvenility and adolescence for the development of social and linguistic skills that are needed in sexual maturity.

Although there is increased independence from family members in childhood, juvenility would have given the young opportunities to prepare themselves, resources – particularly sex and dominance (Locke, 2001a; Locke & Bogin, 2006). Many of the language developments that occur in modern juvenility take place beyond the sentence level, in the quality of extended discourse and narratives. New abilities in pragmatics and verbal performance contribute to a variety of socially relevant activities, from gossiping to joking and storytelling.

Juvenility also accommodates additional syntactic advances (cf. Nippold, 1998), but many of the new developments affect performance. These include an increase in respiratory capacity, which continues into adolescence (Engström, Karlberg, & Kraepellen, 1956; Hoit, Hixon, Watson, & Morgan, 1990), and further increases in fluency and speaking rate. Changes occur beyond the sentence level too, in the quality of extended discourse and narratives (Bamberg, 1987; Burleson, 1982; Karmiloff-Smith, 1985). These advances facilitate a number of socially relevant activities, including gossip and storytelling, and contribute to successful competition and courtship as sexual maturity approaches.

Around ten to 12 years, riddles and jokes become more important. In Turkey, boys engage in verbal duels – ritualistic insults and replies that require "skill in remembering and selecting appropriate retorts to provocative insults" (Dundes, Leach, & Özkök, 1970, p. 135). These duels occur between eight and 14 years, bracketing the transition from juvenility to adolescence.

In a sense, juvenility parallels infancy. Whereas the linguistic knowledge and structure gained in infancy helps to satisfy the informational needs of childhood, juvenility provides opportunities to perfect the persuasive and attractive use of speech, and the ability to manipulate elaborate and socially appropriate utterances, which will be valued in adolescence.

Adolescence

Adolescence is the fourth stage of life history, and the second stage that is uniquely human, since the other primates proceeding directly from juvenility to adulthood (Bogin, 1999b). This stage begins at the end of juvenility and extends to 19 years, when adulthood commences. In modern humans, adolescence is announced by puberty and a simultaneous surge in skeletal growth, strengthening of friendships, and development of new relationships.

In humans, uniquely, there is a distinct skeletal growth spurt in both sexes after several years of gently decreasing juvenile growth. The onset of this spurt, along with puberty or gonadarche marks the onset of two sexes, females revealing negligible changes, males displaying a significant increase in tract length and decrease in fundamental frequency, with further drops in the transition from adolescence to adulthood (Fitch & Giedd, 1999; Lieberman, McCarthy, Hiiemae, & Palmer, 2001; Pedersen, Moller, Krabbe, & Bennett, 1986; Pedersen, MØller, Krabbe, Bennett, & Svenstrup, 1990; Vuorenkoski, Lenko, Tjernlund, Vuorenkoski, & Perheentupa, 1978). The critical variable, testosterone, increases the size of the vocal folds, lowers the fundamental frequency, and changes the vibratory characteristics of the vocal folds (Abitol, Abitol, & Abitol, 1999; Beckford, Rood, & Schaid, 1985; Titze, 1989).

In adolescence – if not sooner – and certainly in adulthood, males also display lung and respiratory superiority over females (Becklake, 1999; Cook & Hamann, 1961; Hibbert, Lannigan, Raven, Landau, & Phelan, 1995; Higgins & Saxman, 1991; Schrader, Quanjer, & Olievier, 1988; Thurlbeck, 1982). Although this variable is often neglected in developmental accounts of language, even in accounts of speech, it undoubtedly has a great deal to do with speaking in a public and competitive way. In humans and a range of other species, respiratory capacity is positively correlated with body size (Engström et al., 1956; Helliesen, Cook, Friedlander, & Agathon, 1958; Stahl, 1967; Tenney & Remmers, 1963), and in the context of mate selection, this ability is likely to have been of considerable interest to ancestral females.

In men, status and dominance are linked to testosterone (Mazur & Booth, 1998), which tends to be higher in men with low vocal pitch (Dabbs & Mallinger, 1999; Pedersen et al., 1986). It comes as no surprise, then, that men with low-pitched voices are judged by female listeners, from vocal samples, to be more dominant and attractive (Collins, 2000; Collins & Missing, 2003; Feinberg, Jones, Little, Burt, & Perrett, 2005; Puts, Gaulin, & Verdolini, 2006). Women also prefer male voices that are low in pitch (Collins, 2000; Oguchi & Kikuchi, 1997), a preference that appears to be enhanced by estrogen (Feinberg et al., 2006; Puts, 2005). Male university students with low voices report slightly more sexual partners than other men (Puts et al., 2006), and baritone opera singers report having more affairs than tenors (Wilson, 1984). In hunter–gatherer societies, men with low voices report fathering more children than men with higher voices (Apicella, Feinberg, & Marlowe, 2007). These findings could be taken to mean that vocal pitch is a fixed trait, but of course men are able to manipulate their voices, and do so when it could alter their perceived dominance (Puts et al., 2006).

Earlier I mentioned increased group size and social complexity as spurs to increased brain size and linguistic behavior. If these pressures applied with unusual force during any one of the stages of life history, adolescence – when the draw of the group is especially strong – would surely be that stage. It is therefore interesting that recent imaging research is now indicating that adolescence, to a surprising degree, is a time of renewed brain development. The volume of cerebral gray matter sharply decreases from childhood to adolescence, evidently due to dendritic pruning, and there are large increases in white matter, caused by myelination, increases in axonal size, and glial proliferation (De Bellis et al., 2001; Giedd, 2005; Giedd et al., 2001; Shaw et al., 2006). This pattern of exuberant growth and pruning is relevant to arguments that adolescence conferred reproductive advantages on our ancestors, partly by giving the young additional opportunities to acquire social and sexual skills before reproducing (Bogin, 1999a,b).

Adolescence provides opportunities to learn the pragmatic and performative skills that are needed to converse and to narrate (Dorval & Eckerman, 1984; Nippold, 1998). It also offers opportunities to learn slang, idioms, and other formulaic expressions, which contribute to group solidarity and enhance the ability to perform, possibly by increasing fluency and rate of speech for that material (Kuiper, 1996). Other performance skills that develop in adolescence include refinements in gossiping, joking, arguing, negotiating, and persuading; and in the rate of speaking (Walsh & Smith, 2002). All these skills stand to impress peers and facilitate the achievement and maintenance of social relationships.

I have emphasized adolescence as an innovative stage with reproductive advantages. The reason, in part, relates to the benefits and pressures associated with group life. Dunbar (1993) has argued that group pressures played a role in the evolution of language. It is reasonable to suppose that the benefits of group affiliation, and the achievement of personal identity and autonomy, have motivated adolescents to invent vocal and verbal behaviors, thereby reinforcing any improvisational abilities carried forward from previous stages. Modern adolescents do not merely learn additional linguistic features and rules of usage. They also modify material learned earlier, and invent new words and constructions. But the changes are not merely lexical. "The relatively high degree of phonological innovation in the adolescent age group," wrote Eckert (1988), "is an indication that the development of adolescent social structure provides a major impetus for phonological change" (p. 197).

Development of other secondary sexual characteristics, and a sharp increase in height and weight, also occur in adolescence. These physical new relationships, i.e., the new affiliations as well as membership in peer groups, facilitate intimacy and mutual support (Whitmire, 2000). Adolescence draws to a close with the attainment of adult stature and the biosocial skills needed for successful reproduction. Typically, this occurs at about 19 years of age in women and 21 to 25 years in men (Bogin, 1999a, 2001).

Concluding remarks

If development occurs in stages, then behaviors that develop owe their existence to some feature of those stages. This implores us to look beyond the development of mechanisms that evolved and explore the evolution of the developmental stages themselves, asking which of many biological factors are responsible for the induction of linguistic systems.

The stages of life history have unique and coherent properties. These properties provide the context for a range of social and cognitive developments, including language. This suggests that there are linguistic discontinuities at stage boundaries. Several have been identified here, but there are likely to be a great many others.

In research on language development, there is a tendency to focus on infancy and childhood, probably because it is during these stages that knowledge of words and grammatical rules is acquired. This accords well with implicit views of language as an object. But knowledge of language enables one to speak, thus to act in social situations, and to express oneself in social groups. By adopting human life history as our theoretical framework, one is encouraged to ask about the contribution of each developmental stage, from infancy and childhood through juvenility and adolescence, and it is during these later stages that this second (social) view of language becomes more salient.

It is for these reasons that developing individuals who speak in accepted ways should experience far more social success than those who do not, and there is no shortage of evidence that this is so. However, the causes of social acceptance (and rejection) at sexual maturity are not as closely linked to linguistic knowledge and structure as to vocal and verbal performance. Clearly, the relevant speaking skills – the perceptible and, from a causal standpoint, proximate behaviors – presuppose prior accomplishment in all areas of language, however inconspicuous these accomplishments might be initially.

Until now, research on language development has emphasized acquisition of a lexicon and linguistic grammar, but other advances in maturation, learning, persuasively, thus competitively. If in evolution, as now, these developments occurred during a stage that follows childhood, communicative ability in preceding stages would have been important. In a treatise on the embryological development of the chick, Wolff wrote, "each part is first of all an effect of the preceding part, and itself becomes the cause of the following part" (Wolff, 1764, in Hall, 1999, p. 112). Since development is continuous, one supposes that infants and children who achieved effective use of sound-meaning signals precociously carried some form of the relevant control behaviors into juvenility and adolescence. The result, on a continuity hypothesis, would have been other exceptional skills in the use of spoken language. These would have facilitated attainment for status, sex, and additional resources, enhancing reproductive success while strengthening the precursory behaviors that had persisted, in some form, from earlier stages.

I have suggested that studies of language development can benefit from a new model – one that explores synergies between evolution and development. Such a model encourages us to think in new ways about development and to explore new issues. These include the fitness-cue value of various components of spoken language. If elements of speech were selected, they may now be supported by special-purpose mechanisms. To the degree that they are, the behaviors enabled by these mechanisms may enjoy a different developmental course than other behaviors.

It is clear that we need a functional account of vocal imitation, one that parallels work on facial and manual activity, and its necessity to develop greater understanding of the proximal mechanisms that are at work in infants' learning of vocal and symbolic activity. Before infants become aware of the communicative value of linguistic material, they absorb and accommodate to it, but on what motivation?

Where the faculty of language is concerned, the biological trait that evolved was the ability to speak, and yet there are no standardized tests of speaking. As a consequence, we have no way to measure the relationship of language-as-code and the ability to speak, where speaking is sensitive to performance variables of the sort mentioned above. There is room for a great deal of research here.

Further reading

Locke, J. L. (2021). The indexical voice: Communication of personal states and traits in humans and other primates. *Frontiers in Psychology, 12*. https://doi.org/10.3389/fpsyg.2021.651108.

Locke, J. L., & Bogin, B. (2022). An unusually human time: Effects of the most social stage on the most social species. In S. L. Hart & D. F. Bjorklund (Eds.), *Evolutionary perspectives on infancy*. Switzerland: Springer Nature.https://www.springer.com/gp/about-springer.

References

Abitol, J., Abitol, P., & Abitol, B. (1999). Sex hormones and the female voice. *Journal of Voice, 13*(3), 424–446.

Akhtar, N. (2005). The robustness of learning through overhearing. *Developmental Science, 8*(2), 199–209.

Apicella, C. L., Feinberg, D. R., & Marlowe, F. W. (2007). Voice pitch predicts reproductive success in male hunter-gatherers. *Biology Letters, 3*(6), 682–684.

Asher, S. R., & Renshaw, P. D. (1981). Children without friends: Social knowledge and social-skill training. In S. R. Asher & J. M. Gottman (Eds.), *The development of children's friendships*. Cambridge: Cambridge University Press, 273–296.

Bamberg, M. (1987). *The acquisition of narratives*. Berlin: Mouton de Gruyter.

Baron-Cohen, S., Tager-Flusberg, H., & Cohen, D. J. (Eds.). (1993). *Understanding other minds: Perspectives from autism*. New York: Oxford University Press.
Bates, E., Dale, P. S., & Thal, D. (1994). Individual differences and their implications for theories of language development. In P. Fletcher & B. MacWhinney (Eds.), *Handbook of child language*. Oxford: Basil Blackwell. https://doi.org/10.1111/b.9780631203124.1996.00005.x.
Bates, E., & Goodman, J. C. (1997). On the inseparability of grammar and the lexicon: Evidence from acquisition, aphasia and real-time processing. *Language and Cognitive Processes, 12*(5–6), 507–584.
Beckford, N. S., Rood, S. R., Schaid, D., & Schanbacher, B. (1985). Androgen stimulation and laryngeal development. *Annals of Otology, Rhinology, and Laryngology, 94*(6 Pt 1), 634–640.
Becklake, M. R., & Kauffmann, F. (1999). Gender differences in airway behaviour over the human life span. *Thorax, 54*(12), 1119–1138.
Bickerton, D. (1984). The language bioprogram hypothesis. *Behavioral and Brain Sciences*, 7(2), 173–188.
Bjorklund, D. F. (1997). The role of immaturity in human development. *Psychological Bulletin, 122*(2), 153–169.
Bogin, B. (1988). *Patterns of human growth*. Cambridge: Cambridge University Press.
Bogin, B. (1990). The evolution of human childhood. *Bio-Science, 40*(1), 16–25.
Bogin, B. (1999a). *Patterns of human growth* (2nd ed.). New York: Cambridge University Press.
Bogin, B. (1999b). Evolutionary perspective on human growth. *Annual Review of Anthropology, 28*, 109–153.
Bogin, B. (2001). *The growth of humanity*. New York: Wiley-Liss.
Bogin, B. (2003). The human pattern of growth and development in paleontological perspective. In J. L. Thompson, G. E. Krovitz, & A. J. Nelson (Eds.), *Patterns of growth and development in the Genus Homo*. Cambridge: Cambridge University Press. DOI: 10.1017/CBO9780511542565.002.
Botting, N., & Conti-Ramsden, G. (2000). Social and behavioural difficulties in children with language impairment. *Child Language Teaching and Therapy, 16*, 105–120.
Botting, N., & Conti-Ramsden, G. (2008). The role of language, social cognition, and social skill in the functional social outcomes of young adolescents with and without a history of SLI. *British Journal of Developmental Psychology, 26*(2), 281–300.
Burleson, B. R. (1982). The development of comforting communication skills in childhood and adolescence. *Child Development, 53*(6), 1578–1588.
Burling, R. (1986). The selective advantage of complex language. *Ethology and Sociobiology*, 7(1), 1–16.
Castro-Caldas, A., Petersson, K. M., Reis, A., Stone-Elander, S., & Ingvar, M. (1998). The illiterate brain: Learning to read and write during a childhood influences the functional organization of the adult brain. *Brain, 121*(6), 1053–1063.
Chomsky, N. (1959). Review of *verbal behavior*, by B. F. Skinner. *Language, 35*, 26–58.
Chomsky, N. (1967). The formal nature of language. Appendix A. In E. Lenneberg (Ed.), *Biological foundations of language*. New York: John Wiley and Sons, 397–442.
Chomsky, N. (1980). *Rules and representations*. Oxford: Basil Blackwell.
Chomsky, N. (2002). *On nature and language*. Cambridge: Cambridge University Press.
Collins, S. A. (2000). Men's voices and women's choices. *Animal Behaviour, 60*(6), 773–780.
Collins, S. A., & Missing, C. (2003). Vocal and visual attractiveness are related in women. *Animal Behaviour, 65*(5), 997–1004.
Conti-Ramsden, G., & Botting, N. (2004). Social difficulties and victimization in children with SLI at 11 years of age. *Journal of Speech, Language, and Hearing Research, 47*(1), 145–161.
Cook, C. D., & Hamann, J. F. (1961). Relation of lung volumes to height in healthy persons between the ages of 5 and 38 years. *Journal of Pediatrics, 59*, 710–714.
Dabbs, J. M., & Mallinger, A. (1999). Higher testosterone levels predict lower voice pitch among men. *Personality and Individual Differences*, 27(4), 801–804.
De Bellis, M. D., Keshavan, M. S., Beers, S. R., Hall, J., Frustaci, K., Masalehdan, A., … Boring, A. M. (2001). Sex differences in brain maturation during childhood and adolescence. *Cerebral Cortex, 11*(6), 552–557.
DeCasper, A., & Fifer, W. P. (1980). On human bonding: Newborns prefer their mothers' voices. *Science, 208*(4448), 1174–1176.
de Laguna, G. A. (1927). *[Speech]: Its function and development*. New Haven, CT: Yale University Press.
Dorval, B., & Eckerman, C. O. (1984). Developmental trends in the quality of conversation achieved by small groups of acquainted peers. *Monographs of the Society for Research in Child Development* (Serial No. 206), *49*(2), 1–91.
Dunbar, R. I. M. (1993). Coevolution of neocortical size, group size and language in humans. *Behavioral and Brain Sciences, 16*(4), 681–694.
Dundes, A., Leach, J. W., & Özkök, B. (1970). The strategy of Turkish boys' verbal dueling rhymes. In J. J. Gumperz & D. Hymes (Eds.), *Directions in sociolinguistics: The ethnography of communication*. New York: Holt, Rinehart and Winston, 325–349.

Durkin, K., & Conti-Ramsden, G. M. (2007). Language, social behaviour, and the quality of friendships in adolescents with and without a history of specific language impairment. *Child Development, 78*(5), 1441–1457.
Eckert, P. (1988). Adolescent social structure and the spread of linguistic change. *Language and in Society, 17*(2), 183–207.
Engström, I., Karlberg, P., & Kraepellen, S. (1956). Respiratory studies in children. *Acta Paediatrica, 46*(3), 277–294.
Feinberg, D. R., Jones, B. C., Law Smith, M. J., Moor, F. R., DeBruine, L. M., Cornwell, R. E., ... Perrett, D. I. (2006). Menstrual cycle, trait estrogen level, and masculinity preferences in the human voice. *Hormones and Behavior, 49*(2), 215–222.
Feinberg, D. R., Jones, B. C., Little, A. C., Burt, M. D., & Perrett, D. I. (2005). Manipulations of fundamental frequency and formant frequencies influence the attractiveness of human male voices. *Animal Behaviour, 69*(3), 561–568.
Fitch, W. T. (2004). Kin selection and "mother tongues": A neglected component in language evolution. In D. K. Oller & U. Griebel (Eds.), *The evolution of communication systems: A comparative approach*. Cambridge, MA: MIT Press, 275–296.
Fitch, W. T., & Giedd, J. (1999). Morphology and development of the human vocal tract: A study using magnetic resonance imaging. *Journal of the Acoustical Society of America, 106*(3 Pt 1), 1511–1522.
Garstang, W. (1922). The theory of recapitulation: A critical re-statement of the biogenetic law. *Journal of the Linnaean Society (Zoology), 35*(232), 81–101.
Giedd, J. N. (2005). Structural magnetic resonance imaging of the adolescent brain. *Annals of the New York Academy of Science, 1021*, 77–85.
Giedd, J. N., Blumenthal, J., Jeffries, N. O., Castellanos, F. X., Liu, H., Zijdenbos, A., ... Rapoport, J. L. (2001). Brain development during childhood and adolescence: A longitudinal MRI study. *Nature Neuroscience, 2*(10), 861–863.
Girolametto, L., Wiigs, M., Smyth, R., Weitzman, E., & Pearce, P. S. (2001). Children with a history of expressive vocabulary delay: Outcomes at 5 years of age. *American Journal of Speech-Language Pathology, 10*(4), 358–369.
Gleason, J. B., & Weintraub, S. (1976). The acquisition of routines in child language. *Language in Society, 5*(2), 129–136.
Goody, J. (1977). *The domestication of the savage mind*. Cambridge: Cambridge University Press.
Gordon, R. G. (Ed.). (2005). *Ethnologue: Languages of the world* (15th ed.). Dallas, TX: SIL International.
Gossen, G. H. (1976a). Verbal dueling in Chamula. In B. Kirshenblatt-Gimblett (Ed.), *Speech play: Research and resources for the study of linguistic creativity*. Philadelphia, PA: University of Pennsylvania Press, 121–146.
Gossen, G. H. (1976b). Chamula genres of verbal behavior. In A. Paredes & R. Bauman (Eds.), *Toward new perspectives in folklore*. Austin, TX: University of Texas Press, 159–179.
Gottlieb, G. (2002). *Individual development and evolution: The genesis of novel behavior*. Mahwah, NJ: Erlbaum.
Gould, S. J. (1977). *Ontogeny and phylogeny*. Cambridge, MA: Harvard University Press.
Hall, B. K. (1999). *Evolutionary developmental biology*. London: Chapman and Hall.
Hart, B., & Risley, T. (1995). *Meaningful differences in everyday parenting and intellectual development in young American children*. Baltimore, MD: Brookes.
Hauser, M. D., Chomsky, N., & Fitch, W. T. (2002). The faculty of language: What is it, who has it, and how did it evolve? *Science, 298*(5598), 1569–1579.
Helliesen, P. J., Cook, C. D., Friedlander, L., & Agathon, S. (1958). Studies of respiratory physiology in children. I. Mechanics of respiration and lung volumes in 85 normal children 5 to 17 years of age. *Pediatrics, 22*(1, Part 1), 80–93.
Hermann, J. (2008). The 'language' problem. *Language and Communication, 28*(1), 93–99.
Hibbert, M., Lannigan, A., Raven, J., Landau, L., & Phelan, P. (1995). Gender differences in lung growth. *Pediatric Pulmonology, 19*(2), 129–134.
Higgins, M. B., & Saxman, J. H. (1991). A comparison of selected phonatory behaviors of healthy aged and young adults. *Journal of Speech and Hearing Research, 34*(5), 1000–1010.
Hockett, C. F. (1960). The origin of speech. *Scientific American, 203*(3), 88–96.
Hogan, J. A. (1988). Cause and function in the development of behavior systems. In E. M. Blass (Ed.), *Handbook of behavioral neurobiology: Developmental psychobiology and behavioral ecology, IX*. New York: Plenum, 63–106.
Hoit, J. D., Hixon, T. J., Watson, P. J., & Morgan, W. J. (1990). Speech breathing in children and adolescents. *Journal of Speech and Hearing Research, 33*(1), 51–69.
Hrdy, S. B. (2006). Evolutionary context of human development. In C. S. Carter, L. Ahnert, K. E. Grossmann, S. B. Hrdy, M. E. Lamb, S. W. Porges, & N. Sachser (Eds.), *Attachment and bonding: A new synthesis*. Cambridge, MA: MIT Press, 9–32.

Janson, C. H., & van Schaik, C. P. (1993). Ecological risk aversion in juvenile primates: Slow and steady wins the race. In M. E. Pereira & L. A. Fairbanks (Eds.), *Juvenile primates: Life history, development, and behavior.* Oxford: Oxford University Press, 57–74.

Jespersen, O. (1924/1963). *The philosophy of grammar.* London: George Allen & Unwin.

Joffe, T. H. (1997). Social pressures have selected for an extended juvenile period in primates. *Journal of Human Evolution, 32*(6), 593–605.

Karmiloff-Smith, A. (1985). Some fundamental aspects of language development after age 5. In P. Fletcher & M. Garman (Eds.), *Language acquisition: Studies in first language development* (2nd ed.). Cambridge: Cambridge University Press.

Kuiper, K. (1996). *Smooth talkers: The linguistic performance of auctioneers and sports-casters.* Mahwah, NJ: Lawrence Erlbaum.

Lakoff, G., & Johnson, M. (1980). *Metaphors we live by.* Chicago, IL: University of Chicago Press.

Lieberman, D. E., McCarthy, R. C., Hiiemae, K. M., & Palmer, J. B. (2001). Ontogeny of postnatal hyoid and larynx descent in humans. *Archives of Oral Biology, 46*(2), 117–128.

Linell, P. (2005). *The written language bias in linguistic: Its nature, origins and transformations.* London and New York: Routledge.

Locke, J. L. (1993a). *The child's path to spoken language.* Cambridge, MA: Harvard University Press.

Locke, J. L. (1993b). The role of the face in vocal learning and the development of spoken language. In B. de Boysson-Bardies, S. de Schonen, P. Jusczyk, P. MacNeilage, & J. Morton (Eds.), *Developmental neurocognition: Speech and face processing in the first year of life.* The Netherlands: Kluwer Academic Publishers, 317–328.

Locke, J. L. (1994). Development of the capacity for spoken language. In P. Fletcher & B. MacWhinney (Eds.), *Handbook of child language.* Oxford: Blackwell Publishers, 277–302.

Locke, J. L. (1996). Why do infants begin to talk? Language as an unintended consequence. *Journal of Child Language, 23*(2), 251–268.

Locke, J. L. (1997). A theory of neurolinguistic development. *Brain and Language, 58*(2), 265–326.

Locke, J. L. (1998a). Social sound-making as a precursor to spoken language. In J. R. Hurford, M. Studdert-Kennedy, & C. Knight (Eds.), *Approaches to the evolution of language: Social and cognitive bases.* Cambridge: Cambridge University Press, 190–201.

Locke, J. L. (1998b). Are developmental language disorders primarily grammatical? Speculations from an evolutionary model. In R. Paul (Ed.), *Exploring the speech-language connection.* Baltimore, MD: Paul H. Brookes.

Locke, J. L. (1999). Towards a biological science of language development. In M. Barrett (Ed.), *The development of language.* Hove (East Sussex): Psychology Press.

Locke, J. L. (2001a). Rank and relationships in the evolution of spoken language. *Journal of the Royal Anthropological Institute,* 7(1), 37–50.

Locke, J. L. (2001b). First communion: The emergence of vocal relationships. *Social Development, 10*(3), 294–308.

Locke, J. L. (2006). Parental selection of vocal behavior: Crying, cooing, babbling and the evolution of spoken language. *Human Nature, 17*(2), 155–168.

Locke, J. L. (2008a). The trait of human language: Lessons from the canal boat children of England. *Biology and Philosophy, 23*(3), 347–361.

Locke, J. L. (2008b). Cost and complexity: Selection for speech and language. *Journal of Theoretical Biology, 251*(4), 640–652.

Locke, J. L. (2009). Evolutionary developmental linguistics: Naturalization of the faculty of language. *Language Sciences, 31*(1), 33–59.

Locke, J. L., & Bogin, B. (2006). Language and life history: A new perspective on the evolution and development of linguistic communication. *Behavioral and Brain Science, 29*(3), 259–325.

Malinowski, B. (1923). The problem of meaning in primitive languages. In C. K. Ogden & I. A. Richards (Eds.), *The meaning of meaning.* London: Routledge and Kegan Paul, 296–336.

Marchman, V. A., & Bates, E. (1994). Continuity in lexical and morphological development: A test of the critical mass hypothesis. *Journal of Child Language, 21*(2), 339–366.

Mazur, A., & Booth, A. (1998). Testosterone and dominance in men. *Behavioral and Brain Sciences, 21*(3), 353–363.

McGhee, P. E. (1979). *Humor: Its origin and development.* San Francisco, CA: W. H. Freeman.

Meltzoff, A. N., & Moore, M. K. (1994). Imitation, memory, and the representation of persons. *Infant Behavior and Development, 17*(1), 83–99.

Miller, G. (2000). *The mating mind: How sexual choice shaped the evolution of human nature.* London: William Heinemann.

Miller, G. A. (1965). Some preliminaries to psycholinguistics. *American Psychologist, 20,* 15–20.

Moon, C., Cooper, R. P., & Fifer, W. P. (1993). Two-day olds prefer their native language. *Infant Behavior and Development, 16*(4), 495–500.
Morais, J. (2001). The literate mind and the universal human mind. In E. Dupoux (Ed.), *Language, brain, and cognitive development: Essays in honor of Jacques Mehler*. Cambridge, MA: MIT Press, 463–480.
Navas, A. L. G. P. (2004). Implications of alphabetic instruction in the conscious and unconscious manipulations of phonological representations in Portuguese-Japanese bilinguals. *Written Language and Literacy*, 7(1), 119–131.
Nelson, K. (1996). Memory development from 4 to 7 years. In A. J. Sameroff & M. M. Haith (Eds.), *The five to seven year shift: The age of reason and responsibility*. Chicago, IL: University of Chicago Press.
Nelson, K. E., Carskaddon, G., & Bonvillian, J. D. (1973). Syntax acquisition: Impact of experimental variation in adult verbal interaction with the child. *Child Development, 44*(3), 497–504.
Newmeyer, F. J. (2003). What can the field of linguistics tell us about the origins of language? In M. H. Christiansen & S. Kirby (Eds.), *Language evolution*. Oxford: Oxford University Press, 58–76.
Nippold, M. A. (1998). *Later language development: The school-age and adolescent years*. Austin, TX: Pro-ED.
Northcutt, R. G. (1990). Ontogeny and phylogeny: A re-evaluation of conceptual relationships and some applications. *Brain, Behavior and Evolution, 36*(2–3), 116–140.
Ochs, E. (1982). Talking to children in Western Samoa. *Language and in Society, 2*(1), 77–104.
Oguchi, T., & Kikuchi, H. (1997). Voice and interpersonal attraction. *Japanese Psychological Research, 39*(1), 56–61.
Oller, D. K. (2004). Underpinnings for a theory of communicative evolution. In D. K. Oller & U. Griebel (Eds.), *The evolution of communication systems: A comparative approach*. Cambridge, MA: MIT Press, 49–65.
Oller, D. K., Eilers, R. E., Neal, A. R., & Schwartz, H. K. (1999). Precursors to speech in infancy: The prediction of speech and language disorders. *Journal of Communication Disorders, 32*(4), 223–245.
Olson, D. (1994). *The world on paper: The conceptual and cognitive implications of writing and reading*. Cambridge: Cambridge University Press.
Ostrosky-Solís, F., Ramirez, M., & Ardila, A. (2004). Effects of culture and education on neuropsychological testing: A preliminary study with indigenous and nonindigenous population. *Applied Neuropsychology, 11*(4), 186–193.
Paul, R., & Jennings, P. (1992). Phonological behavior in toddlers with slow expressive language development. *Journal of Speech and Hearing Research, 35*(1), 99–107.
Paul, R., & Shiffer, M. E. (1991). Communicative initiations in normal and late-talking toddlers. *Applied Psycholinguistics, 12*(4), 419–431.
Pawlby, S. J. (1977). Imitative interaction. In H. R. Schaffer (Ed.), *Studies in mother-infant interaction*. New York: Academic Press, 203–224.
Pedersen, M. F., Moller, S., Krabbe, S., & Bennett, P. (1986). Fundamental voice frequency measured by electroglottography during continuous speech: A new exact secondary sex characteristic in boys in puberty. *International Journal of Pediatric Otorhinolaryngology, 11*(1), 21–27.
Pedersen, M. F., Møller, S., Krabbe, S., Bennett, P., & Svenstrup, B. (1990). Fundamental voice frequency in female puberty measured with electroglottography during continuous speech as a secondary sex characteristic: A comparison between voice, pubertal stages, oestrogens and androgens. *International Journal of Pediatric Otorhinolaryngology, 20*(1), 17–24.
Pinker, S. (1994). *The language instinct: The new science of language and mind*. London: Penguin Press.
Pinker, S., & Bloom, P. (1990). Natural language and natural selection. *Behavioral and Brain Sciences, 13*(4), 707–784.
Plunkett, K., & Marchman, V. (1993). From rote learning to system building: Acquiring verb morphology in children and connectionist nets. *Cognition, 48*(1), 21–69.
Putallaz, M., & Gottman, J. M. (1981). Social skills and group acceptance. In S. R. Asher & J. M. Gottman (Eds.), *The development of children's friendships*. Cambridge: Cambridge University Press, 116–149.
Puts, D. A. (2005). Mating context and menstrual phase affect women's preferences for male voice pitch. *Evolution and Human Behavior, 26*(5), 388–397.
Puts, D. A., Gaulin, S. J. C., & Verdolini, K. (2006). Dominance and the evolution of sexual dimorphism in human voice pitch. *Evolution and Human Behavior, 27*(4), 283–296.
Rescorla, L., & Ratner, T. (1996). Phonetic profiles of toddlers with specific expressive language impairment (SLI-E). *Journal of Speech and Hearing Research, 39*(1), 153–165.
Sanches, M., & Kirshenblatt-Gimblett, B. (1976). Children's traditional speech play and child language. In B. Kirshenblatt-Gimblett (Ed.), *Speech play: Research and resources for studying linguistic creativity*. Philadelphia, PA: University of Pennsylvania Press.
Schleidt, W. M. (1973). Tonic communication: Continual effects of discrete signs in animal communication systems. *Journal of Theoretical Biology, 42*(2), 359–386.

Schrader, P. C., Quanjer, P. H., & Olievier, I. C. (1988). Respiratory muscle force and ventilatory function in adolescents. *European Respiratory Journal, 1*(4), 368–375.

Senghas, A., & Coppola, M. (2001). Children creating language: How Nicaraguan Sign Language acquired a spatial grammar. *Psychological Science, 12*(4), 323–328.

Senghas, A., Kita, S., & Ozyurek, A. (2004). Children creating core properties of language: Evidence from an emerging sign language in Nicaragua. *Science, 305*(5691), 1779–1782.

Seyfarth, R. M., & Cheney, D. L. (2003). Signalers and receivers in animal communication. *Annual Reviews of Psychology, 54*, 145–173.

Shaw, P., Greenstein, D., Lerch, J., Clasen, L., Lenroot, R., Gogtay, N., ... Giedd, J. (2006). Intellectual ability and cortical development in children and adolescents. *Nature, 440*(7084), 676–679.

Sherzer, J. (2002). *Speech play and verbal art*. Austin, TX: University of Texas Press.

Shriberg, L. D., Tomblin, J. B., & McSweeny, J. L. (1999). Prevalence of speech delay in 6-year-old children and comorbidity with language impairment. *Journal of Speech, Language, and Hearing Research, 42*(6), 1461–1481.

Shultz, T. R., & Horibe, F. (1974). Development of the appreciation of verbal jokes. *Developmental Psychology, 10*(1), 13–20.

Simonton, D. K. (1999). Talent and its development: An emergenic and epigenetic model. *Psychological Review, 106*(3), 435–457.

Slomkowski, C. L., Nelson, K., Dunn, J., & Plomin, R. (1992). Temperament and language: Relations from toddlerhood to middle childhood. *Developmental Psychology, 28*(6), 1090–1095.

Smith, A. (2006). Speech motor development: Integrating muscles, movements, and linguistic units. *Journal of Communication Disorders, 39*(5), 331–349.

Stahl, W. R. (1967). Scaling of respiratory variables in mammals. *Journal of Applied Physiology, 22*(3), 453–460.

Starkweather, C. W. (1987). *Fluency and stuttering*. Englewood, NJ: Prentice-Hall.

Studdert-Kennedy, M. (1991). Language development from an evolutionary perspective. In N. Krasnegor, D. Rumbaugh, R. Schiefelbusch, & M. Studdert-Kennedy (Eds.), *Language acquisition: Biological and behavioral determinants*. Hillsdale, NJ: Erlbaum, 5–28.

Studdert-Kennedy, M. (1998). The particulate origins of language generativity: From syllable to gesture. In J. R. Hurford, M. Studdert-Kennedy, & C. Knight (Eds.), *Approaches to the evolution of language: Social and cognitive biases*. Cambridge: Cambridge University Press, 202–221.

Studdert-Kennedy, M. (2005). How did language go discrete? In M. Tallerman (Ed.), *Language origins: Perspectives on evolution*. Oxford: Oxford University Press, 48–67.

Studdert-Kennedy, M., & Goldstein, L. (2003). Launching language: The gestural origin of discrete infinity. In M. Christiansen & S. Kirby (Eds.), *Language evolution*. Oxford: Oxford University Press, 235–254.

Tambiah, S. J. (1983). The magical power of words. *Man, 3*(2), 175–208.

Tenney, S. M., & Remmers, J. E. (1963). Comparative quantitative morphology of the mammalian lung: Diffusing area. *Nature, 197*, 54–56.

Thal, D., Oroz, M., & McCaw, V. (1995). Phonological and lexical development in normal and late-talking toddlers. *Applied Psycholinguistics, 16*(4), 407–424.

Thurlbeck, W. M. (1982). Postnatal human lung growth. *Thorax, 37*(8), 564–571.

Titze, I. (1989). Physiologic and acoustic differences between male and female voices. *Journal of the Acoustical Society of America, 85*(4), 1699–1707.

Tomblin, J. B., Records, N. L., Buckwalter, P., Zhang, X., Smith, E., & O'Brien, M. (1997). Prevalence of specific language impairment in kindergarten children. *Journal of Speech, Language, and Hearing Research, 40*(6), 1245–1260.

Tunmer, W. E., & Cole, P. G. (1991). Learning to read: A metalinguistic act. In C. S. Simon (Ed.), *Communication skills and classroom success: Assessment and therapy methodologies for language and learning disabled students*. Eau Claire, WI: Thinking Publishers, 293–312.

van IJzendoorn, M. H., Kijkstra, J., & Bus, A. G. (1995). Attachment, intelligence, and language: A meta-analysis. *Social Development, 4*(2), 115–128.

Veneziano, E. (1988). Vocal-verbal interaction and the construction of early lexical knowledge. In M. D. Smith & J. L. Locke (Eds.), *The emergent lexicon: The child's development of a linguistic vocabulary*. New York: Academic Press, 109–147.

Vihman, M. M., Macken, M. A., Miller, R., Simmons, H., & Miller, J. (1985). From babbling to speech: A reassessment of the continuity issue. *Language, 61*(2), 397–446.

Vuorenkoski, V., Lenko, H. L., Tjernlund, P., Vuorenkoski, L., & Perheentupa, J. (1978). Fundamental voice frequency during normal and abnormal growth, and after androgen treatment. *Archives of Disease in Childhood, 53*(3), 201–209.

Waldstein, R. S. (1990). Effects of postlingual deafness on speech production: Implications for the role of auditory feedback. *Journal of the Acoustical Society of America, 88*(5), 2099–2114.
Walsh, B., & Smith, A. (2002). Articulatory movements in adolescents: Evidence for protracted development of speech motor control processes. *Journal of Speech, Language, and Hearing Research, 45*(6), 1119–1133.
West-Eberhard, M. J. (2003). *Developmental plasticity and evolution.* Oxford: Oxford University Press.
Whitmire, K. A. (2000). Adolescence as a developmental phase: A tutorial. *Topics in Language Disorders, 20*(2), 1–14.
Wilson, G. D. (1984). The personality of opera singers. *Personality and Individual Differences, 5*(2), 195–201.

2

EMERGENTISM AND LANGUAGE DISORDERS

Brian MacWhinney

Introduction

The human brain is the most complicated structure in the known universe, and language is the most complex mental function, relying on large parts of the cerebral cortex and midbrain. Additional complexity arises from the social and developmental forces that produce continual variation in the shapes of words, sounds, and communications. It is difficult to imagine a full account of language disorders that does not come to grips with this great complexity, both in terms of neural processing and the shape of language itself.

The biggest challenge facing a theory of language disorder is that there are so many alternative forms of language across individuals and so many possible expressions of language disorder. Given the complexity of language, there are good reasons to expect that patterns in language disorders should be at least as complex as disorders of other biological systems, such as the immune system or the skeletal system. Within this complex system, there may well be pivotal mechanisms that trigger a disorder. However, the behavioral and neurological effects of that pivotal mechanism are surely going to be modified by other components of the system.

Traditionally, there have been two competing approaches to explaining language disorders. The nativist approach emphasizes the ways in which variations in genetic structures can lead to language disorder. For example, studies of mutations in the FOXP2 gene in the KE family (Fisher & Scharff, 2009) have been shown to impact aspects of language production, although they also impact motor behaviors and control more generally (Vargha-Khadem, Gadian, Copp, & Mishkin, 2005). Nativist accounts typically view language as controlled by distinct brain modules that function automatically with non-interactive informational encapsulation (Fodor, 1983). They also emphasize the structuring of language through recursive rule systems (Hauser, Chomsky, & Fitch, 2002) which are viewed as the core event in language evolution.

In contrast, empiricist accounts of language disorders emphasize the extent to which language learning and processing rely on general cognitive resources (Christiansen & Chater, 2008; Elman et al., 1996) and environmental inputs. These accounts see neural processing as involving dynamic associations between highly interactive areas (McClelland, Mirman, & Holt, 2006). They view language learning as the acquisition of constructions, rather than rules (Goldberg, 2006), and as being driven by usage (Bybee, 2010) and statistics (Conway, 2020).

These two approaches have made important contributions to our understanding of language, brain, and disorders. However, they also suffer from core weaknesses. The nativist emphasis on modularity fails to account for the dynamic interplay of neural functioning (Hagoort, 2013) during

DOI: 10.4324/9781003204213-4

actual language processing. Nativist emphasis on syntactic rules and recursion as the core features of human language fails to account for the equally important roles of articulation, audition, lexicon, and interaction in language functioning and language evolution (MacWhinney, 2005b).

Empiricist accounts have difficulty assigning a role to genetic and epigenetic causes of language disorders, such as familial inheritance of stuttering (Frigerio-Domingues & Drayna, 2017). Although genetic determination may account for not more that 16% of cases of stuttering, it is still useful to understand these relations and the relations between this type of direct causation and other etiologies. Another weakness of some empiricist accounts is their failure to fully consider developmental or epigenetic changes in language functioning across the lifespan.

Often the opposition between nativism and empiricism is characterized by questions such as "how much of a given behavior is due to nature and how much is due to nurture". This poses the problem as a forced choice between the two approaches. We can avoid this forced choice by saying that we need to take the best insights from each, but then the question is how exactly to do this. The most promising way to achieve this integration involves consideration of both language and the brain as complex dynamic systems (Beckner et al., 2009). To best explore this option, we need consider the theory of emergentism with particular attention to the theory of neuroemergentism (Hernandez et al., 2019). This framework has the great advantage of allowing us to piece together a view that incorporates insights from a diversity of component models.

Emergentism

Scientific approaches to large complex systems rely on the formulation of multiple interlocking component theories. Geological accounts of the past and present of our planet rely on theories about radioactive decay, crystal formation, element separation in magma, state transitions, fluid dynamics, crustal movements, vulcanism, and plate tectonics. Similarly, to understand language processing and language disorders we need to invoke many well-developed theories, ranging from gene expression (Wong, Morgan-Short, Ettlinger, & Zheng, 2012) to the impact of stress on stuttering (Bloodstein & Bernstein Ratner, 2008) or the role of corrective feedback in children's language learning (MacWhinney, 2004). Emergentism provides a way of linking these already developed component theories into a coherent whole. It does this by articulating the role of four core analytic frameworks: competition, mechanisms as constraints on structures, emergent levels, and time/process frames (MacWhinney, 2015).

Competition

The theory of competition builds on Darwin's (1859) vision of evolution and adaptation as arising from the operation of three processes: proliferation, competition, and selection. For individual speakers, proliferation of language forms and functions is driven by the rich language variety to which they are exposed. Learners pick up thousands of sound forms, referents, words, multiword expressions, constructions, syntactic patterns, and conversational practices. These forms and functions vary markedly based on dialect, genre, and speaker variation (Hymes, 1962). The learner's task is to deal with the competition and cooperation created by this great proliferation. This is a task not just for language, but for all cognitive processing (Rosenbaum, 2015).

During both comprehension and production, the learner must rely on a system of cue validity to select winning forms and functions. The component model that articulates this process is the Unified Competition Model (MacWhinney, 2021). This model provides a functionalist account of how languages are learned across the lifespan and how they are processed in real time. Research based on this model has shed light on aspects of first language learning, second language learning, bilingual processing, developmental language disorders, and language loss in aphasia. The model's fundamental claim is that, during comprehension, alternative interpretations compete online in terms of their relative cue validity. Similarly, during production, alternative expressions compete in terms of the validity of their match to intentions. To probe these various competitions, researchers have used multifactorial experimental designs to measure the process of cue competition. As summarized in MacWhinney (2021) and elsewhere, the predictions of the model have been uniformly supported across four decades of research involving 15 different languages (MacWhinney & Bates, 1989).

We can supplement behavioral evidence for competition with evidence from Cognitive Neuroscience. Computational models of brain functioning rely on facts about lateral inhibition (Kohonen, 2001), cell assembly structure (Hebb, 1949; Pulvermüller, 2003), and connectivity (Hickok, 2009; Valiant, 2014) to explain how competition is processed both locally and between cortical areas. These models have been articulated for many levels of language processing, including lexical selection, code-switching, sentence processing, and speech recognition.

Models of neural competition can help us understand both speech errors and stuttering. The fact that speakers can detect and subsequently correct their speech errors (Maclay & Osgood, 1959) has led researchers to postulate a system that monitors or compares candidate output forms with the auditory shape of the intended target (Roelofs, 2011). However, evidence from the ERN (error-related negativity) component of the EEG suggests that the competition between candidate forms arises immediately during the process of initial form activation (Nozari & Novick, 2017). Nozari and Hepner (2019) show how a signal detection model of the competition between lexical forms can account for observed details in the pattern of speech errors. This model views hesitation pauses and retraces as arising from a lower level of confidence regarding the outcome of a competition on the lexical level. The drift-diffusion model (Ratcliff & McKoon, 2008) provides a similar account.

Competition must also be involved in stuttering, although in a way that is more complex than what we see in speech errors from fluent speakers. One possibility is that problems in the cortico-basal ganglia-thalamocortical (cortico-BG) loop for motor activation could further exacerbate problems arising from competitions between lexical items (Chang & Guenther, 2020). The cortico-BG loop account can then be integrated with other component models, including the model for speech errors proposed by Nozari and Hepner (2019), Guenther's DIVA feedback model (Guenther & Vladusich, 2012), the theory of dopamine action on the basal ganglia (Civier, Bullock, Max, & Guenther, 2013), and the model of segregated basal ganglia circuitry (Alexander, DeLong, & Strick, 1986). The need to piece together component models in this way is driven by the complexity of language and the brain.

Mechanisms constraining structures

Human language is structured into a series of interactive levels, including audition, articulation, lexicon, morphology, syntax, discourse, narrative, and conversation. On each of these levels, we find that structures emerge from the impact of mechanisms that impose constraints on possible forms and structural levels.

Nature abounds with examples of emergent structures. Whether we are talking about the shape and properties of water, soap bubbles, ocean tides, honeycomb cells, protein molecules, optical dominance columns, mental representations, neurolinguistic modules, linguistic forms, or social groups, we can view all structures in the natural world as emerging from the force of mechanisms that impose constraints on how these structures can be configured.

As Mill (1859) noted, water provides a perfect example. To produce water from hydrogen and oxygen, one must apply a spark of energy to break the covalent bonds. After that, the process of molecular formation produces its own energy, and the reaction will go to completion. The first emergent property of this new molecule is its polarity, which then responds to constraints on the molecular level to produce hydrogen-bonding of each water molecule with up to four additional water molecules. These new links then produce water's high surface tension as a further emergent property, as well as its high thermal conductivity, specific heat capacity, heat of vaporization, and heat of fusion. As water accumulates in larger bodies like lakes and oceans, these local properties shape new emergent patterns such as snowflakes, rain drops, ocean currents, glaciers, thunderstorms, and many other features of our planet and its climate.

Language is shaped by a wide range of constraints, and researchers have formulated accounts and models for each of these constraints. These models constitute important components of the overall emergentist framework. Here we can list the mechanisms or constraints that have been most thoroughly studied.

1. Functional mapping. Language forms are designed to express communicative functions. As Bates and MacWhinney (1981) noted, "the forms of natural languages are created, governed, constrained, acquired and used in the service of communicative functions." This is a core constraint in accounts such as the Unified Competition Model or Construction Grammar (Goldberg, 2006).
2. Conversational determination. Possible lexical forms are constrained by the possibilities of achieving systematic coreference with other speakers (Goldstone, 2002). Syntactic structures adapt to frequent conversational patterns (Ochs, Schegloff, & Thompson, 1996). Possible conversational patterns are shaped by social practices (Goodwin, 2013) and preference management (Korniol, 1995).
3. Embodied determination. The functions expressed by language forms are grounded on our embodied experiences as human actors (MacWhinney, 2005a).
4. Generalization. Language forms organize into groups or gangs, based on similarity and this organization then produces patterns that can generalize to new forms (McClelland, 2015). Generalization plays a major role in systems as diverse as morphological categories, metaphor, constructions, narrative, and phonotactics.
5. Self-organization and error correction. The formation of groups and new patterns can arise either through self-organization in which forms that behave similarly are grouped together (Kohonen, 2001) or through error correction in which we compare what we say or understand with what we should have said or should have understood (Berwick, 1987).
6. Simplicity and expressiveness. The mapping of forms to functions is governed by the operation of two major competing constraints: simplicity and expressiveness. Language seeks to be simple by creating a minimal number of forms for a function. At the same time, it seeks to be expressive by creating forms for fine-grained differences in meaning. Much of language complexity arises from the competition between these two constraints (MacWhinney, Malchukov, & Moravcsik, 2014).
7. Physical constraints. The formation of articulatory gestures and their linkage into syllables and words are constrained by the mechanics of the vocal system and neural control (Browman & Goldstein, 1992).
8. Item-based patterns. The linking of words into sentences is constrained by the operation of argument slots on lexical forms (MacWhinney, 2014).
9. Incrementality. Possible syntactic patterns are constrained by the incremental "now or never" functioning of sentence processing (Christiansen & Chater, 2016; O'Grady, 2005).
10. Perceptual recording. Both infants and adults can apply general-purpose mechanisms to record and learn sequential patterns (Conway, 2020).
11. Chunking. On each structural level, forms and functions that occur together frequently are treated as a single chunk for memory storage and processing (Hebb, 1949; Newell, 1990).
12. Resonance. Apart from chunking within levels, the integration of new information with old information and across levels can lead to strengthening of associations (Schlichting & Preston, 2015), greater fluency (Dominey & Boussaoud, 1997), and improved recall (Pavlik & Anderson, 2008).

13. Connectivity and localization. The need to communicate information across neural regions constrains the localization of processing levels to areas that are well connected with other areas required for their computations (Dronkers, 2011). Moreover, the detailed shape of cortical areas maintains a topological connection to the body in terms of retinotopic, tonotopic, and somatotopic maps. This principle of topological mapping extends even further to control areas such as the thalamus and hippocampus.
14. Imitation. We can learn both forms and functions by recording speech and then imitating it (Whitehurst & Vasta, 1975). Imitation or copying is a fundamental mechanism for usage-based linguistics (Diessel, 2017).
15. Plasticity. Processes of neural reuse and plasticity permit reorganization of neural functioning (Zerilli, 2022).

As we will see in the next section, these mechanisms and others not listed in this overview operate in different ways across the emergent levels of language structure. A given language disorder could impact relative reliance on any given mechanism. For example, the motor disorder in the KE family caused by SNP (single nucleotide polymorphism) mutations of the Fox2P gene impact phonology, morphology, and syntax, but in different ways for each level. Moreover, these mechanisms interact in different ways for different disorders. For example, problems with syntactic control lead to argument omissions in non-fluent aphasia (Thompson et al., 2013), whereas they lead to disfluencies in stuttering. The fact that some linguistic structures are particularly vulnerable echoes findings from linguistic analysis regarding the emergence of complexity in syntax (Chomsky, 2007; Culicover, 2013).

Emergent levels

Once new forms emerge from the actions of constraints, they become subject to new constraints. This interplay of forms, constraints, and levels can be illustrated by examining the process of protein folding which goes through four structural levels to determine a protein's final folded form. On the primary level, a simple chain of amino acids emerges from the ribosome. This structure is constrained or shaped by the operation of messenger RNA and transfer RNA. On the secondary level, constraints from hydrogen bonding across the amino acid chain serve to create either helices or pleated sheets, based on the nature of the sequences of amino acids derived from the primary level. On the tertiary level, the helices and pleated sheets twist into other forms based on the new constraints of hydrophobic and hydrophilic attractions. On the quaternary level, multiple polypeptide chains formed on the tertiary level combine further to produce still more complex 3-D patterns appropriate for functioning, such as the ability of hemoglobin in transport oxygen, or the ability of antibodies to engulf viruses. On each of these four levels, folding is further guided or constrained by catalysts and molecular chaperones. Once proteins are available for neuronal functioning, they can further determine the structure of neurons, transmitters, and hormones. As neurons group on higher levels, they are subject to constraints from neuronal packing, local and distal connectivity patterns, activation thresholds, gang effects, and other properties of neural assemblies and areas.

This analysis of the emergence of structural levels through the creation of new forms subject to new constraints also applies to language and language learning. In children's language learning, the shape of the basic levels of linguistic structure emerges from the operation of constraints on those levels. One component of the theory of neuroemergentism (MacWhinney, 2019) is that data tends to self-organize into a particular brain area based on the connections of that area with other areas that optimize functioning. For example, the organization of sound patterns into auditory cortex is facilitated by its linkage to medial geniculate body of the thalamus, the planum temporale, and lexical processing in the ventral pathway of the temporal lobe. Auditory cortex is also well connected to the dorsal pathway for support of motor aspects of speech perception (Hickok, 2009). In children with early deafness, this pathway receives only weak input, thereby allowing it to reorganize for visual motion detection (Shiell, Champoux, & Zatorre, 2015).

The emergence of distinct areas for lexical processing is also driven by the connectivity constraints on these areas (Gow, 2012). This leads to a concentration of phonetic information in the inferior parietal, a concentration of core lexical information in the superior temporal sulcus and medial temporal gyrus, and a concentration of item-based syntactic frame information in the anterior temporal lobe. Similar patterns of connectivity determine structuring for the levels of articulation, clausal syntax, mental model processing, and control of conversation. Note that self-organization may occur during neural organization before birth, as the fetus is able to process the mother's voice while in the womb (Webb, Heller, Benson, & Lahav, 2015).

This view of the emergent and adaptable nature of processing areas contrasts with the nativist view of genetically fixed, encapsulated neural modules (Fodor, 1983; Galton, 1883; Pinker, 1994). It also provides us with a fuller understanding of the complex nature of language disorders. During online production, these multiple structural levels interact dynamically. As we listen to messages from our conversational partners, we are also formulating our own contributions. These ideas are shaped into clauses as we activate words bit by bit into phrases and begin to articulate these ideas, even before all the components of the utterance are fully formed. The interactions of these levels involves just-in-time processing (Christiansen & Chater, 2016) along with gating between areas to make sure that articulations are not begun until the underlying message is at least approximately correct. These demands underscore the key role of fluency in language production and comprehension. Preschoolers are still piecing together basic elements for fluency and, even as adults, we can become disfluent when the components of our messages are not well practiced.

Timescale/process constraints

In a process like protein folding, the movement across structural levels occurs within a span varying from an hour to microseconds with larger proteins taking longer to fold (Naganathan & Muñoz, 2005). For language, new structures emerge across three very divergent timescales. One is the timescale of learning in the individual which extends from seconds to decades. The second is the timescale of language change in the community which extends from decades to centuries. The third is the timescale of language evolution which includes thousands and even millions of years.

For understanding language disorders, the most important timescales are those that impact the individual speaker. Here, we can consider ideas from the theory of neuroemergentism (Hernandez et al., 2019) which focuses on three processes leading to cortical reorganization. The first is what Dehaene calls "cultural recycling" (Dehaene & Cohen, 2007). This is the process involved in the reshaping of the left face form area (FFA) to become the visual word form area (VWFA) used in reading. This type of repurposing of an area depends both on the cytoarchitectonic structure of an area and its pattern of connectivity with other areas involved in a type of processing. In the case of learning to read, the ability of the left FFA to encode precise visual patterns, along with its connectivity to the ventral stream of language processing (Hickok & Poeppel, 2004) allow it to take over the function of visual word processing.

An equally remarkable example of recycling involves the use of IFG (inferior frontal gyrus, Broca's area) by signers to support syntactic processing in sign language and the use of STG (superior temporal gyrus, Wernicke's area) to support lexical processing in sign (Hickok, Bellugi, & Klima, 2001). Similar effects arise through increases in the part of the hippocampus dedicated to route finding for London taxicab drivers (Woollett & Maguire, 2011), increases in a variety of auditory areas as a result of musical training (Olszewska, Gaca, Herman, Jednoróg, & Marchewka, 2021), and greater functional connectivity as a result of learning new words in Chinese as a second language (Li, Legault, & Litcofsky, 2014). Recycling may have important consequences for language disorders. On the one hand, inadequate language input could lead to temporary deficits in language functioning (Hart & Risley, 1995). On the other hand, recycling suggest that deficits can be mitigated or reversed through training (Recanzone & Merzenich, 1993) and exposure (Roberts, Rosenfeld, & Zeisel, 2004).

A second neuroemergentist process involves neural reuse. Looking at fMRI activation data for 968 brain regions, Anderson (2010) found that brain regions are often involved in 20 different tasks or more and that, on average, a brain region is active in 4.32 clearly different domains. This pattern of reuse for multiple functions is a fundamental aspect of emergence in biology, as noted by Darwin (1862, p. 348) for organs or West-Eberhard (2003) for processes in epigenetic and phenotypic control of developmental plasticity. The theory of neuronal recycling is highly compatible with the theory of neural reuse. If an area can serve multiple functions in alternative configurations of functional neural circuits, then recycling can be directly supported during ontogenesis and later.

The third neuroemergentist process involves what Johnson (2011) calls "interactive specialization." This framework elaborates on the motto from Bates (1999) that, "modules are made, not born." For example, Edelman (1987) shows how processes of Darwinian neural competition shape emerging cortical areas during embryogenesis and early infancy. Carrying this further into infancy, Johnson (2011) shows how the formation of visual areas in precocial birds involves an interaction between the genetic guidance of vision through CONSPEC and its shaping by the process of CONLEARN. This same process operates in human infants. Johnson shows how the ability of infants to focus on their mother's eyes sets the stage for further development of an interactional and communication bond with the mother which then leads to specialization of visual areas for face perception.

Language disorders

Reacting against his failure to locate the engrams of memory, Lashley (1951) proposed that all cognitive functioning is global. However, given what we now know about the details of neural connectivity (Schmahmann et al., 2007; Van Essen, Felleman, DeYoe, Olavarria, & Knierim, 1990), it is difficult to deny that different neuronal areas have different functions. However, functional differentiation does not fully invalidate Lashley's insight. To understand how specific impairments can lead to general disorders, we can think of language processing as an acrobat who is simultaneously juggling across seven separate dimensions. At any given moment, there is a contribution from attentional areas, lexical processing, links from lexicon to syntax, and often elaboration of a mental model. If processing in any one of these coordinated areas suddenly "crashes" or breaks down, then the larger process is disrupted. In the case of normal speakers, the juggler is so skillful that this seldom happens, and when it does, there is a quick recovery. In a speaker with impairments, problems in any area can impact the whole system. Because of this, the Unified Competition Model (MacWhinney, 2021) places an emphasis on overall patterns of cognitive *cost* or cognitive *load*. If stress to the system causes failure primarily in a highly "vulnerable" or costly area of language, then within a language, there should be a common tendency across disorders for similar structures and processes to be harmed. That is, aphasics and SLI patients may display similar deficits in terms of which elements of language are impaired, either in comprehension or production.

Evidence for the systemic properties of language disorders comes from non-disordered individuals under cognitive load. First, we know that marked increases in cognitive load can impair normal comprehension (Just & Carpenter, 1992). Moreover, varying the type and quality of cognitive load creates a performance profile in normal college students that closely resembles the one found in aphasics (Dick et al., 2001). Because we know there is no systematic physiological or genetic damage to the language system in these control participants, results like these support a model of language as a broad, complex, resource-intensive system that depends on smooth coordination between diverse local resources.

Aphasics and children with SLI have similar deficits in terms of the elements of language that are impaired, both in comprehension and production. This similarity shifts the emphasis in language disorders from specific competency deficits (e.g., inflectional morphology in Broca's aphasics) and moves it to consideration of the relative vulnerability of a linguistic form or process to damage. The resemblance between the areas of language affected under cognitive load in normal speakers and those affected by SLI is a good example of this vulnerability effect.

The Competition Model does not suggest there are no differences among different disorders. Differences and dissociations are very informative in understanding neural specialization and other properties of language. However, the deciding role of the weakest link in a chain leads us to expect many commonalities across disorders. To illustrate this, let us consider two major disorder groups in further detail: SLI (Specific Language Impairment) and aphasia.

Specific Language Impairment

SLI is characterized by normal cognitive function combined with poor performance on language tasks. As such, the disorder is a logical testing ground for hypotheses about the domain-generality of language as well as genetic vs. learning bases of grammatical abilities.

Some researchers have argued that SLI is a genetic disorder resulting in a phenotypically unified competence deficit. For example, the Extended Optional Infinitive Hypothesis (Rice & Wexler, 1996) proposes that SLI involves a failure to develop tense and agreement marking, thereby delaying grammatically correct production. Similarly, the G-SLI model (van der Lely, 2005) proposes that there is a subgroup of SLI patients whose essential deficit involves grammatical processing of canonical linking chains with no problems in word learning, phonology, or working memory.

These analyses advance three main claims: (1) the cause of SLI is genetic in origin, (2) the deficits seen in SLI are fundamentally domain-specific, and (3) there are diagnostic characteristics that mark the fundamental difference between SLI and normally developing individuals. Let us examine each of these claims.

The cause of SLI is genetic in origin

To characterize SLI as a disorder with a genetic cause, several pieces of evidence are needed. First, the argument requires an identifiable genetic source of the disorder. For example, language disorder in the KE family is associated with a mutation in FOXP2 which determines dominant inheritance (Pinker, 1994).

Although we can relate language deficits in this family to a mutation in FOXP2, this does not provide evidence for a general role of FOXP2 in SLI. A large-scale study of 270 four-year-old language-impaired children from a general population sample of 18,000 children (Meaburn, 2002) did not find a FOXP2 mutation in any participants. Therefore, there must be some alternative account for SLI in general. Moreover, mutations of FOXP2 in the KE family are also associated with small-scale orofacial motor control. Thus, behavioral deficits in these individuals extend beyond functional language processing to motor control (including motor control that is necessary for speech). Vargha-Khadem and colleagues (1995) note that the disorder in affected members "indicates that the inherited disorder does not affect morphosyntax exclusively, or even primarily; rather, it affects intellectual, linguistic, and orofacial praxic functions generally" (p. 930). Given the complex range of deficits, it is unclear how a mutation in this area could yield a phenotypically unified disorder such as that proposed by van der Lely (2005).

There are cases in which a disorder can be closely linked to a specific genetic pattern. In the cases of sickle cell anemia or phenylketonuria we know the exact pathways of gene expression that lead to the disorders. No such simple relation has yet been found for any language disorder. We understand the complex genetic determination of chromosomal abnormalities in Downs Syndrome and

Williams Syndrome. But we do not know how the expression of these genetic factors impacts language. For these and other disorders, a complex model, involving interactions between multiple genetic factors with possible epigenetic expression, seems most probable. Recently, Vernes et al. (2008) traced the down-regulation of FOXP2 on CNTNAP2, a gene that encodes a neurexin that influences cortical development. Looking at a British database of 847 individuals from families with at least one child with SLI, this group then focused on nine CNTNAP2 polymorphisms. Each of these had a significant association with non-word repetition scores. The most powerful association was for a haplotype labeled *ht1* linked to a lowering of non-word repetition scores by half a standard deviation. However, this same pattern is also heavily associated with autism. Interactions of this type argue for the emergentist view of language processing as an integrated system with points of failure that are revealed differentially across syndromes and comorbidities.

Van der Lely sought to identify a highly specified subgroup of SLI language users. However, attempts to replicate this selection specificity (Bishop, Bright, James, Bishop, & van der Lely, 2000) have not succeeded. Moreover, even if such a distinct subtype were identified, and if there were an association between that disorder and some genetic mutation or set of mutations, we would still need to construct a cognitive or neural model by which the mutations could be linked mechanistically to the disorder in question.

SLI deficits are domain-specific

Claims of specific competence deficits in children with SLI have been used to support nativist views regarding the "faculty of language" (Hauser et al., 2002). The idea is that the specificity of this disorder implies that language learning and processing depend on a separate linguistic module, rather than on domain-general processes, and that damage to the module causes highly specified symptoms as hypothesized in SLI. However, the comorbidity of non-linguistic task difficulties for children with SLI (Barry, Yasin, & Bishop, 2006) calls this interpretation into question.

Studies have found various deficits in non-linguistic tasks in SLI patients, seemingly disputing the definition of SLI as an exclusively linguistic (or exclusively grammatical) disorder. SLI patients have impaired phonological short-term memory (Evans & MacWhinney, 1999); the KE family and others have comorbid motor problems (Vargha-Khadem et al., 1995); and SLI children take longer to respond in a word gating task (Mainela-Arnold, 2008).

SLI is a deficit in linguistic competence

The strongest form of nativist analysis views SLI as a deficit in linguistic competence. Specific hypothesized failures include non-termination of the Optional Infinitive stage (Rice & Wexler, 1996) or misapplication of canonical linking rules (van der Lely, 1994). Van der Lely and Christian (2000) describe the choice between processing models and competence deficit models as hinging on whether or not "impaired input processes and processing capacity cause SLI" (p. 35). However, for each of the putative competence deficits, there exist plausible processing deficit accounts. For example, crosslinguistic patterns that have been used to support the Optional Infinitive Hypothesis can also be explained through learning models such as MOSAIC (Freudenthal, Pine, Aguado-Orea, & Gobet, 2007). Van der Lely was able to pick out a group to match the criterion that focused on grammatical problems, but this process of careful selective exclusion then leaves us with no explanation for all the remaining SLI sub-types. Nor does it help us understand the status of children that show grammatical deficits along with additional linguistic, cognitive, and motoric impairments.

There is substantial evidence that the SLI diagnosis can be further sub-divided based on whether the impairment in language competence extends to receptive as well as expressive language use (Evans & MacWhinney, 1999). It is difficult to see how a competence account alone can explain this further dissociation. The Competition Model can account for this asymmetry in terms of differences in processing. Expressive SLI functions much like Broca's aphasia. In typical speakers, Broca's area serves to gate the firing of lexical items during production. In expressive SLI, as in Broca's aphasia, disruption in the connectivity between Broca's and Wernicke's areas interrupts the smooth gating of lexical items for production. This gating is only important during production and is much less involved in comprehension. In the case of receptive-expressive SLI, then, we would expect to see a different, more general problem of information exchange between brain areas, affecting connections between IFG, DLPFC, MTG, and attentional areas generally.

Aphasia

Neuroemergentism can also help us understand varying patterns in aphasia. The cause of aphasia is well understood, because it arises when a brain lesion from trauma or stroke produces a linguistic impairment. Traditionally, aphasia has been divided into three main categories: Broca's or nonfluent aphasia; Wernicke's or fluent aphasia; and anomia for problems with word finding. Additional types include global, conduction, transcortical sensory, and transcortical motor. Because the etiology of aphasia is much clearer than that of SLI, and because the injuries are easier to map, aphasia provides a useful counterpoint to SLI. In SLI, the functional deficits are well defined, but etiology remains unclear. In aphasia, the opposite is true.

Although aphasia has a clear etiology, lesion site is not a strong predictor of symptom pattern. Two patients with lesions in very different areas will often have similar linguistic profiles. Similarly, patients with lesions in the same area often end up with very different profiles in language performance (Dronkers, Wilkins, Van Valin, Redfern, & Jaeger, 2004). Moreover, if a person with Wernicke's aphasia is impaired in grammaticality judgment in a way that resembles a person with Broca's aphasia, this does not necessarily mean that Broca's and Wernicke's areas perform the same processing tasks, or that they are neuronally identical. Rather, it means that grammar is a complex computational task with vulnerable components that can be impaired in similar ways through damage to various parts of the language network. In this way, aphasia sometimes teaches us more about language than about the brain (McDonald & MacWhinney, 1989).

Crosslinguistic studies of aphasia (Bates, Wulfeck, & MacWhinney, 1991) have illustrated and validated this approach. There is a rich literature demonstrating differences between Broca's aphasics who are native speakers of different languages. For example, the use of agreement in aphasic patients whose native language is Italian is relatively less impaired than in comparison patients whose native language is English. This result is predictable in a Unified Competition Model framework, given the strength of agreement cues in Italian compared to English. In both fluent and non-fluent aphasics, obligatory structures such as SVO word order in German and Italian patients are preserved (Bates et al., 1988). These structures are also the most valid, least costly (as defaults in the language), and most highly frequent. Similarly, when Turkish speakers become aphasic, they still maintain the use of SOV word order, which is the standard in Turkish. As Bates has said, "You can take the Turks out of Turkey, but you can't take the Turkish out of the Turks." In other words, the major determinant of cue survival in aphasia is the relative strength of the cue in the person's language.

The status of competence accounts in aphasia parallels their status in SLI. In SLI, competence accounts look for a simple causal association between a damaged component (such as a specific mutation) and a language deficit. In aphasia, competence accounts also require that a specific lesioned local area or module be the root cause of the aphasic disability. In both cases, the competence approach fails to consider the broader context of the language system, wherein levels of processing (semantics, syntax, lexicon, audition, comprehension) interact within a distributed functional neural network of brain areas (Dronkers, 2011; Kemmerer, 2015).

In the neuroemergentist analysis, the effects of lesions are understood in terms of the damage inflicted on both grey matter and white matter. Damages to grey matter impact the content of the representational maps that organize structural levels. Damages to white matter tracts impact coordination and gating between areas. Thus, observed patterns of aphasia relate not just to the processing in local maps, but also to disorders in connectivity and processing that occur as two or more maps attempt to work in synchrony.

Gupta et al. (2003) showed that, in children who had had early focal lesions, learning was quantitatively delayed in word learning, non-word repetition, and serial recall tasks. Although the level of performance was impaired overall, the relation between measures of verbal working memory and word learning was maintained, and those relations were like the control group. These data are consistent with the finding that children with focal lesions are able to achieve functional language use, although their overall reaction times are often slower than those of controls (MacWhinney, Feldman, Sacco, & Valdes-Perez, 2000).

A similar, and perhaps even more striking, finding comes from Wilson and Saygun (2004). They report evidence in direct contradiction to models that hypothesize that Broca's area is the unique site for comprehension of maximal trace projections (Grodzinsky, 2000). In Wilson and Saygun's study, all patient groups, including anomics, shared a general impairment pattern, although the quantitative performance of the patients varied, as expected. These results show that different injuries to the language network can create similar performance profiles. These data fit well with the analysis of the emergentist Competition Model.

Summary and conclusion

This chapter has examined ways in which neuroemergentism as expressed in the Unified Competition Model can be used to understand language disorders. Apart from providing a comprehensive theoretical approach, emergentism provides clear methodological guidance through its emphasis on component models. The complexities of language, structural emergence, mechanisms, and the brain make it imperative to rely on multiple component models to understand language disorders. Earlier, we considered the disorder of stuttering as an example. For this, we need to model the time course of language production as it moves through an interconnected functional neural circuit from formulation to articulation. We need models of neural activation and competition to consider whether incomplete gating signals are being transmitted between areas. We need to elaborate models of basal ganglia control of fluency or proceduralization to evaluate the contributions of the cortico-BG loop (Chang & Guenther, 2020) and within that model the relative contributions of the loop to learning vs. processing. We also need to understand the role of dopamine (Civier et al., 2013) in control of the loop. We need to consider neuroemergentist accounts of the ways in which stutterers develop compensatory strategies (Bloodstein & Bernstein Ratner, 2008) across the lifespan, and the extent to which specific linguistic structures can trigger stuttering. By linking component models in this way, we can derive at a fuller understanding of stuttering and other language disorders.

For each language disorder, we need to consider the involvement of mechanisms such as the 16 listed earlier, as well as specific genetic variations that impact these mechanisms as they unfold either in embryogenesis or through epigenesis and interactive specialization. During these explorations, we may discover genetic or processing mechanisms that play a pivotal role in shaping the disorder. However, we can be sure that the effects of these pivotal mechanisms will be further modified by interactions with other constraints and processes across diverse timescales.

Further reading

Bishop, D. (2013). Developmental cognitive genetics: How psychology can inform genetics and vice versa. *Quarterly Journal of Experimental Psychology*, *59*(7), 1153–1168.

MacWhinney, B. (2021). The competition model: Past and future. In J. Gervain (Ed.), *A life in cognition* (pp. 3–16). New York: Springer Nature.

References

Alexander, G. E., DeLong, M. R., & Strick, P. L. (1986). Parallel organization of functionally segregated circuits linking basal ganglia and cortex. *Annual Review of Neuroscience, 9*(1), 357–381.

Anderson, M. L. (2010). Neural reuse: A fundamental organizational principle of the brain. *Behavioral and Brain Sciences, 33*(4), 245–266.

Barry, J., Yasin, I., & Bishop, D. (2006). Heritable risk factors associated with language impairments. *Genes, Brain and Behavior, 6*(1), 66–76.

Bates, E. (1999). Plasticity, localization, and language development. In S. Broman & J. M. Fletcher (Eds.), *The changing nervous system: Neurobehavioral consequences of eary brain disorders* (pp. 213–253). New York: Oxford University Press.

Bates, E., & MacWhinney, B. (1981). Second language acquisition from a functionalist perspective: Pragmatic, semantic and perceptual strategies. In H. Winitz (Ed.), *Annals of the New York academy of sciences conference on native and foreign language acquisition* (pp. 190–214). New York: New York Academy of Sciences.

Bates, E., Wulfeck, B., & MacWhinney, B. (1991). Crosslinguistic research in aphasia: An overview. *Brain and Language, 41*(2), 123–148. Retrieved from https://psyling.talkbank.org/years/1991/overview.pdf.

Beckner, C., Blythe, R., Bybee, J., Christiansen, M., Croft, W., Ellis, N., ... Schoenemann, T. (2009). Language is a complex adaptive system: Position paper. *Language Learning, 59*(s1), 1–26.

Berwick, R. (1987). Parsability and learnability. In B. MacWhinney (Ed.), *Mechanisms of language acquisition.* Hillsdale, NJ: Lawrence Erlbaum Associates.

Bishop, D., Bright, P., James, C., Bishop, S. J., & van der Lely, H. (2000). Grammatical SLI: A distinct subtype of developmental language impairment. *Applied Psycholinguistics, 21*(2), 159–181.

Bloodstein, O., & Bernstein Ratner, N. (2008). *A handbook on stuttering* (6th ed.). Delmar, NY: Cengage.

Browman, C. P., & Goldstein, L. (1992). Articulatory phonology: An overview. *Phonetica, 49*(3–4), 155–180.

Bybee, J. (2010). *Language, usage, and cognition.* New York: Cambridge University Press.

Chang, S.-E., & Guenther, F. (2020). Involvement of the cortico-basal ganglia-thalamocortical loop in developmental stuttering. *Frontiers in Psychology, 10*, 3088.

Chomsky, N. (2007). Approaching UG from below. In U. Sauerland & M. Gaertner (Eds.), *Interfaces + recursion = language?* (pp. 1–30). New York: Mouton de Gruyter.

Christiansen, M., & Chater, N. (2008). Language as shaped by the brain. *Behavioral and Brain Sciences, 31*(5), 489–558.

Christiansen, M., & Chater, N. (2016). The now-or-never bottleneck: A fundamental constraint on language. *Behavioral and Brain Sciences, 39.*

Civier, O., Bullock, D., Max, L., & Guenther, F. H. (2013). Computational modeling of stuttering caused by impairments in a basal ganglia thalamo-cortical circuit involved in syllable selection and initiation. *Brain and Language, 126*(3), 263–278.

Conway, C. M. (2020). How does the brain learn environmental structure? Ten core principles for understanding the neurocognitive mechanisms of statistical learning. *Neuroscience and Biobehavioral Reviews, 112*, 279–299.

Culicover, P. (2013). *Explaining syntax: Representations, structures, and computation.* New York: Oxford University Press.

Darwin, C. (1859). *On the origin of species.* London: John Murray.

Darwin, C. (1862). *On the various contrivances by which orchids are fertilized by insects (1862).* Chicago, IL: University of Chicago Press.

Dehaene, S., & Cohen, L. (2007). Cultural recycling of cortical maps. *Neuron, 56*(2), 384–398.

Dick, F., Bates, E., Wulfeck, B., Utman, J., Dronkers, N., & Gernsbacher, M. A. (2001). Language deficits, localization and grammar: Evidence for a distributive model of language breakdown in aphasics and normals. *Psychological Review, 108*(4), 759–788.

Diessel, H. (2017). Usage-Based Linguistics. *Oxford Research Encyclopedia of Linguistics.* Retrieved 23 Feb. 2023, from https://oxfordre.com/linguistics/view/10.1093/acrefore/9780199384655.001.0001/acrefore-9780199384655-e-363.

Dominey, P. F., & Boussaoud, D. (1997). Encoding behavioral context in recurrent networks of the fronto-striatal system: A simulation study. *Cognitive Brain Research, 6*(1), 53–65.

Dronkers, N. (2011). The neural architecture of the language comprehension network: Converging evidence from lesion and connectivity analyses. *Frontiers in Systems Neuroscience, 5*, 1.

Dronkers, N., Wilkins, D., Van Valin, R., Redfern, B., & Jaeger, J. (2004). Lesion analysis of the brain areas involved in language comprehension. *Cognition, 92*(1–2), 145–177.

Edelman, G. (1987). *Neural Darwinism: The theory of neuronal group selection.* New York: Basic Books.

Elman, J. L., Bates, E., Johnson, M., Karmiloff-Smith, A., Parisi, D., & Plunkett, K. (1996). *Rethinking innateness.* Cambridge, MA: MIT Press.

Evans, J. L., & MacWhinney, B. (1999). Sentence processing strategies in children with expressive and expressive-receptive specific language impairments. *International Journal of Language and Communication Disorders, 34*(2), 117–134. https://doi.org/10.1080/136828299247469.
Fisher, S. E., & Scharff, C. (2009). FOXP2 as a molecular window into speech and language. *Trends in Genetics, 25*(4), 166–177.
Fodor, J. (1983). *The modularity of mind: An essay on faculty psychology*. Cambridge, MA: MIT Press.
Freudenthal, D., Pine, J. M., Aguado-Orea, J., & Gobet, F. (2007). Modeling the developmental patterning of finiteness marking in English, Dutch, German, and Spanish using MOSAIC. *Cognitive Science, 31*(2), 311–341.
Frigerio-Domingues, C., & Drayna, D. (2017). Genetic contributions to stuttering: The current evidence. *Molecular Genetics and Genomic Medicine, 5*(2), 95–102.
Galton, F. (1883). *Inquiries into human faculty and its development*. London: Dent.
Goldberg, A. (2006). *Constructions at work: The nature of generalization in language*. Oxford: Oxford University Press.
Goldstone, R., & Rogosky, B. J. (2002). Using relations within conceptual systems to translate across conceptual systems. *Cognition, 84*(3), 295–320.
Goodwin, C. (2013). The co-operative, transformative organization of human action and knowledge. *Journal of Pragmatics, 46*(1), 8–23.
Gow, D. W. (2012). The cortical organization of lexical knowledge: A dual lexicon model of spoken language processing. *Brain and Language, 121*(3), 273–288.
Grodzinsky, Y. (2000). The neurology of syntax: Language use without Broca's area. *Behavioral and Brain Sciences, 23*(1), 1–21.
Guenther, F., & Vladusich, T. (2012). A neural theory of speech acquisition and production. *Journal of Neurolinguistics, 25*(5), 408–422.
Gupta, P., MacWhinney, B., Feldman, H., & Sacco, K. (2003). Phonological memory and vocabulary learning in children with focal lesions. *Brain and Language, 87*(2), 241–252. https://doi.org/10.1016/s0093-934x(03)00094-4.
Hagoort, P. (2013). MUC (memory, unification, control) and beyond. *Frontiers in Psychology, 4*, 1–13.
Hart, B., & Risley, T. R. (1995). *Meaningful differences in the everyday experience of young American children*. Baltimore, MD: Paul H. Brookes.
Hauser, M., Chomsky, N., & Fitch, T. (2002). The faculty of language: What is it, who has it, and how did it evolve? *Science, 298*(5598), 1569–1579.
Hebb, D. (1949). *The organization of behavior*. New York: Wiley.
Hernandez, A. E., Claussenius-Kalman, H. L., Ronderos, J., Castilla-Earls, A. P., Sun, L., Weiss, S. D., & Young, D. R. (2019). Neuroemergentism: A framework for studying cognition and the brain. *Journal of Neurolinguistics, 49*, 214–223.
Hickok, G. (2009). The functional neuroanatomy of language. *Physics of Life Reviews, 6*(3), 121–143.
Hickok, G., Bellugi, U., & Klima, E. S. (2001). Sign language in the brain. *Scientific American, 284*(6), 58–65.
Hickok, G., & Poeppel, D. (2004). Dorsal and ventral streams: A framework for understanding aspects of the functional anatomy of language. *Cognition, 92*(1–2), 67–99.
Hymes, D. (1962). The ethnography of speaking. *Anthropology and Human Behavior, 13*(53), 11–74.
Johnson, M. (2011). Interactive specialization: A domain-general framework for human functional brain development? *Developmental Cognitive Neuroscience, 1*(1), 7–21.
Just, M., & Carpenter, P. (1992). A capacity theory of comprehension: Individual differences in working memory. *Psychological Review, 99*(1), 122–149.
Kemmerer, D. (2015). *The cognitive neuroscience of language*. New York: Psychology Press.
Kohonen, T. (2001). *Self-organizing maps* (3rd ed.). Berlin: Springer.
Korniol, R. (1995). Stuttering, language, and cognition: A review and model of stuttering as suprasemental sentence plan alignment (SPA). *Psychological Review, 117*, 104–124.
Lashley, K. (1951). The problem of serial order in behavior. In L. A. Jeffress (Ed.), *Cerebral mechanisms in behavior*. New York: Wiley. 112–146.
Li, P., Legault, J., & Litcofsky, K. A. (2014). Neuroplasticity as a function of second language learning: Anatomical changes in the human brain. *Cortex, 58*, 301–324.
Maclay, H., & Osgood, C. E. (1959). Hesitation phenomena in spontaneous English speech. *Word, 25*(1), 19–44. Retrieved from http://search.ebscohost.com/login.aspx?direct=true&db=mzh&AN=1959001726&site=ehost-live.
MacWhinney, B. (2004). A multiple process solution to the logical problem of language acquisition. *Journal of Child Language, 31*(4), 883–914. https://doi.org/10.1017/s0305000904006336.

MacWhinney, B. (2005a). The emergence of grammar from perspective. In D. Pecher & R. A. Zwaan (Eds.), *The grounding of cognition: The role of perception and action in memory, language, and thinking* (pp. 198–223). Mahwah, NJ: Lawrence Erlbaum Associates.

MacWhinney, B. (2005b). Language evolution and human development. In B. Ellis & D. Bjorklund (Eds.), *Origins of the social mind* (pp. 383–410). New York: Guilford.

MacWhinney, B. (2014). Item-based patterns in early syntactic development. In T. Herbst, H.-J. Schmid, & S. Faulhaber (Eds.), *Constructions collocations patterns* (pp. 33–70). Berlin: de Gruyter Mouton.

MacWhinney, B. (2019). Neuroemergentism: Levels and constraints. *Journal of Neurolinguistics*, *49*, 232–234. https://doi.org/10.1016/j.jneuroling.2018.04.002.

MacWhinney, B. (2021). The competition model: Past and future. In J. Gervain (Ed.), *A life in cognition*. New York: Springer Nature, 3–16.

MacWhinney, B., & Bates, E. (Eds.). (1989). *The crosslinguistic study of sentence processing*. New York: Cambridge University Press.

MacWhinney, B., Feldman, H., Sacco, K., & Valdes-Perez, R. (2000). Online measures of basic language skills in children with early focal brain lesions. *Brain and Language*, *71*(3), 400–431. https://doi.org/10.1006/brln.1999.2273.

MacWhinney, B., Malchukov, A., & Moravcsik, E. (Eds.). (2014). *Competing motivations in grammar and usage*. New York: Oxford University Press.

Mainela-Arnold, E., Evans, J. L., & Coady, J. A. (2008). Lexical representations in children with SLI: Evidence from a frequency-manipulated gating task. *Journal of Speech, Language, and Hearing Research*, *51*(2), 381–393.

McClelland, J. (2015). Capturing gradience, continuous change, and quasi-regularity in sound, word, phrase, and meaning. In B. MacWhinney & W. O'Grady (Eds.), *The handbook of language emergence* (pp. 53–80). New York: Wiley.

McClelland, J., Mirman, D., & Holt, L. (2006). Are there interactive processes in speech perception? *Trends in Cognitive Sciences*, *10*(8), 363–369.

McDonald, J., & MacWhinney, B. (1989). Maximum likelihood models for sentence processing research. In B. MacWhinney & E. Bates (Eds.), *The crosslinguistic study of sentence processing* (pp. 397–421). New York: Cambridge University Press.

Meaburn, E., Dale, P. S., Craig, I., & Plomin, R. (2002). Language-impaired children: No sign of the FOXP2 mutation. *NeuroReport*, *13*(8), 1075–1077.

Mill, J. S. (1859). *System of logic, rationative and inductive; being a connected view of the principles of evidence and the methods of scientific investigation. Chapter VI: Of the composition of causes*. New York: Harper and Brothers.

Naganathan, A. N., & Muñoz, V. (2005). Scaling of folding times with protein size. *Journal of the American Chemical Society*, *127*(2), 480–481.

Newell, A. (1990). *A unified theory of cognition*. Cambridge, MA: Harvard University Press.

Nozari, N., & Hepner, C. R. (2019). To select or to wait? The importance of criterion setting in debates of competitive lexical selection. *Cognitive Neuropsychology*, *36*(5–6), 193–207.

Nozari, N., & Novick, J. (2017). Monitoring and control in language production. *Current Directions in Psychological Science*, *26*(5), 403–410.

Ochs, E. A., Schegloff, M., & Thompson, S. A. (1996). *Interaction and grammar*. Cambridge: Cambridge University Press.

O'Grady, W. (2005). *Syntactic carpentry*. Mahwah, NJ: Lawrence Erlbaum Associates.

Olszewska, A. M., Gaca, M., Herman, A. M., Jednoróg, K., & Marchewka, A. (2021). How musical training shapes the adult brain: Predispositions and neuroplasticity. *Frontiers in Neuroscience*, *15*, 204.

Pavlik, P., & Anderson, J. (2008). Using a model to compute the optimal schedule of practice. *Journal of Experimental Psychology: Applied*, *14*(2), 101–117.

Pinker, S. (1994). *The language instinct*. New York: William Morrow.

Pulvermüller, F. (2003). *The neuroscience of language*. Cambridge: Cambridge University Press.

Ratcliff, R., & McKoon, G. (2008). The diffusion decision model: Theory and data for two-choice decision tasks. *Neural Computation*, *20*(4), 873–922.

Recanzone, G., & Merzenich, M. (1993). Functional plasticity in the cerebral cortex: Mechanisms of improved perceptual abilities and skill acquisition. *Concepts in Neuroscience*, *4*, 1–23.

Rice, M., & Wexler, K. (1996). Toward tense as a clinical marker of specific language impairment in English-speaking children. *Journal of Speech and Hearing Research*, *39*(6), 1239–1257.

Roberts, J. E., Rosenfeld, R. M., & Zeisel, S. A. (2004). Otitis media and speech and language: A meta-analysis of prospective studies. *Pediatrics*, *113*(3), e238–e248.

Roelofs, A. (2011). Modeling the attentional control of vocal utterances: From Wernicke to WEAVER+. In J. Guendozi, F. Loncke, & M. Williams (Eds.), *The handbook of psycholinguistic and cognitive processes: Perspectives in communication disorders* (pp. 189–208). New York: Psychology Press.
Rosenbaum, D. (2015). *It's a jungle in there: How competition and cooperation in the mind shape the brain*. New York: Oxford University Press.
Schlichting, M. L., & Preston, A. R. (2015). Memory integration: Neural mechanisms and implications for behavior. *Current Opinion in Behavioral Sciences, 1*, 1–8.
Schmahmann, J., Pandya, D., Wang, R., Dai, G., D'Arceuil, H., de Crespigny, A., & Wedeen, V. (2007). Association fibre pathways of the brain: Parallel observations from diffusion spectrum imaging and autoradiography. *Brain, 130*(3), 630–653.
Shiell, M. M., Champoux, F., & Zatorre, R. J. (2015). Reorganization of auditory cortex in early-deaf people: Functional connectivity and relationship to hearing aid use. *Journal of Cognitive Neuroscience, 27*(1), 150–163.
Thompson, C. K., Meltzer-Asscher, A., Cho, S., Lee, J., Wieneke, C., Weintraub, S., & Mesulam, M. (2013). Syntactic and morphosyntactic processing in stroke-induced and primary progressive aphasia. *Behavioural Neurology, 26*(1–2), 35–54.
Valiant, L. G. (2014). What must a global theory of cortex explain? *Current Opinion in Neurobiology, 25*, 15–19.
van der Lely, H. (1994). Canonical linking rules: Forward vs. reverse linking in normally developing and Specifically Language Impaired children. *Cognition, 51*(1), 29–72.
van der Lely, H. (2005). Domain-specific cognitive systems: Insight from Grammatical-SLI. *Trends in Cognitive Sciences, 9*(2), 53–59.
van der Lely, H., & Christian, V. (2000). Lexical word formation in children with grammatical SLI: A grammar-specific versus an input-processing deficit? *Cognition, 75*(1), 33–63.
Van Essen, D. C., Felleman, D. F., DeYoe, E. A., Olavarria, J. F., & Knierim, J. J. (1990). Modular and hierarchical organization of extrastriate visual cortex in the macaque monkey. *Cold Spring Harbor Symposium on Quantitative Biology, 55*, 679–696.
Vargha-Khadem, F., Gadian, D. G., Copp, A., & Mishkin, M. (2005). FOXP2 and the neuroanatomy of speech and language. *Nature Reviews Neuroscience, 6*(2), 131–138.
Vargha-Khadem, F., Watkins, K., Alcock, K., Fletcher, P., & Passingham, R. (1995). Praxic and nonverbal cognitive deficits in a large family with a genetically transmitted speech and language disorder. *Proceedings of the National Academy of Sciences of the United States of America, 92*(3), 930–933.
Vernes, S., Newbury, D., Abrahams, B., Winchester, L., Nicod, J., Groszer, M., … Fisher, S. (2008). A functional genetic link between distinct developmental language disorders. *New English Journal of Medicine, 359*, 1–9.
Webb, A. R., Heller, H. T., Benson, C. B., & Lahav, A. (2015). Mother's voice and heartbeat sounds elicit auditory plasticity in the human brain before full gestation. *Proceedings of the National Academy of Sciences, 112*(10), 3152–3157.
West-Eberhard, M. J. (2003). *Developmental plasticity and evolution*. Oxford: Oxford University Press.
Whitehurst, G., & Vasta, R. (1975). Is language acquired through imitation? *Journal of Psycholinguistic Research, 4*(1), 37–59.
Wilson, S. M., & Saygin, A. P. (2004). Grammaticality judgments in aphasia: Deficits are not specific to syntactic structures, aphasic syndromes, or lesion sites. *Journal of Cognitive Neuroscience, 16*(2), 238–252.
Wong, P. C., Morgan-Short, K., Ettlinger, M., & Zheng, J. (2012). Linking neurogenetics and individual differences in language learning: The dopamine hypothesis. *Cortex, 48*(9), 1091–1102.
Woollett, K., & Maguire, E. A. (2011). Acquiring "the knowledge" of London's layout drives structural brain changes. *Current Biology, 21*(24), 2109–2114.
Zerilli, J. (2022). *The adaptablel mind: What neuroplasticity and neural reuse tell us about language and cognition*. New York: Oxford University Press.

3

HEALTHY AGING AND COMMUNICATION

The complexities of, um, fluent speech production

Lise Abrams and Katherine White

Introduction

For over 30 years, the topics of perception, comprehension, and production of language in older adulthood have been prominent areas of research (for reviews, see Abrams & Farrell, 2011; Burke & Shafto, 2008; Kemper, 2006; Peelle, 2019). Age-related changes in language processing play a critical role in communication, which is essential to older adults' health and wellbeing (e.g., Hummert & Nussbaum, 2001). Interpersonal communication can be negatively affected by changes in older adults' speech production. For example, proper names are more difficult for older adults to retrieve (e.g., Cohen, 1994), and forgetting a name during a conversation coupled with aging stereotypes about memory can result in negative perceptions of older adults' communicative competence, both from the listener and the speaker (e.g., Hummert et al., 2004; Ryan et al., 1992). However, other speech production changes enhance communication, leading to older adults being viewed as better storytellers than younger adults (e.g., Kemper et al., 1989; Pratt & Robins, 1991). A key contributor to communication is a speaker's fluency, which refers to speech that proceeds continuously without frequent pauses or errors, is produced at an appropriate pace, and is comprehensible to a listener (e.g., Bortfeld et al., 2001; Castro & James, 2014). The purpose of the present chapter is to review the literature on older adults' fluency during speech production, focusing on the ways in which speech fluency contributes to successful communication as we age. The chapter reviews the empirical research that has investigated older adults' fluency and the factors underlying age-related differences, focusing specifically on the measures of disfluencies in connected speech, word retrieval failures, lexical diversity and non-normative word use, off-topic speech and communicative goals, and the role of cognitive factors affecting fluency. The chapter concludes with a discussion of several directions for future research that may help to clarify the mechanisms underlying age-related changes in fluency during communication.

Methods and measures of fluency

In research studies, older adults' speech fluency has been elicited in various ways and contexts (see Kavé & Goral, 2017, for a review). With respect to elicitation, tasks can be *constrained* such that the scope of possible words to be produced is narrowed. For example, studies using a picture description task instruct speakers to describe the events or story represented in the picture, such as the Cookie Theft picture which shows a line drawing of two children stealing cookies behind their

DOI: 10.4324/9781003204213-5

Table 3.1 Measurement of older adults' fluency

Construct	*Description*	*Example Measures*
Continuity	Number, duration, or type of disfluency	Silent pauses; filled pauses (e.g., "um")
Speed	Speech rate or amount of speech produced	Number of words produced per minute; total number of words or utterances
Accuracy	Number or type of errors made	Tip-of-the-tongue (TOT) states
Lexical richness	Unique word use	Lexical diversity and non-normative word use
Coherence	Extent to which discourse represents its intended meaning	Off-topic speech

mother's back (Goodglass et al., 2001). Production tasks can be further constrained to a single word, such as tasks which ask speakers to retrieve one specific word that can be elicited from a picture or a general knowledge question. Alternatively, tasks can induce speech that is *spontaneous*, which does not presuppose the use of specific words by the speaker. Tasks involving spontaneous speech often involve speakers discussing autobiographical topics via stories or narratives, such as their family or a vacation, and the speech can be elicited individually or in conjunction with a partner. Tasks with a partner can involve naturalistic conversations or instructional interactions such as referential communication, in which information such as giving directions or describing differences between pictures is exchanged between two speakers.

The measurement of older adults' fluency has also varied across studies, focusing broadly on the constructs of continuity, speed, accuracy, lexical richness, and coherence of the produced speech (see Table 3.1 for descriptions and measures). It is important to note that speech fluency as discussed in this chapter differs from verbal fluency, a clinical task that has also been used with healthy older adults. Tasks measuring verbal fluency involve word generation, such as naming as many animals as possible in one minute (e.g., Taler et al., 2020). While retrieval of words on verbal fluency tasks and retrieval of words during story recall have been proposed to utilize similar cognitive mechanisms (e.g., Kavé & Sapir-Yogev, 2020), this chapter focuses specifically on the production of words that occurs during connected speech (i.e., sequences of words), as is typical during real-world communication.

Disfluencies

Aging is associated with an increase in disfluencies in a variety of connected speech tasks, including conversational speech (e.g., Horton et al., 2010), picture description (e.g., Castro & James, 2014; Dennis & Hess, 2016), story retelling (e.g., Lee et al., 2019; Saling et al., 2012), and reading aloud (Gollan & Goldrick, 2019). Some research has suggested that older adults produce slower speech (e.g., Horton et al., 2010; Saling et al., 2012), longer pauses (e.g., Castro & James, 2014; Cooper, 1990), and more nonword filled pauses, such as *um* or *uh*, than younger adults (e.g., Dennis & Hess, 2016; Horton et al., 2010; although see Arslan & Göksun, 2022). Filled pauses have been proposed to arise during speech planning (Corley & Stewart, 2008), although they can also reflect word finding difficulties (e.g., Metz & James, 2019). Nonetheless, speakers may also use them to keep the listener's attention and signal the temporary nature of the speech interruption (Clark, 1994).

However, other research suggests that age-related increases in disfluencies occur only in specific circumstances. For example, several studies have shown that older adults pause more than younger adults at non-syntactic boundaries (within a phrase or word) but not syntactic boundaries (between sentences or phrases) (e.g., Bortfeld et al., 2001; James et al., 2018; Lee et al., 2019). Dennis and Hess (2016) found that older adults had more interrupted speech than younger adults when producing words that were less frequently used among participants. Finally, although older adults are typically characterized as more disfluent than younger adults, some studies have found age equivalence in disfluencies (e.g., Beier et al., in press; Castro & James, 2014, for neutral pictures; Duchin & Mysak, 1987), or have found that younger adults are more disfluent overall (Long et al., 2020) or only for select types of disfluencies (e.g., filled pauses, Arslan & Göksun, 2022). These mixed findings could be due to the specific measures of fluency that were used (Beier et al., in press) or to older adults having more variability in their disfluencies (Saryazdi et al., 2019). Alternatively, older adults' disfluencies may be a consequence of tasks that elicit word retrieval difficulties. For example, increased disfluencies may allow older speakers to compensate for word retrieval problems by increasing the time to retrieve an intended word (Kavé & Goral, 2017). Conversely, decreased disfluencies are more likely to occur specifically in the speech of adults after age 70 (Luo et al., 2020), which may reflect a different compensatory strategy of avoiding words that are more susceptible to word retrieval failures (Schmitter-Edgecombe et al., 2000).

More recent research has begun to investigate whether factors such as the content of the speech or the conditions experienced while speaking influence age-related differences in disfluency production. For example, drawing from research showing age-related differences in emotion processing, Castro and James (2014) found that older adults produced more disfluencies than younger adults when describing negative pictures, but had similar disfluency rates when describing neutral pictures. In analyzing speech delivered under stressful vs. less stressful conditions, Metz and James (2019) found that stressful conditions led to more mid-phrase fillers for older adults but not younger adults and more unfilled pauses for both age groups. Independent of emotion, other research has shown that factors that increase cognitive demands, such as greater task complexity or less familiar content, may determine how frequently older adults produce disfluencies (e.g., Bortfeld et al., 2001; Castro & James, 2014; James et al., 2018). Studies investigating specific factors that mediate younger and older adults' disfluencies have potential to further our understanding of age-related differences in disfluencies by targeting specific mechanisms (e.g., regulation of emotion, cognitive load) that may mediate age differences.

It is worth noting that variability in the measurement of specific disfluencies limits conclusions that can be drawn from the data thus far. For example, some studies primarily focus on filled and unfilled pauses, whereas others include additional types of disfluencies, such as repetitions, repairs, stutters, tongue slips, and sentence changes or incompletions. Studies also differ in proportional measures of disfluencies, measured as a function of total words produced (e.g., Castro & James, 2014) or as a function of total number of disfluencies (e.g., Arslan & Göksun, 2022). Furthermore, some disfluency types occur infrequently, which can make it difficult for age differences to emerge. Composite measures that combine multiple disfluency types can offset potential floor effects (e.g., Castro & James, 2014; Dennis & Hess, 2016) and also allow for increased power to detect age differences, but this in turn may gloss over age-related differences in specific types of disfluencies. Instead of investigating disfluencies through a lens of "decline" which assumes disfluencies increase with age, an alternative approach is to focus on their *utility* for communication. For example, Saryazdi et al. (2021) showed that both younger and older listeners use disfluencies to guide referential processing, suggesting that disfluencies can be informative of upcoming speech (Clark & Fox Tree, 2002). The production of disfluencies may be related to social factors such as communicative intentions (e.g., Arslan & Göksun, 2022). For example, Taschenberger et al. (2019) found individual differences irrespective of age in the use of filled pauses during adverse listening conditions, suggesting that speakers may adapt their strategies when communication is challenging. Taken together, these studies suggest that understanding age-related differences in speech continuity requires consideration of both the conditions under which disfluencies disrupt production and the ways in which disfluencies enhance communication.

Word retrieval failures

While disfluencies affect the continuity and speed of speech, word retrieval failures such as TOTs reflect accuracy of speech (see Table 3.1). A TOT state is a temporary and often frustrating word-finding problem, i.e., an inability to retrieve a known word (e.g., Brown & McNeill, 1966). While TOTs are a relatively universal experience among speakers of various languages and ages, older adults have more TOTs, both in laboratory studies and in everyday life (e.g., Burke et al., 1991; Maylor, 1990). Proper names are particularly susceptible to TOTs in older adults (e.g., Burke et al., 1991; Juncos-Rabadán et al., 2010; Ouyang et al., 2020), who report them as their most irritating memory failure (e.g., Lovelace & Twohig, 1990). Although TOTs are often a concern for older adults who view them as a potential indicator of dementia, TOTs in healthy older adults are less frequent than in people with Alzheimer's disease (e.g., Astell & Harley, 1996) and people with mild cognitive impairment or subjective memory/cognitive complaints (e.g., Campos-Magdaleno et al., 2020; Juncos-Rabadán et al., 2011, 2013; Kim et al., 2020).

TOTs are thought to occur when access to a word's phonological representations is incomplete (Burke et al., 1991). Encountering words phonologically related to the TOT (e.g., James & Burke, 2000), specifically words with the TOT's first syllable (e.g., Abrams et al., 2003; White & Abrams, 2002) can increase the likelihood of resolving them. However, older adults are less likely than younger adults to resolve their TOTs in this way (e.g., Abrams et al., 2007; White & Abrams, 2002). Older adults' TOTs are also uniquely affected by factors related to the *frequency* of words phonologically related to them, such as neighborhood frequency (the frequency of words that differ from the TOT by a single phoneme; Vitevitch & Sommers, 2003) and first syllable frequency (the average frequency of words containing the TOT's first syllable; Farrell & Abrams, 2011). Furthermore, adults in their late 70s and 80s relative to those in their 60s and early 70s are particularly susceptible to the factors that affect TOTs (e.g., Abrams et al., 2007; Farrell & Abrams, 2011; White & Abrams, 2002). Despite complex interactions among these variables and age, these findings clarify that older adults consistently experience more TOTs because of difficulty strengthening access to phonological representations, both the TOTs' and words phonologically related to them.

It is worth noting that the majority of laboratory studies assess TOTs through tasks that require production of a single word rather than in the context of connected speech. Even though TOTs are often failures to retrieve a single word, they can have negative implications for older adults' communication in naturalistic contexts of connected speech, such as a withdrawal from social interactions to avoid creating a perception of incompetence (e.g., Cohen, 1994). TOTs can also produce feelings of stress (e.g., Cohen & Faulkner, 1986) and increase physiological arousal as observed with pupil dilation (Ryals et al., 2021). Affective factors associated with arousal, such as anxiety, have been associated with disfluencies (Murray, 1971), but research linking these factors with TOTs is sparse. One study (Shafto et al., 2019) examined the relationship between trait anxiety and TOTs across the life span. They found that older adults who self-reported more anxiety symptoms also had more TOTs, a relationship that did not occur for younger or middle-aged adults. In contrast, no age differences in TOTs emerged when arousal was induced via evaluative observation (Schmank & James, 2020): Giving a speech while being watched and evaluated increased TOTs similarly for younger, middle-aged, and older adults. Further research is needed to clarify the role of affective factors on older adults' TOTs and the mechanisms underlying these effects.

Lexical diversity and non-normative word use

While the previous sections have focused on measures that disrupt communication to some degree, i.e., disfluencies and TOTs, older adults' fluency can also be described with respect to successful word retrieval and the ways in which their word choices differ from younger adults (i.e., are more lexically rich; see Table 3.1). Several studies have shown that older adults' conversational speech is more lexically diverse than younger adults (e.g., Fergadiotis et al., 2011; Kemper & Sumner, 2001), i.e., includes more varied words (for a review of lexical diversity measures, see Kintz et al., 2016). However, a more nuanced analysis shows that age-related differences in lexical diversity depend on the type of discourse. Age-related increases in lexical diversity have been found in conversational speech (e.g., Horton et al., 2010), autobiographical narratives (e.g., Kemper & Sumner, 2001), and referential communication (e.g., Saryazdi et al., 2019). However, age differences are not typically found when the task relies on constrained speech, as when participants are asked to describe or tell stories about pictures (e.g., Capilouto et al., 2016; Fergadiotis et al., 2011; for a review, see Altmann, 2016).

An alternative measure of lexical richness, non-normative word use, has received only limited attention in studies to date. Unlike lexical diversity which measures lexical retrieval processes within one speaker's discourse sample, measures of non-normativeness compare word use across participants in the sample. Aging has been associated with greater non-normative word use, with respect to words produced by less than 5% of the sample (Dennis & Hess, 2016) and nouns that were produced only once across all participants (Kavé et al., 2009). Kavé et al. (2009) also extended findings of non-normative word use to word frequency, demonstrating a negative correlation between speaker age and frequency of nouns produced. Importantly, older adults' greater lexical diversity and non-normative word use were related to a speaker's vocabulary (Kavé & Nussbaum, 2012), which has been proposed to help compensate for retrieval difficulties (e.g., Kavé & Nussbaum, 2012; Kemper et al., 2010). However, older adults' greater non-normative word use has also been found to occur in conjunction with *more* disfluencies (Dennis & Hess, 2016), which could indicate that older speakers are searching for words to increase the richness of their speech, rather than offsetting word-finding problems. Together, these findings suggest the importance of considering the relationship between lexical richness and other fluency measures.

Off-topic speech and its relationship to speakers' goals for communication

Beyond individual word use, any assessment of older adults' fluency should also consider the discourse's focus and coherence (see Table 3.1). Even when connected speech is fluent, speakers can sometimes produce off-topic speech, which is prolonged, unconstrained, and irrelevant to the topic being described (e.g., Arbuckle & Gold, 1993; Gold et al., 1988). Age-related increases in off-topic speech have been demonstrated in various contexts involving discourse, including life-history interviews (e.g., Arbuckle & Gold, 1993; Gold et al., 1988), narratives about autobiographical topics (e.g., James et al., 1998; Trunk & Abrams, 2009), referential communication tasks (e.g., Arbuckle et al., 2000; Yin & Peng, 2016), and picture descriptions or storytelling (e.g., James et al., 1998; Kavé & Nussbaum, 2012). Off-topic speech has been coded in multiple ways, including the number of individual words or blocks of continuous speech judged to be off topic (e.g., Arbuckle et al., 2000; James et al., 1998), relevance ratings of nouns taken from speakers' picture descriptions (Kavé & Nussbaum, 2012), and holistic judgments of a speaker's focus and coherence in their narratives (e.g., Trunk & Abrams, 2009).

Despite having more off-topic speech and reduced coherence in some situations, older adults consistently produce better stories, i.e., stories that are rated as higher-quality, more interesting, clearer, and more informative, than younger adults (e.g., James et al., 1998; Kemper et al., 1989; Pratt & Robins, 1991; Trunk & Abrams, 2009). This narrative quality has been linked to an age-related shift in pragmatic goals for communication (e.g., James et al., 1998). Older speakers may have greater awareness that expressive goals, which produce speech that is elaborative, are necessary to tell a good story (Trunk & Abrams, 2009), and consequently may hold these goals even in tasks where conciseness can be helpful for the listener (see Long et al., 2020, for a related idea of communicative strategies motivating older adults' use of redundant words). For example, research with referential communication tasks (e.g., Beechey et al., 2019; Yule, 1997) has shown that older adults are less successful in adapting their speech to accommodate a listener, a process called audience design. Specifically, they are less likely to use shared labels as a function of the listener's age or knowledge (e.g., Horton & Spieler, 2007; Kemper et al., 1995, 1996; Schubotz et al., 2019) and are more likely to provide superfluous information (Saryazdi et al., 2019). However, older adults are successful in audience design under specific circumstances, such as when speaking to a listener with an intellectual disability (Gould & Shaleen, 1999) or referentially communicating within a live social interaction (Yoon & Stine-Morrow, 2019).

While off-topic speech can be interpreted as an age-related deficit in speech production (e.g., early research in this area used the term "off-topic verbosity"), this conclusion presents an incomplete picture. Older adults' use of off-topic speech may reflect age differences in goals for communication: They prioritize telling a good story over succinctness, which ultimately makes communication more enjoyable. Furthermore, older adults also show sensitivity to their listener's needs when communicating in more naturalistic settings, suggesting that the context in which language use occurs can affect the choice of goals (Schubotz, 2021). Further research is needed to understand the reasons underlying older adults' goal choices, e.g., whether they consciously choose to use expressive goals even in contexts where conciseness is necessary or whether there are cognitive demands that make changing goals more challenging. Nonetheless, similar to lexical diversity and non-normativeness, off-topic speech is another example where age differences in word choices can have some positive effects on communication.

Cognitive factors underlying older adults' speech fluency

The most consistent pattern across the different measures of fluency described thus far is that age differences do not always occur, and various cognitive factors have been proposed to explain these inconsistencies. One of the most reliable findings in the cognitive aging literature is an age-related increase in vocabulary and general knowledge (e.g., Kavé & Yafé, 2014; Keuleers et al., 2015; Verhaeghen, 2003). It has therefore been proposed that older adults' larger lexicons may provide a compensatory mechanism to offset potential fluency declines, which may explain why age differences in disfluencies are not consistently found. However, vocabulary does not predict all measures of fluency. For example, age differences in TOTs still emerge after controlling for vocabulary score (e.g., Heine et al., 1999; Juncos-Rabadán et al., 2010), and more generally research has failed to demonstrate a relationship between larger vocabularies and increased TOTs in older adulthood (e.g., Facal et al., 2012; Salthouse & Mandell, 2013; Shafto et al., 2017). It is also unclear whether the buffering effects of vocabulary would generalize to older adults with smaller vocabularies, a group not commonly included in research studies. Given the importance of vocabulary in language production more broadly and the mixed evidence with respect to its predictive value for explaining age-related changes in various fluency measures, future studies should include vocabulary as a covariate.

Vocabulary is not the only predictor of older adults' fluency, as some measures of fluency are related to other cognitive abilities (e.g., Schubotz, 2021). For example, working memory has been shown to predict lexical diversity (Kemper & Sumner, 2001), and age-related differences in coherence have been linked to changes in executive function that are common in healthy aging (e.g., Hoffman et al., 2018; Wright et al., 2014). However, the contribution of cognitive abilities to fluency varies across studies (e.g., Kemper & Sumner, 2001; Rabaglia & Salthouse, 2011). Some of the conflicting findings may be related to the type of communication task, as some tasks may rely more heavily on specific cognitive processes than others or may have different levels of cognitive demand. For example, tasks that are less constrained, rely on longer discourse segments, or require back-and-forth communication, are likely to depend more on working memory than single-word retrieval (e.g., TOT) tasks. Furthermore, declines in other cognitive abilities such as processing speed (e.g., Facal et al., 2012) and attention (e.g., Roelofs & Piai, 2011) have been linked to speech production more broadly (e.g., Polsinelli et al., 2020) rather than to fluency specifically, which has not consistently been investigated in conjunction with these cognitive factors. Although cognitive abilities are not anticipated to fully explain age-related changes in speech fluency, they may be able to clarify some of the disparate findings and should be included in future studies of fluency in aging.

Future directions

Additional domains for future research should focus on interactions among factors known to influence the fluency of communication but are underexplored in older adults. One possible area of research is the relationship between co-speech gestures and speech fluency, as the limited research on aging and gestures suggests a complex interplay among cognition, fluency, and gesture. Although gestures have been proposed to facilitate language production in younger speakers by decreasing cognitive load (e.g., Goldin-Meadow et al., 2001) or by facilitating conceptual planning (e.g., Kita, 2000) and lexical retrieval (e.g., Rauscher et al., 1996), less is known about whether older speakers benefit from using gestures to enhance speaking. The majority of research on age-related differences in multimodal communication has focused primarily on gesture *use* (but see Arslan & Göksun, 2022), demonstrating relatively few age-related differences in *overall* gesture use during spontaneous speech tasks such as an interview (e.g., Feyereisen & Havard, 1999) and a task that involved describing routes (e.g., Özer et al., 2017).

Other evidence suggests that age differences may be limited to some gesture types. For example, older adults produce fewer representational gestures (i.e., gestures that relate to the semantic elements of speech) than younger adults (e.g., Arslan & Göksun, 2021; Cohen & Borsoi, 1996; Feyereisen & Havard, 1999), a difference that has been attributed to age-related reductions in working memory or mental imagery (e.g., Arslan & Göksun, 2021; Özer & Göksun, 2020). In contrast, age similarity has been found in the production of non-representational gestures (e.g., Cohen & Borsoi, 1996; Feyereisen & Havard, 1999). A more nuanced look at the communicative contexts reveals that age differences in gesture use may depend on the audience (e.g., emerging when older adults speak to an experimenter but not with other participants; Schubotz et al., 2019) or the task (e.g., Arslan & Göksun, 2021; Theocharopoulou et al., 2015), similar to the ways in which contexts influence the occurrence of age differences in fluency measures. For example, younger adults gestured more in a narrative task whereas older adults gestured more during a TOT task (Theocharopoulou et al., 2015). Arslan and Göksun (2021) also reported age differences in representational gesture use only in an address description task, i.e., when a spatial context was given. Future research should aim to understand the conditions in which speakers may use gestures to support fluency as well as the role that cognitive processes play in multimodal communication.

A second underexplored area of research is the relationship between bilingualism and fluency. Bilinguals are another population in which increased disfluencies have been reported relative to monolinguals (e.g., Bergmann et al., 2015), findings which have been interpreted in support of language co-activation influencing bilinguals' fluency. Bilinguals enable the exploration of specific variables such as language proficiency and code switching in both of their languages (e.g., Kang & Lust, 2019), although these variables have yet to be explored within the context of speech fluency. Recent research has linked gestures with disfluency in bilinguals and found that gestures were more likely to occur during fluent rather than disfluent speech, which has been interpreted as contradicting the assumption that gestures are a compensatory strategy to offset disfluencies (Graziano & Gullberg, 2018). However, all of the existing research on bilingual speech disfluency has focused solely on children and younger adults (e.g., Carias & Ingram, 2006; Morin-Lessard & Byers-Heinlein, 2019). The only research with respect to aging, bilingualism, and disfluency, of which we are aware, has investigated TOTs (Gollan & Brown, 2006) or more generally focuses primarily on lexical access rather than fluency (e.g., Goral et al., 2008; Higby et al., 2020). The paucity of research with older adult bilinguals, along with the other future directions described above, provide a number of avenues to further our understanding of the many complexities underlying fluent speech production in healthy aging.

Further reading

Arslan, B., & Göksun, T. (2022). Aging, gesture production, and disfluency in speech: A comparison of younger and older adults. *Cognitive Science*, *46*(2), e13098.

Bergmann, C., Sprenger, S., & Schmid, M. S. (2015). The impact of language co-activation on L1 and L2 speech fluency. *Acta Psychologica*, *161C*, 25–35.

Dennis, P. A., & Hess, T. M. (2016). Aging-related gains and losses associated with word production in connected speech. *Aging, Neuropsychology, and Cognition*, *23*(6), 638–650.

References

Abrams, L., & Farrell, M. T. (2011). Language processing in normal aging. In J. Guendouzi, F. Loncke, & M. J. Williams (Eds.), *The handbook of psycholinguistic and cognitive processes: Perspectives in communication disorders* (pp. 49–73). Psychology Press. https://doi.org/10.4324/9780203848005.ch3

Abrams, L., Trunk, D. L., & Merrill, L. A. (2007). Why a superman cannot help a tsunami: Activation of grammatical class influences resolution of young and older adults' tip-of-the-tongue states. *Psychology and Aging*, *22*(4), 835–845. https://doi.org/10.1037/0882-7974.22.4.835

Abrams, L., White, K. K., & Eitel, S. L. (2003). Isolating phonological components that increase tip-of-the-tongue resolution. *Memory and Cognition*, *31*(8), 1153–1162. https://doi.org/10.3758/bf03195798

Altmann, L. J. P. (2016). Language: Discourse production and communication. In N. A. Pachana (Ed.), *Encyclopedia of geropsychology*. Springer Singapore. https://doi-org.ccl.idm.oclc.org/10.1007/978-981-287-080-3_222-1

Arbuckle, T. Y., & Gold, D. P. (1993). Aging, inhibition, and verbosity. *Journal of Gerontology*, *48*(5), P225–P232. https://doi.org/10.1093/geronj/48.5.P225

Arbuckle, T. Y., Nohara-LeClair, M., & Pushkar, D. (2000). Effect of off-target verbosity on communication efficiency in a referential communication task. *Psychology and Aging*, *15*(1), 65–77. https://doi.org/10.1037//0882-7974.15.1.65

Arslan, B., & Göksun, T. (2021). Ageing, working memory, and mental imagery: Understanding gestural communication in younger and older adults. *Quarterly Journal of Experimental Psychology*, *74*(1), 29–44. https://doi.org/10.1177/1747021820944696

Arslan, B., & Göksun, T. (2022). Aging, gesture production, and disfluency in speech: A comparison of younger and older adults. *Cognitive Science*, *46*(2), e13098. https://doi.org/10.1111/cogs.13098

Astell, A. J., & Harley, T. A. (1996). Tip-of-the-tongue states and lexical access in dementia. *Brain and Language*, *54*(2), 196–215. https://doi.org/10.1006/brln.1996.0071

Beechey, T., Buchholz, J. M., & Keidser, G. (2019). Eliciting naturalistic conversations: A method for assessing communication ability, subjective experience, and the impacts of noise and hearing impairment. *Journal of Speech, Language, and Hearing Research*, *62*(2), 470–484. https://doi.org/10.1044/2018_JSLHR-H-18-0107

Beier, E. J., Chantavarin, S., & Ferreira, F. (in press). Do disfluencies increase with age? Evidence from a sequential corpus study of disfluencies. *Psychology and Aging*.

Bergmann, C., Sprenger, S., & Schmid, M. S. (2015). The impact of language co-activation on L1 and L2 speech fluency. *Acta Psychologica*, *161C*, 25–35. https://doi.org/10.1016/j.actpsy.2015.07.015

Bortfeld, H., Leon, S. D., Bloom, J. E., Schober, M. F., & Brennan, S. E. (2001). Disfluency rates in conversation: Effects of age, relationship, topic, role, and gender. *Language and Speech*, *44*(2), 123–147. https://doi.org/10.1177/00238309010440020101

Brown, R., & McNeill, D. (1966). The "tip of the tongue" phenomenon. *Journal of Verbal Learning and Verbal Behavior*, *5*(4), 325–337. https://doi.org/10.1016/S0022-5371(66)80040-3

Burke, D. M., MacKay, D. G., Worthley, J. S., & Wade, E. (1991). On the tip of the tongue: What causes word finding failures in young and older adults? *Journal of Memory and Language*, *30*(5), 542–579. https://doi.org/10.1016/0749-596X(91)90026-G

Burke, D. M., & Shafto, M. A. (2008). Language and aging. In F. I. M. Craik & T. A. Salthouse (Eds.), *The handbook of aging and cognition* (3rd ed., pp. 373–443). Psychology Press.

Campos-Magdaleno, M., Leiva, D., Pereiro, A. X., Lojo-Seoane, C., Mallo, S. C., Nieto-Vieites, A., Juncos-Rabadán, O., & Facal, D. (2020). Longitudinal patterns of the tip-of-the-tongue phenomenon in people with subjective cognitive complaints and mild cognitive impairment. *Frontiers in Psychology*, *11*, 425. https://doi.org/10.3389/fpsyg.2020.00425

Capilouto, G. J., Wright, H. H., & Maddy, K. M. (2016). Microlinguistic processes that contribute to the ability to relay main events: Influence of age. *Aging, Neuropsychology, and Cognition*, *23*(4), 445–463. https://doi.org/10.1080/13825585.2015.1118006

Carias, S., & Ingram, D. (2006). Language and disfluency: Four case studies on Spanish–English bilingual children. *Journal of Multilingual Communication Disorders*, *4*(2), 149–157. https://doi.org/10.1080/14769670601092663

Castro, N., & James, L. E. (2014). Differences between young and older adults' spoken language production in descriptions of negative versus neutral pictures. *Aging, Neuropsychology, and Cognition, 21*(2), 222–238. https://doi.org/10.1080/13825585.2013.804902
Clark, H. H. (1994). Managing problems in speaking. *Speech Communication, 15*(3–4), 243–250. https://doi.org/10.1016/0167-6393(94)90075-2
Clark, H. H., & Fox Tree, J. E. (2002). Using uh and um in spontaneous speaking. *Cognition, 84*(1), 73–111. https://doi.org/10.1016/s0010-0277(02)00017-3
Cohen, G. (1994). Age-related problems in the use of proper names in communication. In M. L. Hummert, J. M. Wiemann, & J. F. Nussbaum (Eds.), *Interpersonal communication in older adulthood: Interdisciplinary theory and research* (pp. 40–57). Sage Publications, Inc. https://doi.org/10.4135/9781483326832.n3
Cohen, G., & Faulkner, D. (1986). Memory for proper names: Age differences in retrieval. *British Journal of Developmental Psychology, 4*(2), 187–197. https://doi.org/10.1111/j.2044-835X.1986.tb01010.x
Cohen, R. L., & Borsoi, D. (1996). The role of gestures in description-communication: A cross-sectional study of aging. *Journal of Nonverbal Behavior, 20*(1), 45–63. https://doi.org/10.1007/BF02248714
Cooper, P. V. (1990). Discourse production and normal aging: Performance on oral picture description tasks. *Journal of Gerontology, 45*(5), P210–P214. https://doi.org/10.1093/geronj/45.5.p210
Corley, M., & Stewart, O. W. (2008). Hesitation disfluencies in spontaneous speech: The meaning of um. *Language and Linguistics Compass, 2*(4), 589–602. https://doi.org/10.1111/j.1749-818X.2008.00068.x
Dennis, P. A., & Hess, T. M. (2016). Aging-related gains and losses associated with word production in connected speech. *Aging, Neuropsychology, and Cognition, 23*(6), 638–650. https://doi.org/10.1080/13825585.2016.1158233
Duchin, S. W., & Mysak, E. D. (1987). Disfluency and rate characteristics of young adult, middle-aged, and older males. *Journal of Communication Disorders, 20*(3), 245–257. https://doi.org/10.1016/0021-9924(87)90022-0
Facal, D., Juncos-Rabadán, O., Rodríguez, M. S., & Pereiro, A. X. (2012). Tip-of-the-tongue in aging: Influence of vocabulary, working memory and processing speed. *Aging: Clinical and Experimental Research, 24*(6), 647–656. https://doi.org/10.3275/8586
Farrell, M. T., & Abrams, L. (2011). Tip-of-the-tongue states reveal age differences in the syllable frequency effect. *Journal of Experimental Psychology: Learning, Memory, and Cognition, 37*(1), 277–285. https://doi.org/10.1037/a0021328
Fergadiotis, G., Wright, H. H., & Capilouto, G. J. (2011). Productive vocabulary across discourse types. *Aphasiology, 25*(10), 1261–1278. https://doi.org/10.1080/02687038.2011.606974
Feyereisen, P., & Havard, I. (1999). Mental imagery and production of hand gestures while speaking in younger and older adults. *Journal of Nonverbal Behavior, 23*(2), 153–171. https://doi.org/10.1023/A:1021487510204
Gold, D., Andres, D., Arbuckle, T., & Schwartzman, A. (1988). Measurement and correlates of verbosity in elderly people. *Journal of Gerontology, 43*(2), P27–P33. https://doi.org/10.1093/geronj/43.2.P27
Goldin-Meadow, S., Nusbaum, H., Kelly, S. D., & Wagner, S. (2001). Explaining math: Gesturing lightens the load. *Psychological Science, 12*(6), 516–522. https://doi.org/10.1111/1467-9280.00395
Gollan, T. H., & Brown, A. S. (2006). From tip-of-the-tongue (TOT) data to theoretical implications in two steps: When more TOTs means better retrieval. *Journal of Experimental Psychology: General, 135*(3), 462–483. https://doi.org/10.1037/0096-3445.135.3.462
Gollan, T. H., & Goldrick, M. (2019). Aging deficits in naturalistic speech production and monitoring revealed through reading aloud. *Psychology and Aging, 34*(1), 25–42. https://doi.org/10.1037/pag0000296
Goodglass, H., Kaplan, E., & Barresi, B. (2001). *Boston diagnostic aphasia examination–third edition (BDAE-3).* Lippincott Williams & Wilkins.
Goral, M., Libben, G., Obler, L. K., Jarema, G., & Ohayon, K. (2008). Lexical attrition in younger and older bilingual adults. *Clinical Linguistics and Phonetics, 22*(7), 509–522. https://doi.org/10.1080/02699200801912237
Gould, O. N., & Shaleen, L. (1999). Collaboration with diverse partners: How older women adapt their speech. *Journal of Language and Social Psychology, 18*(4), 395–418. https://doi.org/10.1177/0261927X99018004003
Graziano, M., & Gullberg, M. (2018). When speech stops, gesture stops: Evidence from developmental and crosslinguistic comparisons. *Frontiers in Psychology, 9*, Article 879. https://doi.org/10.3389/fpsyg.2018.00879
Heine, M. K., Ober, B. A., & Shenaut, G. K. (1999). Naturally occurring and experimentally induced tip-of-the-tongue experiences in three adult age groups. *Psychology and Aging, 14*(3), 445–457. https://doi.org/10.1037/0882-7974.14.3.445
Higby, E., Donnelly, S., Yoon, J., & Obler, L. (2020). The effect of second-language vocabulary on word retrieval in the native language. *Bilingualism: Language and Cognition, 23*(4), 812–824. https://doi.org/10.1017/S136672891900049X
Hoffman, P., Loginova, E., & Russell, A. (2018). Poor coherence in older people's speech is explained by impaired semantic and executive processes. *eLife*, 7, e38907. https://doi.org/10.7554/eLife.38907

Horton, W. S., & Spieler, D. H. (2007). Age-related differences in communication and audience design. *Psychology and Aging, 22*(2), 281–290. https://doi.org/10.1037/0882-7974.22.2.281

Horton, W. S., Spieler, D. H., & Shriberg, E. (2010). A corpus analysis of patterns of age-related change in conversational speech. *Psychology and Aging, 25*(3), 708–713. https://doi.org/10.1037/a0019424

Hummert, M. L., Garstka, T. A., Ryan, E. B., & Bonnesen, J. L. (2004). The role of age stereotypes in interpersonal communication. In J. F. Nussbaum & J. Coupland (Eds.), *Handbook of communication and aging research* (pp. 91–114). Lawrence Erlbaum Associates Publishers.

Hummert, M. L., & Nussbaum, J. F. (Eds.). (2001). *Aging, communication, and health: Linking research and practice for successful aging*. Lawrence Erlbaum Associates Publishers.

James, L. E., & Burke, D. M. (2000). Phonological priming effects on word retrieval and tip-of-the-tongue experiences in young and older adults. *Journal of Experimental Psychology: Learning, Memory, and Cognition, 26*(6), 1378–1391. https://doi.org/10.1037/0278-7393.26.6.1378

James, L. E., Burke, D. M., Austin, A., & Hulme, E. (1998). Production and perception of "verbosity" in younger and older adults. *Psychology and Aging, 13*(3), 355–367. https://doi.org/10.1037/0882-7974.13.3.355

James, L. E., Chambers, B. N., & Placzek, C. L. (2018). How scenes containing visual errors affect speech fluency in young and older adults. *Aging, Neuropsychology, and Cognition, 25*(4), 520–534. https://doi.org/10.1080/13825585.2017.1337061

Juncos-Rabadán, O., Facal, D., Lojo-Seoane, C., & Pereiro, A. X. (2013). Tip-of-the-tongue for proper names in non-amnestic mild cognitive impairment. *Journal of Neurolinguistics, 26*(3), 409–420. https://doi.org/10.1016/j.jneuroling.2013.01.001

Juncos-Rabadán, O., Facal, D., Rodríguez, M. S., & Pereiro, A. X. (2010). Lexical knowledge and lexical retrieval in ageing: Insights from a tip-of-the-tongue (TOT) study. *Language and Cognitive Processes, 25*(10), 1301–1334. https://doi.org/10.1080/01690961003589484

Juncos-Rabadán, O., Rodríguez, N., Facal, D., Cuba, J., & Pereiro, A. X. (2011). Tip-of-the-tongue for proper names in mild cognitive impairment. Semantic or post-semantic impairments? *Journal of Neurolinguistics, 24*(6), 636–651. https://doi.org/10.1016/j.jneuroling.2011.06.004

Kang, C., & Lust, B. (2019). Code-switching does not predict executive function performance in proficient bilingual children: Bilingualism does. *Bilingualism: Language and Cognition, 22*(2), 366–382. https://doi.org/10.1017/S1366728918000299

Kavé, G., & Goral, M. (2017). Do age-related word retrieval difficulties appear (or disappear) in connected speech? *Aging, Neuropsychology and Cognition, 24*(5), 508–527. https://doi.org/10.1080/13825585.2016.1226249

Kavé, G., & Nussbaum, S. (2012). Characteristics of noun retrieval in picture descriptions across the adult lifespan. *Aphasiology, 26*(10), 1238–1249. https://doi.org/10.1080/02687038.2012.681767

Kavé, G., Samuel-Enoch, K., & Adiv, S. (2009). The association between age and the frequency of nouns selected for production. *Psychology and Aging, 24*(1), 17–27. https://doi.org/10.1037/a0014579

Kavé, G., & Sapir-Yogev, S. (2020). Associations between memory and verbal fluency tasks. *Journal of Communication Disorders, 83,* Article 105968. https://doi.org/10.1016/j.jcomdis.2019.105968

Kavé, G., & Yafé, R. (2014). Performance of younger and older adults on tests of word knowledge and word retrieval: Independence or interdependence of skills? *American Journal of Speech-Language Pathology, 23*(1), 36–45. https://doi.org/10.1044/1058-0360(2013/12-0136)

Kemper, S. (2006). Language in adulthood. In E. Bialystok & F. I. M. Craik (Eds.), *Lifespan cognition: Mechanisms of change* (pp. 223–238). Oxford University Press. https://doi.org/10.1093/acprof:oso/9780195169539.003.0015

Kemper, S., Kynette, D., Rash, S., O'Brien, K., & Sprott, R. (1989). Life-span changes to adults' language: Effects of memory and genre. *Applied Psycholinguistics, 10*(1), 49–66. https://doi.org/10.1017/S0142716400008419

Kemper, S., Othick, M., Warren, J., Gubarchuk, J., & Gerhing, H. (1996). Facilitating older adults' performance on a referential communication task through speech accommodations. *Aging, Neuropsychology, and Cognition, 3*(1), 37–55. https://doi.org/10.1080/13825589608256611

Kemper, S., Schmalzried, R., Hoffman, L., & Herman, R. (2010). Aging and the vulnerability of speech to dual task demands. *Psychology and Aging, 25*(4), 949–962. https://doi.org/10.1037/a0020000

Kemper, S., & Sumner, A. (2001). The structure of verbal abilities in young and older adults. *Psychology and Aging, 16*(2), 312–322. https://doi.org/10.1037/0882-7974.16.2.312

Kemper, S., Vandeputte, D., Rice, K., Cheung, H., & Gubarchuk, J. (1995). Speech adjustments to aging during a referential communication task. *Journal of Language and Social Psychology, 14*(1–2), 40–59. https://doi.org/10.1177/0261927X95141003

Keuleers, E., Stevens, M., Mandera, P., & Brysbaert, M. (2015). Word knowledge in the crowd: Measuring vocabulary size and word prevalence in a massive online experiment. *Quarterly Journal of Experimental Psychology, 68*(8), 1665–1692. https://doi.org/10.1080/17470218.2015.1022560

Kim, J., Kim, M., & Yoon, J. H. (2020). The tip-of-the-tongue phenomenon in older adults with subjective memory complaints. *PLOS ONE, 15*(9), e0239327. https://doi.org/10.1371/journal.pone.0239327

Kintz, S., Fergadiotis, G., & Wright, H. H. (2016). Aging effects on discourse production. In H. H. Wright (Ed.), *Cognition, language and aging* (pp. 81–106). John Benjamins Publishing Company.

Kita, S. (2000). How representational gestures help speaking. In D. McNeill (Ed.), *Language and gesture* (pp. 162–185). Cambridge University Press. https://doi.org/10.1017/CBO9780511620850.011

Lee, J., Huber, J., Jenins, J., & Fredrick, J. (2019). Language planning and pauses in story retell: Evidence from aging and Parkinson's disease. *Journal of Communication Disorders, 79*, 1–10. https://doi.org/10.1016/j.jcomdis.2019.02.004

Long, M., Rohde, H., & Rubio-Fernandez, P. (2020). The pressure to communicate efficiently continues to shape language use later in life. *Scientific Reports, 10*(1), 8214. https://doi.org/10.1038/s41598-020-64475-6

Lovelace, E. A., & Twohig, P. T. (1990). Healthy older adults' perceptions of their memory functioning and use of mnemonics. *Bulletin of the Psychonomic Society, 28*(2), 115–118. https://doi.org/10.3758/BF03333979

Luo, M., Neysari, M., Schneider, G., Martin, M., & Demiray, B. (2020). Linear and nonlinear age trajectories of language use: A laboratory observation study of couples' conflict conversations. *Journals of Gerontology: Series B, Psychological Sciences and Social Sciences, 75*(9), e206–e214. https://doi.org/10.1093/geronb/gbaa041

Maylor, E. A. (1990). Recognizing and naming faces: Aging, memory retrieval, and the tip of the tongue state. *Journal of Gerontology, 45*(6), P215–P226. https://doi.org/10.1093/geronj/45.6.P215

Metz, M. J., & James, L. E. (2019). Specific effects of the Trier social stress test on speech fluency in young and older adults. *Aging, Neuropsychology, and Cognition, 26*(4), 558–576. https://doi.org/10.1080/13825585.2018.1503639

Morin-Lessard, E., Poulin-Dubois, D., Segalowitz, N., & Byers-Heinlein, K. (2019). Selective attention to the mouth of talking faces in monolinguals and bilinguals aged 5 months to 5 years. *Developmental Psychology, 55*(8), 1640–1655. https://doi.org/10.1037/dev0000750

Murray, D. C. (1971). Talk, silence, and anxiety. *Psychological Bulletin, 75*(4), 244–260. https://doi.org/10.1037/h0030801

Ouyang, M., Cai, X., & Zhang, Q. (2020). Aging effects on phonological and semantic priming in the tip-of-the-tongue: Evidence from a two-step approach. *Frontiers in Psychology, 11*, Article 338. https://doi.org/10.3389/fpsyg.2020.00338

Özer, D., & Göksun, T. (2020). Gesture use and processing: A review on individual differences in cognitive resources. *Frontiers in Psychology, 11*, 573555. https://doi.org/10.3389/fpsyg.2020.573555

Özer, D., Tansan, M., Özer, E. E., Malykhina, K., Chatterjee, A., & Göksun, T. (2017, July 16–29). The effects of gesture restriction on spatial language in young and elderly adults. In G. Gunzelmann, A. Howes, T. Tenbrink, & E. J. Davelaar (Eds.), *Proceedings of the 39th annual meeting of the cognitive science society*. https://mindmodeling.org/cogsci2017/papers/0290/index.html

Peelle, J. E. (2019). Language and aging. In G. I. de Zubicaray & N. O. Schiller (Eds.), *The Oxford handbook of neurolinguistics*. Oxford University Press. https://doi.org/10.1093/oxfordhb/9780190672027.013.12

Polsinelli, A. J., Moseley, S. A., Grilli, M. D., Glisky, E. L., & Mehl, M. R. (2020). Natural, everyday language use provides a window into the integrity of older adults' executive functioning. *Journals of Gerontology: Series B, Psychological Sciences and Social Sciences, 75*(9), e215–e220. https://doi.org/10.1093/geronb/gbaa055

Pratt, M. W., & Robins, S. L. (1991). That's the way it was: Age differences in the structure and quality of adults' personal narratives. *Discourse Processes, 14*(1), 73–85. https://doi.org/10.1080/01638539109544775

Rabaglia, C. D., & Salthouse, T. A. (2011). Natural and constrained language production as a function of age and cognitive abilities. *Language and Cognitive Processes, 26*(10), 1505–1531. https://doi.org/10.1080/01690965.2010.507489

Rauscher, F. H., Krauss, R. M., & Chen, Y. (1996). Gesture, speech, and lexical access: The role of lexical movements in speech production. *Psychological Science*, 7(4), 226–231. https://doi.org/10.1111/j.1467-9280.1996.tb00364.x

Roelofs, A., & Piai, V. (2011). Attention demands of spoken word planning: A review. *Frontiers in Psychology, 2*, Article 307. https://doi.org/10.3389/fpsyg.2011.00307

Ryals, A. J., Kelly, M. E., & Cleary, A. M. (2021). Increased pupil dilation during tip-of-the-tongue states. *Consciousness and Cognition, 92*, 103152. https://doi.org/10.1016/j.concog.2021.103152

Ryan, E. B., See, S. K., Meneer, W. B., & Trovato, D. (1992). Age-based perceptions of language performance among younger and older adults. *Communication Research, 19*(4), 423–443. https://doi.org/10.1177/009365092019004002

Saling, L. L., Laroo, N., & Saling, M. M. (2012). When more is less: Failure to compress discourse with re-telling in normal ageing. *Acta Psychologica, 139*(1), 220–224. https://doi.org/10.1016/j.actpsy.2011.10.005

Salthouse, T. A., & Mandell, A. R. (2013). Do age-related increases in tip-of-the-tongue experiences signify episodic memory impairments? *Psychological Science*, *24*(12), 2489–2497. https://doi.org/10.1177/0956797613495881

Saryazdi, R., Bannon, J., & Chambers, C. G. (2019). Age-related differences in referential production: A multiple-measures study. *Psychology and Aging*, *34*(6), 791–804. http://doi.org/10.1037/pag0000372

Saryazdi, R., DeSantis, D., Johnson, E. K., & Chambers, C. G. (2021). The use of disfluency cues in spoken language processing: Insights from aging. *Psychology and Aging*, *36*(8), 928–942. https://doi.org/10.1037/pag0000652

Schmank, C. J., & James, L. E. (2020). Adults of all ages experience increased tip-of-the-tongue states under ostensible evaluative observation. *Aging, Neuropsychology, and Cognition*, *27*(4), 517–531. https://doi.org/10.1080/13825585.2019.1641177

Schmitter-Edgecombe, M., Vesneski, M., & Jones, D. W. (2000). Aging and word-finding: A comparison of spontaneous and constrained naming tests. *Archives of Clinical Neuropsychology*, *15*(6), 479–493. https://doi.org/10.1016/S0887-6177(99)00039-6

Schubotz, L. (2021). *Effects of aging and cognitive abilities on multimodal language production and comprehension in context*. [Unpublished doctoral dissertation]. Radboud University.

Schubotz, L., Holler, J., Drijvers, L., & Özyürek, A. (2021). Aging and working memory modulate the ability to benefit from visible speech and iconic gestures during speech-in-noise comprehension. *Psychological Research*, *85*(5), 1997–2011. https://doi.org/10.1007/s00426-020-01363-8

Schubotz, L., Özyürek, A., & Holler, J. (2019). Age-related differences in multimodal recipient design: Younger, but not older adults, adapt speech and co-speech gestures to common ground. *Language, Cognition and Neuroscience*, *34*(2), 254–271. https://doi.org/10.1080/23273798.2018.1527377

Shafto, M. A., James, L. E., Abrams, L., & Cam, C. A. N. (2019). Age-related changes in word retrieval vary by self-reported anxiety but not depression symptoms. *Aging, Neuropsychology, and Cognition*, *26*(5), 767–780. https://doi.org/10.1080/13825585.2018.1527284

Shafto, M. A., James, L. E., Abrams, L., Tyler, L. K., & Cam, C. A. N. (2017). Age-related increases in verbal knowledge are not associated with word finding problems in the Cam-CAN Cohort: What you know won't hurt you. *Journals of Gerontology: Series B, Psychological Sciences and Social Sciences*, *72*(1), 100–106. https://doi.org/10.1093/geronb/gbw074

Taler, V., Johns, B. T., & Jones, M. N. (2020). A large-scale semantic analysis of verbal fluency across the aging spectrum: Data from the Canadian Longitudinal Study on Aging. *Journals of Gerontology: Series B, Psychological Sciences and Social Sciences*, *75*(9), e221–e230.

Taschenberger, L., Tuomainen, O., & Hazan, V. (2019, September 12–13). Disfluencies in spontaneous speech in easy and adverse communicative situations: The effect of age. In R. L. Rose & R. Eklund (Eds.), *Proceedings of the DiSS 2019, the 9th workshop on disfluency in spontaneous speech*. https://doi.org/10.21862/diss-09-015-tasc-etal

Theocharopoulou, F., Cocks, N., Pring, T., & Dipper, L. T. (2015). TOT phenomena: Gesture production in younger and older adults. *Psychology and Aging*, *30*(2), 245–252. https://doi.org/10.1037/a0038913

Trunk, D. L., & Abrams, L. (2009). Do younger and older adults' communicative goals influence off-topic speech in autobiographical narratives? *Psychology and Aging*, *24*(2), 324–337. https://doi.org/10.1037/a0015259

Verhaeghen, P. (2003). Aging and vocabulary score: A meta-analysis. *Psychology and Aging*, *18*(2), 332–339. https://doi.org/10.1037/0882-7974.18.2.332

Vitevitch, M. S., & Sommers, M. S. (2003). The facilitative influence of phonological similarity and neighborhood frequency in speech production in younger and older adults. *Memory and Cognition*, *31*(4), 491–504. https://doi.org/10.3758/bf03196091

White, K. K., & Abrams, L. (2002). Does priming specific syllables during tip-of-the-tongue states facilitate word retrieval in older adults? *Psychology and Aging*, *17*(2), 226–235. https://doi.org/10.1037/0882-7974.17.2.226

Wright, H. H., Koutsoftas, A. D., Capilouto, G. J., & Fergadiotis, G. (2014). Global coherence in younger and older adults: Influence of cognitive processes and discourse type. *Aging, Neuropsychology, and Cognition*, *21*(2), 174–196. https://doi.org/10.1080/13825585.2013.794894

Yin, S., & Peng, H. (2016). The role of inhibition in age-related off-topic verbosity: Not access but deletion and restraint functions. *Frontiers in Psychology*, 7, Article 544. https://doi.org/10.3389/fpsyg.2016.00544

Yoon, S. O., & Stine-Morrow, E. A. L. (2019). Evidence of preserved audience design with aging in interactive conversation. *Psychology and Aging*, *34*(4), 613–623. https://doi.org/10.1037/pag0000341

Yule, G. (1997). *Referential communication tasks*. Lawrence Erlbaum Associates. https://doi.org/10.4324/9781315044965

4

WORKING MEMORY AND ATTENTION IN LANGUAGE USE

Nelson Cowan

Introduction

Working memory refers to a small amount of information held in the mind, readily accessible for a short time to help an individual comprehend language and solve problems. As such, it is not just any topic, but potentially the key mechanism that organizes and represents one's conscious experience as a human being; James (1890) referred to it as primary memory, which he described as the trailing edge of consciousness. The purpose of this chapter is to alert you to the ways in which scientists in this field have been thinking about working memory and its implications for language, attention, and the mind. The discussion will be based on some important findings from various laboratories to illustrate our notions about working memory. It will come out in the discussion that there is a lot of debate in this field.

Plan for the chapter

We will start with just a touch of history to give us our bearings about where the field came from. Then the discussion turns to the various ways in which working memory could be involved in language processing. This leads to an explanation of a couple of theoretical models that could help in understanding how working memory may operate. Finally, the chapter will focus on a single key issue. It is the issue of whether there is one central working memory function that uses attention and cuts across domains (such as verbal and nonverbal processing) or whether there are specific working memory modules for different types of materials. Research on individual differences and age differences will be woven into the fabric of this discussion about the key issue of the nature of working memory. The field of working memory is rich and diverse, but the aims of the chapter are more focused in order to keep our eye on the ball, which is gaining a useful perspective on what working memory means and what it is worth scientifically.

The history of working memory research in a nutshell

There is a difference between the vast information storehouse of the mind, known as long-term memory, and working memory, the small portion of that memory held in the mind for a brief time. Miller kicked off the field in modern times with his famous article (1956) based on a long conference address he was cajoled into giving despite some reluctance as a young professor (see Miller, 1989). It helped establish this working memory concept and, in the process, helped launch the field

DOI: 10.4324/9781003204213-6

of cognitive psychology that went beyond behavior to draw inferences about how ideas seem to be represented in the mind. His article relayed his entertaining observation that he was being persecuted by a number, the seven or so items that one could barely manage to recall from a just-encountered list. What was most important in Miller's observations was that anything meaningful to the individual—such as a letter, a word, an acronym, or an idiom—could serve as a meaningful unit or chunk among the seven or so apparently held in working memory. (Later the observation would be made that the seven or so items one might recall were themselves grouped into three–five chunks, which more fundamentally defines the working memory limit; see Broadbent, 1975; Cowan, 2001.) Miller, Galanter, and Pribram (1960) coined the term working memory to refer to the use of this brief memory to keep track of one's current goals and subgoals while trying to accomplish them.

Soon afterward, Miller turned his attention to other aspects of language but Baddeley and Hitch picked up the ball where Miller left off (Baddeley & Hitch, 1974), using a rich set of studies on list memory and reasoning to demarcate different aspects of working memory. According to their theory, working memory was a system that included a central and meaningful holding faculty related to consciousness and attention, echoing earlier contemplations by the extraordinary philosopher and armchair psychologist James (1890). Working memory was also said to include some more automatic holding mechanisms supposedly specialized in speech sounds on the one hand, and visual and spatial patterns on the other hand. These faculties were all supposed to be coordinated in their functioning by mechanisms known to be dependent on the frontal lobes of the brain, termed central executive processes. Baddeley (1986) thought he could explain working memory data without the attention-related type of storage and dropped it, in contrast to others, including Cowan (1988), who resembled James (1890) in seeing that type storage and the focus of attention as a key basis of working memory. Baddeley (2000) later seemed to agree, adding an episodic buffer that was said to mediate similarly central, abstract types of storage. There are still vivid discussions about such theoretical topics as just what role attention plays in working memory and how general or specialized the working memory storage devices are in the brain. We will return to these questions after explaining how working memory may be involved in processing language.

Working memory in language processing

Types of information included in working memory for language

The theories of working memory were mostly developed to explain a rather focused body of knowledge in which certain variables were emphasized, such as the number of items in a list to be

Table 4.1 Possible types of verbal working memory and examples of the units for each type

STIMULUS: "I saw the best minds of my generation destroyed by madness…" (Ginsburg, Howl)

Possible Types of Verbal Working Memory	*Example of Units*
SENSORY	(speech sound frequency patterns as perceived)
PHONOLOGICAL	/… dəstrƆId baI madnəs…/
ARTICULATORY	(mouth movement plans to produce the phonemes)
LEXICAL	I, saw, the, best…
SEMANTIC	(self concept) (see + past) (def. article) (superlative)…
GRAMMATICAL	(subject – I) [verb phrase – (verb saw, object phrase the best minds of my generation)]…
CONSTRUCTED SCENE	(conception of intent and implications of the sentence)
PRIMING ACTIVATION	concepts related to I, saw, best, minds…
INTENDED SPEECH	plans for what one intends to say in response to stimulus

recalled, the semantic (meaning-based) or phonological (speech-sound-based) similarity between items in the list, or the presence or absence of a second task during the presentation of the list. Theoretically, though, we have to allow for the possibility that many levels of concepts in memory become active when a new stimulus is presented (or, for that matter, when one's mind wanders among the possibilities in long-term memory). Table 4.1 illustrates many of the levels of units that may become active in memory when one hears the sentence (from Ginsburg's poem *Howl*, 1956, "I saw the best minds of my generation destroyed by madness"). Any of these active units could become part of working memory. One might, for example, remember a bit about the tone of voice in which the sentence was spoken. As a second or so elapses after the stimulus sentence, some of the acoustic and phonological information may drift out of working memory but it may be replaced by an increasing awareness of the meaning of the sentence, which also will leave working memory and awareness as time progresses.

Mechanisms of information loss from working memory

There are several ways in which this temporary information could leave working memory, as shown in Table 4.2. The long history of considering these possibilities was reviewed by Cowan (2005). It is critical to realize that no matter how an item is lost from working memory, it presumably still might be retrieved from long-term memory if sufficient cues are presented, though there is no guarantee that the subject will remember that this particular unit from long-term memory was presented at a certain particular time or within a certain particular event.

In one possible mechanism of loss from working memory, called decay, information is simply lost as a function of time. This mechanism is analogous to radioactive decay, in which a particular element such as uranium has a known period of decay or half-life. This possibility is still a leading contender, for example, in the case of sensory memory, the memory of the way an event looked, sounded, felt, and so on. (Some researchers would not consider this part of working memory but it is according to the rather theory-neutral definition that I gave in the first sentence.) Decay also has been nominated as a mechanism for the forgetting of phonological and visuospatial information by Baddeley (1986). People could recall as much as they could recite in about two seconds (Baddeley, Thomson, & Buchanan, 1975) and that can be explained on the basis that covert verbal rehearsal refreshes the information before it decays from working memory beyond the point at which retrieval becomes impossible, which presumably would happen in about two seconds. This feature of working memory has, however, been hotly contested over the years. As just one example, Lewandowsky, Duncan, and Brown (2004) had subjects recall letters in a list quickly (after saying "super" between each two letters recalled) or slowly (after saying "super, super, super" between

Table 4.2 Possible mechanisms of loss of verbal working memory and descriptions of the mechanisms

Possible Mechanisms of Working Memory Loss	*Description of Mechanism*
DECAY	units are lost over time, in a matter of seconds
CAPACITY LIMITS	units are lost if there are more than a few to be retained at the same time
SPECIFIC INTERFERENCE	units are lost or contaminated if similar units occur afterward
ACID BATH	loss of units in which an interfering item has an effect that depends on the duration of its presentation
LOSS OF CONTEXT	as time elapses and conditions change, the retrieval cues present at encoding of the stimuli are no longer fully present

each two letters). No difference in recall was observed despite the difference in the time course of recall.

Another way in which information could leave working memory is that there could be a limit in how many units can be retained at once. If too many items are presented, the subject may have to make a decision about which ones to retain, or perhaps this decision sometimes occurs automatically in the brain. This notion of capacity limits, too, has been controversial. Although Miller (1956) documented that people could recall lists of about seven items, he also provided enough information to provoke doubt as to whether each item was recalled as a separate chunk or whether subjects group together items to form larger chunks on the fly (for example, grouping seven-digit telephone numbers into a group of three digits followed by a group of four digits, which might be memorized separately). In that case, the important limit may be how many separate chunks are retained, and it may be fewer than seven. In situations in which it is difficult to group items together or rehearse them (because, for example, the items were not attended at the time they were presented or rehearsal was suppressed), normal adults most typically can recall only three to five items, not seven (Cowan, 2001). Nevertheless, as the commentaries at the end of the Cowan reference indicate, not everyone is convinced that there is a constant chunk capacity limit to working memory or some central part of it. Some researchers are just not convinced that the process of chunking has been controlled well enough to tell what the limit in chunks is, or whether that limit is truly constant across situations.

A third way in which information can be lost from working memory is through interference. This means that items replace other items in working memory. In this case, though, the replacement comes not because there is a fixed limit on how many items can be in working memory at once—a capacity limit—but because newly presented items that have features similar to items already in working memory replace or contaminate the representation of those pre-stored items in working memory.

Fourth, there can be a combination of interference and decay, degradation by an interfering stimulus over time, called an acid bath (Posner & Konick, 1966). In this mechanism, there is interference that depends not only on the similarity of the item in memory and the interfering item, but also on the time during which an item is presented. In one good example of this type of forgetting, Massaro (1970) found that memory for the pitch of a tone was lost steadily over time during which another tone was presented; steadily but at a slower rate when a white noise was presented instead; and steadily at a very slow rate when there was no interfering sound.

It is very difficult to tell the difference between decay and an acid bath. Except possibly for sensory memory, it appears that people may prevent memory loss through rehearsal over time if there are no interfering stimuli. In order to prevent rehearsal, it is usually necessary to include stimuli to be recited. In that case, however, any memory loss over time can be attributed to an acid bath from the stimuli used to prevent rehearsal. Reitman (1971, 1974) tried to prevent rehearsal using a condition in which a subject listened carefully for a sound but, on particular trials, did not detect a sound. Some forgetting still seemed to occur. In our laboratory, Zwilling (2008) has replicated this type of experiment using a slightly different procedure, but did not find any forgetting. So it remains uncertain how it would be possible to detect decay.

One way that decay might be observed is by making the stimulus unattended at the time of its presentation. If an unattended stream of sounds is presented, one can present an occasional cue to switch attention to the sensory memory of that sound stream, which presumably will not have been rehearsed. Then it is possible to determine how the sensory memory is lost over time. Eriksen and Johnson (1964) and Cowan, Lichty, and Grove (1990) did this, and did find some loss of memory as a function of the time between the sound and the retrieval cue.

There is, however, one additional mechanism of forgetting that can be confused with decay, loss of context. It is possible that the retrieval of information from working memory depends on retrieval cues that change rather rapidly over time. If one receives a stimulus and later is asked to retrieve it, loss of ability over time may not indicate decay. Instead, it may indicate that the retrieval cues have changed too much as the context has changed. A well-known result that indicates as much is one by Bjork and Whitten (1974). Ordinarily, there is especially good memory for the items at the end of a list to be recalled in a free recall task, in which the items can be recalled in any order. Subjects tend to recall the items at the end of the list first, and then go back and recall other list items. This list-final advantage or recency effect is lost if there is an interfering task lasting several seconds between the list and recall. Traditionally, this loss of the recency effect was attributed to decay of memory for items at the end of the list, with earlier items having been memorized and therefore unaffected by the delay (Glanzer & Cunitz, 1966). Bjork and Whitten, however, considered that it may be the relative rather than the absolute recency of the items at the end of the list that made them easy to recall. They placed an interfering task lasting 12 seconds between each pair of items to be recalled. When items were separated like this, it was found that the recency effect was not lost even after an interfering task between the list and recall. Apparently, the recency effect occurred at least partly because the most recent item was temporally distinct relative to the rest of the list (like a telephone pole that one is standing near compared to other poles down the line, which start to blend together in the distance), not because of decay. However, this "long-term recency effect" of Bjork and Whitten was not as large as the regular recency effect so it remains possible that decay plays a role, too.

Competing models of working memory

It is possible to proceed to consider working memory functioning without worrying overly much about which mechanisms of loss are at play. We will now examine a few simple theoretical models that can help you to conceptualize working memory, and these models assume particular mechanisms of loss or forgetting. It is instructive to think about what is similar between these models and what is different.

Models of Baddeley

Baddeley (1986) presented a model that included three components: the phonological loop, the visuospatial sketchpad, and the central executive. The model was designed to account for the results of various studies, including those of Baddeley and Hitch (1974), but actually beginning earlier, in which verbal or pictorial material was presented for immediate recall. The results suggested that verbal material interfered with other verbal material and that the source of interference was primarily in the sound system of language (as opposed to meaning, for example). This sound-based interference occurred even if the material was visually presented. For example, people have a great deal of difficulty recalling the order of the letters in the list d, b, c, t, v, p, g even if they are visually presented because, mentally, a speech-based code is formed and the rhyming letters cause speech-sound-based confusion (Conrad, 1964). In contrast, there is relatively little interference with working memory of a spatial layout from printed or spoken letters, and little interference with working memory of the letters from a spatial layout. This type of evidence was used to justify the separation of phonological and visuospatial buffers, which presumably each hold information of a particular type for a short time. The information is held automatically but a voluntary-attention-based system, the central executive, is responsible for helping to determine when and how the buffers are used. Certain processes are out of the control of the central executive nevertheless, such as the automatic entry of spoken language into the phonological buffer. A large corpus of evidence contributed to this sort of model.

This model was modified (Baddeley, 2000, 2001) on the grounds that people remember semantic information in working memory and bindings between different sorts of information, such as the association between a shape and a name that was assigned to it. On such grounds, an episodic buffer

A

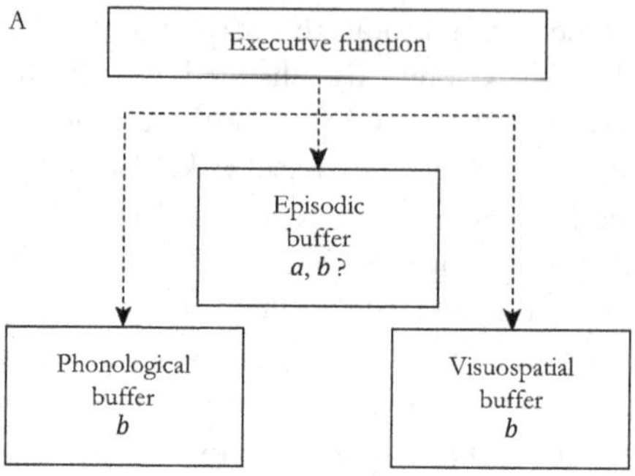

B

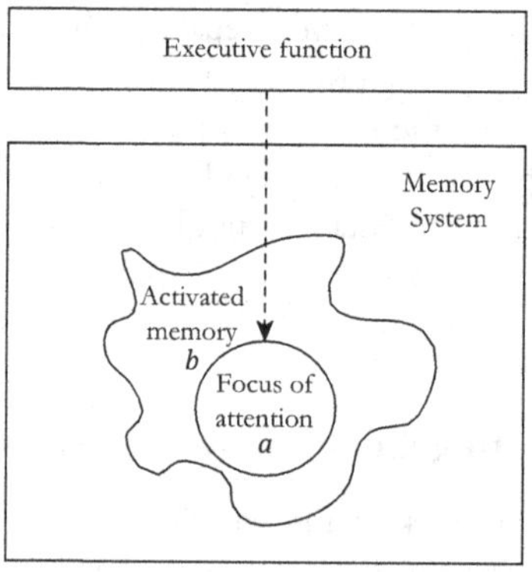

Figure 4.1 Two simple models of working memory. A. The model of Baddeley (2000). B. The model of Cowan (1988, 1999). In both models, a = stores assumed to be capacity-limited; b = stores assumed to be time-limited; a, b ? = store with limits open to debate.

was added to account for information that is neither purely phonological nor purely visuospatial in nature. The resulting model is depicted in Figure 4.1. In this model, it was said that the phono-logical and visuospatial buffers contain information that is subject to decay, which is depicted by the subscript b in the diagram. (As an aside, I think we could substitute an acid bath here without doing terrible damage to the gist of the model.) The mechanism of loss characteristics of the episodic buffer was left for future research and might include both a capacity limit (Baddeley, 2001), a, and possibly decay, b.

Both Baddeley (1986; Baddeley & Hitch, 1974) and Cowan (1988) built their models largely in reaction to the standard information processing models of the early era of the field of cognitive psychology. The most influential of these models were the seminal model of Broadbent (1958) and the elaboration of that sort of model by Atkinson and Shiffrin (1968). The reactions of Baddeley and Cowan were for somewhat different reasons. In these early models, a single sensory memory fed information into a short-term store, which in turn fed information into long-term storage. Processes like the central executive processes governed the transfer of information from one store to the next, at least in the Atkinson and Shiffrin model in which details of processing were explored mathematically. Baddeley and Hitch (1974) reacted to the inclusion of only a single short-term store, regardless of the type of information stored. They found evidence that different types of information seem to be stored separately.

Model of Cowan

Cowan (1988) was not so concerned with that point and was less inclined to like separate modules for the storage of phonological and visuospatial information. The differential interference results cannot be denied but they could be accounted for with the general principle that stimuli sharing features of various sorts are more likely to interfere with one another (cf. Nairne, 1990). Baddeley's postulation of phonological and visuospatial stores seemed to rule out the untested possibility that storage differs in other, perhaps equally important ways: say, in the sensory modality of input, or in the speech versus nonspeech quality of sounds. There was also evidence that semantic information was saved in working memory, even though it was not so important in retaining the serial order of items in a list. In response to these considerations, Cowan (1988, p. 171) suggested that instead of separate buffers, various stimuli activated elements of long-term memory, which served a short-term retention function:

> The spectral, temporal, and spatial properties of sensation would be present as coded features in memory that behave in a way comparable to non-sensory features such as meaning and object categories. At least, this is the simplest hypothesis until evidence to the contrary is obtained. One might hypothesize that premotor and prespeech plans … also consist of activated memory elements.

What Cowan (1988) was reacting to in the early information processing models was not so much the problem of a single storage mechanism, but the problem of the relation between memory and selective attention. In the early models, information from an all-encompassing but short-lived sensory memory was selectively forwarded for further processing and storage in short-term (or working) memory. This arrangement seemed to overlook the point that some features of memory were activated automatically by incoming stimuli. It also overlooked the point that not all information that was readily accessible had the same status. Some information was in the focus of attention and awareness, and this information could be readily integrated and deeply processed (as in the levels-of-processing conception of Craik & Lockhart, 1972). In contrast, other accessible information persisted for a short time in an unintegrated form. Examples might include the stream of sounds or phonemes from someone who just spoke when you were not paying attention, and a sentence to which you attended a few seconds ago but have now stopped attending.

The outcome of these concerns was a model like that developed by Cowan (1988), illustrated in Figure 4.2. Here it was suggested that there are two different working memory mechanisms that lose information in different ways. The temporarily activated elements of long-term memory lose activation through decay, denoted with subscript b (or, again, one could substitute an acid bath). In contrast, the subset of these activated elements that are in the focus of attention are resistant to decay but are limited to a handful of chunks at any one time, denoted with subscript a; about four chunks in normal adults, according to Cowan (2001).

In subsequent writing a further, important detail was discussed. Working memory should not be thought of as only the collection of activated features from long-term memory inasmuch as working memory must also include new links between features. One might have seen many blue objects and many different apples in one's life, but never a blue apple. If one is presented, this new binding between object identity and color must be retained in working memory as well as being stored in long-term memory. Cowan (1995, 1999, 2005) suggested that one function of the focus of attention is to store the bindings between features found in stimuli (or, for that matter, the results of creative thought), some of which may not already exist in long-term memory. It would retain, for example, information about what shape is in what location and what color goes with each shape in each location. At least, it would do so until a capacity limit is reached.

There is a new puzzle for this suggestion that the focus of attention retains binding information. When visual arrays are retained in working memory, retention of the binding between features (e.g., which shape goes with which color) does not differentially depend on attention. If you are distracted while retaining an array of objects, it will hurt your retention of the binding between features such as color and shape, or color and location, but it apparently will not do so more than

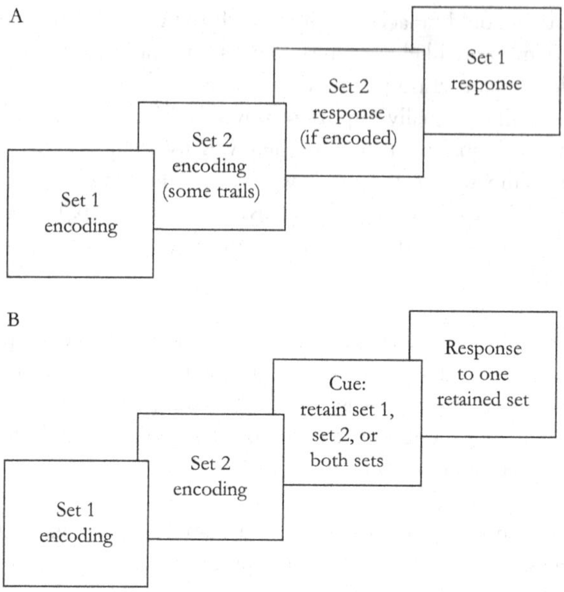

Figure 4.2 Two procedures to examine attention-sharing between tasks. A. Embedded-task procedure. B. Postcue procedure.

it hurts your retention of the features themselves (Allen, Baddeley, & Hitch, 2006; Cowan, Naveh-Benjamin, Kilb, & Saults, 2006). This puzzle can be explained, though, under the premise that attention perceives and retains objects. Attention is needed to put the features together to perceive and retain the object but retaining the bindings between features may be part of that process of retaining the object, at no extra charge to working memory capacity (see Luck & Vogel, 1997). This process of binding between features and its cost to attention has not been examined as carefully in the domain of language.

Mathematical models of working memory

It is important not to leave the impression that the Baddeley (1986, 2001) and Cowan (1988, 2001) models are the only ones that treat working memory, or even the models that predict the results in the most detail. These two models were proposed in a spirit of a general framework for further research, with many details left unsettled. In contrast, many others have devised models with a different aim. These other models have aimed to generate numerical predictions of performance in working memory tasks. To do so, they have had to rely on some assumptions that cannot be verified, so there is a tradeoff in strengths and weaknesses of the methods. Some such models have been constructed to explain results in a certain domain, such as the recall of verbal lists (e.g., Burgess & Hitch, 1999). Some rely on principles different from the ones stressed by Baddeley or Cowan, such as retrieval cues and context changes over time (e.g., Brown, Neath, & Chater, 2007) or effects of interference between items on capacity (e.g., Davelaar, Goshen-Gottstein, Ashkenazi, Haarman, & Usher, 2005). Some were designed to account for memory and information processing as a whole, including working memory processes (e.g., Anderson & Lebiere, 1998; Grossberg, 1978; Newell, 1990). Continuing to refine and test such mathematical models is an important avenue for further research, though it is outside the scope of the present chapter.

A key issue: The domain generality versus specificity of working memory

The models of Baddeley and Cowan seem to differ in a key prediction. (The difference may not hold when the episodic buffer is added to the model, as it may act in a way similar to the focus of attention.) The greater modularity of the Baddeley (1986) model means that there should be little interference between phonological and visuospatial information. In contrast, Cowan (1988) predicts that there can be interference between very different types of information provided that the information has to occupy the focus of attention. Which is it? Is working memory for language a separate faculty or set of faculties of the mind that can be used to comprehend and produce speech without taking into account other ongoing tasks that demand working memory such as, perhaps, keeping in mind what way you are driving? Or do all types of working memory tax a single, central resource such as attention? These are two very different conceptions of the mind.

In the remainder of the chapter, we will discuss the contributions of several types of methods to resolve this basic question. To anticipate, the answer appears to be that there is some working memory mechanism related to attention that cuts across stimulus encoding domains, in addition to some domain-specific mechanisms. The issue can be investigated either by manipulating memory loads and examining the average effect of this, which is an experimental approach; or by determining how much individual difference variance is shared by different types of working memory task, which is a psychometric approach. I will discuss these methods in the abstract and then discuss some research using each method, within the following sections of the chapter. In the final sections, the application of these concepts to working memory for language will be examined in more detail.

The potential contribution of experimental methods

Experimental methods operate by manipulating variables in groups of normal subjects and examining the effects on the means. If two tasks share the same working memory resource, then it should be possible to show that requiring retention in both tasks at once is harmful to the recall in at least one of the tasks. For example, it should be possible to ask whether memory for a word or digit list shares a resource along with memory for an array of visual objects. One way to examine this question is to embed one task within another one on some trials, as shown in Figure 4.2A. This figure illustrates what I will call an embedded task procedure. Suppose, for example, that Set 1 is an array of visual objects and Set 2 is a list of spoken words. On dual-task trials, Set 1 (a visual array) will be presented for perceptual encoding into working memory first, and then Set 2 (a word list) will be presented. After Set 2 is tested, Set 1 can be tested. For example, subjects might be asked to recognize one visual object and/or its location in the array, and then one word and/or its serial position in the list. During the entire task of encoding, retaining, and responding to Set 2, there is a visual memory load from retaining the items in Set 1. Also, during Set 1 retention, there is a memory load from doing all of the Set 2 activities. To measure these tasks, one can compare performance in those dual-task trials with performance in other, single-task trials that include only Set 1 or only Set 2.

If one cannot find interference between two tasks in an embedded task procedure, it seems likely that there is no common working memory resource between the tasks. However, if interference is found, the embedded task procedure is not able to indicate with certainty that it is working memory retention in the two tasks that conflict with one another. An alternative source of interference is that Set 1 retention could be hurt by Set 2 encoding or responding. Conversely, the effect of Set 1 on Set 2 performance could occur because retention of the Set 1 materials interferes with Set 2 encoding or responding.

One way to deal with this problem was developed by Cowan and Morey (2007), who used what we can call a postcue procedure, illustrated in Figure 4.2B. Both sets are presented for encoding. Then there is a cue to retain only the first set, only the second set, or both sets. The test is always on an item from one of the sets that the subject was supposed to retain according to the cue. Encoding of the sets is identical in all trial types because the subject does not know in advance what type of cue will be presented. If retention of either set is hurt by the cue to retain both sets at once, that dual-task interference can only be attributed to interference in working memory maintenance.

There are limitations of the postcue procedure as well. Set 2 encoding might be confined by the fact that Set 1 was already encoded. Therefore, the postcue procedure does not necessarily pick up the entire conflict between maintenance in the two sets. If the two sets are encoded into distinctly different modules with no resource overlap, however, encoding of Set 2 should not be impeded by maintenance of Set 1. At any rate, if an effect of a dual-set postcue is in fact obtained, that effect cannot be attributed to effects taking place at encoding. We will return to these methods with results after explaining a very different, psychometric method of looking at the issue of a common resource between different types of working memory tasks.

The potential contribution of psychometric methods and individual variation

The psychometric method involves careful testing of individual differences in performance, making use of the pattern of correlations (and regressions) between tasks. Fundamentally, if performance on verbal and spatial working memory tasks correlate highly, it is possible that they stem from a common working memory mechanism. If they do not correlate at all, it is highly improbable that they stem from a common mechanism. This logic can also be taken to another level. Many have suggested that working memory is critical for intelligence (e.g., Engle, Tuholski, Laughlin, & Conway, 1999). If two different measures of working memory account for a common pool of variance in intelligence tests, they may be measuring the same working memory mechanism.

I have stated these conclusions about mechanisms based on correlations in a guarded way because one must be careful about the inferences that are drawn. To see this, it helps to go into a little detail about hypothetical research scenarios. Imagine a situation in which there are four task types: verbal memory, verbal perception, nonverbal memory, and nonverbal perception. Imagine further that the perception tasks require the same skills as the memory tasks, except for holding the information in working memory. For example, a verbal memory task could be to hear a series of seven digits and recall the digits from memory; the equivalent perception task could be to hear a series of seven digits and write them down while listening. Suppose there is a common memory faculty, CM, shared between the two memory tasks; a separate verbal memory faculty, VM; a common perceptual faculty shared between the two verbal tasks, VP; a separate nonverbal memory faculty, NM; and a common perceptual faculty shared between the two nonverbal tasks, NP. (For the sake of the argument let us present the items quickly so that perception is not trivial.) Then according to a linear model, each individual i would have performance levels on the four tasks as follows:

Verbal memory, $= CM^i + VM^i + VPi + error^1$ (4.1)
Verbal perception, $= VP^i + error^2$ (4.2)
Nonverbal memory, $= CM^i + NM^i + NP^i + error^3$ (4.3)
Nonverbal perception, $= NP^i + error^4$ (4.4)

In these formulas, error in each case refers to measurement error. If there is a correlation between the types of memory task, it could be either because they both include CMi or because some other terms are correlated. Assuming that the errors are uncorrelated, it could still be that there is a correlation between VMi and NMi even though they are different mechanisms. By analogy, the hands and feet are very different body parts but there is a correlation between the size of one's hands and of one's feet.

It could also be that there is a correlation between VPi and NPi. If we find, however, that verbal and nonverbal perception tasks are uncorrelated, we can be assured that the correlation between memory tasks does not occur for perceptual reasons.

The central question under examination is whether CMi is too large to be neglected, which would indicate that there is a common memory resource across types of task. Even if the memory tasks are correlated it is hard to be sure of that because there is no independent estimate of VMi and NMi and they could correlate with one another. In terms of classifying people, this issue may not be important. By analogy, one might want to classify people into those with large hands and feet, versus those with small hands and feet. Still, one would not want to claim that hands and feet are the same things.

A combination of experimental and correlational findings is most powerful. One can find out whether there is a common working memory mechanism according to a dual-task experimental design, and also whether a common mechanism is possible according to a correlational design. Let us now put these methods to use.

Within-domain and general, cross-domain mechanisms of working memory

Within-domain mechanisms

Baddeley (1986) very clearly described a large body of evidence suggesting that the coding of word lists relies heavily on a specialized, phonological storage mechanism. Semantic similarities between items in a list (e.g., rat, mouse, squirrel, etc.) are of very little consequence when the items must be recalled in order, which is serially, whereas phonological similarities (e.g., rat, mat, hat, etc.) are of great consequence, resulting in poor serial recall. Other phonological factors also play a special role in the serial recall of lists, including the length of words and the presence of irrelevant speech. A person is able to recall about as many items of a certain type as he or she can repeat in about two seconds. These findings were said to point toward a phonological storage mechanism from which information can decay, unless the phonological information is refreshed by the use of covert verbal rehearsal before the two-second period is over.

According to Cowan (1999, 2005), the phonological store is only one type of activated information from long-term memory, which may include newly formed links between items such as the serial order of items in the list. These newly formed links become newly added information in long-term memory. Both theorists agree that covert verbal rehearsal is a very powerful and efficient way to retain phonological information, as one finds in verbal lists.

Unlike Baddeley (1986), Cowan (1988, 1995) emphasized that there are other sorts of activated information contributing to working memory performance as well. This point is underscored, for example, by the work on memory for quickly presented sentences described by Potter and Lombardi (1990). This work indicates that semantic information is constructed and used in working memory tasks. On each trial in the experiments described, a sentence was followed by a list of words presented very rapidly and then a probe, which was to be judged present or absent from the list. One of the unprobed words in the list was a lure item that was semantically related to a word in the sentence. Recall of the sentence turned out to be tainted by intrusion of the lure item on a large number of trials (compared to a small number of substitutions when there was no lure word in the list). For example, the sentence, The knight rode around the palace searching for a place to enter could be mis-remembered with the word castle replacing palace, a type of substitution that was much more likely when castle was among the list items in the probe task (even though this semantically related item was never used as the probe item). These results support the inference that a semantic representation of the sentence was held in working memory, in a vulnerable form. Providing related evidence, Romani and Martin (1999) found neurological patients with a specific deficit in working memory for semantic and lexical information. Potter (1993) summarized additional evidence that people ordinarily construct semantic representations in short-term (or working) memory.

It is not yet clear whether this sort of evidence can be accounted for best by the revised model of Baddeley (2000, 2001) or Cowan (1988, 1999). Baddeley's episodic buffer can hold semantic or lexical information but, in the 2001 paper, it was said to be subject to a capacity limit. In contrast, Cowan envisions semantic information as possibly present in the activated region of long-term memory with no capacity limit, just a time limit. (The focus of attention may be needed to make the semantic information active but that activated information was supposed to stay active for some time after it leaves the focus of attention.) Until we know how much semantic information can be active outside of the focus of attention, we cannot tell the model that works better in this regard.

General, cross-domain mechanisms

Some recent research seems to suggest that there is a common working memory mechanism across modalities or domains that might be based on the focus of attention as proposed, for example, by Cowan (1988, 1999, 2001, 2005). Much of it has relied on the embedded task procedure as described in Figure 4.2. Cocchini, Logie, Della Sala, MacPherson, and Baddeley (2002) carried out such a procedure using either verbal or spatial tasks as the first and second tasks and reported little interference between tasks. Morey and Cowan (2004, 2005) found somewhat different results in a study based on the visual array comparison procedure of Luck and Vogel (1997). In this procedure, an array of differently colored squares at haphazard locations is presented. In the version we used, a second array is presented but one item in the array is circled. Either the second array is identical to the first (except for the presence of the circle cue in the second array) or else the circled item has changed color. The task is to indicate whether that color has changed. This task becomes increasingly difficult when more than four items are in the array. Morey and Cowan sometimes required that a random list of six or seven spoken digits be retained in memory during the same period when the first array also had to be retained. The visual and verbal memory tasks interfered with one another substantially, provided that the digit list was recited aloud during this retention period. It was not simply verbal coding that interfered with the visual array memory, inasmuch as a simple recitation of the subject's known seven-digit telephone number had little effect on that memory. Stevanovski and Jolicoeur (2007) carried out a study with the visual array comparison task in which a tone identification task was presented between the arrays, and they included repetition of a single word ("banana") to prevent rehearsal. The finding was that the tone identification task impaired memory of the visual array; more so when the identification task included four tones rather than two and therefore was more difficult. These results suggest that there is a common capacity shared between verbal and visual materials.

Saults and Cowan (2007) took this conclusion further by suggesting that with sensory memory out of the way, all of the remaining capacity seemed to be central rather than modular in nature. Along with visual arrays they presented an array of spoken digits from four loudspeakers arranged around the subject. Each of the four digits was in a different voice (male or female adult or child). There was only one test, either a repetition of the visual array that might contain a change in one color or a repetition of the spoken array that might contain a change in one digit. In the best experiment, the auditory test involved digits that had been rearranged, so that the only potential cue that the subject could use was the link between the voice and the digit produced in that voice. Therefore, it did not allow the use of spatial information as in the visual stimuli. In other trial blocks, the subject knew they should attend only to the visual arrays or only to the spoken digits.

Saults and Cowan (2007) found that the results depended on whether there was a mask, a combination of complex squares and combined speech sounds to eliminate the sensory afterimage of the stimuli to be remembered. The mask was placed long enough after the arrays to allow good encoding of the abstract information. When there was no such mask, the two sets of stimuli interfered with one another but, still, subjects could remember more items when two modalities were to be remembered than when only one modality was to be remembered. However, when there was a mask, the amount that could be remembered if only visual items had to be remembered (about three-and-a-half visual items) was almost exactly the same as the amount that could be remembered if both modalities had to be remembered (about three-and-a-half items in all, some visual and some auditory). This suggests that any separate visual or verbal storage mechanism (possibly sensory in nature) can be masked out and that what remains when it is masked out is a substantial, remaining component that applies across modalities and holds three to four items in an abstract manner.

One nagging problem with these embedded task studies is that it is difficult to tell whether the conflict between tasks occurs in the process of retaining items from both modalities in working memory, or from the conflict between retention in one modality and encoding, or responding in the other modality. Cowan and Morey (2007) addressed this question using a postcue procedure as illustrated in Figure 4.2. On some trials, a visual array and a spoken list of digits or letters were presented, in either order. On other trials, two different visual arrays were presented (one with colored circles and one with colored squares) and, on still other trials, two different spoken lists were presented (one with digits and one with letters). After the presentation, there was a cue to keep remembering only the first set (array or list), only the second set (array or list), or both sets. The test was on one array item or one list item. In both cases, the item was shown in the correct location or in the wrong location; it was the correct or wrong spatial location for the visual item, or the correct or wrong serial position in the list for the spoken item. Overall, the cost of retaining a second visual set along with the visual set that was then tested (0.61 items) was about the same as the cost of retaining a verbal set along with the visual set that was then tested (0.58 items). Visual memory storage seems to occur in a form abstract enough that it can be interrupted equally by another set of visual items or a set of verbal items. For tests of verbal items, the cost of retaining a second verbal set along with the verbal set that was then tested was 0.65 items, versus 0.36 items for retention of a visual set along with the verbal set that was then tested. Although this difference did not reach significance, perhaps verbal working memory storage does include a modality-specific component, as we will discuss in a following section. Overall, though, these results tend to reinforce the notion from embedded task studies that there is a central, attention-demanding component of working memory retention.

Confirmation of this notion of a central, attention-demanding component of working memory retention comes also from a psychometric type of study conducted by Kane et al. (2004). They administered a variety of working memory tasks in which processing and storage were combined, including some verbally based and some spatially based tasks. It also included some simple span tasks that required storage and repetition of multiple items (e.g., a list of words or a series of spatial locations) but no separate processing component. The method of evaluation was structural equation modeling, a type of confirmatory factor analysis that produces a model of the various sources of variance that could contribute to the results. The best-fitting model did not need separate verbal and spatial working memory tasks of the complex, storage-and-processing sort. A single component fit the data across modalities and correlated well with both verbal and nonverbal intelligence measures. In contrast, the simple span tasks divided into more separate components for verbal versus spatial storage, with verbal span tasks accounting for some variance in intelligence tests using verbal materials and spatial span tasks accounting for some variance in intelligence tests using spatial materials.

The general factor for working memory tasks that include both storage and processing could reflect the contribution of an attention-demanding aspect of working memory storage, such as the focus of attention of Cowan (1999) or the episodic buffer of Baddeley (2000). Attention can be used to save information and to process it, and the attention-based mechanism deals with information in the abstract rather than tying it closely to the modality or code in which the information arrived. In contrast, the separation between simple verbal versus spatial span tasks could reflect skill in dealing with verbal versus spatial information. Although there is some correlation between an individual's ability to handle information in one modality and another, these specific skills are probably automatic and the profile of skills across modalities and codes can differ from one individual to the next; some people may be more interested in, experienced with, and/or naturally capable with verbal materials, and others with spatial materials.

Working memory structure and the levels of language

What we have discussed to this point could be consistent with either of the models shown in Table 4.1. Many or all of the levels of language shown in Table 4.1 are activated by the incoming speech or printed stimuli. If one has to remember a string of phonological information, an advantage is that the human mind is well-suited to rehearse the material. According to the model of Baddeley (2000), other forms of language information must be held in the episodic buffer and therefore would be limited to a few items (Baddeley, 2001).

According to the model of Cowan (1999, 2005), there is a slightly different analysis. Activated elements of long-term memory could include all sorts of language codes; but the focus of attention would be able to provide more integrated, analyzed information of up to a few items. As mentioned above, we do not yet know what model is correct. They differ in the mechanisms whereby nonphono-logical language information can be held in working memory.

Another hypothesis, beyond both of these theories, is that there is a specialized module that holds one type of grammatical information, namely the way in which words are combined to form sentences, or syntax (Caplan, Waters, & DeDe, 2007). That type of theory is in line with the theoretical work of Noam Chomsky, in which he suggests that the language acquisition device in children includes some innate syntactical information that can cut down on the possible grammars that have to be considered (Piattelli-Palmarini, 1980). Caplan et al. summarized a great deal of research looking at whether memory for syntax is affected by a memory load. That research included both dual task and psycho-metric factors. The conclusion was that syntactical working memory is separate, in that people with poor working memory are not impaired in syntactic analysis compared to people with good working memory, and that syntactic memory load and other types of memory load result in different patterns of activation in brain imaging studies.

A study by Fedorenko, Gibson, and Rohde (2007) may warrant a revision in all of these approaches. They compared easier, subject-extracted sentences (e.g., The janitor who frustrated the plumber lost the key on the street) to more difficult, object-extracted sentences (e.g., The janitor who the plumber frustrated lost the key on the street). The greater difficulty of the latter sentence type was attributed to the need to retrieve the subject of the sentence (janitor) as the object of the verb within the dependent clause (frustrated). Reading a sentence was combined with a math problem. For example, the subject might see the words The janitor with 12 above it, who frustrated the plumber with + 4 above it, and lost the key with + 5 above it, and on the street with + 4 above it. The math problem was either relatively easy or relatively hard; the one shown here is easy, involving small numbers. Subjects reported the sum and then answered questions about the sentence.

The most important dependent variable in the study of Fedorenko et al. (2007) was the speed with which subjects advanced through the parts of the problem. These reaction times were slower for object- than for subject-extracted sentences, mainly in the part of the sentence in which the interpretation of the relative clause was involved (who frustrated the plumber versus who the plumber frustrated). Moreover, this sentence type effect interacted with the difficulty of the math problem in that the added effect of difficult problems was larger for object-extracted sentences than for subject-extracted sentences. The result was replicated in two experiments.

So far, this result could be explained in at least two different ways. It could be that verbal information processing for the harder math problems interfered with difficult syntactic processing, or it could be that the drain on attention from the harder math problems interfered with difficult syntactic processing. A second pair of experiments, however, distinguished between these hypotheses by using spatial tasks instead of math. For example, one of them involved adding pie chart sections together visually. This visual task affected reaction times related to syntactic processing but there was no interaction between the difficulty of syntactic processing and the difficulty of the secondary task problem. The secondary task difficulty effect was the same for subject- and object-extracted sentences.

From these data, it seems possible to conclude that one part of the difficulty of working memory for syntax is specific to verbal materials. This is the part that causes the syntactic difficulty by math difficulty interaction. Additionally, the main effect of secondary task difficulty even with a spatial secondary task suggests that syntactic processing may require attention, to a comparable extent for each sentence type. Perhaps attention is needed in this procedure to discriminate whether the sentence is a subject- or object-extracted one, whereas subject-extracted sentence processing in ordinary life might not require as much attention as it does in this experimental setting with mixed sentence types.

The results of Fedorenko et al. (2007) seem to confirm that there is a specific verbal working memory component that depends on verbal processing. In contrast to the theoretical assertion of Caplan et al. (2007), though, it is not syntax-specific. It may well be a covert articulation component that is involved in both syntax processing and math. The finding, discussed by Caplan et al., that individual differences in working memory capacity tend not to affect syntactic processing may have a simple explanation. This may be found because most normal adults can use covert articulatory processes sufficiently well to process syntax. In fact, span tasks that allow articulation do not correlate very well with intelligence in adults (Cowan et al., 2005). One could predict, though, that individuals with impairment in articulatory processes may well display impaired syntax, as well as some impairment on working memory. Clearly, this question of whether there is a separate working memory for syntax is heating up and there is no agreement on it yet.

Tradeoff between storage and processing of language

Last, it is important to acknowledge that the amount that can be retrieved in a working memory task depends on what other storage and processing is taking place (e.g., Bunting, Cowan, & Colflesh, 2008). Within an attention-based model, attention devoted to processing is used at the expense of some storage. A number of authors have suggested that the individuals who can store the most information and do the best processing are those who can inhibit the processing or storage of irrelevant information so that working memory can be devoted to the relevant information (e.g., Gernsbacher, 1993; Hasher, Stolzfus, Zacks, & Rypma, 1991; Kane, Bleckley, Conway, & Engle, 2001). On the other hand, at least one study suggests that the ability to control attention and the capacity of working memory are partly independent of one another among adults (Cowan, Fristoe, Elliott, Brunner, & Saults, 2006).

Conclusion

Working memory is a surprisingly encompassing concept that is involved in most information processing, including most language comprehension and production. This makes it important but also difficult to analyze. I have suggested that working memory for language depends on an ensemble of attention-dependent and automatic activation processes. The exact best model is not yet known but I have indicated several types of evidence that would help to clarify it. The goal was to sketch a model or set of models (see Figure 4.1) simple enough to be helpful in thinking about language processing, yet accurate enough to make useful predictions.

Further reading

Cowan, N., Morey, C. C., & Naveh-Benjamin, M. (2021). An embedded-processes approach to working memory: How is it distinct from other approaches, and to what ends? In R. H. Logie, V. Camos, & N. Cowan (Eds.), *Working memory: State of the science*. Oxford: Oxford University Press.

Gray, S., Lancaster, H., Alt, M., Hogan, T., Green, S., Levy, R., & Cowan, N. (2020). The structure of word learning in young school-age children. *Journal of Speech, Language, and Hearing Research, 63*(5), 1446–1466.

Greene, N. R., Naveh-Benjamin, M., & Cowan, N. (2020). Adult age differences in working memory capacity: Spared central storage but deficits in ability to maximize peripheral storage. *Psychology and Aging, 35*(6), 866–880.

Guitard, D., & Cowan, N. (2020). Do we use visual codes when information is not presented visually? *Memory and Cognition, 48*(8), 1522–1153. https://doi.org/10.3758/s13421-020-01054-0

Jiang, Q., & Cowan, N. (2020). Incidental learning of list membership is affected by serial position in the list. *Memory, 28*(5), 669–676.

References

Allen, R. J., Baddeley, A. D., & Hitch, G. J. (2006). Is the binding of visual features in working memory resource-demanding? *Journal of Experimental Psychology: General, 135*(2), 298–313.

Anderson, J. R., & Lebiere, C. (1998). *Atomic components of thought*. Hillsdale, NJ: Erlbaum.

Atkinson, R. C., & Shiffrin, R. M. (1968). Human memory: A proposed system and its control processes. In K. W. Spence & J. T. Spence (Eds.), *The psychology of learning and motivation: Advances in research and theory* (Vol. 2, pp. 89–195). New York: Academic Press.

Baddeley, A. (2000). The episodic buffer: A new component of working memory? *Trends in Cognitive Sciences, 4*(11), 417–423.

Baddeley, A. (2001). The magic number and the episodic buffer. *Behavioral and Brain Sciences, 24*(1), 117–118.

Baddeley, A. D. (1986). *Working memory*. Oxford: Clarendon Press.

Baddeley, A. D., & Hitch, G. (1974). Working memory. In G. H. Bower (Ed.), *The psychology of learning and motivation* (Vol. 8, pp. 47–89). New York: Academic Press.

Baddeley, A. D., Thomson, N., & Buchanan, M. (1975). Word length and the structure of short-term memory. *Journal of Verbal Learning and Verbal Behavior, 14*(6), 575–589.

Bjork, R. A., & Whitten, W. B. (1974). Recency-sensitive retrieval processes in long-term free recall. *Cognitive Psychology, 6*(2), 173–189.

Broadbent, D. E. (1958). *Perception and communication*. New York: Pergamon Press.

Broadbent, D. E. (1975). The magic number seven after fifteen years. In A. Kennedy & A. Wilkes (Eds.), *Studies in long-term memory* (pp. 3–18). Oxford: John Wiley & Sons.

Brown, G. D. A., Neath, I., & Chater, N. (2007). A temporal ratio model of memory. *Psychological Review, 114*(3), 539–576.

Bunting, M. F., Cowan, N., & Colflesh, G. H. (2008). The deployment of attention in short-term memory tasks: Tradeoffs between immediate and delayed deployment. *Memory and Cognition, 36*(4), 799–812.

Burgess, N., & Hitch, G. J. (1999). Memory for serial order: A network model of the phonological loop and its timing. *Psychological Review, 106*(3), 551–581.

Caplan, D., Waters, G., & Dede, G. (2007). Specialized verbal working memory for language comprehension. In A. R. A. Conway, C. Jarrold, M. J. Kane, A. Miyake, & J. N. Towse (Eds.), *Variation in working memory* (pp. 272–302). New York: Oxford University Press.

Cocchini, G., Logie, R. H., Della Sala, S., MacPherson, S. E., & Baddeley, A. D. (2002). Concurrent performance of two memory tasks: Evidence for domain-specific working memory systems. *Memory and Cognition, 30*(7), 1086–1095.

Conrad, R. (1964). Acoustic confusion in immediate memory. *British Journal of Psychology, 55*(1), 75–84.

Cowan, N. (1988). Evolving conceptions of memory storage, selective attention, and their mutual constraints within the human information processing system. *Psychological Bulletin, 104*(2), 163–191.

Cowan, N. (1995). Attention and memory: An integrated framework. In *Oxford psychology series, no. 26*. New York: Oxford University Press. (Paperback edition: 1997).

Cowan, N. (1999). An embedded-processes model of working memory. In A. Miyake & P. Shah (Eds.), *Models of working memory: Mechanisms of active maintenance and executive control* (pp. 62–101). Cambridge: Cambridge University Press.

Cowan, N. (2001). The magical number 4 in short-term memory: A reconsideration of mental storage capacity. *Behavioral and Brain Sciences, 24*(1), 87–185.

Cowan, N. (2005). *Working memory capacity*. Hove, East Sussex: Psychology Press.

Cowan, N., Elliott, E. M., Saults, J. S., Morey, C. C., Mattox, S., Hismjatullina, A., & Conway, A. R. A. (2005). On the capacity of attention: Its estimation and its role in working memory and cognitive aptitudes. *Cognitive Psychology, 51*(1), 42–100.

Cowan, N., Fristoe, N. M., Elliott, E. M., Brunner, R. P., & Saults, J. S. (2006). Scope of attention, control of attention, and intelligence in children and adults. *Memory and Cognition, 34*(8), 1754–1768.

Cowan, N., Lichty, W., & Grove, T. R. (1990). Properties of memory for unattended spoken syllables. *Journal of Experimental Psychology: Learning, Memory, and Cognition, 16*(2), 258–269.

Cowan, N., & Morey, C. C. (2007). How can dual-task working memory retention limits be investigated? *Psychological Science, 18*(8), 686–688.

Cowan, N., Naveh-Benjamin, M., Kilb, A., & Saults, J. S. (2006). Life-span development of visual working memory: When is feature binding difficult? *Developmental Psychology, 42*(6), 1089–1102.

Craik, F. I. M., & Lockhart, R. S. (1972). Levels of processing: A framework for memory research. *Journal of Verbal Learning and Verbal Behavior, 11*(6), 671–684.

Davelaar, E. J., Goshen-Gottstein, Y., Ashkenazi, A., Haarman, H. J., & Usher, M. (2005). The demise of short-term memory revisited: Empirical and computational investigations of recency effects. *Psychological Review, 112*(1), 3–42.

Engle, R. W., Tuholski, S. W., Laughlin, J. E., & Conway, A. R. A. (1999). Working memory, short-term memory, and general fluid intelligence: A latent-variable approach. *Journal of Experimental Psychology: General, 128*(3), 309–331.

Eriksen, C. W., & Johnson, H. J. (1964). Storage and decay characteristics of nonattended auditory stimuli. *Journal of Experimental Psychology, 68*, 28–36.

Fedorenko, E., Gibson, E., & Rohde, D. (2007). The nature of working memory in linguistic, arithmetic and spatial integration processes. *Journal of Memory and Language, 56*(2), 246–269.

Gernsbacher, M. A. (1993). Less skilled readers have less efficient suppression mechanisms. *Psychological Science, 4*(5), 294–298.

Glanzer, M., & Cunitz, A. R. (1966). Two storage mechanisms in free recall. *Journal of Verbal Learning and Verbal Behavior, 5*(4), 351–360.

Grossberg, S. (1978). A theory of human memory: Self-organization and performance of sensory-motor codes, maps, and plans. In R. Rosen & F. Snell (Eds.), *Progress in theoretical biology* (Vol. 5, pp. 500–639). New York: Academic Press.

Hasher, L., Stolzfus, E. R., Zacks, R. T., & Rypma, B. (1991). Age and inhibition. *Journal of Experimental Psychology: Learning, Memory, and Cognition, 17*(1), 163–169.

James, W. (1890). *The principles of psychology*. New York: Henry Holt.

Kane, M. J., Bleckley, M. K., Conway, A. R. A., & Engle, R. W. (2001). A controlled-attention view of working-memory capacity. *Journal of Experimental Psychology: General, 130*(2), 169–183.

Kane, M. J., Hambrick, D. Z., Tuholski, S. W., Wilhelm, O., Payne, T. W., & Engle, R. E. (2004). The generality of working-memory capacity: A latent-variable approach to verbal and visuo-spatial memory span and reasoning. *Journal of Experimental Psychology: General, 133*(2), 189–217.

Lewandowsky, S., Duncan, M., & Brown, G. D. A. (2004). Time does not cause forgetting in short-term serial recall. *Psychonomic Bulletin and Review, 11*(5), 771–790.

Luck, S. J., & Vogel, E. K. (1997). The capacity of visual working memory for features and conjunctions. *Nature, 390*(6657), 279–281.

Massaro, D. W. (1970). Retroactive interference in short-term recognition memory for pitch. *Journal of Experimental Psychology, 83*(1), 32–39.

Miller, G. A. (1956). The magical number seven, plus or minus two: Some limits on our capacity for processing information. *Psychological Review, 63*(2), 81–97.

Miller, G. A. (1989). George A. Miller. In L. Gardner (Ed.), *A history of psychology in autobiography* (Vol. VIII, pp. 391–418). Stanford, CA: Stanford University Press.

Miller, G. A., Galanter, E., & Pribram, K. H. (1960). *Plans and the structure of behavior*. New York: Holt, Rinehart and Winston, Inc.

Morey, C. C., & Cowan, N. (2004). When visual and verbal memories compete: Evidence of cross-domain limits in working memory. *Psychonomic Bulletin and Review, 11*(2), 296–301.

Morey, C. C., & Cowan, N. (2005). When do visual and verbal memories conflict? The importance of working-memory load and retrieval. *Journal of Experimental Psychology: Learning, Memory, and Cognition, 31*(4), 703–713.

Nairne, J. S. (1990). A feature model of immediate memory. *Memory and Cognition, 18*(3), 251–269.

Newell, A. (1990). *Unified theories of cognition*. Cambridge, MA: Harvard University Press.

Piattelli-Palmarini, M. (1980). *Language and learning: The debate between Jean Piaget and Noam Chomsky*. London: Routledge and Kegan Paul.

Posner, M. I., & Konick, A. F. (1966). On the role of interference in short-term retention. *Journal of Experimental Psychology, 72*(2), 221–231.

Potter, M. C. (1993). Very short-term conceptual memory. *Memory and Cognition, 21*(2), 156–161.
Potter, M. C., & Lombardi, L. (1990). Regeneration in the short-term recall of sentences. *Journal of Memory and Language, 29*(6), 633–654.
Reitman, J. S. (1971). Mechanisms of forgetting in short term memory. *Cognitive Psychology, 2*(2), 185–195.
Reitman, J. S. (1974). Without surreptitious rehearsal, information in short-term memory decays. *Journal of Verbal Learning and Verbal Behavior, 13*(4), 365–377.
Romani, C., & Martin, R. (1999). A deficit in the short-term retention of lexical-semantic information: Forgetting words but remembering a story. *Journal of Experimental Psychology: General, 128*(1), 56–77.
Saults, J. S., & Cowan, N. (2007). A central capacity limit to the simultaneous storage of visual and auditory arrays in working memory. *Journal of Experimental Psychology: General, 136*(4), 663–684.
Stevanovski, B., & Jolicoeur, P. (2007). Visual short-term memory: Central capacity limitations in short-term consolidation. *Visual Cognition, 15*(5), 532–563.
Zwilling, C. E. (2008). *Forgetting in short-term memory: The effect of time.* [Unpublished master's thesis], University of Missouri, Columbia, MO.

5

NEUROBIOLOGICAL BASES OF THE SEMANTIC PROCESSING OF WORDS

Karima Kahlaoui, Bernadette Ska, Clotilde Degroot, and Yves Joanette

Introduction

Language is defined as a brain-based system allowing for interpersonal communication using sounds, symbols, and words to express a meaning, idea, or abstract thought. Human beings' ability to understand and produce language involves a considerable amount of brain resources. For over a century, our understanding of brain mechanisms for language came mainly from lesion studies; essentially, lesion studies pointed to the existence of some association between a damaged brain region and a given set of language deficits (e.g., Broca, 1865; Wernicke, 1874). In recent decades, imaging methods—which permit one to measure various indirect indices of ongoing neural activities arising from the brain "in action"—have revolutionized cognitive neuropsychology and neurolinguistics, providing a new way of mapping language abilities and, in particular, much better evidence about both the anatomical and temporal aspects of brain processes. Currently, a fundamental question in cognitive neuroscience concerns where and how the normal brain constructs meaning, and how this process takes place in real time (Kutas & Federmeier, 2000). Imaging methods have been highly successful in investigating semantic information processing, revealing cortical area networks that are certainly plausible, given our previous knowledge of cerebral anatomy and lesion studies. Several imaging methods allow one to explore different aspects of the brain: spatial distribution (using hemodynamic methods), temporal deployment (using electrophysiological methods), or both (using emerging imaging methods). This chapter focuses on the convergent contribution of different imaging methods to our understanding of the neural bases of the semantic processing of words. First, an overview of imaging methods will be presented. Then, the converging results concerning the neurobiological bases of semantic processes will be reported for each method mentioned above. Since the number of publications on language processing and, more specifically, on the neurobiological bases of the semantic processing of words exceeds what can be reviewed here, this chapter focuses on the most representative papers in each area.

An overview of imaging methods

Notwithstanding the existence of specific imaging approaches using Positron Emission Tomography (PET) along with specific neurochemical markers, the noninvasive methods currently available for human brain research are most frequently divided into two general approaches: hemodynamic and electrophysiological.

DOI: 10.4324/9781003204213-7

The most important of the methods based on hemodynamic principles are PET and functional magnetic resonance imaging (fMRI). Although both PET and fMRI present an approximation of neural activation by detecting the locally specific changes in blood composition and flow that accompany brain activity, there are some subtle differences between them. PET detects blood flow changes relatively directly using labeled oxygen as a marker, while fMRI, which is based on the principle of blood oxygenation level dependent (BOLD) measures blood flow via changes in the magnetization properties linked with the relative concentration of deoxyhemoglobin (HHb) on the venous side of the capillary bed. Overall, these methods have a very good spatial resolution and, in the case of fMRI, have the advantage of being able to provide a functional map that can be plotted on the anatomical image collected during the same session. The main limitation of these methods is their poor temporal resolution (>1 second). This is because of the intrinsic nature of the hemodynamic signal, which lags behind the corresponding neuronal signal by several seconds (for a thorough review, see Shibasaki, 2008).

Methods based on electrophysiological principles include event-related potentials (ERPs) and magnetoencephalography (MEG). These methods measure the neuronal activity of the brain, in particular postsynaptic discharges that can be recorded at the scalp in response to specific stimuli or events (e.g., a sound). The most important advantage of ERPs and MEG is their excellent temporal resolution (milliseconds) of brain neural activity, which makes it possible to investigate the whole sequence of cognitive processes occurring from sensory signal arrival to meaning comprehension. However, their major limitation is their poor spatial resolution.

Since the pioneering work of Jöbsis (1977), a third class of noninvasive brain imaging techniques has begun to emerge: optical imaging methods. These methods—which provide spatial and/or time course resolution—are based on the absorption and scattering properties of near-infrared light, which allow users to measure the functional activity occurring in the brain tissue (Gratton, Fabiani, Elbert, & Rockstroh, 2003). The principle is simple: the near-infrared light penetrates the head and permits one to measure some of the optical properties of the cortical tissue. The two main optical imaging methods are near-infrared spectroscopy (NIRS, estimating hemodynamic signals) and event-related optical signal (EROS, estimating neuronal signals). With the NIRS technique, one can assess changes in both oxyhemoglobin (O2Hb) and deoxyhemoglobin (HHb), in contrast to fMRI, which makes use of only the relative changes in HHb and cerebral blood volume. Oxygen consumption during brain activation results in a decrease in HHb and an increase in O2Hb and total hemoglobin (Hb-tot; i.e., the sum of O2Hb and HHb). In contrast, the EROS technique allows the identifying of fast optical signals in cortical tissue. The advantages of optical methods include good portability, low cost, and the possibility of executing acquisitions in a natural setting. Since these methods are light, low-cost, and do not require strict motion restriction, they are particularly suitable for research and applications in newborns, children, and healthy or sick adults.

Neurobiological bases of word semantic processing

Since the advent of the various imaging methods, the exploration of the neural substrates of semantic memory and semantic processes has become a frequent focus of investigation, in both neurologically healthy individuals and patients. Semantic memory is usually described as our organized general world knowledge, which includes meanings of words, properties of objects, and other knowledge that is not dependent on particular time and space contexts (Tulving, 1972). An important cognitive tool for investigating the structure of semantic memory, and particularly the mental representations of word meanings and their interrelationships in the brain, is the semantic priming paradigm. In behavioral studies, a semantic priming effect occurs when participants are faster at recognizing a target word, as indicated by lexical decision or semantic categorization, for example (e.g., nurse), when it is preceded by a related word (e.g., doctor) than when it is preceded by an unrelated word (e.g., bread; Meyer & Schvaneveldt, 1971). Such priming effects reflect the fact that lexical concepts in semantic memory are clustered according to a network of semantic similarity (Collins & Loftus, 1975). According to the spreading activation model, the activity in semantic networks spreads quickly between strongly connected nodes (as in the case of related words) and decays exponentially as the distance between nodes increases (as in the case of unrelated words). By modulating the time period between prime and target presentation (i.e., stimulus onset asynchrony (SOA)), it is possible to distinguish at least two different types of mechanisms underlying semantic priming effects: automatic spreading activation and controlled semantic processing (Neely, 1991). When the SOA is short, automatic processing is generally believed to take place because not enough time is available to develop a strategy. In contrast, a longer SOA gives participants enough time to consciously process the relationship between prime and target, including both facilitation and inhibition components, and thus leads to attentional or strategic processing. Priming effects can also be influenced by the relatedness of prime–target pairs and by the instructions given to participants; a lower proportion of relatedness pairs and instructions that avoid any allusion to related pairs in a stimulus set influence automatic processes (Neely, 1991).

Hemodynamic-based neuroimaging of the semantic processing of words

Historically, the retrieval of semantic information has been associated with the left temporal lobe, based mainly on the evidence of clinical data from patients with aphasia, Alzheimer's disease, or semantic dementia (Hodges & Gurd, 1994; Hodges, Salmon, & Butters, 1990, 1992). This pattern has been supported by neuroimaging PET and fMRI studies showing that semantic knowledge is represented in a distributed manner and its storage and retrieval depend primarily on the inferior and lateral temporal cortical regions (Damasio, Tranel, Grabowski, Adolphs, & Damasio, 2004; Démonet, Thierry, & Cardebat, 2005). Usually, semantic priming effects are reflected by a decrease in the amount of brain activation ("response suppression") for related compared to unrelated pairs of stimuli (Mummery, Shallice, & Price, 1999). It has been suggested that this phenomenon reflects the decrease in neural activity required to recognize targets, given that these words are easier to process because they have lower recognition thresholds as a result of spreading activation (Copland et al., 2003). However, a so-called inverse pattern (i.e., an increase in brain activity for related compared to unrelated prime–target pairs) has also been observed in some imaging studies. Using PET, Mummery et al. (1999) investigated the neural substrates of semantic priming by manipulating the proportion of related prime–target word pairs from 0% to 100%. The results showed a decrease in activity in the left anterior temporal lobe with increasing relatedness, except for the highest proportion of pairs, where an increase in activity was observed. This complex pattern was explained as the result of two processes: automatic (reflected in the decrease in activity) and strategic (reflected in the increase in activity) priming. More recently, Copland et al. (2003; Copland, de Zubicaray, McMahon, & Eastburn, 2007) also observed a decrease in brain activity for related compared to unrelated prime–target pairs of words using a short SOA (150 ms) but an increase in brain activity in the same condition using a long SOA (1,000 ms). One suggested explanation is that the increased brain activity may reflect either postlexical semantic integration (Kotz, Cappa, von Cramon, & Friederici, 2002) or the detection of the semantic relationships between words (Copland et al., 2007; Rossell, Price, & Nobre, 2003).

Other brain regions are activated during semantic processing, such as the left inferior prefrontal gyrus (LIPG). Evidence for the involvement of the LIPG during semantic processing came from an fMRI study that demonstrated that repeated access to semantic knowledge is associated with a decrease of LIPG activity. Demb et al. (1995) investigated repetition priming effects in both semantic (abstract/concrete judgment) and perceptual (uppercase/lowercase) decision tasks. Activation of the LIPG decreased as a function of item repetition but only in the semantic task, suggesting that the LIPG is a part of a semantic executive system that participates in the retrieval of semantic information. This reduced activation during repetition priming has been interpreted as indicating more efficient or faster word processing because lower thresholds activate existing representations (Henson, Shallice, & Dolan, 2000). In line with these data, several fMRI and PET studies have shown an activation of the LIPG in different semantic processing tasks, including the generation of semantically similar words, word classification (Gabrieli et al., 1996), and semantic monitoring (Démonet et al., 1992). The manipulation of the number of semantic items has also been reported to influence LIPG activation (Gabrieli, Poldrack, & Desmond, 1998; Wagner, Pare-Blagoev, Clark, & Poldrack, 2001). In addition, clinical data showed that patients with lesions to the LIPG, although impaired on some semantic tasks, do not typically present semantic deficits such as those seen following a temporal lobe lesion (Swick & Knight, 1996). Based on these observations, it has been argued that the LIPG mediates either central executive retrieval of semantic knowledge (Wagner et al., 2001) or semantic working memory processes (Gabrieli et al., 1998).

Challenging these hypotheses, a different interpretation of the contribution of the LIPG to the semantic processing of words emerges from a series of fMRI and neuropsychological studies. According to Thompson-Schill, Aguirre, D'Esposito, and Farah (1999) and Thompson-Schill, D'Esposito, Aguirre, and Farah (1997), the LIPG is involved in the selection of semantic knowledge from among competing alternative responses. To test their hypothesis, Thompson-Schill et al. (1997) compared high- and low-selection conditions in three different semantic tasks (generation vs. classification vs. comparison tasks) using fMRI. For example, in the classification task, participants classified line drawings of common objects. In the high-selection condition, the classification of items was based on a specific attribute of the object's representation (e.g., a line drawing of a car was associated with the word "expensive"). In the low-selection condition, the classification was based on the object's name (e.g., a line drawing of a fork was associated with the corresponding word: "fork"). Overall, the results showed that activation occurs in a similar region of the LIPG for high- and low-selection conditions, suggesting that it is the selection process, not retrieval of semantic knowledge that triggered activity in the LIPG. Similarly, Thompson-Schill et al. (1999) investigated the effects of repeated word generation under different conditions during whole-brain echoplanar fMRI. Participants performed a word generation task. During the second presentation of a word stimulus, participants were asked to generate either the same response as with the first presentation ("same" condition) or a different response than with the first presentation ("different" condition). At the behavioral level, priming effects were found for both relevant ("same") and irrelevant ("different") information. At the brain activation level, relevant primes produced a decrease in LIPG activation, while irrelevant primes produced an increase in LIPG activation. The authors attributed the LIPG decrease to a reduction in competition and, hence, in selection demands. The LIPG increase has been interpreted as an increase in the selection of competing responses because the word has already been retrieved once. In other words, the selection of a semantic representation is more demanding in the irrelevant than the relevant condition, because the generation of a target word in the latter condition was facilitated by relevant priming. The pattern of activation is different in the left temporal lobe: item repetition produced a decrease in activation in the left temporal cortex for both relevant and irrelevant conditions, suggesting a decrease in retrieval of the semantic information. According to Thompson-Schill et al. (1999), this dissociation suggests that selection of competing responses and retrieval are separate processes subserved by different regions, namely the LIPG and the left temporal cortex, respectively. Nevertheless, studies have recently shown that the temporal cortex may also be sensitive to the presence of semantic competitors in some conditions (Noppeney, Phillips, & Price, 2004; Spalek & Thompson-Schill, 2008), restarting the debate.

The LIPG has also been reported to be involved in the phonological processing of words (e.g., Fiez, 1997). Indeed, the LIPG, and in particular the posterior part, has been associated with speech production for a long time (Broca, 1865). Individuals with lesions in this area are characterized by motor and phonological deficits affecting language production (Damasio & Damasio, 1992). Thus, some researchers have suggested that there is a functional dissociation between the anterior and posterior parts of the LIPG, which play a specific role in semantic and phonological processing, respectively. This dissociation between anatomical regions in the LIPG for phonological and semantic processes is supported by numerous clinical and functional neuroimaging studies (Bookheimer, 2002; Costafreda et al., 2006; Démonet et al., 2005). These observations, however, are not unanimously accepted. In some studies, similar activations have been reported for both phonological and semantic processes in the anterior and posterior LIPG (Devlin, Matthews, & Rushworth, 2003; Gold & Buckner, 2002), suggesting that some common underlying cognitive processing is involved.

While a number of variables appear to influence semantic processes, one important factor is the categorization of objects. Semantic categorization is a basic property of the semantic information organization process that permits the recognition of semantic items and relates them to other familiar entities, but also needs to classify new objects into the existing knowledge structure. Classically, most models of semantic knowledge organization are based on hierarchical or taxonomic categories (e.g., natural categories, such as animals or fruits; and artifact categories, such as furniture or tools). Studies of category-specific effects have become increasingly important in revealing the organization of semantic memory. This field of research originated in neuropsychological studies with brain-damaged patients (e.g., Warrington & McCarthy, 1994). Most reports of category-specific deficits describe patients with impaired recognition of natural objects (e.g., animals, fruits) rather than artifacts (e.g., furniture, tools); the opposite pattern is reported much less frequently (for reviews, see Capitani, Laiacona, Mahon, & Caramazza, 2003; Laws, 2005). Three main explanations have been advanced to account for these dissociations: the sensory-functional (Humphreys & Forde, 2001; Warrington & Shallice, 1984), domain-specific (Caramazza & Shelton, 1998), and correlated feature hypotheses (Tyler & Moss, 2001).

- The sensory-functional hypothesis suggests that conceptual knowledge is organized according to semantic object features. Sensory features are claimed to be more relevant for distinguishing natural items, while functional features are critical for recognizing artifacts. Hence, the loss of sensory or functional knowledge impairs natural or artifact categories.
- The domain-specific hypothesis assumes that evolutionary pressure has segregated the neural systems dedicated to natural and artifact objects.
- Finally, the correlated feature account suggests that category effects need not always reflect segregation within the semantic system because the conceptual features are stored in a single semantic system in which natural objects share more features than artifacts.
- Each of these hypotheses makes different assumptions about the underlying neuroanatomy, which can be evaluated by different functional neuroimaging methods.

Several reports using PET and fMRI have provided anatomical confirmation of the natural object/artifact dissociation in the brain. Brain activations related to semantic categories have been observed during different semantic tasks (e.g., picture naming, semantic decisions; Chao & Martin, 2000; Mummery, Patterson, Hodges, & Price, 1998; Perani et al., 1999). Classically, natural objects (e.g., animals) produced stronger activation in visual association areas of the occipito-temporal cortex, while artifacts (e.g., tools) elicited relatively stronger activation in brain areas involved in action representation, namely the pre-motor areas, left middle temporal cortex, and parietal cortex. A meta-analysis based on seven PET studies reported on the influence of an experimental task in probing the stored semantic knowledge (Devlin et al., 2002). This review demonstrated specific activations for each category: while natural objects activated the bilateral anterior temporal cortex, artifacts activated the left posterior middle temporal region. Most of these neuroanatomical dissociations are in agreement with the sensory-functional hypothesis. Importantly, Devlin et al. (2002) showed that category-specific effects were found for semantic decision (i.e., location, color, action, real-life size) and word retrieval tasks (i.e., category fluency, picture naming, and word reading) but not for perceptual tasks (e.g., screen size judgment). Consequently, category effects seem to be specific to semantic context.

Other models proposed that the organization of semantic knowledge is based on thematic representation. These models propose that categories are held together by a context (scene or event) in which certain objects are encountered (e.g., dog and leash). Sachs, Weis, Krings, Huber, and Kircher (2008a) recently compared categorical and thematic representation using fMRI. Their results showed that both kinds of representations activated similar neural substrates: the left inferior frontal, middle temporal, and occipital regions, suggesting that comparable mechanisms may be involved in the processing of taxonomic and thematic conceptual relations. Interestingly, the same authors (Sachs et al., 2008b) again investigated the neural substrates of these categories but this time under automatic processing conditions (i.e., with SOA of 200 ms), in order to minimize the effect of strategic processes on categorical processing. Participants performed a lexical decision task with four different experimental conditions: thematically related prime-target pairs (e.g., jacket: button), taxonomically related pairs (e.g., jacket: vest), unrelated pairs (e.g., jacket: bottle), and pairs with pseudoword targets (e.g., jacket: neuz). The behavioral data show that the size of a priming effect is greater for thematic than taxonomic categories, arguing that members of thematic categories share a stronger and more salient conceptual relationship. The neuroimaging data show activations mainly located in the right hemisphere: while taxonomic priming effects involve activation in the right precuneus, posterior cingulate, right middle frontal, superior frontal, and postcentral gyrus, thematic priming effects are observed in the right middle frontal gyrus and anterior cingulate. Strangely, no activation is reported in the LIPG or the middle temporal gyrus. Another important result reported by the authors is the involvement of the right precuneus, which was only observed for taxonomic categories, suggesting that these categories require increased effort to resolve semantic ambiguity because they are considered to be less salient. Considering both behavioral and neuroimaging data, and data from other neuroimaging studies (e.g., Cavanna & Trimble, 2006), the authors argue that episodic memory—which has previously been found to be associated with the precuneus—is likely to be more involved in taxonomic categories. According to Sachs et al. (2008b), "it seems much more likely to have an episodic memory of a car in a garage or a button in a coat, than a dog and a goat or a cup and a glass" (p. 201).

Another way to investigate semantic networks is by analyzing the pattern of activation while the individual is engaged in word production. The verbal fluency task (also referred to as oral naming) is a classical language production paradigm in which participants are asked to generate as many words as possible. The most common measures of verbal fluency are orthographic (letter-based, such as "F" or "L") and semantic (category-based, such as "animals" or "sports"). To successfully perform this task, participants need to have intact lexical and semantic knowledge, efficient word access and retrieval, and well-organized semantic networks (Posner & DiGirolamo, 1998). Most neuroimaging studies of verbal fluency have shown that orthographic and semantic fluency tasks activate different brain regions. For example, using PET, Mummery, Patterson, Hodges, and Wise (1996) demonstrated that letter fluency activated left frontal regions, while semantic fluency yielded activation in left temporal regions (including the anteromedial region and inferior temporal gyrus). These early data were replicated by other studies using fMRI, PET and, more recently, voxel-based lesion symptom mapping (e.g., Baldo, Schwartz, Wilkins, & Dronkers, 2006). Similar clinical data were also reported (e.g., Troyer, Moscovitch, Winocur, Alexander, & Stuss, 1998). These dissociations can be explained by the use of different retrieval strategies for words associated with different criteria in the fluency tasks. For example, for letter-based fluency, the retrieval of words on the basis of their initial letter is not a natural component of language processing; consequently, unlike semantic retrieval, participants have to use an unfamiliar access route to the lexicon (Wood, Saling, Abbott, & Jackson, 2001) and a strategic search across graphophonemic or lexical memory. Thus, letter fluency can be harder because lexical stores are broader and less well defined than semantic stores. In contrast, semantic verbal fluency is more dependent on semantic memory because participants have to search for semantic associations within a given category; thus, this task depends mainly on the integrity of the semantic memory. For this reason, deficits in the semantic fluency task reflect semantic memory impairments and not executive dysfunctions.

These findings are not uncontroversial. Indeed, Gourovitch et al. (2000) investigated the neural substrates of both letter and semantic fluency in healthy participants using PET. A relatively greater activation of the inferior frontal cortex and temporo-parietal cortex was observed during letter fluency tasks, while greater activation of the left temporal cortex was observed during semantic fluency tasks. However, relative to the control task (i.e., participants had to generate days of the week and months of the year), this study showed that similar brain regions were activated during both fluency tasks, including the anterior cingulate and left prefrontal regions. It is also relevant that a meta-analysis by Henri and Crawford (2004) has demonstrated that focal frontal lesions are associated with equivalent letter and semantic impairments, suggesting that the frontal lobes are involved in executive control processes and effortful retrieval of semantic knowledge. However, temporal damage was found to be associated with more deficits on semantic than letter fluency. The involvement of the LIPG has also been reported during verbal fluency tasks. Recently, a meta-analysis of fMRI studies demonstrated that the two kinds of verbal fluency tasks activate different parts of the LIPG. While semantic fluency tasks tend to activate a more ventral-anterior portion of the IFG, orthographic fluency appeared to involve a more dorsal posterior part (Costafreda et al., 2006), in line with previous neuroimaging studies (e.g., Fiez, 1997). Given that verbal fluency tasks involve the monitoring of several items in working memory, it has been suggested that these activations reflect working memory rather than semantic processes (Cabeza & Nyberg, 2000). To explain these contradictory data, some authors suggest that semantic and graphophonemic processes might be closely related. It may be the case that some graphophonemic processes are involved in semantic fluency and, similarly, some semantic processes might be involved in orthographic fluency. According to Costafreda et al. (2006), this "noise" would fail to detect spatial differences in brain activations. Although this meta-analysis is significant, none of the fMRI studies included by the authors was conducted with the same participants. The comparison of experimental tasks in a single group of participants is a powerful tool allowing the precise assessment of activation differences. A recent study by Heim, Eickhoff, and Amunts (2008) compared three different types of verbal fluency (orthographic vs. semantic vs. syntactic, i.e., generating nouns in the masculine gender) in the same participants using fMRI. Activations were found in both anterior and posterior parts of the LIPG for all verbal fluency tasks, suggesting that certain unspecific aspects—and not condition-specific demands—of verbal fluency are similar for three tasks. These data, which are in line with Gold and Buckner's (2002) results, may reflect the controlled retrieval of lexical information. In addition, these results are in accordance with the hypothesis whereby the LIPG mediates lexical selection processes (Snyder, Feigenson, & Thompson-Schill, 2007).

Troyer et al. (1998) and, more recently, Hirshorn and Thompson-Schill (2006) proposed that letter/semantic fluency dissociation can be described in terms of clustering (i.e., words produced inside the same subcategory) and switching (i.e., ability to change subcategory). When participants have to produce as many words as possible as a function of a given category or letter, they spontaneously tend to produce more clusters of semantically or phonetically related items. This approach can provide information on the structure of semantic memory, but also on the dynamic interaction between different semantic links. Such spontaneous clusters of words are consistent with the spreading activation model (Collins & Loftus, 1975), according to which a prime word can automatically activate a local network of related concepts. A series of clinical studies demonstrated that the switching is sustained by the frontal lobes whereas clustering is sustained by temporal regions (Troyer et al., 1998). In a recent fMRI study, Hirshorn and Thompson-Schill (2006) demonstrated that the LIPG is involved in the switching of subcategories during semantic fluency. The involvement of the LIPG in switching is due to the high semantic selection demands underlying this process. The switching/clustering dissociation echoes the selection/retrieval dissociation (Hirshorn & Thompson-Schill, 2006).

Electrophysiological neuroimaging of the semantic processing of words

Functional neuroimaging studies provide crucial insights into the neurobiological bases of the semantic processing of words. However, given that neural activity occurs very fast, electrophysiological measures are essential to gain a better understanding of the time course of language processing. In ERP studies, the N400 component, which is a negative deflection that emerges at about 250 ms and peaks approximately 400 ms after word onset, is highly sensitive to semantic processing and, in particular, to semantic priming. The N400 component was first reported to be sensitive to the integration of words in a sentence context (Kutas & Hillyard, 1980). The amplitude of the N400 response to the sentence's final word is reduced if that word is semantically expected in the sentence context (e.g., "The pizza was too hot to eat") compared to an unexpected word (e.g., "The pizza was too hot to cry"). Consequently, it is inversely proportional to the ease with which the stimulus may be integrated into the current semantic context. An N400 component has also been reported during semantic priming paradigms with words (in both visual and auditory modalities: Federmeier & Kutas, 2001; Holcomb, 1993) and pictures of objects (McPherson & Holcomb, 1999), as well as for the processing of other meaningful or potentially meaningful stimuli, such as faces, odors, environmental sounds, and pronounceable pseudowords (Gunter & Bach, 2004; Koelsch et al., 2004). The N400 amplitude has been found to decrease with repetition priming and high word frequency (Kutas & Federmeier, 2000). It has been argued that the N400 component reflects the access and integration of a semantic representation into a current context (Holcomb, 1993).

Similarly to fMRI and PET studies, electrophysiological data have confirmed the importance of the involvement of the temporal cortex in semantic memory and semantic processing in general. Field potentials from intracranial electrodes in patients have demonstrated that the N400 is generated in the temporal cortex (in the area of the collateral sulcus and the anterior fusiform gyrus), confirming the crucial role this area plays in the storage and/or retrieval of semantic knowledge (Nobre, Allison, & McCarthy, 1994). Similar areas have been identified in MEG studies showing that the N400 generators are localized in bilateral fronto-temporal areas (left more than right hemisphere), as well as in the hippocampus, the parahippocampal gyri, the amygdala, and the superior and middle temporal gyri (e.g., Halgren et al., 2002; Marinkovic et al., 2003). Such convergences were explored simultaneously in combined fMRI/ERP studies. For example, Matsumoto, Iidaka, Haneda, Okada, and Sadato (2005) found a significant correlation between BOLD signal and N400 semantic priming effect in the left superior temporal gyrus but not in the LIPG. Interestingly, clinical data show that lesions in the left temporal lobe and temporo-parietal junction produce both decreased amplitudes and delayed latencies for N400 component, whereas LIPG lesions have little or no impact on the N400 (see Van Petten & Luka, 2006). Overall, these data confirm that the left temporal cortex is involved in the retrieval of semantic knowledge and suggest that, although the frontal lobe is required for some aspects of language processing, it does not appear to be involved in the semantic context effects. Matsumoto et al. (2005) proposed that the processes linked to the LIPG (i.e., selection or working memory) could be associated with another ERP component, possibly the Late Positive Component (LPC), which seems to underlie many aspects of language processing such as working memory, episodic memory retrieval, response selection, and reallocation of cognitive resources.

At the same time, the mechanisms underlying the N400 priming effect are still a matter of debate. Comparing short and long SOAs (200 vs. 1,000 ms) during lexical decision tasks, Rossell et al. (2003) found an N400 semantic priming effect for both conditions. Surprisingly, though, this effect starts significantly earlier in the long-SOA condition (300–320 ms) than in the short-

SOA condition (360–380 ms). The authors interpret that result as indicating a facilitation effect of semantic processing by controlled expectancies. In contrast, other ERP studies suggest that the difference in N400 reflects either automatic processes (Kellenbach, Wijers, & Mulder, 2000) or both automatic and controlled processes (Kutas & Federmeier, 2000).

Among the word semantic properties that modulate ERP components, one that is often reported is the object category. A series of ERP studies conducted by Kiefer (2001, 2005) generated some important insights into the temporal aspects of category-specific effects. Kiefer (2001) investigated the time course of both perceptual and semantic aspects of natural and artifact objects during superordinate object categorization (e.g., animal: cat) with pictures and words. At the early—perceptual—level (around 160–200 ms), the ERP data show greater perceptual processing for pictures of natural objects than artifacts. In contrast, at the later—semantic—level (around 300–500 ms), category-specific effects were observed in both modalities and associated with a reduction of N400 amplitude in specific electrodes (i.e., occipito-temporal areas for natural and fronto-central areas for artifact objects). In particular, the second study by Kiefer (2005) demonstrates that category-specific effects are obtained in lexical tasks and not only on semantic tasks, as was previously reported in the fMRI literature (e.g., Devlin et al., 2002). More specifically, the aim of his study was to track the time course of brain activation associated with category-specific effects during a lexical decision task. In order to test the relevance of these effects for semantic memory, a repetition priming paradigm was used. In line with Kiefer (2001), the ERP data showed a greater positive component over occipito-parietal areas in the N400 (about 350–450 ms) and LPC (about 500–600 ms) time windows for natural objects, and a greater positive component over fronto-central regions for artifact objects in the N400 time window for a lexical decision task. Overall, these scalp distribution data are in line with previous PET and fMRI studies, which demonstrate that the occipito-temporal regions subserve visual semantic knowledge, which is more specific to natural objects. Conversely, the frontal cortex, and especially the motor areas, is involved in action-related knowledge, which is more specific to artifacts (Chao & Martin, 2000; Perani et al., 1999). Another important result reported by Kiefer (2005) concerns repetition effects. Consistent with the ERP literature, repetition produces less category-related activity than the initial presentation of words; this reduction occurs over the occipito-parietal and frontal areas for both natural and artifact objects in the N400 and LPC time windows. In addition, an earlier onset of repetition effects is observed for natural than for artifact categories, suggesting that there is a specific temporal dynamic for different types of knowledge and supporting the hypothesis that there are multiple cortical semantic systems. This finding is particularly interesting because it highlights some of the weaknesses related to hemodynamic methods, and in particular concerning the temporal aspects of information processing. Indeed, if the neural signal decays rapidly, hemodynamic methods, due to the relatively slow changes in blood flow, can fail to detect reliable brain activations for specific processes (e.g., Devlin et al., 2002).

In addition, the high temporal resolution of electrophysiological methods is crucial for understanding the interhemispheric dynamics underlying various aspects of language processing. For example, using the ERP method, Bouaffre and Faïta-Ainseba (2007) have recently demonstrated that semantically associated word pairs are activated with delay in the right compared to the left hemisphere, highlighting the left hemisphere's primacy for this kind of processing. Similarly, by using MEG, some researchers (Dhond, Witzel, Dale, & Halgren, 2007; Liu et al., 2008) showed that there are spatio-temporal differences in concrete versus abstract word processing. Combining MEG and synthetic aperture magnetometry (i.e., analysis that volumetrically localizes language processing), Liu et al. (2008) found no neuromagnetic differences between abstract and concrete words in the primary visual and auditory cortices. However, significant differences were observed over the frontal regions: more neurons were activated in the left frontal areas for abstract words, while more neurons were activated in the right frontal areas for concrete words. Neuromagnetic changes were also observed in the left posterior temporal areas and LIPG for all words but as a function of specific frequency band. The authors suggest that processing of abstract words is lateralized in the left hemisphere, whereas processing of concrete words is bilateral (with the right hemisphere sustaining imagistic processing). Dhond et al. (2007) observed differences between processing of abstract and concrete words in the fronto-temporal regions from 300 to 400 ms, arguing that, although the encoding of both concrete and abstract words seems similar, different parts of the network are more specialized for concrete versus abstract words.

Data from emerging imaging methods

The new imaging methods now emerging are likely to complement current approaches exploring the physiological substrates of cognitive processes and the time course of their involvement. In addition, analysis methods are becoming increasingly well developed, allowing us to address such fundamental issues as the connectivity (i.e., functional or effective) and the interaction (how and in which direction) between different neural networks. For example, fMRI or functional neuroimaging data can now be analyzed in such a way as to allow for the description of putative networks associated with a given ability or task. Those networks are said to be functional or effective depending on whether or not they include causality indications. The nature of the information they provide is complementary to those of traditional activation pattern data. They can even offer converging evidence such as the results from Walter, Jbabdi, Marrelec, Benali, and Joanette (2006) showing that the functional connectivity associated with the semantic processing of words (semantic categorization decision task) includes a neural network involving both right- and left-hemisphere-based loci, whereas the network associated with graphophonological processing (rhyme decision task) is limited to the left hemisphere.

Regarding emerging imaging techniques, NIRS has been successfully used to detect brain activation related to a number of language tasks. Among cognitive tasks known to activate the prefrontal cortex, the verbal fluency task is often reported on in the literature about NIRS use. During semantic and orthographic fluency tasks, activations (i.e., increased O2Hb and decreased HHb) are reported in inferior and dorsolateral prefrontal areas in healthy individuals (Herrmann, Ehlis, & Fallgatter, 2003; Quaresima et al., 2005), as well as patients with neurological (Hermann, Langer, Jacob, Ehlis, & Fallgatter, 2008) or psychiatric diseases (Ehlis, Herrmann, Plichta, & Fallgatter, 2007; Quaresima, Giosuè, Roncone, Casacchia, & Ferrari, 2009). The data concerning lateralization effects are contradictory. Activation in the bilateral prefrontal cortex is observed in most NIRS studies (Hermann et al., 2003; Herrmann, Walter, Ehlis, & Fallgatter, 2006; Kameyama, Fukuda, Uehara, & Mikuni, 2004; Kameyama et al., 2006; Matsuo, Watanabe, Onodera, Kato, & Kato, 2004; Watanabe, Matsuo, Kato, & Kato, 2003). This bilateral activation has been interpreted as underlying executive processes related to verbal fluency and not to specific language processes. However, other NIRS studies have reported a clear lateral effect, with higher oxygenation in the left hemisphere, according to most fMRI studies on verbal fluency (Fallgatter et al., 1997; Hermann et al. 2006). Why are there such discrepancies between studies? Several possible explanations can be put forward, such as number of NIRS channels (very limited in many studies), position of NIRS optodes on scalp, number of participants, and data analysis method. Recently, Quaresima et al. (2009) found high variability between participants performing verbal fluency and visuospatial working memory tasks. In particular, single-subject analysis demonstrated bilateral prefrontal activation for only a few participants. In addition, significant inter-individual variations in O2Hb and HHb were reported in response to both tasks. The authors proposed some explanations of these phenomena and emphasized the importance of single-subject analysis, which provides more anatomical information about the changes in brain activity. In addition, to improve the poor spatial resolution related to single- or two-channel studies, multichannel NIRS systems have been introduced (e.g., Schecklmann, Ehlis, Plichta, & Fallgatter, 2008).

Using high spatial and temporal sampling, the EROS approach allows users to obtain brain images with very good spatial and temporal resolution: on the order of a few millimeters and a few milliseconds, respectively (Tse et al., 2007). The first EROS study of language processing has recently been carried out by Tse et al. (2007), who reported on the spatial and temporal dynamics in processing semantic and syntactic anomalies in sentences. A rapid interaction between left superior/middle temporal cortices and the IFC was obtained during semantically and syntactically anomalous sentence processing using both EROS and ERP. Remembering that semantic and syntactic anomalies induce typical ERP patterns at the N400 and P600 components, respectively, it is interesting to note that EROS data show an increase in activation first in the left superior/middle temporal cortices then in the inferior frontal cortices, suggesting that activation moves from posterior (temporal) to anterior (frontal) regions in the course of sentence processing.

Conclusion

The emergence of imaging methods has had a tremendous impact for the development of cognitive neurosciences over the last decades. In particular, they have allowed a unique understanding of the spatial and/or temporal aspects of the neurobiological bases of the semantic processing of words. However, because of the large number of intrinsic (e.g., nature of semantic features) and extrinsic (e.g., characteristics/limitations of a given neuroimaging acquisition and/or data analysis technique) factors that can influence the results, one should not be surprised to find nonconverging—and sometimes contradictory—results in the literature. Thus, direct comparisons between studies are difficult because of differences in the kind of method used but also because of the nature of stimuli, experimental tasks that reflect different levels of semantic processing, the way the data were analyzed, and the methodology used. In fact, we are only starting to unveil the neurobiological bases of the semantic processing of words. The present review shows that this question is very complex since the semantic processing of words appears to result from a large and distributed neural network of which components are modulated by a myriad of semantic features, characteristics, and representations. The addition of new emerging imaging methods, along with the quest for converging evidence across the different neuroimaging approaches, will reveal new and important insights regarding language processing in general and the semantic processing of words in particular.

Further reading

Ferre, P., Jarret, J., Brambati, S., Bellec, P., & Joanette, Y. (2020). Functional connectivity of successful picture-naming: Age-specific organization and the effect of engaging in stimulating activities. *Frontiers in Aging Neuroscience, 12*.

Fonseca, R. S., Marcotte, K., Hubner, L. C., Zimmerman, N., Netto, T. M., Joannette, Y., … Ansaldo, A. I. (2021). The impact of age and education on phonemic and semantic verbal fluency: Behavioral and fMRI correlates. *BioRxiv*. https://doi.org/10.1101/2021.01.14.426642.

Haitas, N., Amiri, M., Wilson, M., Joanette, Y., & Steffener, J. (2021). Age-preserved semantic memory & the CRUNCH effect manifested as differential semantic control networks: An fMRI study. *PLOS ONE, 16*(6), e0249948. https://doi.org/10.1371/journal.pone.0249948.

References

Baldo, J.V., Schwartz, S., Wilkins, D., & Dronkers, N. F. (2006). Role of frontal versus temporal cortex in verbal fluency as revealed by voxel-based lesion symptom mapping. *Journal of the International Neuropsychological Society, 12*(6), 896–900.

Bookheimer, S. (2002). Functional MRI of language: New approaches to understanding the cortical organization of semantic processing. *Annual Review of Neuroscience, 25*, 151–188.

Bouaffre, S., & Faïta-Ainseba, F. (2007). Hemispheric differences in the time-course of semantic priming processes: Evidence from event-related potentials (ERPs). *Brain and Cognition, 63*(2), 123–135.
Broca, P. (1865). Du siège de la faculté du langage articulé. *Bulletin de la Société d'Anthropologie, 6*, 337–393.
Cabeza, R., & Nyberg, L. (2000). Imaging cognition II: An empirical review of 275 PET and fMRI studies. *Journal of Cognitive Neuroscience, 12*(1), 1–47.
Capitani, E., Laiacona, M., Mahon, B., & Caramazza, A. (2003). What are the facts of semantic category-specific deficits? A critical review of the clinical evidence. *Cognitive Neuropsychology, 20*(3), 213–261.
Caramazza, A., & Shelton, J. R. (1998). Domain-specific knowledge systems in the brain the animate-inanimate distinction. *Journal of Cognitive Neuroscience, 10*(1), 1–34.
Cavanna, A. E., & Trimble, M. R. (2006). The precuneus: A review of its functional anatomy and behavioural correlates. *Brain, 129*(3), 564–583.
Chao, L. L., & Martin, A. (2000). Representation of manipulable man-made objects in the dorsal stream. *Neuroimage, 12*(4), 478–484.
Collins, A. M., & Loftus, E. F. (1975). A spreading-activation theory of semantic processing. *Psychological Review, 82*(6), 407–428.
Copland, D. A., de Zubicaray, G. I., McMahon, K., & Eastburn, M. (2007). Neural correlates of semantic priming for ambiguous words: An event-related fMRI study. *Brain Research, 1131*(1), 163–172.
Copland, D. A., de Zubicaray, G. I., McMahon, K., Wilson, S. J., Eastburn, M., & Chenery, H. J. (2003). Brain activity during automatic semantic priming revealed by event-related functional magnetic resonance imaging. *Neuroimage, 20*(1), 302–310.
Costafreda, S. G., Fu, C. H., Lee, L., Everitt, B., Brammer, M. J., & David, A. S. (2006). A systematic review and quantitative appraisal of fMRI studies of verbal fluency: Role of the left inferior frontal gyrus. *Human Brain Mapping, 27*(10), 799–810.
Damasio, A. R., & Damasio, H. (1992). Brain and language. *Scientific American, 267*(3), 88–95.
Damasio, H., Tranel, D., Grabowski, T., Adolphs, R., & Damasio, A. R. (2004). Neural systems behind word and concept retrieval. *Cognition, 92*(1–2), 179–229.
Demb, J. B., Desmond, J. E., Wagner, A. D., Vaidya, C. J., Glover, G. H., & Gabrieli, J. D. (1995). Semantic encoding and retrieval in the left inferior prefrontal cortex: A functional MRI study of task difficulty and process specificity. *Journal of Neuroscience, 15*(9), 5870–5878.
Démonet, J. F., Chollet, F., Ramsay, S., Cardebat, D., Nespoulous, J. L., Wise, R., ... Frackowiak, R. (1992). The anatomy of phonological and semantic processing in normal subjects. *Brain, 115*(6), 1753–1768.
Démonet, J. F., Thierry, G., & Cardebat, D. (2005). Renewal of the neurophysiology of language: Functional neuroimaging. *Physiological Reviews, 85*(1), 49–95.
Devlin, J. T., Matthews, P. M., & Rushworth, M. F. (2003). Semantic processing in the left inferior prefrontal cortex: A combined functional magnetic resonance imaging and transcranial magnetic stimulation study. *Journal of Cognitive Neuroscience, 15*(1), 71–84.
Devlin, J. T., Moore, C. J., Mummery, C. J., Gorno-Tempini, M. L., Phillips, J. A., Noppeney, U., ... Price, C. J. (2002). Anatomic constraints on cognitive theories of category specificity. *Neuroimage, 15*(3), 675–685.
Dhond, R. P., Witzel, T., Dale, A. M., & Halgren, E. (2007). Spatiotemporal cortical dynamics underlying abstract and concrete word reading. *Human Brain Mapping, 28*(4), 355–362.
Ehlis, A. C., Herrmann, M. J., Plichta, M. M., & Fallgatter, A. J. (2007). Cortical activation during two verbal fluency tasks in schizophrenic patients and healthy controls as assessed by multi-channel near-infrared spectroscopy. *Psychiatry Research, 156*(1), 1–13.
Fallgatter, A. J., Roesler, M., Sitzmann, L., Heidrich, A., Mueller, T. J., & Strik, W. K. (1997). Loss of functional hemispheric asymmetry in Alzheimer's dementia assessed with near-infrared spectroscopy. *Cognitive Brain Research, 6*(1), 67–72.
Federmeier, K. D., & Kutas, M. (2001). Meaning and modality: Influences of context, semantic memory organization, and perceptual predictability on picture processing. *Journal of Experimental Psychology: Learning Memory and Cognition, 27*(1), 202–224.
Fiez, J. A. (1997). Phonology, semantics, and the role of the left inferior prefrontal cortex. *Human Brain Mapping, 5*(2), 79–83.
Gabrieli, J. D. E., Desmond, J. E., Demb, J. B., Wagner, A. D., Stone, M. V., Vaidya, C. J., & Glover, G. H. (1996). Functional magnetic resonance imaging of semantic memory processes in the frontal lobes. *Psychological Science*, 7(5), 278–283.
Gabrieli, J. D. E., Poldrack, R. A., & Desmond, J. E. (1998). The role of left prefrontal cortex in language and memory. *Proceedings of the National Academy of Sciences of the USA, 95*(3), 906–913.
Gold, B. T., & Buckner, R. L. (2002). Common prefrontal regions coactivate with dissociable posterior regions during controlled semantic and phonological tasks. *Neuron, 35*(4), 803–812.
Gourovitch, M. L., Kirkby, B. S., Goldberg, T. E., Weinberger, D. R., Gold, J. M., Esposito, G., ... Berman, K. F. (2000). A comparison of rCBF patterns during letter and semantic fluency. *Neuropsychology, 14*(3), 353–360.

Gratton, G., Fabiani, M., Elbert, T., & Rockstroh, B. (2003). Seeing right through you: Applications of optical imaging to the study of the human brain. *Psychophysiology, 40*(4), 487–491.

Gunter, T. C., & Bach, P. (2004). Communicating hands: ERPs elicited by meaningful symbolic hand postures. *Neuroscience Letters, 372*(1–2), 52–56.

Halgren, E., Dhond, R. P., Christensen, N., Van Petten, C., Marinkovic, K., Lewine, J. D., & Dale, A. M. (2002). N400-like magnetoencephalography responses modulated by semantic context, word frequency, and lexical class in sentences. *Neuroimage, 17*(3), 1101–1116.

Heim, S., Eickhoff, S. B., & Amunts, K. (2008). Specialisation in Broca's region for semantic, phonological, and syntactic fluency? *Neuroimage, 40*(3), 1362–1368.

Henri, J. D., & Crawford, J. R. (2004). A meta-analytic review of verbal fluency performance following focal cortical lesions. *Neuropsychology, 18*(2), 284–295.

Henson, R., Shallice, T., & Dolan, R. (2000). Neuroimaging evidence for dissociable forms of repetition priming. *Science, 287*(5456), 1269–1272.

Herrmann, M. J., Ehlis, A. C., & Fallgatter, A. J. (2003). Frontal activation during a verbal-fluency task as measured by near-infrared spectroscopy. *Brain Research Bulletin, 61*(1), 51–56.

Herrmann, M. J., Langer, J. B., Jacob, C., Ehlis, A. C., & Fallgatter, A. J. (2008). Reduced prefrontal oxygenation in Alzheimer disease during verbal fluency tasks. *American Journal of Geriatric Psychiatry, 16*(2), 125–135.

Herrmann, M. J., Walter, A., Ehlis, A. C., & Fallgatter, A. J. (2006). Cerebral oxygenation changes in the prefrontal cortex: Effects of age and gender. *Neurobiology of Aging, 27*(6), 888–894.

Hirshorn, E. A., & Thompson-Schill, S. L. (2006). Role of the left inferior frontal gyrus in covert word retrieval: Neural correlates of switching during verbal fluency. *Neuropsychologia, 44*(12), 2547–2557.

Hodges, J. R., & Gurd, J. M. (1994). Remote memory and lexical retrieval in a case of frontal Pick's disease. *Archives of Neurology, 51*(8), 821–827.

Hodges, J. R., Salmon, D. P., & Butters, N. (1990). Differential impairment of semantic and episodic memory in Alzheimer's and Huntington's diseases: A controlled prospective study. *Journal of Neurology, Neurosurgery, and Psychiatry, 53*(12), 1089–1095.

Hodges, J. R., Salmon, D. P., & Butters, N. (1992). Semantic memory impairment in Alzheimer's disease: Failure of access or degraded knowledge? *Neuropsychologia, 30*(4), 301–314.

Holcomb, P. J. (1993). Semantic priming and stimulus degradation: Implications for the role of the N400 in language processing. *Psychophysiology, 30*(1), 47–61.

Humphreys, G. W., & Forde, E. M. (2001). Hierarchies, similarity, and interactivity in object recognition: "Category-specific" neuropsychological deficits. *Behavioral and Brain Sciences, 24*(3), 453–476.

Jöbsis, F. F. (1977). Noninvasive, infrared monitoring of cerebral and myocardial oxygen sufficiency and circulatory parameters. *Science, 198*(4323), 1264–1267.

Kameyama, M., Fukuda, M., Uehara, T., & Mikuni, M. (2004). Sex and age dependencies of cerebral blood volume changes during cognitive activations: A multichannel near-infrared spectroscopy study. *Neuroimage, 22*(4), 1715–1721.

Kameyama, M., Fukuda, M., Yamagishi, Y., Sato, T., Uehara, T., Ito, M., ... Mikuni, M. (2006). Frontal lobe function in bipolar disorder: A multichannel near-infrared spectroscopy study. *Neuroimage, 29*(1), 172–184.

Kellenbach, M. L., Wijers, A. A., & Mulder, G. (2000). Visual semantic features are activated during the processing of concrete words: Event-related potential evidence for perceptual semantic priming. *Cognitive Brain Research, 10*(1–2), 67–75.

Kiefer, M. (2001). Perceptual and semantic sources of category-specific effects: Event-related potentials during picture and word categorization. *Memory and Cognition, 29*(1), 100–116.

Kiefer, M. (2005). Repetition-priming modulates category-related effects on event-related potentials: Further evidence for multiple cortical semantic systems. *Journal of Cognitive Neuroscience, 17*(2), 199–211.

Koelsch, S., Kasper, E., Sammler, D., Schulze, K., Gunter, T., & Friederici, A. D. (2004). Music, language and meaning: Brain signatures of semantic processing. *Nature Neuroscience*, 7(3), 302–307.

Kotz, S. A., Cappa, S. F., von Cramon, D. Y., & Friederici, A. D. (2002). Modulation of the lexical-semantic network by auditory semantic priming: An event-related functional MRI study. *Neuroimage, 17*(4), 1761–1772.

Kutas, M., & Federmeier, K. D. (2000). Electrophysiology reveals semantic memory use in language comprehension. *Trends in Cognitive Sciences, 4*(12), 463–470.

Kutas, M., & Hillyard, S. A. (1980). Reading senseless sentences: Brain potentials reflect semantic incongruity. *Science, 207*(4427), 203–205.

Laws, K. R. (2005). "Illusions of normality": A methodological critique of category-specific naming. *Cortex, 6*(6), 842–851.

Liu, Y., Xiang, J., Wang, Y., Vannest, J. J., Byars, A. W., & Rose, D. F. (2008). Spatial and frequency differences of neuromagnetic activities in processing concrete and abstract words. *Brain Topography, 20*(3), 123–129.

Marinkovic, K., Dhond, R. P., Dale, A. M., Glessner, M., Carr, V., & Halgren, E. (2003). Spatio-temporal dynamics of modality-specific and supramodal word processing. *Neuron, 38*(3), 487–497.

Matsumoto, A., Iidaka, T., Haneda, K., Okada, T., & Sadato, N. (2005). Linking semantic priming effect in functional MRI and event-related potentials. *Neuroimage*, *24*(3), 624–634.

Matsuo, K., Watanabe, A., Onodera, Y., Kato, N., & Kato, T. (2004). Prefrontal hemodynamic response to verbal-fluency task and hyperventilation in bipolar disorder measured by multi-channel near-infrared spectroscopy. *Journal of Affective Disorders*, *82*(1), 85–92.

McPherson, W. B., & Holcomb, P. J. (1999). An electophysiological investigation of semantic priming with pictures of real objects. *Psychophysiology*, *36*(1), 53–65.

Meyer, D. E., & Schvaneveldt, R. W. (1971). Facilitation in recognizing pairs of words: Evidence of a dependence between retrieval operations. *Journal of Experimental Psychology*, *90*(2), 227–234.

Mummery, C. J., Patterson, K., Hodges, J. R., & Price, C. J. (1998). Functional neuroanatomy of the semantic system: Divisible by what? *Journal of Cognitive Neuroscience*, *10*(6), 766–777.

Mummery, C. J., Patterson, K., Hodges, J. R., & Wise, R. J. S. (1996). Generating 'tiger' as an animal name or a word beginning with T: Differences in brain activation. *Proceedings Biological Sciences/Royal Society*, *263*(1373), 989–995.

Mummery, C. J., Shallice, T., & Price, C. J. (1999). Dual-process model in semantic priming: A functional imaging perspective. *Neuroimage*, *9*(5), 516–525.

Neely, J. H. (1991). Semantic priming effects in visual word recognition: A selective review of current findings and theory. In D. Besner & G. W. Humphreys (Eds.), *Basic processes in reading: Visual word recognition* (pp. 264–336). Hillsdale, NJ: Erlbaum.

Nobre, A. C., Allison, T., & McCarthy, G. (1994). Word recognition in the human inferior temporal lobe. *Nature*, *37*(6503), 260–263.

Noppeney, U., Phillips, J., & Price, C. (2004). The neural areas that control the retrieval and selection of semantics. *Neuropsychologia*, *42*(9), 1269–1280.

Perani, D., Schnur, T., Tettamanti, M., Gorno-Tempini, M., Cappa, S. F., & Fazio, F. (1999). Word and picture matching: A PET study of semantic category effects. *Neuropsychologia*, *37*(3), 293–306.

Posner, M. I., & DiGirolamo, G. J. (1998). Executive attention: Conflict, target detection, and cognitive control. In R. Parasuraman (Ed.), *The attentive brain*. Cambridge, MA: MIT Press.

Quaresima, V., Ferrari, M., Torricelli, A., Spinelli, L., Pifferi, A., & Cubeddu, R. (2005). Bilateral prefrontal cortex oxygenation responses to a verbal fluency task: A multichannel time-resolved near-infrared topography study. *Journal of Biomedical Optics*, *10*(1), 11012.

Quaresima, V., Giosuè, P., Roncone, R., Casacchia, M., & Ferrari, M. (2009). Prefrontal cortex dysfunction during cognitive tests evidenced by functional near-infrared spectroscopy. *Psychiatry Research: Neuroimaging*, *171*(3), 252–257.

Rossel, S. L., Price, C. J., & Nobre, A. C. (2003). The anatomy and time course of semantic priming investigated by fMRI and ERPs. *Neuropsychologia*, *41*(5), 550–564.

Sachs, O., Weis, S., Krings, T., Huber, W., & Kircher, T. (2008a). Categorical and thematic knowledge representation in the brain: Neural correlates of taxonomic and thematic conceptual relations. *Neuropsychologia*, *46*(2), 409–418.

Sachs, O., Weis, S., Zellagui, N., Hubert, W., Zvyagintsev, M., Mathiak, K., & Kircher, T. (2008b). Automatic processing of semantic relations in fMRI: Neural activation during semantic priming of taxonomic and thematic categories. *Brain Research*, *1218*, 194–205.

Schecklmann, M., Ehlis, A. C., Plichta, M. M., & Fallgatter, A. J. (2008). Functional near-infrared spectroscopy: A long-term reliable tool for measuring brain activity during verbal fluency. *Neuroimage*, *43*(1), 147–155.

Shibasaki, H. (2008). Human brain mapping: Hemodynamic response and electrophysiology. *Clinical Neurophysiology*, *119*(4), 731–743.

Snyder, H. R., Feigenson, K., & Thompson-Schill, S. L. (2007). Prefrontal cortical response to conflict during semantic and phonological tasks. *Journal of Cognitive Neuroscience*, *19*(5), 761–775.

Spalek, K., & Thompson-Schill, S. L. (2008). Task-dependent semantic interference in language production: An fMRI study. *Brain and Language*, *107*(3), 220–228.

Swick, D., & Knight, R. T. (1996). Is prefrontal cortex involved in cued recall? A neuropsychological test of PET findings. *Neuropsychologia*, *34*(10), 1019–1028.

Thompson-Schill, S. L., Aguirre, G. K., D'Esposito, M., & Farah, M. J. (1999). A neural basis for category and modality specific of semantic knowledge. *Neuropsychologia*, *37*(6), 671–676.

Thompson-Schill, S. L., D'Esposito, M., Aguirre, G. K., & Farah, M. J. (1997). Role of left inferior prefrontal cortex in retrieval of semantic knowledge: A reevaluation. *Proceedings of the National Academy of Sciences of the USA*, *94*(26), 14792–14797.

Troyer, A. K., Moscovitch, M., Winocur, G., Alexander, M. P., & Stuss, D. (1998). Clustering and switching on verbal fluency: The effects of focal frontal- and temporal-lobe lesions. *Neuropsychologia*, *36*(6), 499–504.

Tse, C.Y., Lee, C. L., Sullivan, J., Garnsey, S. M., Dell, G. S., Fabiani, M., & Gratton, G. (2007). Imaging cortical dynamics of language processing with the event-related optical signal. *Proceedings of the National Academy of Sciences of the USA, 104*(43), 17157–17162.

Tulving, E. (1972). Episodic and semantic memory. In E. Tulving & W. Donaldson (Eds.), *Organization of memory*. New York: Academic Press.

Tyler, L. K., & Moss, H. E. (2001). Towards a distributed account of conceptual knowledge. *Trends in Cognitive Sciences, 5*(6), 244–252.

Van Petten, C., & Luka, B. J. (2006). Neural localization of semantic context effects in electromagnetic and hemodynamic studies. *Brain and Language, 97*(3), 279–293.

Wagner, A. D., Pare-Blagoev, E. J., Clark, J., & Poldrack, R. A. (2001). Recovering meaning: Left prefrontal cortex guides controlled semantic retrieval. *Neuron, 31*(2), 329–338.

Walter, N., Jbabdi, S., Marrelec, G., Benali, H., & Joanette, Y. (2006, March 1–4). Carl Wernicke was essentially right: FMRI brain interactivity analysis of phonological and semantic processing of isolated word. Communication presented at the World Federation of Neurology: Aphasia and Cognitive Disorders Research Group, Buenos Aires (Argentina).

Warrington, E. K., & McCarthy, R. A. (1994). Multiple meaning systems in the brain: A case of visual semantics. *Neuropsychologia, 32*(12), 1465–1473.

Warrington, E. K., & Shallice, T. (1984). Category specific semantic impairments. *Brain, 107*(3), 829–854.

Watanabe, A., Matsuo, K., Kato, N., & Kato, T. (2003). Cerebrovascular responses to cognitive tasks and hyperventilation measured by multi-channel near-infrared spectroscopy. *Journal of Neuropsychiatry and Clinical Neurosciences, 15*(4), 442–449.

Wernicke, C. (1874). *Der aphasische Symptomenkomplex. Eine psychologische Studie auf anatomischer Basis*. Breslau: Max Cohn & Weigert.

Wood, A. G., Saling, M. M., Abbott, D. F., & Jackson, G. D. (2001). A neurocognitive account of frontal lobe involvement in orthographic lexical retrieval: An fMRI study. *Neuroimage, 14*(1 Pt 1), 162–169.

6

FROM PHONEMES TO DISCOURSE

Event-related brain potentials (ERPs) and paradigms for investigating normal and abnormal language processing

Marta Kutas and Michael Kiang

Introduction

Over the past few decades technological advances have made it possible to characterize typical, atypical, or compromised language comprehension and production by eliciting and then "reading" patterns of voltage differences between electrodes on the human scalp. Indeed, electrical brain activity (or "brainwaves") triggered by written, spoken, signed, gestured, or depicted events in the physical world can serve as windows on the brain's responsivities, representations, and computations. Such event-related brain potentials (ERPs) can be recorded throughout the lifespan, at various levels of consciousness (from alert or sleeping healthy individuals to comatose or vegetative state patients), and in populations diverse in their abilities to respond motorically. These electrical "snapshots" of neocortical activity concomitant with comprehension and production of language offer a relatively sensitive and temporally precise look at the factors that influence human communication.

In this review we examine normal linguistic and communicative processes via scalp-recorded brainwave studies of reading, listening, signing, and gesturing. The topics range from how brains respond to small linguistic units (e.g., phonemes) to higher levels of linguistic analysis (e.g., pragmatic aspects of discourse comprehension). We introduce robust paradigms, describe the concomitant patterns of electrical brain activity, and explain what sorts of questions about language they can answer, even if little indicates that either the dependent measures or answers are language specific.

Electrophysiological measures of brain activity

The electroencephalogram (EEG) reflects ongoing, so-called background electrical activity of the brain, which is typically decomposed into frequency bands (delta, theta, alpha, beta, gamma), and analyzed as power in these bands as a function of recording site and task conditions (though see Donoghue et al., 2020, for a principled method of quantifying the neural power spectrum and increasing analytical power by separating oscillations from aperiodic activity).

Of importance for researchers – even if background EEG is presumably averaged out in the calculation of an average ERP – are changes in EEG with age (at different rates in different cortical areas) and clinical condition. Clinical groups, for example, often show less power in the higher frequencies, suggesting a maturational lag, given that normal maturation is characterized by decreased

DOI: 10.4324/9781003204213-8

power in lower frequencies and increased power in higher ones (Clarke et al., 2001). EEG can be used to assess cognitive functions across a lifetime. In the past few decades, electrophysiologists also have analyzed spectral changes of power and phase in different frequency bands in response to stimuli/events (known as event-related synchronization or desynchronization; Pfurtscheller & Lopes da Silva, 1999), and the systematic relationships between evoked and induced rhythms and various cognitive processes.

Oscillations (rhythmic activity within a narrow band frequency) have been hypothesized to coordinate interregional information transfer. Oscillations support neural networks that bias exchange of spike volleys between brain regions using phase locking and local phase amplitude coupling (PAC) where lower frequencies modulate high-frequency actvity (HFA), and directional PAC where a region sends a low-frequency oscillation to modulate the occurrence of HFA activity in another. These network dynamics operate on a background of neural activity (traditionally viewed as noise) with a characteristic 1/f function (power falling off exponentially with frequency). EEG research is currently being turned topsy-turvy by findings showing that the 1/f slope is not noise, may track changes in excitatory/inhibitory balance, changes with advancing age, and seems to play an important role in cognition and various disorders and diseases (Molina et al., 2020; Voytek et al., 2015).

ERPs are the electrical brain activity synchronized in time to a stimulus, response, event, or its absence. ERPs can be recorded intracranially with depth electrodes (typically in individuals with intractable epilepsy, aka intracranial EEG or iEEG), or with "wet" electrodes at the scalp surface or "dry" electrodes, embedded in a cap, net, helmet, or band. Electrocorticography (ECOG) is a type of iEEG recorded from exposed cortex that has played an increasingly greater role in language studies because it is relatively large absent the attenuating power of the skull, has millimeter-scale spatial resolution, and has a frequency bandwidth up to 200 Hz, providing unfettered access to high frequency activity (gamma plus) linked to speech. Because of ECOG's invasiveness, however, its use is typically restricted to individuals with epilepsy being prepared for surgery (Vakani & Nair, 2019).

ERPs are presumed to be the neocortical region's response to eliciting events, comprised of millisecond-by-millisecond time series of voltages at individual recording sites. ERPs are typically extracted via averaging across multiple repetitions of an eliciting event. The eliciting events need not be the same physical stimulus as long as they are conceptually similar within the experiment: e.g., averaging the responses to anomalies across 40 different, but similarly anomalous, sentences. The ERP waveform tracks information processing (post-synaptic potentials) as "sensory inputs" travel from the eye or ear to the brain/mind for comprehension, or in reverse, as "outputs" travel from mind to tongue or hand for production. The scalp ERP, at each recording site, is an instantaneous reflection of the sum of all the electrical brain activity that meets criteria for being recordable at the scalp (see Kutas & Dale, 1997). Measuring how such signals change over (ab)normal development, as a function of healthy or pathological aging, or due to brain damage, offers a few applications for which ERPs are advantageous, as they can be elicited even without any overt behavior or explicit task demand.

ERPs offer an image of neocortical brain activity at multiple timescales, from milliseconds to seconds recorded in a continuous, relatively non-invasive manner. All studies reviewed here rely on the ERP method, using well-known paradigms with stimuli or responses occurring at a predetermined or self-paced rate. The moment of stimulus or movement onset – or at which the (missing) item (would have) occurred – is considered "zero" on the time axis; in this way the ERP is temporally synchronized to an eliciting event. What exactly these ERPs or voltage waveforms represent, however, is a matter of debate. On one view, the electrical brain activity synchronized to stimulus onset reflects the subset of summed post-synaptic potentials associated with neural analysis of that item at that moment that can be seen at the scalp. On an alternative view, each item merely perturbs (and re-aligns) the ongoing EEG rhythms. In either case, these recordings are a time series of potentials generated by the brain in response to events, which can be interpreted within the context of an experimental design to reveal how brains construe or produce language.

While this methodology has much to recommend it for the study of cognitive or language phenomena, "reading" ERP waveforms is neither straightforward nor intuitive. Although electrical brain activity is sensitive to a variety of factors (e.g., recency of last meal, tiredness, or a person's mood during recording, among many others), these potentials do not come with a legend. At any given moment, the ERP waveform is negative, positive, or neutral in voltage relative to some baseline, but these peaks and troughs have no intrinsic meaning as to their neural generators. Nonetheless, cognitive ERPers have been compiling a glossary of ERP components and effects by developing manipulations that *usually* elicit and modulate them. These in turn are defined by their polarity, shape, amplitude topography across the scalp, and latency relative to zero. The patterns – which by convention derive their names from their polarity and/or approximate latency (e.g., N400, P600), location (left anterior negativity), or hypothesized functional significance (e.g., lateralized readiness potential, mismatch negativity, mismatch response, NoGo N200, error-related negativity) – serve as proxies for various constructs or information processing operations (e.g., response preparation, sensory discrimination, auditory pattern regularity violation, focused selective attention, error processing, semantic processing, working memory updating, grammatical processing, etc.) and can sometimes adjudicate alternative theoretical accounts of some psychological phenomenon. We hedge in noting that certain manipulations *usually* lead to particular brainwave patterns, because sometimes they do not, contrary to well-conceived hypotheses and published findings (a case in point being the N400 discovered in a study designed to elicit a posterior P300). There are few, if any, linguistic/cognitive processes under neocortical purview that cannot benefit from ERP analyses. That said, the language ERP literature is vast and we are limited by space to a selective overview beginning with production followed by a few levels of language comprehension.

Investigating production via response preparation and monitoring

ERP investigations of language "production" have been relatively scarce compared to those of comprehension, primarily because ERPs, like most neuroimaging methods, are not tolerant of bodily movements. However, certain advances over the last 30 years or so have led to an upswing in such studies: development of analytic procedures (e.g., independent components analysis and Second Order Blind Identification) for decomposing scalp-recorded signals and extracting relevant and discarding irrelevant (artifactual) subcomponents (Delorme et al., 2007; Romero et al., 2008); the use of tasks such as picture naming which is slower than reading words aloud, thereby leaving almost the first half-second after picture onset free of speech-related contamination; or using tasks that call for delayed or covert naming. Of course, these solutions eliminate scrutiny of names produced so quickly that they would contaminate the artifact-free zone of the waveform (or limit the analysis epoch to the shortest response latency), or so slowly that the relevant processes fall beyond the 500-ms analysis epoch.

Picture-naming ERP studies are typically electrophysiological versions of naming-time studies designed to delineate stages of word production (lexical selection, lemma retrieval, morphological and phonological code retrieval, articulation); the majority rely on naming isolated pictures in contexts known to yield well-established behavioral effects in monolingual and/or bilingual speakers (e.g., picture-word interference task, cumulative semantic interference paradigm, language switching, translation from one language to another).

Most picture-naming ERP studies have been focused on the time course of word selection during single word production. One of the more consistent findings is the modulation of a posterior P2 (150-200 ms), larger for lexical items that are harder to access (Strijkers et al., 2010). Overall, ERP data suggest that lexical selection/access takes place by at least 200 ms post-picture onset (e.g., Aristei et al., 2011), phonological encoding between 275 and 400 ms (Eulitz et al., 2000), and morphological processes starting at ~350 ms (Koester & Schiller, 2008) – a timecourse broadly in line with Indefrey and Levelt's (2000) model. A few studies have ventured beyond single word production (Lange et al., 2015; Timmers et al., 2013).

Much also has been learned from clever experimental paradigms for monitoring preparation to produce, even when no production occurs. ERP effects used to delineate stages of information processing, in general, and language production, in particular, include the lateralized readiness potential (LRP); the NoGo-N200 (a frontocentral negative stimulus-locked ERP peaking around 200 ms, or later depending on information availability, reflecting response inhibition); and the error-related negativity or ERN (also known as the Ne), a potential linked to performance monitoring, error processing (peaking around 100 ms post-response onset), conflict/inhibition, or to a feedback stimulus, with an amplitude sensitive to mood and personality (Luu et al., 2000).

The readiness potential (RP), from which the LRP is derived, is a gradually increasing negativity beginning about 500 ms to 1 sec prior to a prepared movement (onset defined by switch closure or muscle activity), whether voluntary (Deecke et al., 1969) or elicited by an "imperative" stimulus (Rohrbaugh et al., 1976). RPs can be initiated by body limbs as well as swallowing and speaking. The initial symmetric portion of the RP is contingent on supplementary motor area functioning; its later asymmetric portion, generated in the primary motor cortex, is contingent on cerebello-thalamo-cortical loop functioning. Besides its characterization in individuals with motor problems, the RP has been employed with healthy people in studies of "free will," because it begins before individuals indicate awareness of their intent to move (Libet et al., 1983; Sirigu et al., 2004). As RPs are not seen preceding speeded responses to stimuli at unpredictable intervals for which individuals cannot prepare (Papa et al., 1991), it is taken to reflect movement preparation, rather than movement per se. This in combination with (a) its contralateral, somatotopic topography – more negative over right central sites preceding left finger, hand, or arm movements, and vice versa, and (b) its identifiability in stimulus-locked (not just response-locked) ERP waveforms, have made the RP a useful index of the timing of mental events (mental chronometry).

The LRP – derived from RPs elicited in paradigms wherein the response-related asymmetry over central sites is a proxy for response activation (de Jong et al., 1988; Gratton et al., 1988) – has been of great utility in analyzing the stimulus versus response aspects of information processing. The LRP can be derived in several ways (e.g., double subtraction method or subtraction averaging method), which are equivalent as long as within a given experimental condition, a right-hand response is correct for half the trials and a left-hand response for the other half. In the subtraction averaging procedure, the ERP from the central site ipsilateral to the responding hand is subtracted from the ERP on the contralateral site, separately for each hand, and the two are averaged. The resultant LRP, if any, reflects lateralization due to motor preparation with direction (polarity) indicating which response has been preferentially activated, magnitude indicating degree of activation, and latency indicating when activation occurred.

Accordingly, LRPs have been used to investigate the dynamics of information processing (e.g., partial information transmission), the order in which different stimulus attributes are extracted, the processing locus of various experimental effects, and individual differences. Whenever a question can be phrased in terms of the relative activation of the two responses (right and left hands), an LRP analysis can provide an answer. The most common methods of eliciting RPs for LRP derivation are via the conflict and Go-NoGo paradigms as long as the experimental stimuli have multiple attributes which can be mapped onto different responses (hands) or different aspects of a response (respond or not). In the conflict paradigm, the different attributes are mapped onto the same hand in some conditions and different hands in others, with critical inferences drawn from the direction of the LRP on conflict trials. In the Go-NoGo paradigm one attribute determines which hand will respond, if a response is required, which is determined by the other attribute; critical inferences are then drawn from the presence and timing of the LRP on NoGo trials. This Go-NoGo paradigm is also the experimental milieu for eliciting a NoGo N2 (an index of response inhibition), whose timing affords inferences about the timepoint by which information for a (prepared) response must have been available. The Go-NoGo paradigm has been used to adjudicate language production accounts.

Schmitt, Münte, and Kutas (2000) used the LRP and NoGo N200 to determine the relative timing of access to semantic and phonological information during tacit picture naming. Participants viewed pictures of animals or inanimate objects (the semantic attribute) whose names began with a vowel or a consonant (the phonological attribute). In one condition, the Go-NoGo decision was contingent on the semantic attribute, and the response hand on the phonological; in the other, with reversed mapping the Go-NoGo decision was contingent on the phonological attribute, and the response hand on the semantic. Regardless of condition, all Go trials should be associated with large indistinguishable LRPs (as long as the isolated semantic and phonological decisions are equally difficult). Of critical interest are LRPs on NoGo trials. Reliable presence of LRPs – even a short-lived one – on NoGo trials implies that the information indicating which hand to prepare is available before that indicating whether to respond at all. LRP duration provides an upper limit on the time by which the information not to respond has become available. By contrast, the absence of LRPs on NoGo trials implies that the information on which the response hand hinges is available coincident with or after the information on which responding hinges. Schmitt et al. found reliable LRPs on NoGo trials when contingent on phonology but not when contingent on semantics, suggesting prior access to semantic compared to phonological information (see Figure 6.1a).

In these types of experiments, participants do not voice the picture's name, thereby minimizing muscle artifacts due to speech. It is assumed (although not universally) that participants engage the same semantic and phonological processes for tacit as for overt naming. LRP analyses in dual-choice Go-NoGo tasks of this type demonstrate that semantic information (animal versus object) is available before phonological information (van Turennout et al., 1997) and that semantic information (an object's weight) is also available before syntactic gender in German or Dutch (Schmitt et al., 2001). Using a slightly different design, Abdel Rahman, van Turennout and Levelt (2003) showed that phonological retrieval is not contingent on retrieval of semantic information – as proposed by serial models of language production (e.g., Levelt et al., 1999); but, rather, can occur before semantic access, consistent with parallel processing of the two (e.g., Dell & O'Seaghdha, 1992).

To date, the potential of the LRP (and NoGo N200, which is the more robust of these ERP effects) to examine whether, and if so how, clinical (cognitive or motor) disorders might affect the timing of language processes has remained largely untapped. By identifying the time points at which semantic and phonological information are accessed, for example, LRPs in a Go-NoGo paradigm could provide data on the impact of diminished availability of semantic information on naming deficits in individuals with Alzheimer's dementia.

Language comprehension

The bulk of the ERP language literature has focused on investigating comprehension of language – written, spoken (with and without gesture), and signed. ERPs have proven especially useful for this purpose because their exquisite temporal sensitivity spans the analysis of language signals from phonemes to discourse.

Language or not? Early sensory components

Evoked potentials (EPs) within the 200 ms following stimulus onset are considered obligatory and are presumed to reflect sensory processing, occasionally with attentional modulation. These sensory EPs are modality-specific; their amplitudes and/or latencies vary with physical parameters (intensity, frequency, timing) of the stimuli. Abnormalities in these EPs are routinely used to assess

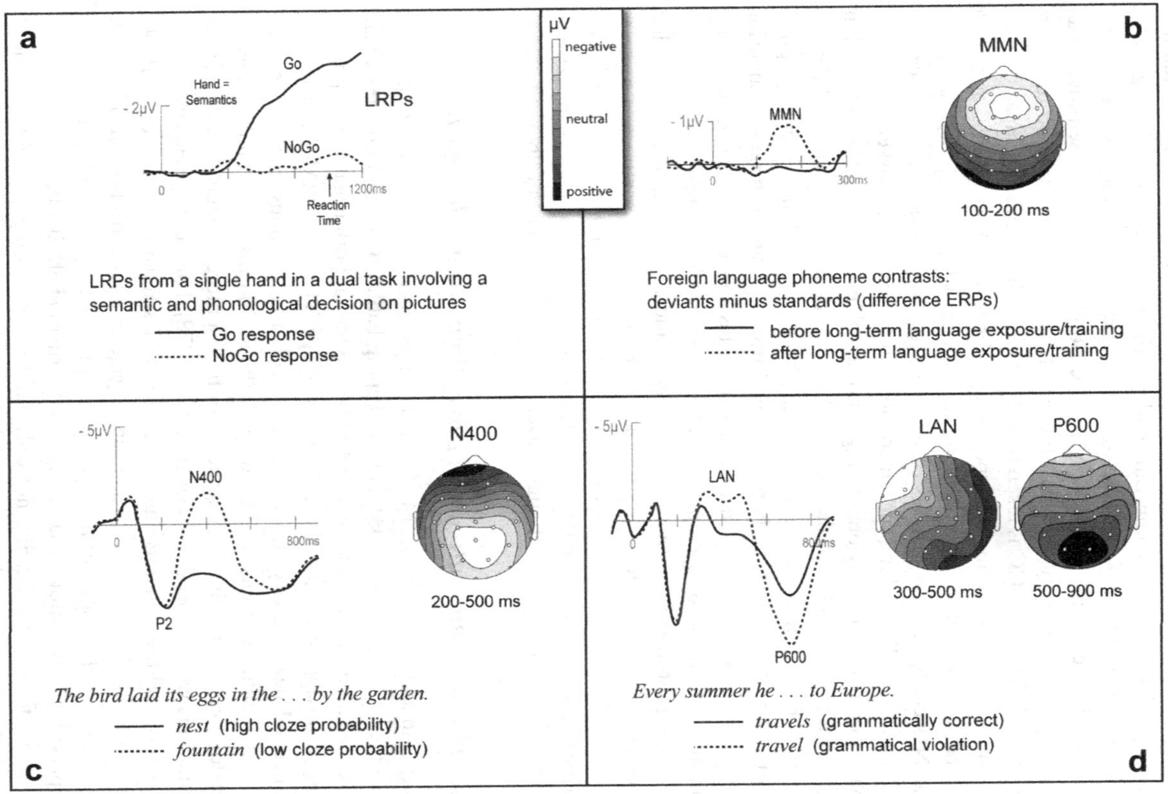

Figure 6.1 Idealized versions of five ERP effects (waveforms and scalp topography) used for investigating language. By convention, negative voltage is plotted upward. (a) LRPs (see text for derivation) in a dual task Go-NoGo paradigm, with responding hand determined by outcome of a semantic decision and whether to respond (go) or not (nogo) determined by outcome of a phonological decision. There is a large LRP on go trials, but also a reliable nogo response (~400 ms), indicating response activation, on nogo trials. (b) The MMN created by subtracting ERPs to standards from ERPs to deviants; compared are MMNs to the same phoneme contrasts salient in a second – but not native – language, prior to and following long-term language exposure/training. The large, fronto-central MMN indicates perceptual sensitivity to the phoneme distinction as a result of training. (c) A centro-parietal N400 effect for more versus less contextually expected continuations within a written sentence. (d) The left anterior negativity (LAN) and P600 elicited by subject-verb agreement errors in written sentences. The LAN (as shown here) has a frontal and left-lateralized focus and the P600 has a centro-parietal focus, though the scalp distributions of both effects vary across studies.

the integrity of the evoking sensory system. For instance, the auditory brainstem response (ABR, aka BER) is a highly replicable response occurring within 10 ms post-click onset used to screen hearing in newborns, children, and individuals with brainstem lesions; it is impervious to attention, sleep, or sedation. Given infinite resources, every ERP investigation of language and non-language auditory processing would begin with audiometric and ABR assessments to rule out peripheral abnormalities coincident with auditory language deficits.

The P1-N1-P2 complex elicited by a brief stimulus reflects the neural processing of sound at the auditory cortex. Longer-lasting stimuli comprising multiple time-varying acoustic changes, e.g., speech, elicit multiple overlapping P1-N1-P2 responses time-locked to stimulus onset, change(s), and offset. This "acoustic change complex" (ACC; Martin & Boothroyd, 1999) is sensitive to all manner of acoustic changes in speech, even in the absence of attention, and has good test-retest reliability (Tremblay et al., 2003). The ACC is taken to index speech discrimination capacity.

Early EP componentry can be used to monitor speech segmentation and detection. Comparing EPs before and after training on multisyllabic nonsense words (e.g., *babupu* or *bupada*), Sanders et al. (2003) found that N1s could serve as markers of word onsets in continuous speech (see also Tremblay & Kraus, 2002 for N1-P2 tracking speech-sound training). Such EP markers can monitor learning in individuals for whom behavioral testing is not a viable option (e.g., infants), and in individuals with dyslexia, autism, or delayed talking, as well as second language learners. The N1 is comprised of three functionally distinct subcomponents: the N1a generated in the supratemporal plane of auditory cortex, and N1b and N1c, both generated from the lateral surface of superior temporal gyri, albeit with different maturational trajectories. This suggests caution generalizing across studies (within or across individuals) employing different electrode montages.

As surface reflections of post-synaptic activity, ERPs are good indices of synaptic plasticity (due to experience, learning). Changes in auditory- and/or speech-triggered ERPs can be used to assess the functional reorganization of the central auditory system after introduction of hearing aids or a cochlear implant. Critically, auditory EPs can be reliably recorded with equal sensitivity in a variety of clinical groups from infancy to old age (although waveforms change systematically with age).

Phonemic discrimination and categorical perception: mismatch negativities

A case in point is the mismatch negativity (MMN) which can be recorded not only in neonates (including those born preterm at 30–35 weeks), but in sleeping babies (Cheour-Luhtanen et al., 1995); in infants, it is called a mismatch response (MMR) because it has both negative and positive aspects, with the positive disappearing around seven years of age. The adult MMN is a fronto-central negativity generated near primary auditory cortex (with a contentious frontal lobe contribution), which in early studies was recorded between 100 and 300 ms post-stimulus onset to infrequent tones that deviated in pitch, intensity, or duration from a more frequent "standard" tone stream in which the deviants were embedded (Naatanen et al., 1978). The greater the deviance, the larger the MMN amplitude and the earlier its onset, given the same standard (Tiitinen et al., 1994). Critically, the MMN can be elicited even as participants engage in a cognitively demanding task (e.g., playing a video game, watching a silent movie) and need not overtly respond to any sounds, although it is not impervious to attentional manipulations (Sussman et al., 2014).

MMNs have proven useful for investigating not only auditory processing capabilities in neuropsychiatric, neurological, and neurodevelopmental disorders (Sussman et al., 2014) but also typical and atypical speech perception. Once a representation of a standard (a repeating regularity) exists, violations of that regularity elicit an MMN as long as it is a pattern that the individual's brain can detect. Standards can be created by stimulus-driven and/or top-down control at any level, e.g., phonemes, syllables, words, and abstract patterns such as complex regularities where the commonality of the "standard" lies in a "rule-like" association (e.g., the MMN is elicited by a descending tone pair (deviant) in a stream of ascending tone pair standards; Paavilainen et al., 1999). Thus, the initial proposal that the MMN is strictly an index of sensory discrimination has been replaced by the view that it is an involuntary memory-based brain response to change in an auditory stream (more generally, a regularity violation response). MMN findings are revealing what sorts of auditory patterns are stored in the auditory cortex, and since the late 1990s have shown how these patterns (e.g., speech) can be altered by exposure and training (for trends in MMN research, see Special Issue in *Brain Topography*, 2014).

The MMN has been used to monitor the acquisition of native and non-native, real and artificial, speech contrasts in infants, children, and adults. For example, Cheour et al. (1998) adapted an MMN paradigm for a cross-linguistic analysis with Finnish and Estonian infants to demonstrate that language-specific memory traces develop at 6–12 months of age. Their standard stimulus was a vowel prototype in both languages (/e/), as was one of the deviants (/ö/); the other deviant occurred only in Estonian (/õ/). Both infant groups showed larger amplitude MMNs to the Finnish-Estonian /ö/ deviant at one year than at six months. However, only Estonian infants showed a similar age-related increase to the Estonian /õ/ deviant; Finnish infants, by contrast, showed a decrease. Thus, within the first year, infants' ability to discriminate native vowel sounds improves as their discrimination of non-native speech sounds diminishes. Winkler et al. (1999) used a similar paradigm with adult monolingual and bilingual speakers to demonstrate categorization of second-language phonemes with language experience. Finns and "Finnish-fluent" Hungarians, but not "Finnish-naïve" Hungarians, showed increased MMNs to vowel categories perceptually distinctive in Finnish, but not in Hungarian (see Figure 6.1b). Such results argue for long-term changes in the adult brain regions involved in phonetic analysis.

The MMN also has been used to assess the relationship between general auditory processing and language deficits in children with dyslexia or specific language impairment (SLI) as well as auditory, language, and/or cognitive abilities in individuals with acquired aphasia, or autism spectrum disorders (reviewed by Naatanen et al. 2014). For example, Baldeweg et al. (1999) explored the hypothesis that specific low-level auditory perceptual deficits are implicated in dyslexia. Specifically, they predicted (and found) that the N1 and MMNs to duration-based deviants would be normal, whereas MMNs to pitch-based deviants would not. These results highlight how the multi-dimensional nature of the ERP (voltage waveform in time linked to different processes) affords a look at multiple processing operations and their interplay in supporting perception and behavior. This study also highlights an important design decision to support specificity – namely, including a comparison expected to yield normal data along with the one expected to be problematic.

Another example of this can be seen in an investigation of whether auditory discrimination difficulties exhibited by children diagnosed with SLI are specific to speech (phonological) or are of a more general auditory nature. Speech and non-speech contrasts, matched in the complexity of acoustic changes (unlike much of the extant literature), served as stimuli in active behavioral tasks and passive MMN paradigms (Davids et al., 2011). The SLI group of five-year-olds (with attested receptive and production speech and language problems) was impaired in behaviorally discriminating the linguistic contrasts compared to age, gender, and non-verbal IQ-matched controls (with typical speech and language development); unlike typical adults, neither group of children could behaviorally discriminate the non-linguistic contrast, presumably due to immature metacognitive (attentional) skills. Children in the SLI group did not exhibit MMNs to the linguistic or non-linguistic contrasts whereas the controls did. Taken together with the worse performance of the SLI group (vs. controls) on all pre-tests of language and attention, it seems that children with SLI have both a phonological deficit and general auditory processing difficulties. Whether the phonological deficit is caused by the general auditory problem cannot be answered by these data, but demonstrating that the control five-year-olds elicit MMNs to a non-linguistic contrast they cannot yet distinguish behaviorally has therapeutic implications given the apparently greater sensitivity of neural (versus behavioral) discrimination, which can be assessed with a passive task.

In sum, the MMN offers an index of the functioning of the auditory memory system that is sensitive to long-term perceptual learning. Critically for diagnostic purposes, the MMN is easy to record, and does not require participant engagement, which neither infants nor others with communication limitations could readily accommodate. As noted, the MMN paradigm has found numerous clinical applications, e.g., in studies of developmental speech, language and literacy impairments, auditory perceptual auditory memory and/or processing deficits in individuals with aphasia, dementia, Parkinson's disease, epilepsy, and other neurological disorders (Naatanen et al., 2014). Given the MMN's sensitivity to long-term experience with the perceptual properties of language, its utility as an analytic tool is limited only by the cleverness of the experimenter in choosing repeating patterns to violate – even though it is not language-specific.

A final note: to date, there are no data to support any substantive relationship between the MMN and the phonological mismatch negativity (PMN), so named by Connolly and Phillips (1994) because it was elicited by a mismatch between the word-initial phoneme of a contextually expected sentence ending and that of other sentence-final words, regardless of semantic congruity. While others have reported similar (albeit not identical) effects with phonological manipulations, explanations range from the PMN being the initial phase of an N400 congruity effect (Van Petten et al., 1999) to its being an N200, distinct from a later N400 effect (van den Brink et al., 2001). Attempts to localize the PMNm (magnetic counterpart of the electrical PMN) to phonological mismatches for words in a lexical decision task have implicated at least partially non-overlapping brain areas with the N400m (Kujala et al., 2004). The issue, however, remains unresolved. Using word lists designed to separate phonological (alliterative) and semantic (category) constraints and sentences with phonological and/or semantic congruency manipulations, Diaz and Swaab (2007) found that both context and task were relevant to the ERP patterns observed. Early negativities to a phonological mismatch at the end of an alliterative word list versus a semantically (in)congruent sentence context had different amplitude maxima at the scalp; in sentences, its topography resembled that of the semantic congruity N400 effect and was thus taken to reflect (early) semantic goodness of fit. In any case, the data from these laboratories all show that context affects word processing and contextual integration quite early, sometimes before a spoken word is fully identified.

Word, sentence, and discourse level comprehension

Although ERPs can be used to explore language comprehension at multiple levels of granularity, most of the work to date has focused on words in isolation, word pairs, sentences, and short discourses. The latter is important, because the presence or absence of certain ERP responses to semantic anomalies or lexical prediction violations appears to be contingent on the comprehender's goal(s) as well as the constraint, length, and semantic richness of the discourse context in which the violations occur (Brothers et al., 2020). The most robust ERP comprehension-sensitive effects – like the N400 and posterior post-N400 positivities (pPNP) – are observed whether the eliciting stimuli are written, spoken, signed, or depicted. Arguably, the most likely ERP effect to be language-specific is the early left anterior negativity (eLAN) often seen in response to violations of word class (i.e., to a word from one lexical class when another is expected, e.g., to a verb when a preposition is more likely to occur).

Measures of meaning: from words to pragmatics

ERP research with words, pseudowords, pictures, gestures, acronyms, environmental sounds, and other potentially meaningful items has revealed that the interval between approximately 200 and 500 ms post-stimulus onset (i.e., the N400 time window) is sensitive to many of the factors that influence ease of lexical access such as frequency of occurrence, repetition, semantic relations, orthographic and phonological neighborhood size, and world knowledge, among others; and factors that reduce the number of likely continuations or increase the probability (and thus predictability) of the next stimulus (see Table 6.1). The average electrical brain activity during this window to such items in relative isolation is typically negative (relative to a pre-stimulus baseline and mastoid reference) or negative-going, peaking ~400 ms. This is what is meant by N400 as the default response to any potentially meaningful item; ERPs to illegal non-words or non-environmental sounds in isolation, for instance, do not typically exhibit an N400, although they may in a sentence context (Laszlo & Federmeier, 2008), like acronyms, e.g., IBM, NASA, etc., do. Many types of context generally reduce N400 amplitude with increasing contextual fit. For instance, the N400 to the second of a pair of words is smaller if the words are semantically associated or related (e.g., cat-dog) than if they are not (table-dog). Likewise, the N400 to a sentence-medial or sentence-final word is smaller if the word is semantically congruent with the preceding sentence fragment than if it is not (*I take coffee with cream and* *<u>sugar</u>* *vs.* *<u>dog</u>*). These examples illustrate two classic N400-eliciting paradigms. Word pairs embedded within a variety of tasks (e.g., lexical decision) have revealed that N400 activity is sensitive to phonological, orthographic, morphological, semantic, associative, and conceptual relations (see Kutas & Hillyard, 1989, for task-related issues). The anomalous sentence or sentence congruity paradigm similarly has been combined with different tasks, although reading or listening and comprehending suffice to assess N400 modulations. This paradigm is an excellent psycholinguistic tool for all types of individuals, including those with compromised or atypical brains, because while semantic anomalies usually elicit large N400s, smaller but reliable N400s also can be seen to words in garden-variety sentences – sans complex structure, anomalies, or ambiguities of any sort (e.g., *He was soothed by the gentle* *<u>wind</u>*.). All else being constant, N400 amplitude is inversely correlated ($r = -.90$) with the eliciting word's offline cloze probability, a proxy for item predictability (see Kutas & Hillyard, 1984; DeLong et al., 2005; Figure 6.1c), although there are circumstances where the relation does not hold.

In young adults, the N400 has a 400 ms peak latency that is relatively stable across experimental paradigms, with a centro-posterior scalp maximum varying slightly with the modality (visual or auditory) and/or nature (pictorial, linguistic, or nonlinguistic) of the eliciting stimuli. N400 amplitudes decrease and latencies increase with normal aging (e.g., Kutas & Iragui, 1998), and even more with dementia.

It is primarily N400 amplitude, not latency, that varies with experimental manipulations that have been found to influence word recognition times (Laszlo & Federmeier, 2009), leading to Federmeier's (2021) proposal that N400 is not specific to semantic access of a specific item upon recognition but rather the activity across the distributed network (semantic long-term memory)

Table 6.1 Some linguistic and physical factors that influence N400 amplitude

	Influence on N400 amplitude
Lexical association	Semantically related primes reduce N400 amplitude to target words
Repetition	Reduced negativity to repeated words
Frequency	Smaller negativity to more frequent than rare words
Word class (open/closed)	Larger negativity to open-class words over posterior sites
Concreteness	Larger negativity to isolated concrete compared to abstract words over frontal sites
Offline expectancy (cloze probability)	Reduced negativity to more versus less predictable words within a sentence/ discourse context
Sentence position	Reduced negativity for open class words across sentence position: larger effect for initial words than approaching sentence end; at least for isolated sentences
Orthographic neighborhood	Larger negativity to items with many (rather than few) neighbors, all else constant

with which the perceptual analysis of the eliciting item makes initial contact; the more new information that is activated in the network, the larger the N400 to the eliciting item. N400 amplitude to a word is thought to reflect the retrieval of or access to its semantic features that have not been pre-activated. More generally, Federmeier unleashes N400 processes from recognition and ties them to time.

While most factors that affect recognition times do not alter N400 latency, some other factors do: e.g., in young adults presentation rates of ten words/s elicit an N480 (Kutas, 1987), bilinguals have slightly longer latency N400s in their weaker (than stronger) language (Kutas et al., 2009), and auditory N400s are delayed for incongruous words whose initial sound overlaps with that of the expected word, e.g., *DOLLARS* when *DOLPHINS* is expected (Van Petten et al., 1999). Dambacher et al. (2012) suggest that the time course of word recognition is best studied at moderate (near typical reading) rates (~280 ms/word).

The utility of N400s comes from using the factors to which it is reliably sensitive to ask well-specified research questions. McLaughlin et al. (2004), for example, used a word pair paradigm to determine how many hours of second language (L2) exposure it took for a second-language learner's processing of L2 words to resemble that of a native speaker (L1). French learners were tested at the beginning, middle, and end of an introductory course with a lexical decision on the second of a pair of written items including semantically related and unrelated word pairs, and word-pseudoword pairs. Compared to a control group receiving no French instruction, L2 learners showed N400 amplitude differences between nonwords and words after only 14 hours of instruction, indicating a sensitivity to lexicality within L2 (prior to reliable sensitivity in any overt response). Additionally, after three hours of instruction, L2 learners exhibited smaller N400s to related than unrelated words, paralleling the typical L1 pattern indicative of some comprehension.

Both the word pair and sentence paradigms have been crossed with the visual half-field paradigm (presenting stimuli ~two degrees to the right or left of fixation, exclusively exposing the contralateral hemisphere to that stimulus for 10 ms or so, before it crosses to the other hemisphere via a commissure). Remarkably, a 10-ms processing headstart yields reliable ERP effects, reflecting differences in the way(s) the two hemispheres deal with semantic relationships, sentential constraint, predictive processing in language, event knowledge activation, linguistic expectancies, jokes, etc. (Coulson & Williams, 2005; Metusalem et al., 2016; Wlotko & Federmeier, 2013). From such studies, Federmeier (2007) proposed that the left hemisphere relies on top-down processes rooted in the neural system supporting language production to predict, while the right hemisphere patiently awaits input to begin integrating it with the representation of the ongoing context to construct meaning.

Intuitively it may seem that sentence processing and discourse-level processing would use the same brain areas and the same mechanisms. Psycholinguists, however, have traditionally distinguished the two, especially regarding timing; e.g., on serial accounts, word-level effects precede sentence-level effects which precede discourse-level effects. Likewise, the neuropsychological literature has implicated the right hemisphere to a greater degree than the left in discourse-level versus word- or sentence-level processing. ERPs have long shown that language processing is not strictly serial: lexical, sentential, and discourse factors all impact a word's processing as reflected in N400 amplitude modulation at about the same time in the same way. A semantically, categorically, or associatively related word, a congruent sentence context, and a constraining discourse context all yield graded reductions in N400 amplitude to the "primed" word. Indeed, the electromagnetic brain activity during the N400 time window is also sensitive to world knowledge, concurrent information in the visual environment, and speaker information (e.g., mismatch between what a message says and who says it). N400 amplitudes, e.g., to *married* in '*Last year I got married in a beautiful castle.*' are reliably smaller if spoken by an adult female voice than a pre-teen's (Van Berkum et al., 2008). Nieuwland and van Berkum (2006) further demonstrated that global context can overrule local pragmatic anomalies. They contrasted animacy violations (e.g., '*The peanut was in love.*') legitimized by discourse context (*'A woman saw a dancing peanut with a big smile…'*) to discourse-anomalous but pragmatically congruent completions (*'The peanut was salted.'*), and found larger N400s to discourse-anomalous completions. Such findings are solid evidence against Gricean semantics-before-pragmatics models.

N400 amplitudes apparently are also sensitive to what a participant believes another person in their presence during a recording session understands, because a so-called "social N400" is only seen in a participant when s/he is not alone in the recording chamber. This social N400 was elicited by the word (*gills*) which the participant and a confederate sitting alongside both read (*'The boy had gills.'*), but which the participant would think the confederate would consider anomalous because they had not worn headphones (as the participant had) and heard an expository context (*'In the boy's dream, he could breathe under water.'*) (Jouravlev et al., 2019; Rueschemeyer et al., 2015). It would be remarkable if the N400 were a sign of participants' mentalizing as proposed and not just a matter of dividing their attention, e.g., between a language comprehension task and a social encounter with a stranger. The ERP methodology also has been fruitfully used to investigate non-literal (figurative) language processing such as jokes, sarcasm, irony, and indirect requests (jokes and metaphor reviewed by Coulson, 2012; indirect requests by Coulson & Lovett, 2010).

ERPs also have been used to investigate processing of static and moving gestures which are an integral part of formal sign language (including hand, face, and body movements). Sign languages utilize visuo-spatial contrasts at phonological, morphological, syntactic, and discourse levels. These languages are remarkably similar to spoken languages in many respects, e.g., requiring an intact left hemisphere for comprehension and production. Electrophysiological studies of spoken language and American (or Dutch) sign languages have focused on their processing similarities, and differences due to their distinct modalities and characteristics. Like written and spoken words, signs elicit larger N400s when semantically anomalous than when contextually congruent, larger P600s for syntactic violations compared to correct combinations, and a left anterior negativity (LAN) linked to early, automatic syntactic analysis, e.g., in response to reversed verb agreement (Capek et al., 2009), with similar time courses and sensitivities. By comparing the ERPs elicited by signs in congenitally deaf and hearing individuals whose first language was a signed language (due to having deaf parents) and deaf individuals who were not exposed to sign until later in life, it has been possible to study neural plasticity and distinguish effects due to differences in input modality versus early language experience (Neville et al., 1997).

ERPs also have proven useful in research on the communicative role of gestures, especially co-speech gestures (Coulson, 2004; Emmorey & Özyürek, 2014). These studies have focused on whether, and if so, how and when, information conveyed by a manual gesture and accompanying speech are integrated. Wu and Coulson (2005), e.g., found that whether participants judged the congruency of a TV cartoon followed by a person gesturing, or the relatedness of a probe word following a cartoon-gesture pair, the N400 time-locked to gesture onset was smaller when semantically congruent than incongruent. Wu and Coulson (2011) showed that speech-gesture congruency effects are positively correlated with kinesthetic working memory capacity, inferred from a test of an individual's memory for body movements. While the time courses of the integration of meaning (indexed by congruity N400s) derived from gestures and spoken words are indistinguishable (Özyürek et al., 2007), the temporal relation between gestures and speech is critical. When the speech and gesture are simultaneous or very close (speech 160 ms after gesture onset), a canonical N400 congruity effect is elicited whereas after a 360-ms delay, no N400 congruity effect appears (Habets et al., 2011). These findings open the door wide to studies of gesture and co-speech gesture in individuals with various acquired aphasias.

Its undeniable use in resolving language issues notwithstanding, even a well-established component like the N400 is not immune to controversy. One debate centers on the degree to which N400s can be modulated by information occurring outside the focus of attention or conscious awareness, operationally defined as verbal report (e.g., during masked priming, attentional blink, sleep, or coma). The exact nature of the neural and/or mental operation(s) that N400s index remain under discussion (Federmeier, 2021). In a scholarly review of the neuropsychological, intracranial, and magnetoencephalography literatures, van Petten and Luka (2006) concluded that a large portion of the temporal lobes – especially in the left hemisphere – is responsible for the scalp-recorded N400 component, at least the canonical N400 elicited by visual words in isolation, word pairs, or anomalous sentences. However, as they note, little is known about generators of N400s in other modalities or by other types of stimulus conditions, because researchers have yet to look. Taken together, studies using a number of different imaging techniques and populations implicate a large network engaged during the N400 time window including mid- and superior temporal gyrus, superior temporal sulcus, inferior frontal gyrus, and dorsolateral prefrontal cortex (Halgren et al., 2002; Lau et al., 2008). Likewise, despite the general consensus on what factors modulate N400 amplitude, there is as of yet no consensus on what "computation" or "process" electrical activity during the N400 window reflects. Some computational models mimic the N400 potential (Laszlo & Plaut, 2012), others the behavior of the N400 to certain manipulations; these have led to the proposal that the N400 reflects the retrieval of word meaning from semantic memory (Brouwer et al., 2017), a prediction error signal (Fitz & Chang, 2019), or semantic network error (Rabovsky & McRae, 2014). Each of these positions has its limitations (see Federmeier, 2021).

Many different types of information widely distributed in the brain are coming together – whether literally onto some common representation or in space or in temporal coincidence – during the time window of the N400 to influence what information is "active" in the comprehender's mind/brain and to influence what is understood implicitly and with attention. Some refer to this process as contextual integration or semantic unification (Hagoort et al., 2009); others link N400 to semantic access/recognition, or to the initial loose binding between the eliciting stimuli and the associative information in semantic memory that begins meaning construction (Federmeier, 2021).

A potentially incisive set of questions about what aspect of semantic analysis N400 activity reflects has been raised by N400 modulations to seemingly grammatical violations (e.g., Hopf et al., 1998) and P600 modulations to seemingly semantic violations (so-called semantic P6, reviewed in Leckey & Federmeier, 2020). Another set of discomfiting results in this regard highlights individual differences to morphosyntactic violations, with some participants showing a P6 and others an N400+P600 complex (Tanner & Van Hell, 2014). These studies raise fundamental questions not only about the components per se, but also about the juxtaposition of the clear distinctions between semantics and syntax drawn by researchers and the messy divide manifest by the activity in their brains.

Because much is known about the factors that influence N400 parameters in specific paradigms, it has great potential for researching special language populations. Researchers have exploited N400 sensitivity to word class to examine open versus closed class processing in aphasics (ter Keurs et al., 1999), semantic categorization in normal and abnormal aging (Iragui et al., 1996), abnormal semantic activation and individuals with schizophrenia (Kiang et al., 2008), and longitudinal N400 patterns in children at risk for developmental language disorders such as specific language impairment (Friedrich & Friederici, 2006), inter alia. The N400 is an excellent diagnostic tool for assessing semantic analysis and meaning construction in humans of all ages and all languages, regardless of input modality.

Effects of structure and syntax

With history as our guide, we know that almost every violation – be it physical, orthographic, phonological, syntactic, pragmatic, etc. – elicits some sort of ERP difference compared to its non-deviant counterpart, although violations are neither necessary nor sufficient to elicit ERP effects. Linguists have documented many regularities at multiple levels of language in remarkably nuanced and formal ways. Nonetheless, there is no consensus on how best to partition linguistic representations and processes, much less for syntax. Thus, it is not surprising there is no single electrical brain manifestation of a violation or processing of syntax, defined loosely as a system of "rules governing sentence structure." The ways, degrees, and timing with which the brain is sensitive to such rules during online comprehension are matters for empirical testing, with due consideration given to working memory, sequencing, inhibition, attention, and monitoring operations, among others.

Kutas and Hillyard (1983) demonstrated that morphosyntactic violations were associated with a frontally distributed negativity and/or a later positivity, not a posterior N400. More linguistically sophisticated ERP studies since have highlighted three main effects (in order of reliability): the P600 (briefly referred to as syntactic positive shift or SPS), the LAN, and an eLAN. The P600 is a positivity beginning around 450–500 ms after the onset of a syntactically anomalous, ambiguous, or complex word, with a waveform shape that ranges between peaked and broad. Its relative amplitude distribution across the scalp also varies considerably, though P600 identification is often tied to a centro-parietal maximum (see Figure 6.1d). Auditory and/or visual P600s have been observed to violations of subject-verb number agreement, pronoun case, pronoun gender or number agreement, verb inflection, and phrase structure (see Swaab et al., 2012, for review).

P600s in response to violations of phrase structure or word order/lexical class are also preceded by a negativity largest over left frontal sites, labelled the eLAN (Figure 6.1d). Some researchers have argued that eLANs are unique to this type of violation, reflecting automatic, first-pass parsing processes, by contrast to the strategically controlled, second-pass parsing processes reflected by the parietal P600 (e.g., Friederici & Mecklinger, 1996). This view of the eLAN, however, has not withstood the test of time empirically or methodologically. An eLAN is not automatically elicited whenever there is a grammatical category violation, and has been observed for different physical forms of words from the same lexico-grammatical category. Moreover, a devastating argument states that the eLANs seen in response to a grammatical category violation are likely artifacts (Steinhauer & Drury, 2012). Among several methodological concerns raised, the most problematic (here and more generally) is the difference in baselines for the two critical words compared in order to isolate the eLAN because each is preceded by a word from a different lexical class (with corresponding differences in their elicited ERPs).

The late positivities variously called P600s, late positivity, late positive complex, and the SPS are typically elicited by grammatical/syntactic violations, syntactic complexity, or regions of syntactic processing difficulty. P600s were observed to the word *to* in '*The woman persuaded to…*' versus '*The woman struggled to…*' (Osterhout & Holcomb, 1992). As *persuaded* could introduce a passivized reduced relative clause, as in '*The woman persuaded to make a donation opened her checkbook*', "*to*" is not grammatically incorrect, although it is less predictable than one in which *persuaded* is followed by its direct object, as in '*The woman persuaded her husband to make a donation.*' P600s also have been observed to grammatical errors in senseless prose composed of real words – e.g., '*Two mellow graves *sinks by the litany*' compared to '*Two mellow graves sink by the litany*,' but not by apparent grammatical errors in pseudoword prose, e.g., '*The slithy toves *gimbles in the wabe*' versus '*The slithy toves gimble in the wabe*,' which elicited a negativity instead (Munte, Matzke, et al., 1997).

P600s are reportedly also elicited by some manipulations that are typically not considered "syntactic", e.g., by what would be traditionally considered N400-eliciting semantic violations, such as thematic role animacy violations: '*Every morning at breakfast the eggs would eat…*' (Kuperberg et al., 2003); anomalous verb forms: '*The hearty meal was devouring…*' (Kim & Osterhout, 2005); and semantically anomalous verb and arguments: '*The javelin has thrown the athletes…*' and '*The cat that fled from the mice…*', respectively (Hoeks et al., 2004; Kolk et al., 2003).

Proposals about the functional significance of the P600 are contentious and run the gamut from language-specific to domain-general. Some researchers take the P600 as some form of syntactic reanalysis, based on demonstrations: (a) that the P600 is decomposable (using principal-components analysis) into subcomponents distinguishing it from a late posterior positivity variously known as the P3, P3b, or P300 in the literature on general information processing, categorization, or decision-making (Friederici et al., 2001), and (b) that P600 amplitude is proportional to the difficulty of syntactic re-analysis (Munte, Szentkuti, et al., 1997). Other researchers have argued, on the basis of experimental results suggesting that both are sensitive to the same probabilistic parameters, that the P600 is a P3 in language contexts – a response to unexpected, infrequent syntactic anomalies or irregularities (Coulson et al., 1998; Gunter et al., 1997). Depending on the research question, whether or not the P600 is a member of the P3 family, or even if the two components are the same thing, may not matter.

For Broca's aphasia patients, characterized by difficulties producing and comprehending grammatical structures, P600s are reduced or absent in response to subject-verb number agreement violations (Wassenaar et al., 2004) and word-class (noun versus verb) violations (Wassenaar & Hagoort, 2005). Moreover, across patients, poorer performance on neuropsychological tests of syntactic comprehension correlates with smaller P600s. These results imply that deficits in syntactic comprehension in Broca's aphasia patients stem from disruption of processes that must be intact to elicit normal P600s; this could be any process prior to and including those manifest by the P600. It remains to be investigated whether P600 testing could have diagnostic or research utility in profiling aphasic patients' impairments in comprehending various grammatical structures, or in predicting patients' prognoses for improvement. Again, it is not obvious to what extent it matters whether the P600 is syntax-specific or not.

Over the past decade, effort has been directed at distinguishing the posterior post-N400 positivity (pPNP) from the anterior post-N400 positivity (aPNP) by their eliciting conditions and functional significances (see Brothers et al., 2020, for the importance of comprehension goals and linguistic context; DeLong et al., 2011; Federmeier, 2007; Kuperberg et al., 2020; Moreno et al., 2002; Ness & Meltzer-Asscher, 2018). These two post-N400 positivities can, at times, be seen in the same experiment, typically in different experimental conditions, and not necessarily in the same or even in all participants (reviewed by Van Petten & Luka, 2012). An aPNP is seen following the N400 to an unexpected, but plausible, word in a strongly constraining context, when compared to the same word of equal cloze probability in a weakly constraining context (and with the same amplitude N400); an implausible word in this situation would elicit a pPNP. The aPNP has been variously linked to inhibitory processes, violation of a specific lexical (versus semantic) expectancy, a revision process after an incorrect prediction, and additional processing of an unexpected word. Whatever the correct functional account, the aPNP is sensitive to individual skills (such as verbal fluency) and task requirements.

The left anterior negativity (LAN)

The LAN, originally considered a specific response to syntactic violations (e.g., Osterhout & Holcomb, 1992), has been observed to various morphosyntactic violations. What looks like the same potential also has been seen in association with long-distance dependencies, grammatical or ungrammatical, and linked to working memory (e.g., Vos, Gunter, Kolk, & Mulder, 2001). These conflicting findings have left its functional significance in limbo. An appealing solution to this conundrum is that the LAN to morphosyntactic violations is an illusion that emerges from temporal and/or spatial overlap and summation of N400 and/or P600 potentials, in an experimental condition (Tanner & Van Hell, 2014). Indeed, component overlap is not unusual and is at times offered as an explanation of observed ERP waveforms, and has impacted how the waveforms were measured, analyzed, and interpreted.

The LAN is more consistently seen in studies with long-distance dependencies and has revealed much about how the brain deals with "discontinuous but linked syntactic positions" (see Kluender, 2021, for review). LANs have been observed with *wh*-questions, relative clauses, topicalization, and long-distance scrambling, in West Germanic head-initial languages and non-Indo-European head-final languages such as Japanese and Korean. King and Kutas (1995) observed LAN effects following introduction of the relative pronoun, *wh*-filler, and the location of its gap at the main clause verb to object relative clauses ('*The reporter [who the senator harshly attacked] admitted the error.*') versus subject relative clauses ('*The reporter [who harshly attacked the senator] admitted the error.*'). A similar negativity also has been reported for referentially ambiguous words in texts, e.g., a pronoun with two possible referents versus only one (Van Berkum et al., 2008), and thus linked to referential ambiguity and called an Nref. Here again, however, it has been argued that the Nref is another instance of a LAN elicited by a retrieval process from working memory, in this case, that of the antecedent of a pronoun, just as takes place when a filler is retrieved to fill a gap. This interpretation remains controversial but tempting.

A final note on the use of ERPs to study language processing. If the electrophysiological study of language processing were contingent on violations and anomalies, ERP researchers would be hard-pressed to argue that their findings and inferences generalize to normal language comprehension. Whether this is a reasonable conclusion depends on what is meant by a violation, whether violations are all-or-none or can be graded, the extent to which comprehenders must be "aware" that a violation occurred, etc. We believe a good argument can be made that as a (predictive) neural machine, the brain is continually generating (mostly unconsciously) expectancies and experiencing violations of these expectancies to varying degrees. However, the beauty of ERP research is that overt violation manipulations are not necessary. Just ask participants to read, listen, gesture, and make sense of the world around them, and then monitor the electrical reflections of these activities at the scalp surface!

Concluding remarks

The background and examples detailed herein paint a diverse picture of the types of language processing questions that ERP paradigms have addressed. Some of the paradigms are tried and true (e.g., the N400 semantic anomaly, the LRP in a Go/NoGo or conflict paradigm, and the MMN oddball). This means that we can be fairly certain that if we follow the "paradigm recipe," we know what ERP effects we are likely to observe, and that we can interpret systematic deviations in overall amplitudes, relative amplitudes across the scalp, and/or latencies in meaningful ways. Of course, we may obtain unexpected findings even in "typical" populations, presumably because an aspect of the paradigm thought irrelevant is not. In that case, we learn more about the factors leading to a particular ERP effect in a particular paradigm, and the design-inference cycle starts again. Moreover, it is not always possible to use or to adapt an extant paradigm to the question at hand. In that case we start the slow process of finding out if a new paradigm elicits any reliable ERP effects, and if so, discovering what modulates these effects, and thus what they may index. This process is the bread and butter of cognitive ERPers' existence. For other researchers, it may be more rewarding to understand the ins and outs of each paradigm and the sorts of questions that each is suited to answer, and then to choose the right one to investigate a specific question, ever mindful that most cognitive ERP paradigms are not language-specific, but can nonetheless be useful to psycholinguists and neurolinguists, particularly researchers interested in communicative disorders.

Acknowledgements

M. Kutas (and some of the work reported herein) was supported by grants AG08313 and HD22614. M. Kiang is supported by the Canadian Institutes of Health Research (#PJT-168989) and the Social Sciences and Humanities Research Council of Canada (#430-2018-0019).

Further Reading

Abdel Rahman, R., van Turennout, M., & Levelt, W. J. (2003). Phonological encoding is not contingent on semantic feature retrieval: An electrophysiological study on object naming. *Journal of Experimental Psychology: Learning, Memory, and Cognition, 29*(5), 850–860.

Aristei, S., Melinger, A., & Abdel Rahman, R. (2011). Electrophysiological chronometry of semantic context effects in language production. *Journal of Cognitive Neuroscience*, *23*(7), 1567–1586.

Baldeweg, T., Richardson, A., Watkins, S., Foale, C., & Gruzelier, J. (1999). Impaired auditory frequency discrimination in dyslexia detected with mismatch evoked potentials. *Annals of Neurology*, *45*(4), 495–503.

Brothers, T., Wlotko, E. W., Warnke, L., & Kuperberg, G. R. (2020). Going the extra mile: Effects of discourse context on two late positivities during language comprehension. *Neurobiology of Language*, *1*(1), 135–160.

Brouwer, H., Crocker, M. W., Venhuizen, N. J., & Hoeks, J. C. J. (2017). A neurocomputational model of the N400 and the P600 in language processing. *Cognitive Science*, *41*(Suppl 6), 1318–1352.

Capek, C. M., Grossi, G., Newman, A. J., McBurney, S. L., Corina, D., Roeder, B., & Neville, H. J. (2009). Brain systems mediating semantic and syntactic processing in deaf native signers: Biological invariance and modality specificity. *Proceedings of the National Academy of Sciences of the USA*, *106*(21), 8784–8789.

Cheour, M., Ceponiene, R., Lehtokoski, A., Luuk, A., Allik, J., Alho, K., & Naatanen, R. (1998). Development of language-specific phoneme representations in the infant brain. *Nature Neuroscience*, *1*(5), 351–353.

Cheour-Luhtanen, M., Alho, K., Kujala, T., Sainio, K., Reinikainen, K., Renlund, M., Aaltonen, O., Eerola, O., & Naatanen, R. (1995). Mismatch negativity indicates vowel discrimination in newborns. *Hearing Research*, *82*(1), 53–58.

Clarke, A. R., Barry, R. J., McCarthy, R., & Selikowitz, M. (2001). Age and sex effects in the EEG: Development of the normal child. *Clinical Neurophysiology*, *112*(5), 806–814.

Connolly, J. F., & Phillips, N. A. (1994). Event-related potential components reflect phonological and semantic processing of the terminal word of spoken sentences. *Journal of Cognitive Neuroscience*, *6*(3), 256–266.

Coulson, S. (2004). Electrophysiology and pragmatic language comprehension. In I. Noveck & D. Sperber (Eds.), *Experimental pragmatics* (pp. 187–206). Palgrave.

Coulson, S. (2012). Cognitive neuroscience of figurative language. In M. J. Spivey, K. McRae, & M. Joanisse (Eds.), *The Cambridge handbook of psycholinguistics* (pp. 523–537). Cambridge University Press.

Coulson, S., King, J. W., & Kutas, M. (1998). Expect the unexpected: Event-related brain response to morpho-syntactic violations. *Language and Cognitive Processes*, *13*(1), 21–58.

Coulson, S., & Lovett, C. (2010). Comprehension of non-conventional indirect requests. *Italian Journal of Linguistics*, *22*(1), 107–124.

Coulson, S., & Williams, R. F. (2005). Hemispheric asymmetries and joke comprehension. *Neuropsychologia*, *43*(1), 128–141.

Dambacher, M., Dimigen, O., Braun, M., Wille, K., Jacobs, A. M., & Kliegl, R. (2012). Stimulus onset asynchrony and the timeline of word recognition: Event-related potentials during sentence reading. *Neuropsychologia*, *50*(8), 1852–1870.

Davids, N., Segers, E., van den Brink, D., Mitterer, H., van Balkom, H., Hagoort, P., & Verhoeven, L. (2011). The nature of auditory discrimination problems in children with specific language impairment: An MMN study. *Neuropsychologia*, *49*(1), 19–28.

de Jong, R., Wierda, M., Mulder, G., & Mulder, L. J. (1988). Use of partial stimulus information in response processing. *Journal of Experimental Psychology: Human Perception and Performance*, *14*(4), 682–692.

Deecke, L., Scheid, P., & Kornhuber, H. H. (1969). Distribution of readiness potential, pre-motion positivity, and motor potential of the human cerebral cortex preceding voluntary finger movements. *Experimental Brain Research*, 7(2), 158–168.

Dell, G. S., & O'Seaghdha, P. G. (1992). Stages of lexical access in language production. *Cognition*, *42*(1–3), 287–314.

DeLong, K. A., Urbach, T. P., Groppe, D. M., & Kutas, M. (2011). Overlapping dual ERP responses to low cloze probability sentence continuations. *Psychophysiology*, *48*(9), 1203–1207.

DeLong, K. A., Urbach, T. P., & Kutas, M. (2005). Probabilistic word pre-activation during language comprehension inferred from electrical brain activity. *Nature Neuroscience*, *8*(8), 1117–1121.

Delorme, A., Sejnowski, T., & Makeig, S. (2007). Enhanced detection of artifacts in EEG data using higher-order statistics and independent component analysis. *Neuroimage*, *34*(4), 1443–1449.

Diaz, M. T., & Swaab, T. Y. (2007). Electrophysiological differentiation of phonological and semantic integration in word and sentence contexts. *Brain Research*, *1146*, 85–100.

Donoghue, T., Haller, M., Peterson, E. J., Varma, P., Sebastian, P., Gao, R., Noto, T., Lara, A. H., Wallis, J. D., Knight, R. T., Shestyuk, A., & Voytek, B. (2020). Parameterizing neural power spectra into periodic and aperiodic components. *Nature Neuroscience*, *23*(12), 1655–1665.

Emmorey, K., & Özyürek, A. (2014). Language in our hands: Neural underpinnings of sign language and co-speech gesture. In M. S. Gazzaniga (Ed.), *The cognitive neurosciences* (pp. 657–666). MIT Press.

Eulitz, C., Hauk, O., & Cohen, R. (2000). Electroencephalographic activity over temporal brain areas during phonological encoding in picture naming. *Clinical Neurophysiology*, *111*(11), 2088–2097.

Federmeier, K. D. (2007). Thinking ahead: The role and roots of prediction in language comprehension. *Psychophysiology*, *44*(4), 491–505.
Federmeier, K. D. (2021). Connecting and considering: Electrophysiology provides insights into comprehension. *Psychophysiology*, *59*(1), e13940.
Fitz, H., & Chang, F. (2019). Language ERPs reflect learning through prediction error propagation. *Cognitive Psychology*, *111*, 15–52.
Friederici, A. D., & Mecklinger, A. (1996). Syntactic parsing as revealed by brain responses: First-pass and second-pass parsing processes. *Journal of Psycholinguistic Research*, *25*(1), 157–176.
Friederici, A. D., Mecklinger, A., Spencer, K. M., Steinhauer, K., & Donchin, E. (2001). Syntactic parsing preferences and their on-line revisions: A spatio-temporal analysis of event-related brain potentials. *Brain Research: Cognitive Brain Research*, *11*(2), 305–323.
Friedrich, M., & Friederici, A. D. (2006). Early N400 development and later language acquisition. *Psychophysiology*, *43*(1), 1–12.
Gratton, G., Coles, M. G., Sirevaag, E. J., Eriksen, C.W., & Donchin, E. (1988). Pre- and poststimulus activation of response channels: A psychophysiological analysis. *Journal of Experimental Psychology: Human Perception and Performance*, *14*(3), 331–344.
Gunter, T. C., Stowe, L. A., & Mulder, G. (1997). When syntax meets semantics. *Psychophysiology*, *34*(6), 660–676.
Habets, B., Kita, S., Shao, Z., Ozyurek, A., & Hagoort, P. (2011). The role of synchrony and ambiguity in speech-gesture integration during comprehension. *Journal of Cognitive Neuroscience*, *23*(8), 1845–1854.
Hagoort, P., Baggio, G., & Wlllems, R. M. (2009). Semantic unification. In M. S. Gazzaniga, E. Bizzi, L. M. Chalupa, S.T. Grafton, T. F. Heatherton, C. Koch, J. E. LeDoux, S. J. Luck, G. R. Mangan, J. A. Movshon, H. Neville, E. A. Phelps, P. Rakic, D. L. Schacter, M. Sur, & B. A. Wandell (Eds.), *The cognitive neurosciences* (4th ed., pp. 819–835). Massachusetts Institute of Technology.
Halgren, E., Dhond, R. P., Christensen, N., Van Petten, C., Marinkovic, K., Lewine, J. D., & Dale, A. M. (2002). N400-like magnetoencephalography responses modulated by semantic context, word frequency, and lexical class in sentences. *Neuroimage*, *17*(3), 1101–1116.
Hoeks, J. C., Stowe, L. A., & Doedens, G. (2004). Seeing words in context: The interaction of lexical and sentence level information during reading. *Brain Research: Cognitive Brain Research*, *19*(1), 59–73.
Hopf, J. M., Bayer, J., Bader, M., & Meng, M. (1998). Event-related brain potentials and case information in syntactic ambiguities. *Journal of Cognitive Neuroscience*, *10*(2), 264–280.
Indefrey, P., & Levelt, W. J. M. (2000). The neural correlates of language production. In M. S. Gazzaniga (Ed.), *The new cognitive neurosciences* (2nd ed., pp. 845–865). MIT Press.
Iragui, V., Kutas, M., & Salmon, D. P. (1996). Event-related brain potentials during semantic categorization in normal aging and senile dementia of the Alzheimer's type. *Electroencephalography and Clinical Neurophysiology*, *100*(5), 392–406.
Jouravlev, O., Schwartz, R., Ayyash, D., Mineroff, Z., Gibson, E., & Fedorenko, E. (2019). Tracking Colisteners' knowledge states during language comprehension. *Psychological Science*, *30*(1), 3–19.
Kiang, M., Kutas, M., Light, G. A., & Braff, D. L. (2008). An event-related brain potential study of direct and indirect semantic priming in schizophrenia. *American Journal of Psychiatry*, *165*(1), 74–81.
Kim, A., & Osterhout, L. (2005). The independence of combinatory semantic processing: Evidence from event-related potentials. *Journal of Memory and Language*, *52*(2), 205–225.
King, J. W., & Kutas, M. (1995). Who did what and when? Using word- and clause-level ERPs to monitor working memory usage in reading. *Journal of Cognitive Neuroscience*, 7(3), 376–395.
Kluender, R. (2021). Nothing entirely new under the sun: ERP responses to manipulations of syntax. In G. Goodall (Ed.), *The Cambridge handbook of experimental syntax*. (pp. 641–686). Cambridge University Press.
Koester, D., & Schiller, N. O. (2008). Morphological priming in overt language production: Electrophysiological evidence from Dutch. *Neuroimage*, *42*(4), 1622–1630.
Kolk, H. H., Chwilla, D. J., van Herten, M., & Oor, P. J. (2003). Structure and limited capacity in verbal working memory: A study with event-related potentials. *Brain and Language*, *85*(1), 1–36.
Kujala, A., Alho, K., Service, E., Ilmoniemi, R. J., & Connolly, J. F. (2004). Activation in the anterior left auditory cortex associated with phonological analysis of speech input: Localization of the phonological mismatch negativity response with MEG. *Brain Research: Cognitive Brain Research*, *21*(1), 106–113.
Kuperberg, G. R., Brothers, T., & Wlotko, E. W. (2020). A tale of two positivities and the N400: Distinct neural signatures are evoked by confirmed and violated predictions at different levels of representation. *Journal of Cognitive Neuroscience*, *32*(1), 12–35.
Kuperberg, G. R., Sitnikova, T., Caplan, D., & Holcomb, P. J. (2003). Electrophysiological distinctions in processing conceptual relationships within simple sentences. *Brain Research: Cognitive Brain Research*, *17*(1), 117–129.

Kutas, M. (1987). Event-related brain potentials (ERPs) elicited during rapid serial visual presentation of congruous and incongruous sentences. *Electroencephalography and Clinical Neurophysiology. Supplement, 40*, 406–411.
Kutas, M., & Dale, A. (1997). Electrical and magnetic readings of mental functions. In M. D. Rugg (Ed.), *Cognitive neuroscience* (pp. 197–242). Psychology Press.
Kutas, M., & Federmeier, K. D., (2011). Thirty years and counting: finding meaning in the N400 component of the event-related brain potential (ERP). *Annual Review of Psychology, 62*, 621–647.
Kutas, M., & Hillyard, S. A. (1983). Event-related brain potentials to grammatical errors and semantic anomalies. *Memory and Cognition, 11*(5), 539–550.
Kutas, M., & Hillyard, S. A. (1984). Brain potentials during reading reflect word expectancy and semantic association. *Nature, 307*(5947), 161–163.
Kutas, M., & Hillyard, S. A. (1989). An electrophysiological probe of incidental semantic association. *Journal of Cognitive Neuroscience, 1*(1), 38–49.
Kutas, M., & Iragui, V. (1998). The N400 in a semantic categorization task across 6 decades. *Electroencephalography and Clinical Neurophysiology, 108*(5), 456–471.
Kutas, M., Moreno, E., & Wicha, N. (2009). Code-switching and the brain. In B. E. Bullock & A. J. Toribio (Eds.), *The Cambridge handbook of linguistic code-switching* (pp. 289–306). Cambridge University Press.
Lange, V. M., Perret, C., & Laganaro, M. (2015). Comparison of single-word and adjective-noun phrase production using event-related brain potentials. *Cortex, 67*, 15–29.
Laszlo, S., & Federmeier, K. D. (2008). Minding the PS, queues, and PXQs: Uniformity of semantic processing across multiple stimulus types. *Psychophysiology, 45*(3), 458–466.
Laszlo, S., & Federmeier, K. D. (2009). A beautiful day in the neighborhood: An event-related potential study of lexical relationships and prediction in context. *Journal of Memory and Language, 61*(3), 326–338.
Laszlo, S., & Plaut, D. C. (2012). A neurally plausible parallel distributed processing model of event-related potential word reading data. *Brain and Language, 120*(3), 271–281.
Lau, E. F., Phillips, C., & Poeppel, D. (2008). A cortical network for semantics: (de)constructing the N400. *Nature Reviews: Neuroscience, 9*(12), 920–933.
Leckey, M., & Federmeier, K. D. (2020). The P3b and P600(s): Positive contributions to language comprehension. *Psychophysiology, 57*(7), e13351.
Levelt, W. J., Roelofs, A., & Meyer, A. S. (1999). A theory of lexical access in speech production. *Behavioral and Brain Sciences, 22*(1), 1–38; discussion 38–75.
Libet, B., Gleason, C. A., Wright, E. W., & Pearl, D. K. (1983). Time of conscious intention to act in relation to onset of cerebral activity (readiness-potential). The unconscious initiation of a freely voluntary act. *Brain, 106*(3), 623–642.
Luck, S. J. (2014). *An introduction to the event-related potential technique* (2nd ed.). MIT Press.
Luu, P., Collins, P., & Tucker, D. M. (2000). Mood, personality, and self-monitoring: Negative affect and emotionality in relation to frontal lobe mechanisms of error monitoring. *Journal of Experimental Psychology: General, 129*(1), 43–60.
Martin, B. A., & Boothroyd, A. (1999). Cortical, auditory, event-related potentials in response to periodic and aperiodic stimuli with the same spectral envelope. *Ear and Hearing, 20*(1), 33–44.
McLaughlin, J., Osterhout, L., & Kim, A. (2004). Neural correlates of second-language word learning: Minimal instruction produces rapid change. *Nature Neuroscience, 7*(7), 703–704.
Metusalem, R., Kutas, M., Urbach, T. P., & Elman, J. L. (2016). Hemispheric asymmetry in event knowledge activation during incremental language comprehension: A visual half-field ERP study. *Neuropsychologia, 84*, 252–271.
Molina, J. L., Voytek, B., Thomas, M. L., Joshi, Y. B., Bhakta, S. G., Talledo, J. A., Swerdlow, N. R., & Light, G. A. (2020). Memantine effects on electroencephalographic measures of putative excitatory/inhibitory balance in schizophrenia. *Biological Psychiatry: Cognitive Neuroscience and Neuroimaging, 5*(6), 562–568.
Moreno, E. M., Federmeier, K. D., & Kutas, M. (2002). Switching languages, switching palabras (words): An electrophysiological study of code switching. *Brain and Language, 80*(2), 188–207.
Munte, T. F., Matzke, M., & Johannes, S. (1997). Brain activity associated with syntactic incongruencies in words and pseudo-words. *Journal of Cognitive Neuroscience, 9*(3), 318–329.
Munte, T. F., Szentkuti, A., Wieringa, B. M., Matzke, M., & Johannes, S. (1997). Human brain potentials to reading syntactic errors in sentences of different complexity. *Neuroscience Letters, 235*(3), 105–108.
Naatanen, R., Gaillard, A. W., & Mantysalo, S. (1978). Early selective-attention effect on evoked potential reinterpreted. *Acta Psychologica, 42*(4), 313–329.
Naatanen, R., Sussman, E. S., Salisbury, D., & Shafer, V. L. (2014). Mismatch negativity (MMN) as an index of cognitive dysfunction. *Brain Topography, 27*(4), 451–466.
Ness, T., & Meltzer-Asscher, A. (2018). Lexical inhibition due to failed prediction: Behavioral evidence and ERP correlates. *Journal of Experimental Psychology: Learning, Memory, and Cognition, 44*(8), 1269–1285.

Neville, H. J., Coffey, S. A., Lawson, D. S., Fischer, A., Emmorey, K., & Bellugi, U. (1997). Neural systems mediating American sign language: Effects of sensory experience and age of acquisition. *Brain and Language, 57*(3), 285–308.

Nieuwland, M. S., & Van Berkum, J. J. (2006). When peanuts fall in love: N400 evidence for the power of discourse. *Journal of Cognitive Neuroscience, 18*(7), 1098–1111.

Osterhout, L., & Holcomb, P. J. (1992). Event-related brain potentials elicited by syntactic anomaly. *Journal of Memory and Language, 31*(6), 785–806.

Özyürek, A., Willems, R. M., Kita, S., & Hagoort, P. (2007). On-line integration of semantic information from speech and gesture: Insights from event-related brain potentials. *Journal of Cognitive Neuroscience, 19*(4), 605–616.

Paavilainen, P., Jaramillo, M., Naatanen, R., & Winkler, I. (1999). Neuronal populations in the human brain extracting invariant relationships from acoustic variance. *Neuroscience Letters, 265*(3), 179–182.

Papa, S. M., Artieda, J., & Obeso, J. A. (1991). Cortical activity preceding self-initiated and externally triggered voluntary movement. *Movement Disorders, 6*(3), 217–224.

Pfurtscheller, G., & Lopes da Silva, F. H. (1999). Event-related EEG/MEG synchronization and desynchronization: Basic principles. *Clinical Neurophysiology, 110*(11), 1842–1857.

Rabovsky, M., & McRae, K. (2014). Simulating the N400 ERP component as semantic network error: Insights from a feature-based connectionist attractor model of word meaning. *Cognition, 132*(1), 68–89.

Rohrbaugh, J. W., Syndulko, K., & Lindsley, D. B. (1976). Brain wave components of the contingent negative variation in humans. *Science, 191*(4231), 1055–1057.

Romero, S., Mananas, M. A., & Barbanoj, M. J. (2008). A comparative study of automatic techniques for ocular artifact reduction in spontaneous EEG signals based on clinical target variables: A simulation case. *Computers in Biology and Medicine, 38*(3), 348–360.

Rueschemeyer, S. A., Gardner, T., & Stoner, C. (2015). The social N400 effect: How the presence of other listeners affects language comprehension. *Psychonomic Bulletin and Review, 22*(1), 128–134.

Sanders, L. D., & Neville, H. J. (2003). An ERP study of continuous speech processing. I. Segmentation, semantics, and syntax in native speakers. *Brain Research: Cognitive Brain Research, 15*(3), 228–240.

Schmitt, B. M., Münte, T. F., & Kutas, M. (2000). Electrophysiological estimates of the time course of semantic and phonological encoding during implicit picture naming. *Psychophysiology, 37*(4), 473–484.

Schmitt, B. M., Schiltz, K., Zaake, W., Kutas, M., & Münte, T. F. (2001). An electrophysiological analysis of the time course of conceptual and syntactic encoding during tacit picture naming. *Journal of Cognitive Neuroscience, 13*(4), 510–522.

Sirigu, A., Daprati, E., Ciancia, S., Giraux, P., Nighoghossian, N., Posada, A., & Haggard, P. (2004). Altered awareness of voluntary action after damage to the parietal cortex. *Nature Neuroscience*, 7(1), 80–84.

Steinhauer, K., & Drury, J. E. (2012). On the early left-anterior negativity (ELAN) in syntax studies. *Brain and Language, 120*(2), 135–162.

Strijkers, K., Costa, A., & Thierry, G. (2010). Tracking lexical access in speech production: Electrophysiological correlates of word frequency and cognate effects. *Cerebral Cortex, 20*(4), 912–928.

Sussman, E. S., Chen, S., Sussman-Fort, J., & Dinces, E. (2014). The five myths of MMN: Redefining how to use MMN in basic and clinical research. *Brain Topography, 27*(4), 553–564.

Swaab, T. Y., Ledoux, K., Camblin, C. C., & Boudewyn, M. A. (2012). Language-related ERP components. In S. J. Luck & E. S. Kappenman (Eds.), *The Oxford handbook of event-related potential components* (pp. 397–439). Oxford University Press.

Tanner, D., & Van Hell, J. G. (2014). ERPs reveal individual differences in morphosyntactic processing. *Neuropsychologia, 56*, 289–301.

ter Keurs, M., Brown, C. M., Hagoort, P., & Stegeman, D. F. (1999). Electrophysiological manifestations of open- and closed-class words in patients with Broca's aphasia with agrammatic comprehension. An event-related brain potential study. *Brain, 122*(5), 839–854.

Tiitinen, H., May, P., Reinikainen, K., & Naatanen, R. (1994). Attentive novelty detection in humans is governed by pre-attentive sensory memory. *Nature, 372*(6501), 90–92.

Timmers, I., Gentile, F., Rubio-Gozalbo, M. E., & Jansma, B. M. (2013). Temporal characteristics of online syntactic sentence planning: An event-related potential study. *PLOS ONE, 8*(12), e82884.

Tremblay, K. L., Friesen, L., Martin, B. A., & Wright, R. (2003). Test-retest reliability of cortical evoked potentials using naturally produced speech sounds. *Ear and Hearing, 24*(3), 225–232.

Tremblay, K. L., & Kraus, N. (2002). Auditory training induces asymmetrical changes in cortical neural activity. *Journal of Speech, Language, and Hearing Research, 45*(3), 564–572.

Vakani, R., & Nair, D. R. (2019). Electrocorticography and functional mapping. *Handbook of Clinical Neurology, 160*, 313–327.

Van Berkum, J. J., van den Brink, D., Tesink, C. M., Kos, M., & Hagoort, P. (2008). The neural integration of speaker and message. *Journal of Cognitive Neuroscience, 20*(4), 580–591.

van den Brink, D., Brown, C. M., & Hagoort, P. (2001). Electrophysiological evidence for early contextual influences during spoken-word recognition: N200 versus N400 effects. *Journal of Cognitive Neuroscience, 13*(7), 967–985.

Van Petten, C., Coulson, S., Rubin, S., Plante, E., & Parks, M. (1999). Time course of word identification and semantic integration in spoken language. *Journal of Experimental Psychology: Learning, Memory, and Cognition, 25*(2), 394–417.

Van Petten, C., & Luka, B. J. (2006). Neural localization of semantic context effects in electromagnetic and hemodynamic studies. *Brain and Language, 97*(3), 279–293.

Van Petten, C., & Luka, B. J. (2012). Prediction during language comprehension: Benefits, costs, and ERP components. *International Journal of Psychophysiology, 83*(2), 176–190.

van Turennout, M., Hagoort, P., & Brown, C. M. (1997). Electrophysiological evidence on the time course of semantic and phonological processes in speech production. *Journal of Experimental Psychology: Learning, Memory, and Cognition, 23*(4), 787–806.

Vos, S. H., Gunter, T. C., Kolk, H. H., & Mulder, G. (2001). Working memory constraints on syntactic processing: An electrophysiological investigation. *Psychophysiology, 38*(1), 41–63.

Voytek, B., Kramer, M. A., Case, J., Lepage, K. Q., Tempesta, Z. R., Knight, R. T., & Gazzaley, A. (2015). Age-related changes in 1/f neural electrophysiological noise. *Journal of Neuroscience, 35*(38), 13257–13265.

Wassenaar, M., Brown, C. M., & Hagoort, P. (2004). ERP effects of subject-verb agreement violations in patients with Broca's aphasia. *Journal of Cognitive Neuroscience, 16*(4), 553–576.

Wassenaar, M., & Hagoort, P. (2005). Word-category violations in patients with Broca's aphasia: An ERP study. *Brain and Language, 92*(2), 117–137.

Winkler, I., Kujala, T., Tiitinen, H., Sivonen, P., Alku, P., Lehtokoski, A., Czigler, I., Csepe, V., Ilmoniemi, R. J., & Naatanen, R. (1999). Brain responses reveal the learning of foreign language phonemes. *Psychophysiology, 36*(5), 638–642.

Wlotko, E. W., & Federmeier, K. D. (2013). Two sides of meaning: The scalp-recorded n400 reflects distinct contributions from the cerebral hemispheres. *Frontiers in Psychology, 4*, 181.

Wu, Y. C., & Coulson, S. (2005). Meaningful gestures: Electrophysiological indices of iconic gesture comprehension. *Psychophysiology, 42*(6), 654–667.

Wu, Y. C., & Coulson, S. (2011). Are depictive gestures like pictures? Commonalities and differences in semantic processing. *Brain and Language, 119*(3), 184–195.

7

EARLY WORD LEARNING

Reflections on behavior, connectionist models, and brain mechanisms indexed by ERP components

Manuela Friedrich

Introduction

From the neurobiological perspective, learning consists in pre- and postsynaptic molecular changes and in structural modifications of synaptic connectivity within specific brain areas, which are triggered by the previous processing of external signals, and in turn affect future signal transmission between neurons. At the behavioral level, learning allows an organism to modify and fine-tune its behavior to the requirements of the environment. It is, however, largely unknown, how the molecular and structural changes at the neural level alter the systemic behavior at the psychological level.

Mathematical models, in principle, have the potential to bridge the gap between learning at the neural level and learning at the behavioral level, and to comprise the complex interplay of neuronal, systemic, and environmental effects. Massively parallel architectures, called artificial neural networks or connectionist models, provide an idea of how the complex interactions of a great many individual neuronal units result in systemic behavior. In these systems learning is studied by simulations, by which the "behavior" of a net, that is, its output under certain internal and environmental learning conditions is compared with the behavior in animals or humans observed experimentally. But even though the simulation results are often compatible with behavioral data and the basic principles of neural network dynamics are copied from biological neuronal signal transmission, most connectionist models are designed architectures and their specific mechanisms described mathematically may not necessarily have a neurobiological basis.

On the other hand, brain imaging techniques and electrophysiological methods such as event-related brain potentials (ERPs) allow observation of the activity within certain brain structures or the related spatio-temporal voltage fluctuations at the scalp surface during perception, cognition, attention, and learning. The ERP, especially, has a high temporal resolution and is therefore particularly suitable for separating successive stages of stimulus processing. It consists of so-called components that systematically vary with certain experimental manipulations and that are assumed to reflect specific neural processes. ERP components mark the presence or absence of certain perceptual, cognitive, or linguistic processing stages; they indicate processing speed, the amount of resources allocated, or the effort necessary to realize the processing. ERP components also reflect learning-related changes of stimulus processing and are therefore used as brain signatures of a certain ability or a specific developmental stage. However, we do not know the brain mechanisms that cause the responses and what kind of neural interaction involved in the perceptual, cognitive, or linguistic processing stages is responsible for the activity patterns observed.

DOI: 10.4324/9781003204213-9

The present chapter is an attempt to bridge the levels of description in the case of early word learning by bringing together findings on behavioral development, ERP research, and neural network dynamics. In particular, the mechanism responsible for the elicitation of the N400 component of the ERP, interpreted as an index of context-dependent semantic memory use (Kutas & Hillyard, 1980), is proposed to be functionally similar to an artificial mechanism that has been developed to stabilize learning within a flexible connectionist memory system (Carpenter & Grossberg, 1987). The implications of the assumed real existence of such a mechanism will be discussed with respect to the development of categorization and word learning abilities in young children.

The structure of the chapter is the following: First, behavioral aspects of early word acquisition are described, particularly with regard to the flexibility of the human lexical–semantic system. This part comprises the reformulating of basic questions of early word learning with respect to neural functioning. In a second step, ERP findings on lexical–semantic processing in infants and toddlers are reviewed. The course of N400 development observed in these studies and its interrelation with the children's language outcome raise questions about the nature of the N400 component and its direct involvement in the process of word learning. In connection with the nature of the N400, the term semantic focus is introduced as a concept to refer to the flexible use of the representations established within the human lexical–semantic system and to the adjustment of these representations to internal needs and environmental requirements. The next paragraph describes the neural network model ART 1 (Carpenter & Grossberg, 1987) that provides a mathematical description of how the setting and the change of the semantic focus could be realized by neural dynamics. Finally, such a mechanism involved in changing the semantic focus is proposed to be reflected in the N400 component of the ERP. This assumption is further used to explain both the developmental course of the N400 and behavioral findings of early word acquisition.

Generally, the chapter is intended to encourage multidisciplinary work in developmental research, and in particular, the relation proposed here might lead to a deeper understanding of how words and their meanings are acquired by the infant brain.

Behavioral findings of early word learning

Word learning includes the acquisition of phonological word forms, the extraction of relevant meanings, and the mapping between word form and word meaning memory representations. In order to learn words and their meanings, the infant has to handle the variability of the environment in a response-appropriate manner. Basically, the infant brain must learn to differentiate what kind of variability is relevant for word learning and needs to be included into lexical–semantic memory representations and what is irrelevant and can be ignored.

Word form and word meaning acquisition

It has been found that infants early tune into the acoustic properties relevant in their native language; they acquire native language phoneme categories, prosodic features like typical word stress patterns, and the statistic distributions of phoneme combinations occurring in their target language (e.g., Friederici, Friedrich, & Christophe, 2007; Friederici & Wessels, 1993; Jusczyk, Cutler, & Redanz, 1993; Jusczyk, Friederici, Wessels, & Svenkerud, 1993; Kuhl, Williams, Lacerda, Stevens, & Lindblom, 1992; Werker & Lalonde, 1988; Werker & Tees, 2002). These skills facilitate the segmentation of the speech stream into single words, and they provide a basis for word form acquisition. Those variations of acoustic properties that are lexically relevant are included as features into the word form representations, whereas changes in the phonetic realization caused by the talker's age, gender, speech rate, or emotional state do not signal linguistic distinction and should therefore not be stored within lexical representations though they contain information relevant for social communication.

The acquisition of concepts and the mapping of words and concepts render word learning much more complex than word form acquisition alone. The infant brain must figure out what kind of meaningful information is relevant and what is not. In general, concept formation occurs spontaneously without supervision by naming. This spontaneous structuring is influenced by words and behavioral relevant information, both guiding the formation and modification of concepts. For example, cats and dogs are initially seen as four-legged mammals, but naming cats as cat and dogs as dog facilitates the acquisition of separate concepts for cats and dogs. Similarly, the unexpected acerbity of a green apple may trigger the finer differentiation of different types of apples by the formation of representations that include color as a distinctive feature. Thus, information that first appeared to be nonmeaningful may become meaningful in new situations, and different weightings of certain features are relevant in different contexts. During the course of development, the human semantic system learns to semantically view a certain object or event in very different ways. The system becomes able to task-dependently switch between different points of view (i.e., between several semantic memory representations), and almost at each moment it must be able to create a new representation if the already acquired representations are not sufficiently appropriate. This enormous capacity enables the semantic system to handle very different objects or events as if they were the same, thereby broadly generalizing and transferring associated knowledge and expected outcomes, as well as discriminating between very similar objects or events if this is behaviorally relevant. The potential availability of the various memory representations with different weighting of semantic features makes the semantic system flexible and powerful allowing effective and optimal responses to the requirements of the environment. The knowledge about the neural basis of the ability to task-dependently adjust the threshold determining equality and dissimilarity in the external or internal environment would mainly contribute to our understanding of how the human lexical–semantic system can be stable, flexible, and constructive in parallel.

Categorization and the degree of generalization

In general, categorization realizes the balance between dissimilarity and equality by considering relevant features and abstracting from irrelevant information. Relevant features of a category are not represented in an all-or-none manner. Rather, the feature representation within a category depends on statistic properties such as the frequency of feature occurrence within exemplars that are considered as instances of the category. This leads to a graded prototypical structure of naturally acquired categories, including the effect that the prototype of a category is rated as a better exemplar than other category members and, even if never seen before, the prototype appears to be more familiar than previously observed exemplars that have constituted the category (e.g., Posner & Keele, 1968; Rosch, 1973). Such a prototypical structure of categories develops very early, it has been observed even in three- to four-month-old infants (Bomba & Siqueland, 1983; Quinn, 1987).

Categories differ extremely in their level of inclusiveness; that is, their degree of generalization. The degree of generalization is often described by three levels of abstraction, by global categories such as animals, basic level categories like dogs, and subordinate categories like poodles. However, there are a lot of categories at various intermediate levels of generality, such as, for example, mammals, four-legged mammals, fur-bearing animals, or several subspecies of poodles. The developmental course of categorization abilities appears to undergo a shift from a global to basic level to subordinate categories (e.g., Younger & Fearing, 2000). However, results on categorization in infancy strongly depend on the behavioral method used (for a review, see Mareschal & Quinn, 2001). In studies that do not require a familiarization phase, infants categorize into broad global categories from about seven months on, and they show first signs of basic level knowledge at the end of their first year of life, although not consistently within the first two years. These broad categories cause overgeneralizations (e.g., a cat is referred to as a dog) that are massively observed in one- to two-year-olds, both in comprehension and production (e.g., McDonough, 2002). In contrast, in studies that require a familiarization phase, when infants have the possibility to form the categories during familiarization within the experiment, infants tune their category width in response to the requirements of the task, they form either global or basic level categories depending on the material used. In visual preference studies, even three- to four-month-old infants are able to form narrow, basic-level categories. The categorization results of these young infants sometimes display asymmetries (i.e., dogs are discriminated from the cat category, but cats are not discriminated from the dog category), which has been shown to depend on the overlap of the feature value distributions of the categories (French, Mareschal, Mermillod, & Quinn, 2004).

The results of behavioral studies clearly indicate that short lasting basic level categories can be acquired at a very early age, but the representations in long-term memory are much broader, and they are broader for a relatively long time. Although, in principle, the different results obtained with different behavioral methods can be attributed to the amount of information that is acquired by short-term learning during the experiment, the interaction of short- and long-term memory mechanisms involved in the formation of categories at varying levels of abstraction is completely unknown. Generally, little is known about how information is transferred from short-term memory into long-term memory and, even less, we know how a certain part of that information resulting in short-term basic level category formation is selected for consolidation and how this consolidation process leads to the establishment of more general categories in long-term memory.

Mapping of words and meanings: Two modes of early word learning

Full word learning requires the mapping of word form and word meaning memory representations and their reciprocal activation. Already at six months, infants associate the words mama and papa with the faces of their mother and father (Tincoff & Jusczyk, 1999). Around eight–ten months, infants comprehend their first words (Bates, Thal, & Janowsky, 1992; Benedict, 1979). Thus, infants are able to establish associative links between phonological and semantic representations well before their first birthday. During this early stage, word learning appears to be a slow and time-consuming process that requires very frequent exposure to the word form within the appropriate context. Some weeks after the children's first birthday, however, infants become able to quickly learn a novel word for a novel meaning on the basis of only a few exposures (Schafer & Plunkett, 1998; Werker, Cohen, Lloyd, Casasola, & Stager, 1998; Woodward, Markman, & Fitzsimmons, 1994).

This fast mapping ability that develops between 12 and 14 months is assumed to be the basis of the rapid increase in vocabulary, the so-called vocabulary spurt that sets in at around 18 months. A main question and an ongoing debate in developmental research are related to the causes that underlie the qualitative change in infants' word learning ability. Several cognitive and sociocommunicative factors are discussed to affect the infant word learning rate (for an overview, see Nazzi & Bertoncini, 2003; Woodward et al., 1994). The assumption that before the vocabulary spurt children are not able to use the principle of linguistic reference is seen as the primary causation of the initial word learning restrictions in infants. According to this account, young children are able to slowly associate objects and words, but they learn a word as an associative context for an object instead of learning a word as symbolic reference that stands for an object even if this object is actually not present. Independent of whether the behaviorally observed qualitative change in the infant's word learning capacity is caused by the development of cognitive, linguistic, or social abilities, the decoding and consolidation of words and concepts appears to be radically changed when children become able to perform fast mapping. It is, however, completely unknown, what kind of changes in the neural mechanisms of perceptual, lexical–semantic, and memory processes are associated with the development of the fast mapping ability, and whether these changes are indeed qualitative or still quantitative in their nature. If assuming that the main developmental step is the ability to acquire and use referential knowledge, then the question will be, in which way the neural coding of referential connections and their involvement in specific stages of perceptual and cognitive stimulus processing differ from those of associative connections.

Hierarchical knowledge and constraints in early word learning

Once children have learned an initial meaning for a word, they must reach the appropriate level of generalization that the word refers to, they expand and refine their lexicon by learning other words with similar meanings, and they begin to reorganize the acquired concepts and to integrate them into hierarchically interpretable (but not necessarily hierarchically stored) knowledge structures.

Behavioral researchers have proposed several constraints that guide the acquisition of new word meanings. Some of these constraints are developed to explain the finding that one- to three-year-old children consistently map a novel word to a novel object when presented with two objects, one familiar and one unfamiliar, and asked for the referent of the novel word (disambiguation effect). It has been proposed that young children assume that an object can have only one name (Mutual Exclusivity Constraint, Markman & Wachtel, 1988), that they are motivated to label an unnamed category (Novel Name-Nameless Category Principle, Golinkoff, Mervis, & Hirsh-Pasek, 1994), or that they assume the meaning of a new word differs from the meaning of previously known words (Contrast Principle, Clark, 1987). However, the early age at which the disambiguation effect is observed suggests that it is not triggered by meta-cognitive abilities (e.g., pragmatic strategies), and therefore, it is not realized by intentional top-down guided neurocognitive processes. For this reason, the primary question is what neural mechanisms generate the behavior that results in the disambiguation effect and that can be described by constraints at the psycholinguistic level. More generally, one could ask what constraints in the maturing and developing brain cause the constraint behavior observed in young children.

Behavioral research has moreover shown that young children have particular difficulties in acquiring conceptual hierarchies. When two- to four-year-old children are trained with a new word for a subset of objects belonging to a known concept and having a known name (i.e., a word for a flower subcategory like rose), after successful learning, many children do not anymore consider the objects of the subcategory to be members of the known concept. That is, for these children, roses are not flowers anymore, even though, before learning, children considered all target objects to be flowers. Goede and Friedrich (1995) showed that this temporary exclusion of category members that follows the acquisition of a subcategory depends on exemplar typicality and is not caused by one of the above-mentioned constraints of early word learning. Rather, the exclusion of objects from a known, more general concept after learning a specific concept suggests that competition or inhibition processes are involved in the acquisition of new words and new concepts for already known objects. However, the neural processes of semantic specification and reorganization, which allow flexibly considering an object as belonging to several different concepts within a conceptual hierarchy, are largely unknown.

ERP components related to lexical–semantic processing

Besides advancements in behavioral methods, during the last decade, electro-physiological and brain imaging methods have been established in developmental research. By early pioneering studies, the electrophysiological responses on acoustic and visual stimuli were explored in infants. Here, researchers have observed several infant-specific ERP components that have no clear adult equivalent (e.g., the P100-N250 complex on acoustic stimulation instead of the obligatory N1 and P2 components in adults), the positive mismatch response instead of the adult mismatch negativity, and the Nc as an infant attentional response (e.g., Courchesne, Ganz, & Norcia, 1981; Dehaene-Lambertz & Dehaene, 1994; Kushnerenko et al., 2002). Recent research has moreover focused on the development of adult-like ERP components, particularly on those that are related to the development of certain language abilities, such as components reflecting semantic or syntactic processing stages (for an overview, see Friederici, 2005).

The N400 component in adults

Semantic processing in adults is reflected in the N400 component of the ERP. The N400 is a centro-parietally distributed negative wave with peak latency at around 400 ms, which was first observed in response to semantically incorrect sentence endings, for example in response to the word socks in the sentence "He spread the warm bread with socks" (Kutas & Hillyard, 1980). Initially the N400 was assumed to reflect lexical search and access, but a number of studies have shown that the N400 is not only elicited by words but also in response to other potentially meaningful stimuli, such as pictures, pseudowords, and natural sounds when they do not match an expectation established by a word, a sentence, a picture story, or even by an odor prime (Barrett & Rugg, 1990; Federmeier & Kutas, 2001; Ganis, Kutas & Sereno, 1996; Holcomb & McPherson, 1994; Nigam, Hoffman, & Simons, 1992; Sarfarazi, Cave, Richardson, Behan, & Sedgwick, 1999; Van Petten & Rheinfelder, 1995; West & Holcomb, 2002). Today the common view is that the N400 amplitude reflects the cognitive effort involved in integrating a non-expected or inappropriate meaningful stimulus into a given semantic context held in working memory (Holcomb, 1993). A relative reduction in the N400 amplitude indicates that a semantic expectation triggered by a prime, a sentence, or any other context, is matched and has facilitated subsequent semantic processing of a target stimulus.

The matching of incoming semantic information with a semantic expectation is not the only factor that affects N400 amplitude. It moreover depends on the general frequency of item usage (e.g., word frequency), on the specific frequency of an item within the experiment (the number of repetitions), on the overlap of physical, functional, and situational features of meaningful items (semantic similarity), and on the overlap of these features with those coded within semantic representations (typicality; for a review see Kutas & Federmeier, 2000). Therefore, the N400 has been proposed to reflect the recognition of meaningful stimuli and the structure and organization of semantic long-term memory, even though it is not known how the mechanisms that underlie N400 generation operate on semantic long-term memory.

The N200-500 component in infants and toddlers

In infants and toddlers, two ERP components have been found to vary in response to lexical–semantic processing, the adult-like N400 and the infant-specific N200-500.

The N200-500 is a fronto-laterally distributed negativity in the 200-500 ms range, which reflects a processing stage involved in word form recognition, such as acoustic-phonological or lexical processing. In 11- to 20-month-olds it is enhanced to known or familiar words as compared to unknown or unfamiliar words, and it is more negative to unknown words than to backward presented words (Mills, Coffey-Corina, & Neville, 1993, 1997; Thierry, Vihman, & Roberts, 2003). A study with ten-month-olds, moreover, demonstrated that, within an experimental session, the N200-500 emerges during online familiarization with repeatedly presented, initially unfamiliar words (Kooijman, Hagoort, & Cutler, 2005).

The N200-500 is not only affected by word familiarity depending on the current number of repetitions or on previous word frequency. It is, moreover, sensitive to the expectation of a word form, which can be induced by priming within a picture–word priming paradigm (Friedrich & Friederici, 2004, 2005a, 2005b, 2006; for a review see Friedrich, 2008). This cross-modal experimental design was particularly developed to explore the neural correlates of lexical–semantic processing in one-year-olds, their developmental course during early word learning, and the role that semantic priming and semantic integration mechanisms play in the progression of word learning in infants and toddlers. In this priming paradigm, pictures of known objects represent a simple, early acquired, and easily accessible context for words. During the experimental session, children sat in front of a monitor, they looked at sequentially presented objects (e.g., a sheep) and listened to words or nonsense words presented acoustically 1,900 ms post picture onset, when primary visual processing was finished but the object was still visible on the screen. Words were either congruous (i.e., named the objects correctly, sheep), or incongruous (i.e., named a semantically unrelated concept, ball). Nonsense words were either pseudowords that are legal according to the rules of German, and thus sound like a real German word (e.g., Fless), or nonwords that had a phonotactically illegal word-onset; that is, a phoneme combination that never occurs at the onset of a German word (e.g., Rlink). Each word and each nonsense word was preceded by the German indefinite article ein that represented an attentional cue and prepared the infant perception for noun onset (i.e., it temporally triggered word form processing).

In all age groups investigated with this cross-modal design so far, the N200-500 was increased in response to congruous words as compared to either incongruous words (Figure 7.1) or nonsense words (Friedrich & Friederici, 2004, 2005a, 2005b). Since congruous and incongruous words, and thus the infants' familiarity with them, were the same in this design (they were physically identical, only the picture–word pairings varied between conditions), prior experience or acoustic variations could not have caused the N200-500 amplitude differences between the word conditions. Therefore, the N200-500 effect is attributed to the matching or nonmatching of the expectation that has been set by the pictured object. This ERP result shows that even in 12-month-olds, the first lexical–semantic knowledge established in memory affects the processing of word forms by cross-modal priming.

In 19-month-olds, moreover, the N200-500 amplitude displayed a gradual differentiation (Friedrich, 2008; Friedrich & Friederici, 2005b). In this age group, congruous words elicited the most negative responses, relative to the other words. Incongruous words and phonotactically legal pseudowords, which both consisted of familiar phoneme combinations but were not primed by the pictured objects, elicited moderately positive responses, while nonsense words, which contain phonotactically illegal phoneme combinations that were unfamiliar to the children, elicited the most positive responses. Thus, in these older children, the N200-500 was affected by priming and familiarity in parallel. This result indicates that the children's early experience with the legal phoneme combinations of their native language differentially affects their processing of novel word forms.

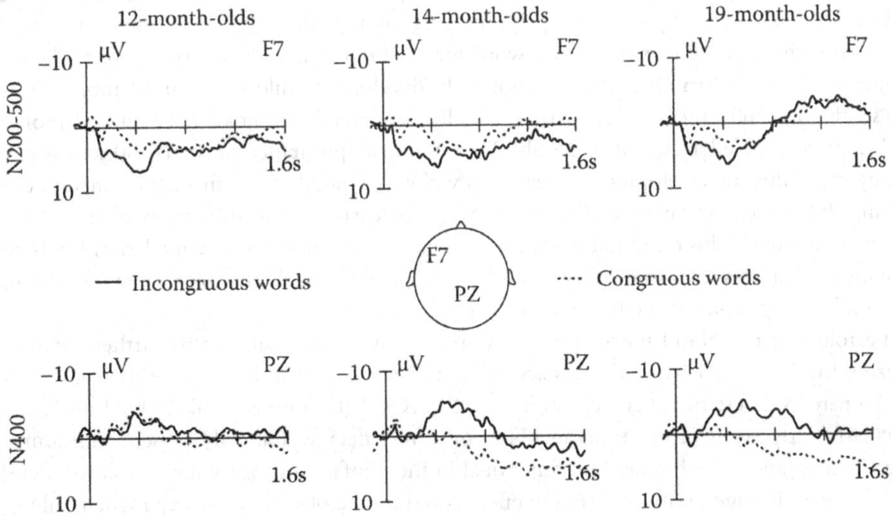

Figure 7.1 The N200-500 word form priming effect and the N400 semantic priming effect in different age groups.

The N400 component in infants and toddlers

In the same picture–word priming paradigm, an N400 semantic priming effect was observed in 14- and 19-month-olds (Figure 7.1), but this effect failed to appear in 12-month-olds (Friedrich & Friederici, 2004, 2005a, 2005b; for a review see Friedrich, 2008). In children of the two older age groups, incongruous words elicited more negative responses than congruous words, which indicates that the processing of picture meanings primed the processing of word meanings. Moreover, the initiation of N400 semantic integration mechanisms was found to depend on the regularity of the phonotactic properties of nonsense words. Whereas semantic mechanisms indexed by the N400 are triggered by both words and legal pseudo-words, these mechanisms were not triggered by phonotactically illegal nonwords. This result indicates that 19-month-old children consider phonotactically legal but not phonotactically illegal nonsense words as potential words of their native language (Friedrich & Friederici, 2005b).

By use of a longitudinal design, we further investigated how the N400 development is related to the children's language development later on. For this purpose, ERP data of the 19-month-old children were retrospectively analyzed according to the children's verbal language skills at two years six months as measured by a German language development test SETK-2 (Grimm, 2000). Children with age-adequate expressive language skills later on displayed an N400 priming effect at 19 months, whereas children with later, poorer language skills who are at risk for a developmental language disorder did not show it at that age (Friedrich & Friederici, 2006). This finding of a relation between the early functioning of the mechanisms underlying N400 generation and children's subsequent success in behavioral language development suits to the result of a study with 20-month-olds. Torkildsen and colleagues found that picture–word matches elicited an N400 priming effect in typically developing 20-month-olds, but not in 20-month-olds at familial risk for dyslexia, who also had lower productive vocabularies than the typically developing children (Torkildsen, Syversen, Simonsen, Moen, & Lindgren, 2007). Recently these findings were extended to the acquisition of new object-word associations. After training with novel pairs of pictures and words, 20-month-olds with high productive vocabularies displayed an N400 priming effect for trained picture–word associations, whereas 20-month-olds with low productive vocabularies did not (Torkildsen et al., 2008).

In both 12-month-olds and 19- to 20-month-olds with delayed language development, the mechanisms of semantic integration that cause N400 generation appear to be either not yet developed or not yet affected by semantic priming, even though the N200-500 effect indicates that, in the same children, objects do prime word forms (Friedrich & Friederici, 2005b, 2006). The presence of an N400 priming effect in normally developing children from 14 months upward suggests that the full functionality of these mechanisms develops between 12 and 14 months of age (Friedrich & Friederici, 2005a, 2005b). Thus, the first appearance of the N400 semantic word priming effect during development is temporally closely related to the first appearance of the fast mapping ability (i.e., the capacity of children to rapidly learn new words for new objects after only a few presentations). This temporal co-occurrence points to a possibly causal relationship between the brain mechanisms responsible for N400 elicitation and the qualitative shift from the slow to the fast word learning mode at the behavioral level.

The role that the N400 mechanisms play in early word acquisition was further explored by analyzing the ERPs of 12-month-olds according to their word production at this age, which was rated by parents in a standardized questionnaire ELFRA-1 (Grimm & Doil, 2000). In infants with particularly early word production, an N400 priming effect was already present indicating that semantic integration mechanisms are functional in these infants. In normally and slowly developing children at that age, an N400 priming effect could not be observed, not even when only words that parents rated to be comprehended by their child were included in the analyses (Friedrich & Friederici, 2009).

In order to find out whether the missing N400 in slowly and normally developing 12-month-olds is caused by the general immatureness of the brain structures mediating the N400 response or by the fact that these mechanisms are not yet triggered by word stimuli, a picture–sound paradigm was developed as analog of the picture–word priming paradigm. Here, 12-month-old infants were presented with pictures of objects (e.g., a dog) and congruous or incongruous natural sounds (e.g., a barking or a ringing). In this study, we found an N400 priming effect on incongruous sounds, indicating that the mechanisms of semantic integration are already functional at 12 months. This result leads to the interpretation that the missing N400 priming effect on words is not caused by immature brain structures or immature N400 neural mechanisms at that age (Babocsai, Friedrich, & Pauen, 2007).

Overall, the studies reviewed here provide evidence that the early functioning of the N400 neural mechanisms interact with children's language development, but we do not know what kind of interaction this is. Although it might be the case that the N400 elicitation and the fast mapping ability are independent but require a similar state of brain development, the result of the picture–sound study argues against this hypothesis and provides evidence for a more direct interrelation. It rather appears that those brain structures realizing semantic integration are mature from early infancy on, but that the N400 neural mechanisms cannot operate on weakly established memory representations acquired in the slow word learning mode. It might even be possible that fast mapping requires the functioning of the mechanisms underlying N400 generation, and that these mechanisms are involved in the process of word learning. However, in order to understand the relation between the mechanisms responsible for N400 elicitation and the infant's word learning capacity, we would have to know what the N400 actually reflects and how semantic integration is realized at a neural level.

Semantic focus: The current view of the semantic system

The mechanisms reflected in the N400 component are involved in primary or secondary semantic processing stages, most likely in setting or changing the semantic focus. Here the term semantic focus means the selective activation of certain aspects of semantic knowledge, which are coded as assemblies of semantic features and stored in (one or more) semantic representations. The semantic focus is the current choice of the semantic system in a certain situation and it represents the context-dependent view of an object or event. That means, from the possible representations available by the semantic system, only a subset is selected within a certain situation. But how does the neural system select the semantic knowledge that is appropriate in a situation?

In principle, selection can be realized by different mechanisms. One is the pre-activation of memory structures either by long-lasting motivations and intentions, or by short-lasting representations currently active in working memory. This short-lasting priming of certain semantic aspects is caused by the activation of memory structures that are semantically related to the ongoing context. Priming is well known to affect response time by realizing faster stimulus processing, but it also modifies the quality of stimulus processing by preventing the unaffected, spontaneous focus of the corresponding neural system. Thus, priming as a semantic selection mechanism sets the focus according to the current semantic context and the organization of this semantic information in long-term memory. Although the N400 is extremely sensitive to semantic priming and it also depends on the organization of semantic memory, it does not reflect the priming process itself (i.e., the semantic preactivation) but rather the effect of semantic preactivation on the semantic processing of a subsequent stimulus.

Another way of selection that more directly depends on memory, is the differentiated modification of activity during neuronal signal transmission. An object that is perceived (or generally, any incoming meaningful information) always activates several possible semantic representations with which the object shares common features. One (or some) of these representations sets the semantic focus, which means it is activated strongest and remains temporally stable in short-term memory. In addition to semantic priming, this focus mainly depends on the overlap of features activated by the object with features coded within potentially relevant representations and on the selective strengths of features (i.e., the weighting of features within these representations). Thus, this kind of selection mainly sets the current semantic focus according to previously acquired knowledge that has been affected by the frequency of activations and the quality of consolidation. N400 amplitude has been shown to depend on semantic similarity and on the typicality of an exemplar as member of a category, both reflected in the overlap of semantic features, as well as on item frequency and previous exposure to items (Kutas & Federmeier, 2000). Therefore, it might be involved in the primary activation of semantic representations and in a potential competition between relevant representations. Since these basic mechanisms of neuronal signal transmission are essential for any further semantic processing, one would expect that they are mature very early and that they are present even in infants. The missing N400 in 12-month-olds suggest that the N400 does not represent a mechanism that is involved in such an obligatory semantic processing stage.

With respect to behavioral relevance a third mechanism of knowledge selection would be necessary in the case of an inappropriate semantic focus. If the current focus does not match the expectation of the ongoing semantic context, or if the consequences associated with this focus (such as the predicted lexical–semantic context or the expected emotional impact) are not matched by the actual consequences, then the current semantic focus caused by priming and previous knowledge should be inhibited. This inhibition should trigger the memory search for a more appropriate semantic focus, and in doing so would realize semantic integration. If existing representations cannot be successfully integrated, this should lead to the acquisition of a new semantic representation that better fits the current contextual situation, and refines, corrects, or complements the representations available within the lexical–semantic system. Such a mechanism would moreover automatically be applied to pseudowords as potential references of meaning; therefore, pseudowords would also "reset" the current state of activity of the semantic system. This supposed selection mechanism would set a new focus according to the evaluation of the previous focus with respect to behavioral consequences, emotional relevance, and both the previous and the forthcoming semantic context. A mismatch of a semantic focus with the semantic context is exactly what the N400 triggers. Like the N400, such an evaluation mechanism would moreover be affected by the organization of semantic memory, and its functioning might depend on a certain developmental state of the representations established within the semantic system.

The stability–plasticity dilemma

But how is the semantic system able to evaluate its own current focus? How does it overcome inappropriate activations? Moreover, how does it know whether the knowledge it already has acquired is appropriate or whether it should rather form a new semantic representation? An even more general question is, how is the human neural system able to learn new semantic representations for objects or events while holding in memory old representations acquired for similar objects or events? With respect to artificial learning systems, this question is called the stability–plasticity dilemma (Grossberg, 1987). It refers to the fact that during training artificial neural networks adjust their weight patterns to the environmental statistics, and a changing environment (i.e., changing probabilities of feature occurrence) can erase previously learned knowledge. Moreover, if neural networks are trained with a new output for an input pattern that has already been trained in another learning environment, then most systems either do not learn the new classification or they "forget" the first learned mapping. This means that these systems are unable to learn new classifications for the same input set while preserving already established knowledge; they are either stable or flexible, but they are not both stable and flexible in parallel. Thus, they cannot acquire hierarchical semantic knowledge without having an explicitly designed hierarchical structure. A predefined hierarchical architecture, however, would strongly limit the flexibility of abstraction. For example, if there are predefined levels to categorize a certain rose as rose, as flower, and as plant, additional levels would be necessary to code it as cut flower, as ornamental plant, as cultivated plant, or as any other category exemplar. The human semantic system does not appear to rely on such hard-wired hierarchies, since it can create and store an unlimited number of partly overlapping representations that, moreover, do not erase each other.

Adaptive Resonance Theory

Adaptive Resonance Theory (ART) was particularly developed to resolve the stability–plasticity dilemma (e.g., Grossberg, 1976a, 1976b, 1980, 1987). This advanced theory provides sophisticated artificial neural mechanisms for stable prototype formation and self-adjusted attention switching, which are mathematically formalized and incorporated into powerful neural network models (e.g., Carpenter & Grossberg, 1987; Carpenter, Grossberg, & Reynolds, 1991; Carpenter, Martens, & Ogas, 2005). The network dynamic fully relies on neurobiologically plausible local and real-time computations, and it incorporates attentional mechanisms, such as attentional gain control, attentional priming, vigilance regulation, and orienting, which realize self-evaluation, self-adjusted memory search, and the stable formation of memory representations, even of those with strongly overlapping features.

The basic model of the ART family, the ART 1 (Carpenter & Grossberg, 1987), is an unsupervised neural network, which means that the net is not given explicit information of the categorical membership of an input exemplar or of the mapping of an input to a certain output. Rather, the net creates its own category structures depending on the feature frequency distributions and the feature correlation structure within the learning environment. This unsupervised learning produces prototypes based on similarity. In contrast, supervised learning models enable arbitrary mappings and the formation of categories that are sensitive to other distinctions such as culturally mediated or linguistically triggered categorizations. In the supervised ARTMAP (Carpenter et al., 1991), the output of an unsupervised ART 1 module is used to determine the categorization of a second ART 1 module. Thus, one ART 1 supervises the other ART 1, which represents a kind of self-supervising as is the case in natural learning systems. This supervised ARTMAP can particularly be used to study the interaction of spontaneous and word guided concept formation and its developmental course.

ART 1 architecture and the concept of adaptive resonance

The ART 1 (Figure 7. 2) consists of an input layer (I) and two representational layers: one coding features (F1) and the other coding categories (F2). Categories are represented by their bidirectional weighted connections from and to the feature representations. Gain control and orienting subsystem are additional components complementing the basic network design. As common in neural networks, the artificial neurons within the layers are called nodes or populations. ART 1 short- and long-term dynamics (i.e., activation and learning) are described by differential equations that allow the simulation of real-time processing. A specific characteristic of ART systems is that short- and long-term dynamics operate on different time scales. This main feature is inspired by the fact that the electro-chemical communication between real neurons is relatively fast as compared to the molecular and structural modifications of synaptic connections, which correspond to learning. With other words, learning needs time, and sufficiently stable learning can only take place in a temporally stable internal state. In ART systems this relative stability is given by the resonant state, in which short-term processing results and which is called adaptive resonance. The resonant state is characterized by the matching and the sustained reciprocal activation of bottom-up input and top-down learned expectations.

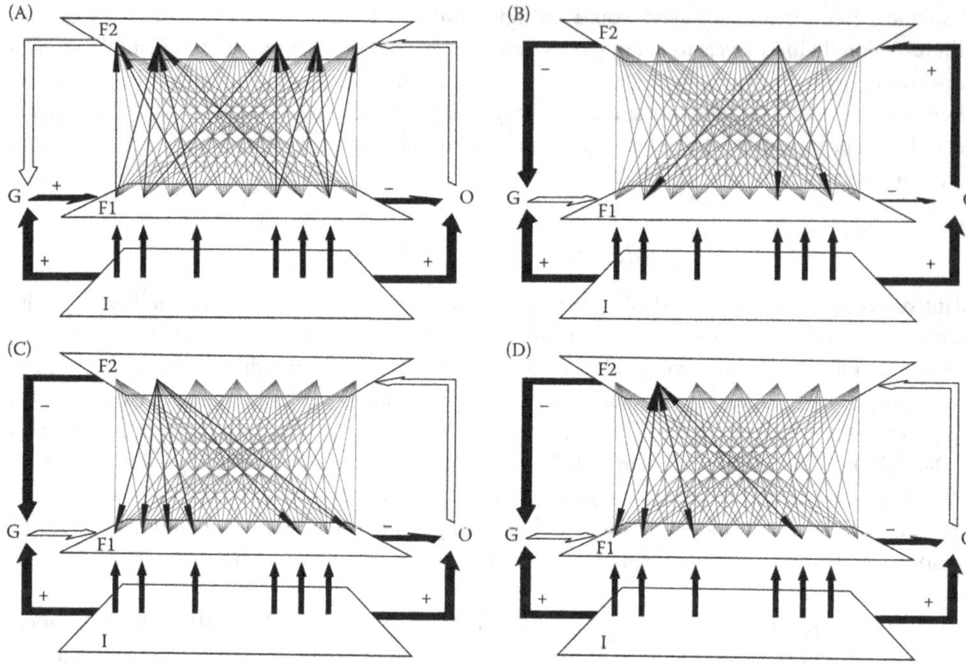

Figure 7.2 ART 1 architecture and the concept of adaptive resonance.

ART 1 short-term dynamics

The short-term dynamics of the ART 1 determines how the activation of the system changes in response to input activity that arises from a certain preprocessing stage. Figure 7.2 provides a slightly simplified illustration of the ART 1 short-term dynamics (for a detailed mathematical description, see Carpenter & Grossberg, 1987). A: An input pattern activates gain control (G), orienting subsystem (O), and specific feature detection nodes in F1. Gain control nonspecifically activates all nodes in F1. Those F1 nodes that receive activation of both input layer and gain control exceed a threshold and generate an output. Activity in F1 inhibits the orienting subsystem and prevents the activity of this subsystem by balancing the activation by the input pattern. The bottom-up signals from F1 to F2 are filtered by adaptive long-term weights, and the input that an F2 node receives is the sum of all weighted signals from F1 to the F2 node. Mathematically this is the scalar product between the F1 output vector and the weight vector to the F2 node, which can be interpreted as similarity of the input exemplar with the prototype of the category coded in F2. B: Competition between F2 nodes results in suprathreshold activity of that F2 node (or of several nodes) that has received the highest signal, whereas the activity of all other F2 nodes is suppressed. Note that strong weights of a few features may lead to the highest signal even though the whole feature pattern of the input might not be matched by the winning F2 node. Output of F2 inhibits gain control, such that F1 is no longer activated nonspecifically. Instead, F1 receives a specific signal from F2; namely, the output of the winning F2 node multiplied with the top-down weight vector from F2 to F1, which represents the feature pattern expectation read out by the category momentarily active in F2. Suprathreshold activity in F1 is now possible if a node receives specific signals from both input and F2. Since normally the category expectation differs from the input pattern, total F1 activity is attenuated and likewise the inhibition of the orienting subsystem decreases. If this decrease is too strong with respect to the criterion set by the value of the vigilance parameter (p), mathematically, if the ratio of the inhibition by the total activity in F1 and the activation by the total input activity is smaller than p, then the orienting system becomes active and resets short-term activity by nonspecific activation of F2. This reset temporary inhibits the category node currently active in F2 and, as a consequence, inhibition of the gain control is removed. C: Thus, (if the input is still present) the system returns into state A, except that the first-pass attracting category is temporary, not sensitive to signals from F1, and therefore it does not win competition again. This enables another F2 category to win competition and to release an expectation in F1. Again, the associated activity decrease in F1 and the attenuated inhibition of the orienting subsystem is evaluated according to the current vigilant state of the system, which possibly leads to further memory search. D: If a category expectation sufficiently matches the input pattern, then the inhibition of the orienting subsystem remains strong enough, and a reset is prevented. Sustained reciprocal activation between F1 and F2 now constitutes the resonant state in which learning takes place.

ART 1 long-term dynamics

The long-term dynamics of the ART 1 determines how the weights of connections change, that is, how the system learns. In ART systems, learning is only possible in the resonant state, in which bottom-up and top-down information is matched. In adaptive resonance the F1 activity of those features that are both present in the input and expected by the category is sustained by reciprocal activation between F1 and F2. Therefore, the connections between these feature nodes and the active category node are strengthened during learning. Moreover, the weights to those features that are expected by the category but not present in the input are reduced.

Learning in ART 1 is time-dependent, and the differential equations can be used to simulate learning for several temporal conditions (Friedrich, 1994, 1997). In the case of fast learning, sufficient time is available for weight changing such that the state of dynamic equilibrium is reached and no further weight change occurs. In this case, weights are fully adapted to the information in resonance; therefore, categories contain only features that are present in each exemplar. In contrast, if there is not enough time for learning (i.e., if the resonant state is interrupted or the rate of leaning is low), then only a certain amount of information is transferred into weights. In this case of slow learning, categories represent features according to their frequency distribution within the category exemplars. Thus, slow learning within ART 1 leads to the formation of prototypical categories with a pronounced graded structure.

Vigilance and the level of generalization

In ART systems, category inclusiveness (i.e., the level of generalization) depends on the value of the vigilance parameter that models the internal evaluation criterion involved in the sensitivity control mechanism of the orienting subsystem. Low vigilance represents a relaxed state, in which the system tolerates high variability between category exemplars. This state leads to the formation of broad, general categories. In contrast, if vigilance is high, then the system is in a state of low tolerance, which enables the fine discrimination between similar exemplars and the formation of narrow, specific categories. As a result of varying vigilance, categories at different levels of inclusiveness, which range from a very global level of abstraction up to representations of individual exemplars, coexist in ART systems.

The effect of vigilance, however, depends on the present learning state of the system, or more specifically, on the learning state of a certain category. The ART reset is only triggered by a mismatch between bottom-up input and the top-down expectations of the currently winning category, and thus, it requires sufficiently specified memory structures coded in that category. When learning is slow due to time or processing limitations, initially the system forms broad global categories that code a lot of features. These very fuzzy categories act as attractors, and they match lots of input patterns, thus, even in the case of maximal vigilance, reset is prevented and specific categories are not acquired. During the course of further learning, categories become sharper and more specified. Now if vigilance is sufficiently high then reset will initiate memory search and specific categories can be formed (Friedrich, 1995, 1997).

Implications for early word learning and N400 development

The ART neural networks are the first artificial neural memory system that can be stable, flexible, and constructive in parallel. They achieve these properties by incorporating a neural mechanism that enables the systems to evaluate their own categorization behavior, to suppress a current focus chosen by priming and first-pass competition of memory representations, and to adjust their category inclusiveness according to internal and external requirements. Since the human memory system is stable, flexible, and constructive in reality, the question can be posed, whether a functionally similar mechanism is actually working in the human brain. Here it is shown what the basic assumptions of ART and the real presence of an ART-like evaluation mechanism would imply with respect to early word learning. It is, moreover, suggested that if such a mechanism would actually exist, then it would have been reflected in the N400 component of the ERP.

The slow learning mode

If following the assumption that a temporally stable state is required for natural learning too, one could further assume that this temporal stability is limited during early development, since the input from preprocessing stages might temporally not be stable, some activity loss during resonance might not be compensated by weak synaptic connections, and molecular and structural synaptic changes might require more time during early than later developmental states. Similar to ART simulations (Friedrich, 1994, 1997), such temporal constraint in the maturing brain would result in behavioral constraints for category formation and word learning. According to ART, first naturally acquired categories would be very global with a fuzzy and pronounced prototypical structure that would cause massive overgeneralizations. The formation of specific categories would depend on the amount of previous learning of more global categories, and it would involve the inhibition of global categories. A frequent successive presentation of exemplars of a certain subcategory (as in behavioral tests that include a familiarization phase) would shift the global category toward the specific features of the subcategory, such that exemplars of another subcategory could initiate reset and constitute its own category. This categorization behavior predicted by simulations is exactly what has been found for natural and experimentally induced categorizations in infants and toddlers (e.g., Bomba & Siqueland, 1983; Goede & Friedrich, 1995; Mareschal & Quinn, 2001; McDonough, 2002; Quinn, 1987; Younger & Fearing, 2000).

Moreover, temporally limited learning would not only result in constraint categorizations but also in weak associations between words and concepts, such as is the case in the slow word learning mode before children acquire the fast mapping ability. At the neural level, the shift from the slow to the fast word learning mode would then be associated with quantitative rather than qualitative changes, such as longer temporal stability and therefore more time for synaptic modifications, or with a higher rate of learning-related changes.

Overcoming errors by ART reset

The advantage of slow learning is that it is relatively robust with respect to the effect of errors. A few errors will be automatically erased by the representation of features according to their frequency distribution. Even false mappings between words and concepts are of no consequence for the whole learning process if the most frequent mappings are correct. Thus, an explicit mechanism for error correction is not required in the slow learning mode.

However, as infants become able to rapidly associate new words with newly built concepts, they may establish inappropriate conceptual representations or wrong associations between words and concepts, such that mechanisms for correcting them would need to develop. Without an explicit error correction mechanism, wrong associations could only be resolved by unspecific forgetting, that is, some kind of synaptic weight decrease that is not specific to the invalid memory representation. The ART reset, however, represents an error correction mechanism that specifically detects wrong associations and enables the formation of new semantic concepts and the correct mappings between words and concepts. According to ART, the functioning of this mechanism actually sets in at the point in development at which it is necessary; that is, when learning becomes faster and therefore error correction becomes crucial.

N400 as the reflection of a semantic short-term reset

It is proposed here that the mechanisms underlying the elicitation of the N400 component of the ERP are involved in a memory search process that is triggered to reinterpret a meaningful stimulus in a way that matches the whole contextual situation, whereby semantic integration of that stimulus into the meaningful context takes place. ART is the first theory that provides a model for real-time memory search in a massively parallel neural architecture. According to this model, memory search is realized by successive nonspecific arousal waves that reset short-term activity. This neural reset mechanism temporally inhibits the activity pattern of the first preferred representations and therefore it enables the system to focus on those aspects of the stimulus that are relevant in the present context.

In the unsupervised basic ART 1 model, memory search is triggered by a nonmatching expectation read out from the currently active category representation. In the supervised ARTMAP model (Carpenter et al., 1991), reset is triggered in the same way, but vigilance regulation and therefore reset is moreover mediated by nonmatching outputs of the two ART 1 modules, such as a word active in one module, which does not match a concept active in the other module, as is the case in the picture–word ERP study with infants and young children.

Dissociation of N200-500 and N400 priming during early development

In both ART 1 and ARTMAP, reset and therefore the memory search for an appropriate semantic focus not only depends on the sensitivity parameter vigilance but also on the expectation read out by the currently active category, which must be sufficiently specified in order to cause a mismatch. If assuming that an ART-like reset mechanism (i.e., the inhibition of the current semantic focus) is reflected in the N400 component of the ERP, this behavior of the model can be used to explain the dissociation of N400 semantic priming and N200-500 word priming observed in the ERP of 12-month-old infants.

Suppose, for instance, an infant has not yet established specific cat or dog categories, but it has an unspecific global mammal representation that is (possibly weakly) associated with the word dog perceived most often in this context. If now, the infant sees a dog (or a cat), then, according to ART, the global mammal category would win first-pass competition and would release an expectation. If vigilance is low, this category is chosen for resonance and would prime the word dog such that the subsequent perceptual processing of the word dog is facilitated. In the infant ERP, this would be reflected as an N200-500 word priming effect; that is, an increased N200-500 amplitude in response to the word dog. If, in contrast, the infant either hears the unexpected word cat or a semantically unrelated word like car, vigilance increases. If the expectation of the mammal representation is sufficiently specified, then this vigilance increase leads to ART reset, which would be reflected as N400 in the ERP. However, ART reset will be prevented and activation will not be removed from the initially winning mammal representation, as long as the expectation of this global category is too unspecific to cause a clear mismatch. Consequently, memory search would not be initiated and the N400 would be missing in the ERP. According to this interpretation, the N400 could, however, be elicited very early in development, if a sufficiently specified memory representation has first been established during a familiarization phase and is then violated in a subsequent test phase.

Conclusions

The ART neural networks provide an idea of how the developmental constraints at the neural level, such as the strength of synaptic connections, the global vigilant state of the system, and the time available for the learning of individual items may cause the systemic constraints observed in the categorization and word learning behavior of infants and toddlers. Most of the neural constraints that are crucial for the systemic behavior are related to ART reset, a mechanism that enables both the formation of new semantic memory representations and the task-dependent switch between several representations already available for an object or event. Here, ART reset is supposed to have a real natural equivalent that is reflected in the N400 component of the ERP. This identification theoretically relates the elicitation of the N400 to the learning state of semantic representations. Moreover, it interprets the developmental course of the N400 as depending on the frequency and the amount of learning. The identification of ART reset and N400 as proposed in the present chapter offers a general explanation for how the mechanisms that underlie N400 generation operate on semantic long-term memory, and how their functioning is related to the categorization and word learning capacities in infants and toddlers.

Further reading

Friedrich, M., & Friederici, A. D. (2017). The origins of word learning: Brain responses of three-month-olds indicate their rapid association of objects and words. *Developmental Science, 20*(2), e12357.

Friedrich, M., Mölle, M., Friederici, A. D., & Born, J. (2019). The reciprocal relation between sleep and memory in infancy: Memory-dependent adjustment of sleep spindles and spindle-dependent improvement of memories. *Developmental Science, 22*(2), e12743.

Friedrich, M., Mölle, M., Friederici, A. D., & Born, J. (2020). Sleep-dependent memory consolidation in infants protects new episodic memories from existing semantic memories. *Nature Communications, 11*(1), 1298.

Friedrich, M., Wilhelm, I., Born, J., & Friederici, A. D. (2015). Generalization of word meanings during infant sleep. *Nature Communications, 6*, 6004.

Friedrich, M., Wilhelm, I., Mölle, M., Born, J., & Friederici, A. D. (2017). The sleeping infant brain anticipates development. *Current Biology, 27*(15), 2374–2380.

References

Babocsai, L., Friedrich, M., & Pauen, S. (2007, March 29–April 1). Neural evidence for 12-month-olds' ability to integrate sight and sound in object categories. Biennial Meeting of the Society for Research in Child Development (SRCD), Boston, Massachusetts.

Barrett, S. E., & Rugg, M. D. (1990). Event-related potentials and the semantic matching of pictures. *Brain and Cognition, 14*(2), 201–212.

Bates, E., Thal, D., & Janowsky, J. S. (1992). Early language development and its neural correlates. In I. Rapin & S. Segalowitz (Eds.), *Handbook of neuropsychology, child neurology* (Vol. 6, pp. 69–110). Amsterdam, the Netherlands: Elsevier.

Benedict, H. (1979). Early lexical development: Comprehension and production. *Journal of Child Language, 6*(2), 183–200.

Bomba, P. C., & Siqueland, E. R. (1983). The nature and structure of infant form categories. *Journal of Experimental Child Psychology, 35*(2), 294–328.

Carpenter, G. A., & Grossberg, S. (1987). A massively parallel architecture for a self-organizing neural pattern recognition machine. *Computer Vision, Graphics, and Image Processing, 37*(1), 54–115.

Carpenter, G. A., Grossberg, S., & Reynolds, J. H. (1991). ARTMAP: Supervised real-time learning and classification of nonstationary data by a self-organizing neural network. *Neural Networks, 4*(5), 565–588.

Carpenter, G. A., Martens, S., & Ogas, O. J. (2005). Self-organizing information fusion and hierarchical knowledge discovery: A new framework using ARTMAP neural networks. *Neural Networks, 18*(3), 287–295.
Clark, E. V. (1987). The principle of contrast: A constraint on language acquisition. In B. MacWhinney (Ed.), *Mechanisms of language acquisition* (pp. 1–33). Hillsdale, NJ: Erlbaum.
Courchesne, E., Ganz, L., & Norcia, A. M. (1981). Event-related brain potentials to human faces in infants. *Child Development, 52*(3), 804–811.
Dehaene-Lambertz, G., & Dehaene, S. (1994). Speed and cerebral correlates of syllable discrimination in infants. *Nature, 370*(6487), 292–294.
Federmeier, K. D., & Kutas, M. (2001). Meaning and modality: Influence of context, semantic memory organization, and perceptual predictability on picture processing. *Journal of Experimental Psychology: Learning, Memory, and Cognition, 27*(1), 202–224.
French, R. M., Mareschal, D., Mermillod, M., & Quinn, P. C. (2004). The role of bottom-up processing in perceptual categorization by 3- to 4-month-old infants: Simulations and data. *Journal of Experimental Psychology: General, 133*(3), 382–397.
Friederici, A. D. (2005). Neurophysiological markers of early language acquisition: From syllables to sentences. *Trends in Cognitive Sciences, 9*(10), 481–488.
Friederici, A. D., Friedrich, M., & Christophe, A. (2007). Brain responses in 4-month-old infants are already language specific. *Current Biology, 17*(14), 1208–1211.
Friederici, A. D., & Wessels, J. M. I. (1993). Phonotactic knowledge of word boundaries and its use in infant speech-perception. *Perception and Psychophysics, 54*(3), 287–295.
Friedrich, M. (1994). *Modellierung und Simulation kategorialer Strukturbildung: Eine Anwendung der Adaptiven Resonanztheorie auf die Begriffsbildung.* [Unpublished doctoral thesis].
Friedrich, M. (1997). Der Erwerb hierarchisch ordenbarer Kategorien in einem neuronalen Netz der Adaptiven Resonanztheorie. *ZASPIL, 8*, 57–80.
Friedrich, M. (2008). Neurophysiological correlates of picture-word priming in one-year-olds. In A. D. Friederici & G. Thierry (Eds.), *Early language development: Bridging brain and behaviour. Series "Trends in language acquisition research" (TiLAR)* (Vol. 5, 137–160). Amsterdam, the Netherlands: John Benjamins.
Friedrich, M., & Friederici, A. D. (2004). N400-like semantic incongruity effect in 19-month-olds: Processing known words in picture contexts. *Journal of Cognitive Neuroscience, 16*(8), 1465–1477.
Friedrich, M., & Friederici, A. D. (2005a). Lexical priming and semantic integration reflected in the ERP of 14-month-olds. *NeuroReport, 16*(6), 653–656.
Friedrich, M., & Friederici, A. D. (2005b). Phonotactic knowledge and lexical-semantic processing in one-year-olds: Brain responses to words and nonsense words in picture contexts. *Journal of Cognitive Neuroscience, 17*(11), 1785–1802.
Friedrich, M., & Friederici, A. D. (2006). Early N400 development and later language acquisition. *Psychophysiology, 43*(1), 1–12.
Friedrich, M., & Friederici, A. D. (2009). Maturing brain mechanisms and developing behavioral language skills. *Developmental Science.* Retrieved from http://doi.org/10.1016/j.bandl.2009.07.004.
Ganis, G., Kutas, M., & Sereno, M. (1996). The search for "common sense": An electro-physiological study of the comprehension of words and pictures in reading. *Journal of Cognitive Neuroscience, 8*(2), 89–106.
Goede, K., & Friedrich, M. (1995). Roses but not flowers: Phenomena of the development and the naming of concepts. In M. Verrips & F. Wijnen (Eds.), *Papers from the Dutch-German colloquium on language acquisition* (Vol. 66, pp. 41–63). Amsterdam, the Netherlands: University of Amsterdam.
Golinkoff, R. M., Mervis, C. B., & Hirsh-Pasek, K. (1994). Early object labels: The case for lexical principles. *Journal of Child Language, 21*(1), 125–155.
Grimm, H. (2000). *SETK-2: Sprachentwicklungstest für zweijährige Kinder (2.0–2.11). Diagnose rezeptiver und produktiver Sprachverarbeitungsfähigkeiten.* Göttingen: Hogrefe.
Grimm, H., & Doil, H. (2000). *ELFRA: Elternfragebögen für die Früherkennung von Risikokindern (ELFRA-1, ELFRA-2).* Göttingen: Hogrefe.
Grossberg, S. (1976a). Adaptive pattern classification and universal recoding, I: Parallel development and coding of neural feature detectors. *Biological Cybernetics, 23*(3), 121–134.
Grossberg, S. (1976b). Adaptive pattern classification and universal recoding: II. Feedback, expectation, olfaction, illusions. *Biological Cybernetics, 23*(4), 187–202.
Grossberg, S. (1980). How does a brain build a cognitive code? *Psychological Review, 87*(1), 1–51.
Grossberg, S. (1987). Competitive learning: From interactive activation to adaptive resonance. *Cognitive Science, 11*(1), 23–63.
Holcomb, P. J. (1993). Semantic priming and stimulus degradation: Implications for the role of the N400 in language processing. *Psychophysiology, 30*(1), 47–61.
Holcomb, P. J., & McPherson, W. B. (1994). Event-related brain potentials reflect semantic priming in an object decision task. *Brain and Cognition, 24*(2), 259–276.

Jusczyk, P.W., Cutler, A., & Redanz, N. J. (1993). Infant's sensitivity to the predominant stress pattern of English words. *Child Development, 64*(3), 675–687.

Jusczyk, P.W., Friederici, A. D., Wessels, J. M. I., Svenkerud, V.Y., & Jusczyk, A. M. (1993). Infant's sensitivity to the sound patterns of native language words. *Journal of Memory and Language, 32*(3), 402–420.

Kooijman, V., Hagoort, P., & Cutler, A. (2005). Electrophysiological evidence for prelinguistic infants' word recognition in continuous speech. *Cognitive Brain Research, 24*(1), 109–116.

Kuhl, P. K., Williams, K. A., Lacerda, F., Stevens, K. N., & Lindblom, B. (1992). Linguistic experience alters phonetic perception in infants by 6 months of age. *Science, 255*(5044), 606–608.

Kushnerenko, E., Ceponiene, R., Balan, P., Fellman, V., Huotilainen, M., & Näätänen, R. (2002). Maturation of the auditory event-related potentials during the first year of life. *NeuroReport, 13*(1), 47–51.

Kutas, M., & Federmeier, K. D. (2000). Electrophysiology reveals semantic memory use in language comprehension. *Trends in Cognitive Sciences, 4*(12), 463–470.

Kutas, M., & Hillyard, S. A. (1980). Reading senseless sentences: Brain potentials reflect semantic incongruity. *Science, 207*(4427), 203–205.

Mareschal, D., & Quinn, P. (2001). Categorization in infancy. *Trends in Cognitive Sciences, 5*(10), 443–450.

Markman, E. V., & Wachtel, G. F. (1988). Children's use of mutual exclusivity to constrain the meaning of words. *Cognitive Psychology, 20*(2), 121–157.

McDonough, L. (2002). Basic-level nouns: First learned but misunderstood. *Journal of Child Language, 29*(2), 357–377.

Mills, D. L., Coffey-Corina, S. A., & Neville, H. J. (1993). Language acquisition and cerebral specialization in 20-month-old infants. *Journal of Cognitive Neuroscience, 5*(3), 317–334.

Mills, D. L., Coffey-Corina, S. A., & Neville, H. J. (1997). Language comprehension and cerebral specialization from 13 to 20 months. *Developmental Neuropsychology, 13*(3), 397–445.

Nazzi, T., & Bertoncini, J. (2003). Before and after the vocabulary spurt: Two modes of word acquisition? *Developmental Science, 6*(2), 136–142.

Nigam, A., Hoffman, J. E., & Simons, R. F. (1992). N400 to semantically anomalous pictures and words. *Journal of Cognitive Neuroscience, 4*(1), 15–27.

Posner, M. I., & Keele, S. W. (1968). On the genesis of abstract ideas. *Journal of Experimental Psychology, 77*(3), 353–363.

Quinn, P. C. (1987). The categorical representation of visual pattern information by young infants. *Cognition, 27*(2), 145–179.

Rosch, E. H. (1973). Natural categories. *Cognitive Psychology, 4*(3), 328–350.

Sarfarazi, M., Cave, B., Richardson, A., Behan, J., & Sedgwick, E. M. (1999). Visual event related potentials modulated by contextually relevant and irrelevant olfactory primes. *Chemical Senses, 24*(2), 145–154.

Schafer, G., & Plunkett, K. (1998). Rapid word learning by fifteen-month-olds under tightly controlled conditions. *Child Development, 69*(2), 309–320.

Thierry, G., Vihman, M., & Roberts, M. (2003). Familiar words capture the attention of 11-month-olds in less than 250 ms. *NeuroReport, 14*(18), 2307–2310.

Tincoff, R., & Jusczyk, P. W. (1999). Some beginnings of word comprehension in 6-month-olds. *Psychological Science, 10*(2), 172–175.

Torkildsen, J. V. K., Svangstu, J. M., Friis Hansen, H., Smith, L., Simonsen, H. G., Moen, I., & Lindgren, M. (2008). Productive vocabulary size predicts ERP correlates of fast mapping in 20-month-olds. *Journal of Cognitive Neuroscience, 20*, 1266–1282.

Torkildsen, J. V. K., Syversen, G., Simonsen, H. G., Moen, I., & Lindgren, M. (2007). Brain responses to lexical–semantic priming in children at-risk for dyslexia. *Brain and Language, 102*(3), 243–261.

Van Petten, C., & Rheinfelder, H. (1995). Conceptual relationships between spoken words and environmental sounds: Event-related brain potential measures. *Neuropsychologia, 33*(4), 485–508.

Werker, J. F., Cohen, L. B., Lloyd, V. L., Casasola, M., & Stager, C. L. (1998). Acquisition of word-object associations by 14-month-old infants. *Developmental Psychology, 34*(6), 1289–1309.

Werker, J. F., & Lalonde, C. E. (1988). Cross-language speech perception: Initial capabilities and developmental change. *Developmental Psychology, 24*(5), 1–12.

Werker, J. F., & Tees, R. C. (2002). Cross-language speech perception: Evidence for perceptual reorganization during the first year of life. *Infant Behavioral Development, 25*(1), 121.

West, W. C., & Holcomb, P. J. (2002). Event-related potentials during discourse-level semantic integration of complex pictures. *Cognitive Brain Research, 13*(3), 363–375.

Woodward, A. L., Markman, E., & Fitzsimmons, C. M. (1994). Rapid word learning in 13- and 18-month-olds. *Developmental Psychology, 30*(4), 553–566.

Younger, B. A., & Fearing, D. D. (2000). A global-to-basic trend in early categorization: Evidence from a dual-category habituation task. *Infancy, 1*(1), 47–58.

8

CONNECTIONIST MODELS OF APHASIA REVISITED

Grant Walker

Introduction

This chapter is an update to the original chapter by Dell and Kittredge (2011). The original chapter covered foundational topics and several examples for understanding connectionist models of aphasia and other language disorders. In this chapter, we will revisit some of these topics and examine several of the more recent applications of connectionist models to the study of aphasia since then, with particular attention given to investigations of neurocognitive mechanisms that support human language. This is a developing area of research, with a variety of approaches that incorporate connectionist models to aid our understanding of language disorders that result from neurological injury.

To review, a model is a simplified imitation of a more complex system. A model provides a link between a theoretical understanding of how the world works and the data we gather from the world around us. By mirroring the interesting relationships that exist in the world and dispensing with the irrelevant details, a model allows an investigator to selectively manipulate and control specific features of a subject of inquiry to understand their function and importance, and to generate predictions about how manipulating their real-world counterparts is likely to affect experimental outcomes. Because the brain and the mind process many types of information in complex ways, researchers often try to simplify and focus on a limited set of mechanisms or processes.

Connectionist models are information processing models that are inspired by the functioning of the nervous system. They are sometimes called artificial neural networks. A connectionist model is a computer program that simulates the spreading activation between interconnected units (sometimes called nodes), much like electrical activity spreads from neuron to neuron via synapses in the nervous system. But the degree of similarity to real neural networks can vary from one connectionist model to another, with some models being highly abstract descriptions of the mind and other models being strongly grounded in the physiology and biological constraints found in real brains. This is especially true for connectionist models of aphasia, which, on the one hand, may focus more on the abstract mental representations and processes of human language or, on the other hand, may focus more on the neurobiological mechanisms of impairment and recovery.

At their most abstract, connectionist models are simply a collection of real-valued variables that are iteratively updated according to specific rules. There are at least two types of variables in a connectionist model: variables representing the activation of units and variables representing the connection strength (also called connection weight) between units. Activation variables typically range from 0 to 1 or from -1 to 1, and the activations of all units are updated on each timestep according

DOI: 10.4324/9781003204213-10

to an activation rule. The activation for a given unit on a given timestep generally depends on: (1) the unit's activation on the previous timestep, (2) the activation of the other units that are connected to it, (3) the connection strengths between the units, (4) a rate of decay of activation over time, and, sometimes, (5) random noise. Units are typically grouped into three subtypes: (1) input units receive activation values that are pre-determined by the modeler or the simulated environment to initiate the flow of activation through the network; (2) output units are monitored to evaluate the decision-making behavior of the network; and (3) hidden units participate in directing the flow of activation through the network from input units to output units.

Units are also typically grouped into layers (sometimes called pools) based on their connections with other units or layers. For example, separate input layers may correspond to different sensory modalities. Sometimes, multiple layers of hidden units are stacked in between input and output units, creating a series of filters that can detect hierarchical features of the input stimulus. These are called deep neural networks. For example, activation in the input layer may correspond to the pattern of light projecting an image onto a retina, with the first hidden layer detecting edges and shadows, the next hidden layer detecting body parts like the eyes or lips, the next hidden layer detecting faces at different viewing angles, and the final output layer detecting the unique identity of the face. The arrangement of units, connections, and layers within a connectionist model is called the model's architecture. When the model's parameters are defined (i.e., the inputs, the architecture, the activation rule, and the connection strengths), a connectionist network embodies a mapping from a pattern of activation in the input units to a pattern of activation in the output units.

Many connectionist models also include a learning rule, such that connection strengths are iteratively updated in an effort to reduce the difference between the observed activation in output units and some target activation for the output units given the input activation. For example, an initial run of a connectionist model could erroneously map an input image of a cat to an output label DOG. The error then signals that connection strengths from the input image to the output label DOG should be reduced and the connection strength from the input image to the output label CAT should be increased. In this way, after many trials and errors, a particular weighting of the network can be discovered that reliably maps a set of input representations each to their corresponding output representations, though, due to the element of chance that is involved in learning network weightings, the degree of reliability may vary from mapping to mapping. These representational mappings can be applied quite generally to many different problems, for example, mapping from an individual's list of previously viewed entertainment to a list of options that are most likely to be viewed next. For commercial or industrial purposes such as these, the nature of the representations or the architectural details of the network may be of little importance compared with the accuracy of the model's output. In the context of aphasia research, by contrast, connectionist models may represent a mapping from a concept to a phonological word form, or a mapping from an auditory stimulus to a motor control program for the speech articulators. Rather than merely representing a person's predicted behavior in its output units, the connectionist model is typically assumed to simulate the process that generated the behavior. To the extent that the model is successful, it can provide powerful insights about the nature of mental representations or mechanisms that may be targeted by interventions to modify the behavior.

Dell and Kittredge (2010) wrote, "Despite the affinity between connectionist models and neural systems, though, connectionist modelers rarely do what Lichtheim did; that is, link model parts with brain regions. Rather, as we will see, connectionist modelers aim to correctly characterize the cognitive mechanisms of language processing, with the hopes that eventually these mechanisms can be identified with brain areas." While this was true at the time of writing, the explicit inclusion of brain areas into connectionist models of aphasia has become more prevalent since then, as we will see. Let's begin, though, by examining how the hopes of identifying cognitive mechanisms in the brain have fared. Dell et al. (2013) explored how a relatively simple connectionist model of word production relates to specific brain areas.

The interactive two-step model of lexical retrieval and the dual-route model of repetition in aphasia

The interactive two-step model of lexical retrieval is a simplified model derived from a larger theory of speech production that posits that retrieval and composition of psycholinguistic representations is achieved through a process of spreading activation (Dell, 1986; Dell et al., 1997; Foygel & Dell, 2000). The simulated lexical network consists of three, consecutive layers of units representing semantic, lexical, and phonological information, respectively. The semantic units represent the meanings of words. A semantic unit can be thought of as a localized representation of a semantic feature, where each unit is associated with a single feature such as a visual or a functional feature. Each concept that is linked with a word is represented by a set of ten semantic units; this is called a distributed representation. When the concept of a word is used to drive speech production, as in the picture naming task, its associated feature units are activated. Words that have similar meanings share features, and thus words for similar concepts will receive activation during a word retrieval attempt. The lexical units, in the middle layer, are localized representations (one unit = one word) that act as hidden units connecting semantic features to phonological forms. The phonological units are also localized representations (one unit = one phoneme) that act as output units, indicating which phoneme will be produced in each syllable position of a CVC target word.

Connections between units are excitatory and bidirectional, meaning that activation flows in both directions between layers. For example, a word unit in the hidden layer activates its constituent phonemes in the output layer, which, in turn, activate other words in the hidden layer that contain the same phonemes. The connections are defined manually by the modeler to represent a lexical neighborhood; there is no learning rule in this model. For example, the lexical unit for CAT would be connected to ten arbitrary semantic units, as well as the /k/, /a/, and /t/ phoneme units in the onset, vowel, and coda positions, respectively. The lexical unit for DOG would be connected to three of the same semantic units that the lexical unit for CAT is connected to and seven of its own unique semantic units. Varying degrees or types of semantic relatedness are not represented in the model. For example, DOG and RAT have different semantic relations to CAT, but these semantic relations would be treated equally by the model. The strength of all connections between two layers are equal. This means, for example, that the prominence of distinguishing features, like MEOW for CAT, is not represented in the model either. Similarly, the retrieval advantage for the phonological onset of words is not represented in the model. The key tenets of this model are: (1) the interactivity between hierarchical psycholinguistic representations during retrieval for production, and (2) the sequential selection of a lexical unit followed by phonological units.

During a simulated picture naming attempt, the model assumes that the person recognizes the picture perfectly and activates the correct semantic features. The target semantic units each receive a jolt of activation that spreads throughout the network. After several timesteps, the most activated lexical unit is selected and receives another jolt of activation. This is the first selection step. After several more timesteps, the most activated units in the onset, vowel, and coda positions of the phonological layer are selected to create a phonological word form. This is the second selection step. Because the activation rule includes decay and inherently random fluctuations, it is possible for selection errors to occur during either selection step, when the target units are unable to receive or maintain their activation levels relative to non-target units. The phonological word form that is ultimately selected in a simulated naming attempt can be compared with the target word form to categorize the type of response that was generated: (1) correct (matches the target), (2) semantic (real word that shares only semantic units with the target), (3) formal (real word that shares only phonological units with the target), (4) mixed (real word that shares semantic and phonological units with the target), (5) unrelated (real word that shares neither semantic nor phonological units with the target), and (6) neologism (a non-word that may or may not share phonological units with the target). When all the parameters of the model (e.g., connection strengths and decay rates) have been set, the network defines the expected rates of these six response types over repeated naming attempts.

With strong connection strengths and low decay rates, the activation flows from semantic features to phonological forms with a high degree of accuracy, mimicking the speech production patterns of neurologically healthy individuals: Mainly correct responses with occasional errors that typically bear a semantic relation to the target. The effect of brain lesions on a speech production network can be simulated by "damaging" the connectionist model. There are several ways to disrupt the normal flow of activation through the network: Reducing the connection strengths between layers or increasing the rate of decay within units are common approaches that have been used with the interactive two-step model. Alternatively, increasing the amount of random activation within units or removing a proportion of units or connections would also disrupt network performance, although modelers tend to apply these manipulations more commonly in larger connectionist networks that rely primarily on distributed representations. While the correspondence between these modeled impairments and disruptions within real biological systems typically remains unspecified, the choice is non-trivial for the effects of simulated lesions on network processing. Both the mechanism of damage (e.g., modifying connection strengths versus decay rates) and the location within the network architecture (e.g., modifying lexical-phonological connections versus lexical-semantic connections) can influence the mapping between concepts and phonological forms in appreciably different ways (Dell et al., 1997; Foygel & Dell, 2000; Martin & Dell, 2019).

The simulations explored by Dell et al. (2013) used localized connection strength reductions to implement lesions. When fitting a patient's naming data with the model, pieces of the model are adjusted to find a setting that makes the model behave as similarly as possible to the patient. Specifically, many naming attempts were generated with the model using a given weighting of the lexical-semantic connections (s-weight) and the lexical-phonological connections (p-weight). Reductions in s-weight tend to result in real-word errors, while reductions in p-weight tend to result in non-word errors. The resulting distribution of response types from the model was compared with the observed distribution of response types from a patient performing a naming task that included 175 common nouns, yielding a prediction error. Then, a new distribution of response types from a new model setting of s-weight and p-weight was compared with the patient's observed distribution of response types in an iterative procedure until the model setting with the least discrepancy between response type distributions was found. Due to the simplicity of the model, there is a one-to-one correspondence between distributions of errors and optimal model settings, enabling this procedure to converge on a single model setting for each patient. This model setting was assumed to characterize the integrity of the patient's word retrieval network.

This approach to simulating word production in aphasia explains a wide range of observed phenomena associated with this task (Abel et al., 2009; Dell et al., 1997; Foygel & Dell, 2000; Schwartz et al., 2006; Schwartz & Dell, 2010; but see Goldrick, 2011). For example, the model explains why mixed errors occur more frequently than would be expected if they were merely independent semantic and phonological errors that coincidentally occurred simultaneously. This bias toward mixed errors arises because the interactive feedback from phonologically related and semantically related words accumulates to give these lexical neighbors an advantage during selection. The model also explains how formal errors can arise at either the lexical level (via whole word substitution) or the phonological level (via segment substitution that results in another word). The relative co-occurrence of formal errors with non-word errors, as well as the phonological neighborhood density of the target word, can help determine the psycholinguistic source, and thus the component of the cognitive processing network, that is responsible for an individual's speech errors. In a group of 94 participants with aphasia, Schwartz et al. (2006) found that the model accounted well for the error rates of most, but not all participants. The model's failures were attributable to acknowledged limitations and simplifications of the model. For example, the underprediction of semantic errors in some participants could be traced to the fallibility of the model's perfect recognition assumption, because these participants exhibited problems understanding pictures in other contexts that did not require speech production. Overall, given the simplicity of the model, its fit to aphasic naming data was judged favorably.

Being able to appropriately fit the data is an important feature for a model, but the real value of a model comes from predicting new data that was not used to estimate the model's parameters. In a group of 65 participants with aphasia, Dell et al. (2007) found that, for most participants, their word repetition scores could be predicted from their p-weight estimates that had been derived from the picture naming task. Essentially, by assuming perfect recognition of auditory stimuli, word repetition was equated with the second step in picture naming. Some participants did worse than expected on repetition tasks given their naming ability, and this could be traced to faulty auditory processing. Notably, some participants did better than would be expected given their phonological impairment during naming. This finding suggests that another route may be available during repetition to transmit the target activation from auditory brain areas to motor brain areas that augments the lexical route that is used during naming. Presumably, this is the same route that is used for repeating non-words, since these are not represented in the lexical retrieval network.

The nl-weight parameter was added to the interactive two-step model of lexical selection to create a dual-route model of repetition that explains non-word repetition performance as well as surprisingly intact word repetition performance in some patients (Baron et al., 2008; Hanley et al., 2004; Nozari et al., 2010). After estimating the s-weight and p-weight using the picture naming task, a new layer representing auditory input was added to the model, along with a separate set of connections that directly activated the phoneme units from this auditory input layer. The strength of these connections was estimated using a non-word repetition task. During word repetition, both the lexical route, driven by the meaning of the word, and the non-lexical route, driven by the auditory features of the word, contributed to activation in the phonological output layer. This dual-route model of repetition is similar to those proposed for reading (Coltheart et al., 2001). Multiple linear regression analyses revealed that both the p-weight and the nl-weight were independently, significantly associated with word repetition scores (Dell et al., 2013). The p-weight was additionally associated with impairments of motor speech planning, while the nl-weight was additionally associated with impairments in auditory processing.

Taken together, the interactive two-step model of lexical retrieval and the dual-route model of repetition propose at least three distinct types of cognitive impairment that can affect speech production, corresponding to reductions in s-weight, p-weight, or nl-weight. A reduction in s-weight has a strong impact on naming and a weak impact on word and non-word repetition. A reduction in p-weight has a strong impact on naming, a potentially strong impact on word repetition that can be moderated, and a weak impact on non-word repetition. A reduction in nl-weight has no impact on naming, a potentially strong impact on word repetition that can be moderated, and a strong impact on non-word repetition. Is it also the case that these distinct impairment types are associated with damage to distinct areas of the brain? If so, that would support the validity of the model by bolstering the claim that these different types of variation are truly observed in this population and can be explained by variations in damage to functionally specific areas of the brain. Before answering this question though, it will be helpful to briefly review what is known about the functional organization of language in the brain.

The dual stream model of language processing in the brain

Speech processing involves perceiving sounds, coordinating the movement of articulators, and thinking effable thoughts. Neurologists have been aware of evidence for the separability of these systems in the brain since at least the late 1800s. For example, Broca's aphasia presents with severe speech production problems marked by dysfluency while speech comprehension remains largely intact and is associated with damage to the inferior frontal lobe. On the other hand, Wernicke's aphasia presents with speech comprehension problems while speech fluency remains intact and is associated with damage to the posterior superior temporal lobe. The schematic model presented by Lichtheim (1885) posited that these areas were "centers" in the brain for motor and auditory knowledge of language, respectively, and that these centers were connected by a fiber bundle (i.e., long-range neuronal axons). The pairing of auditory words with motor speech acts during development was proposed to create a "reflex arc" in the brain, such that heard speech can be repeated automatically. A different pathway was proposed to pair auditory words with their meaning, though it was less clear at the time which brain areas were responsible for semantic processing. Later research revealed that many brain areas are involved with different aspects of semantic processing, though the anterior temporal lobes appear to function as a "center" of sorts for tying together complex, abstract concepts (Binder & Desai, 2011; Jefferies & Lambon Ralph, 2006; Martin & Chao, 2001; Wong & Gallate, 2012).

The dual stream model (Hickok & Poeppel, 2000, 2004, 2007) was proposed to resolve an apparent paradox within the Wernicke-Lichtheim model. There are patients that can comprehend speech but cannot discriminate syllables, and vice versa. If the posterior superior temporal lobe is the seat of auditory knowledge of language, then participants with damage here should not be able to discriminate syllables or comprehend speech. Rather than a single center for auditory language knowledge, the dual stream model proposes that primary auditory information can be translated either into a sensorimotor code that interfaces with motor systems (via the dorsal route, supported by an area of the planum temporale near the termination of the Sylvian fissure, called Spt) or into a phonological code that interfaces with conceptual systems (via the ventral route, supported by the superior temporal sulcus). The dorsal and ventral routes for speech processing are somewhat analogous to those found in the visual system (Goodale & Milner, 1992), sometimes called the "where" (dorsal) and "what" (ventral) pathways. Different speech processing tasks exert different demands on these processing streams. The syllable discrimination task relies on the dorsal route to rehearse and compare word forms, while the speech comprehension task relies on the ventral route to compare word meanings. Because these routes can be independently damaged, the performance on these tasks can doubly dissociate. The dorsal route largely corresponds to Lichtheim's sensorimotor reflex arc, while the ventral route largely corresponds to the link between auditory word images and their meanings.

The Hierarchical State Feedback Control model (Guenther & Hickok, 2015; Hickok, 2014; Hickok et al., 2011) elaborates on the implications of the dual stream model for speech production, since the original proposal was focused on speech perception and comprehension. Again, much of the inspiration comes from the visuomotor domain. Like the coordination of vision and motor systems for reaching and grasping at a target, speech production requires the coordination of motor systems to achieve auditory goals. But this coordination does not merely happen at the lowest levels of sensory perception and motor planning divorced from psycholinguistic representation. Rather, the phonological representations that are described by the interactive two-step model are proposed to arise through the coordination of analogous sensory and motor representations. The model also includes coordination of sensory and motor representations at the syllable level. During picture naming, the ventral stream maps concepts into phonological codes and auditory targets, while the dorsal stream maps auditory targets into motor movements. The picture-naming task is thus proposed to rely on both streams.

Finding the connection weights in the brain

Dell et al. (2013) tested the hypothesis that the s-weight, p-weight, and nl-weight parameters, which are used to simulate different types of damage to a cognitive network, correspond with damage to different brain areas. They approached this question using a technique called voxel-based lesion symptom mapping (Bates et al., 2003), where symptoms were characterized in terms of lesions to the cognitive model. In this technique, a lesion mask is created for each participant from neuroimaging studies (e.g., MRI or CT scans) that indicates where the participant has damage in his or her brain. To compare the locations of damage across different participants, each lesion mask is warped into a standardized space representing an approximately average brain. The standardized space (sometimes called a volume) is divided into very small regions called voxels, much like a digital picture is composed of pixels. Within each one of these voxels, a proportion of the participants will have damage and the remainder of the participants will not have damage. The average effect of damage in that location can be evaluated by comparing the behavioral scores from people with and without damage there. For Dell et al. (2013), the behavioral scores were simply the connection strength estimates from the model.

Lesion masks and connection strength estimates were collected for 103 participants with aphasia. Analyses revealed significant differences in connection strengths between people with and without damage to specific locations in the brain. The s-weight, p-weight, and nl-weight parameters were mostly associated with different brain areas, although there were notable regions of overlap. In accordance with the dual stream model of language organization, the p-weight and nl-weight were associated with dorsal stream regions, and the s-weight was associated with ventral stream regions. Lesions in the anterior portion of the dorsal stream including supramarginal gyrus, precentral and postcentral gyri, and the insula implicated reductions in p-weight. Lesions in the dorsal stream that were more proximal to the auditory input regions including superior temporal gyrus and Spt, as well as the supramarginal and the postcentral gyri, implicated reductions in nl-weight. There were many regions of the brain where damage implicated reductions in s-weight, including the anterior temporal lobe, a key ventral route area which was not associated with p-weight or nl-weight. While there was a notable area of overlap between s-weight and p-weight associations within the core p-weight region, it was argued that this may have been an indirect artifact of lesion volume; that is, lesions in this location were more likely to be large and extend widely into other locations that disrupt semantic processing, rather than damage here directly disrupting semantic processing itself. The anatomical findings supported the behavioral and neural distinction between the model's s-weight and p-weight parameters, while also prompting the authors to reconsider the functional distinctness of p-weight and nl-weight. Instead, p-weight and nl-weight parameters were proposed to represent different functional aspects of the same dorsal route for sensorimotor speech coordination.

Overall, this approach of searching for model parameters in the brain had mixed success. On the one hand, certain model assumptions were supported by independent data while conflicting results motivated a revision of the model's interpretation. These are positive outcomes that move the science forward and improve our understanding of these models. On the other hand, there are some outstanding concerns about the reliability and utility of these results. For example, accounting for the effects of lesion volume essentially negated most of the significant effects of localized damage on any of the model parameters in this study, not just the effect of damage within the p-weight region on the s-weight parameter, although the effect was relatively stronger for this problematic result. There are also concerns about the replicability of the results. For example, Tochadse et al. (2018) also examined the associations between lesion location and s-weight and p-weight parameters estimated from picture naming in 53 participants with chronic stroke aphasia. The general pattern was successfully replicated, with damage to dorsal stream regions implicating reductions in p-weight and damage to ventral stream regions implicating reductions in s-weight. However, the specific areas that were implicated by the two studies were largely non-overlapping: A more anterior and inferior area was identified for p-weight, while a more posterior and circumscribed area of the temporal lobe was identified for s-weight. There was also an area of overlap between s-weight and p-weight in the middle and superior temporal gyri, that is, in the ventral stream. No overlap was found in dorsal stream regions, and the overlapping results survived correction for lesion volume. This result stands in contrast to the findings of Dell et al. (2013). Finally, it is worth noting that the anatomical results of investigating model parameters are strikingly similar to the anatomical results of investigating the overt error type rates (Schwartz et al., 2012). In fact, the error type rates provided a cleaner separation of anatomical associates, specifically, for semantic errors versus non-word errors. That is, it's not clear how much the quantitative assessments provided by the connectionist model have improved our understanding of the brain's architecture beyond the ultimate symptoms themselves. This is certainly not the end of the story, as research continues into this approach, but it is also not the only way to use connectionist models to investigate the neuro-computational mechanisms of speech and language disorders.

Building the brain's architecture into connectionist models

An alternative approach to modeling cognitive processing and searching for its correlates in the brain is to go in the reverse direction, modeling the brain's architecture and investigating its constraints or implications for cognitive processing. Walker and Hickok (2016) investigated the implications of the architecture proposed by the Hierarchical State Feedback Control model for lexical retrieval in aphasia, by modifying the architecture of the interactive two-step model. Specifically, auditorily guided coordination of phonological production was instantiated in the model by adding a duplicate layer of phonological units, called auditory units, and designating the original output layer as motor units. Connections between lexical and auditory units were, likewise, duplicates of the connections between lexical and motor units, while connections between auditory and motor units were one-to-one. Recall that the dual route model for repetition included a similar layer of auditory units connecting to output units, but, unlike the new model, this route was not connected to the lexical layer and was not used in naming because, from a purely linguistic or cognitive perspective, it was not necessary. An additional constraint was placed on the new model such that the lexical-auditory connection weights were always greater than or equal to the lexical-motor connection weights. This architectural constraint reflects the dominance of the auditory-lexical link that arises early in development and continues to guide the production process throughout the lifespan in healthy speakers. This model is called the semantic-lexical-auditory-motor (SLAM) model, reflecting the primary route of activation flow through the model during a naming attempt.

The SLAM model was fit to naming data in the same way as the interactive two-step model, iteratively searching for a set of weights that makes the model produce a similar rate of each type of error as a human participant does. The two additional weight parameters in the SLAM model required a technical upgrade to the fitting procedure to handle the increased number of parameter combinations, but the procedure and convergence on a single setting was essentially the same. It is also worth noting that, unlike with classical statistical models such as regression that rely on partitioning variance in the data according to each parameter, adding parameters to a connectionist model in no way guarantees an improvement in accounting for variance in the data. This means that models of different complexity can be compared straightforwardly in terms of fit statistics. Walker and Hickok (2016) fit naming data from 255 participants with aphasia using both the SLAM model and the interactive two-step model. When the fits to patient data were compared between the two models, they were quite similar for most participants, but it was clear that the SLAM model provided better explanations for the naming patterns of a subgroup of participants.

SLAM fit improvements were most dramatic and reliable for people with conduction aphasia, and were also noticeable, but less so, for people with Wernicke's aphasia. As far back as 1874, conduction aphasia was proposed by Wernicke to arise from disconnection of the auditory and motor centers for speech (Wernicke, 1969). In accordance with this view, the best fitting SLAM weights for conduction aphasia included strong lexical-auditory connections and weak auditory-motor connections. The strong feedback from auditory representations to the lexical units, coupled with weak connections to the motor units, created more opportunities for formal errors to be produced. These errors also occurred alongside neologisms, somewhat obscuring their original source in the overt data, but the formal errors occurred at rates that were higher than would be expected given a purely lexical-phonological disconnection. In summary, the neuroanatomical architecture was able to combine with the psycholinguistic interactivity of the connectionist model to improve our understanding of speech production behaviors in aphasia.

This approach of constructing connectionist models to conform with neuroanatomical or neurophysiological constraints has been applied to more complex connectionist models than SLAM as well. For example, Ueno et al. (2011) presented a connectionist model called Lichtheim2 that adopted a parallel distributed processing approach (McClelland & Rogers, 2003), and they investigated the necessity of the brain's dual pathways (dorsal and ventral) to explain the many patterns of language test results that can emerge in the context of aphasia. They focused specifically on naming, repetition, and comprehension tasks. The connectionist network consisted of layers that were associated with specific functional brain regions. The meanings of words were represented by units associated with the anterior temporal lobe, the sounds of words were represented by units associated with primary auditory area, and the production of words were represented by units in the primary motor and insular cortex. These regions were connected to one another through a series of hidden layers, each associated with a specific brain area, and the connections between layers were learned through training. Comprehension involved mapping a time-varying pattern of activation in the auditory units to a static, distributed pattern of activation in the word meaning units; naming involved mapping from the word meaning units to the motor units; and repetition involved mapping from the auditory units to the motor units.

The different computational natures of the language tasks guided the network to learn different types of mappings that were embedded along different paths through the network. When damage was simulated by removing connections or units at specific places in the network, the resulting deficits across different tasks matched the known patterns of cases described in the literature. When only the dorsal pathways of the network were used, however, the limited variety of computations available to perform the tasks resulted in a poor match to human performance. The investigators concluded that the brain's architecture serves a critical computational function, which was clearly understandable through their connectionist model.

Conclusion

The application of connectionist models to aphasia continues to aid our understanding of both human behavior and the human brain. In this chapter, we have reviewed a few of the models that have been used in this regard, to provide a sampling of the growing research on this topic. While technological, methodological, and theoretical challenges abound, there are many opportunities for connectionist models to highlight mechanisms and processes that may someday provide targets for clinical interventions.

Further reading

Dell, G. S., & Kittredge, A. (2011). Connectionist models of aphasia and other language impairments. In *The handbook of psycholinguistic and cognitive processes: Perspectives in communication disorders* (pp. 169–188). Psych Press.

Walker, G. M., & Hickok, G. (2016). Bridging computational approaches to speech production: The semantic–lexical–auditory–motor model (SLAM). *Psychonomic Bulletin and Review*, *23*(2), 339–352. https://doi.org/10.3758/s13423-015-0903-7

References

Abel, S., Huber, W., & Dell, G. S. (2009). Connectionist diagnosis of lexical disorders in aphasia. *Aphasiology*, *23*(11), 1353–1378. https://doi.org/10.1080/02687030903022203

Baron, R., Hanley, J. R., Dell, G. S., & Kay, J. (2008). Testing single- and dual-route computational models of auditory repetition with new data from six aphasic patients. *Aphasiology*, *22*(1), 62–76. https://doi.org/10.1080/02687030600927092

Bates, E., Wilson, S. M., Saygin, A. P., Dick, F., Sereno, M. I., Knight, R. T., & Dronkers, N. F. (2003). Voxel-based lesion–symptom mapping. *Nature Neuroscience*, *6*(5), 448–450. https://doi.org/10.1038/nn1050

Binder, J. R., & Desai, R. H. (2011). The neurobiology of semantic memory. *Trends in Cognitive Sciences*, *15*(11), 527–536. https://doi.org/10.1016/J.TICS.2011.10.001

Coltheart, M., Rastle, K., Perry, C., Langdon, R., & Ziegler, J. (2001). DRS: A dual route cascaded model of visual word recognition and reading aloud. *Psychological Review*, *108*(1), 204–256. https://doi.org/10.1037/0033-295X.108.1.204

Dell, G. S. (1986). A spreading-activation theory of retrieval in sentence production. *Psychological Review*, *93*(3), 283–321. http://www.ncbi.nlm.nih.gov/pubmed/3749399

Dell, G. S., & Kittredge, A. (2011). Connectionist models of aphasia and other language impairments. In *The handbook of psycholinguistic and cognitive processes* (pp. 169–188). Routledge. https://doi.org/10.4324/9780203848005.ch8

Dell, G. S., Martin, N., & Schwartz, M. F. (2007). A case-series test of the interactive two-step model of lexical access: Predicting word repetition from picture naming. *Journal of Memory and Language*, *56*(4), 490–520. https://doi.org/10.1016/j.jml.2006.05.007

Dell, G. S., Schwartz, M. F., Martin, N., Saffran, E. M., & Gagnon, D. A. (1997). Lexical access in aphasic and nonaphasic speakers. *Psychological Review*, *104*(4), 801–838. http://www.ncbi.nlm.nih.gov/pubmed/9337631

Dell, G. S., Schwartz, M. F., Nozari, N., Faseyitan, O., & Branch Coslett, H. (2013). Voxel-based lesion-parameter mapping: Identifying the neural correlates of a computational model of word production. *Cognition*, *128*(3), 380–396. https://doi.org/10.1016/j.cognition.2013.05.007

Foygel, D., & Dell, G. S. (2000). Models of impaired lexical access in speech production. *Journal of Memory and Language*, *43*(2), 182–216. https://doi.org/10.1006/JMLA.2000.2716

Goldrick, M. (2011). Theory selection and evaluation in case series research. *Cognitive Neuropsychology*, *28*(7), 451–465. https://doi.org/10.1080/02643294.2012.675319

Goodale, M. A., & Milner, A. D. (1992). Separate visual pathways for perception and action. *Trends in Neurosciences*, *15*(1), 20–25. https://doi.org/10.1016/0166-2236(92)90344-8

Guenther, F. H., & Hickok, G. (2015). Role of the auditory system in speech production. In *Handbook of Clinical Neurology* (Vol. 129, pp. 161–175). Elsevier. https://doi.org/10.1016/B978-0-444-62630-1.00009-3

Hanley, R. J., Dell, G. S., Kay, J., & Baron, R. (2004). Evidence for the involvement of a nonlexical route in the repetition of familiar words: A comparison of single and dual route models of auditory repetition. *Cognitive Neuropsychology*, *21*(2–4), 147–158. https://doi.org/10.1080/02643290342000339

Hickok, G. (2014). The architecture of speech production and the role of the phoneme in speech processing. *Language, Cognition and Neuroscience*, *29*(1), 2–20. https://doi.org/10.1080/01690965.2013.834370

Hickok, G., Houde, J., & Rong, F. (2011). Sensorimotor integration in speech processing: Computational basis and neural organization. *Neuron*, *69*(3), 407–422. https://doi.org/10.1016/j.neuron.2011.01.019

Hickok, G., & Poeppel, D. (2000). Towards a functional neuroanatomy of speech perception. *Trends in Cognitive Sciences*, *4*(4), 131–138. https://doi.org/10.1016/S1364-6613(00)01463-7

Hickok, G., & Poeppel, D. (2004). Dorsal and ventral streams: A framework for understanding aspects of the functional anatomy of language. *Cognition*, *92*(1–2), 67–99. https://doi.org/10.1016/J.COGNITION.2003.10.011

Hickok, G., & Poeppel, D. (2007). The cortical organization of speech processing. *Nature Reviews Neuroscience*, *8*(5), 393–402. https://doi.org/10.1038/nrn2113

Jefferies, E., & Lambon Ralph, M. A. (2006). Semantic impairment in stroke aphasia versus semantic dementia: A case-series comparison. *Brain*, *129*(8), 2132–2147. https://doi.org/10.1093/brain/awl153

Lichtheim, L. (1885). On aphasia. *Brain*, 7(4), 433–484.

Martin, A., & Chao, L. L. (2001). Semantic memory and the brain: Structure and processes. *Current Opinion in Neurobiology*, *11*(2), 194–201. https://doi.org/10.1016/S0959-4388(00)00196-3

Martin, N., & Dell, G. S. (2019). Maintenance versus transmission deficits: The effect of delay on naming performance in aphasia. *Frontiers in Human Neuroscience*, *13*, 406. https://doi.org/10.3389/FNHUM.2019.00406

McClelland, J. L., & Rogers, T. T. (2003). The parallel distributed processing approach to semantic cognition. *Nature Reviews. Neuroscience*, *4*(4), 310–322. https://doi.org/10.1038/nrn1076

Nozari, N., Kittredge, A. K., Dell, G. S., & Schwartz, M. F. (2010). Naming and repetition in aphasia: Steps, routes, and frequency effects. *Journal of Memory and Language*, *63*(4), 541–559. https://doi.org/10.1016/j.jml.2010.08.001

Schwartz, M. F., & Dell, G. S. (2010). Case series investigations in cognitive neuropsychology. In *Cognitive Neuropsychology* (Vol. 27, Issue 6, pp. 477–494). https://doi.org/10.1080/02643294.2011.574111

Schwartz, M. F., Dell, G. S., Martin, N., Gahl, S., & Sobel, P. (2006). A case-series test of the interactive two-step model of lexical access: Evidence from picture naming. *Journal of Memory and Language, 54*(2), 228–264. https://doi.org/10.1016/J.JML.2005.10.001

Schwartz, M. F., Faseyitan, O., Kim, J., & Coslett, H. B. (2012). The dorsal stream contribution to phonological retrieval in object naming. *Brain, 135*(12), 3799–3814. https://doi.org/10.1093/brain/aws300

Tochadse, M., Halai, A. D., Lambon Ralph, M. A., & Abel, S. (2018). Unification of behavioural, computational and neural accounts of word production errors in post-stroke aphasia. *NeuroImage: Clinical, 18*, 952–962. https://doi.org/10.1016/J.NICL.2018.03.031

Ueno, T., Saito, S., Rogers, T. T., & Lambon Ralph, M. A. (2011). Lichtheim 2: Synthesizing aphasia and the neural basis of language in a neurocomputational model of the dual dorsal-ventral language pathways. *Neuron, 72*(2), 385–396. https://doi.org/10.1016/j.neuron.2011.09.013

Walker, G. M., & Hickok, G. (2016). Bridging computational approaches to speech production: The semantic–lexical–auditory–motor model (SLAM). *Psychonomic Bulletin and Review, 23*(2), 339–352. https://doi.org/10.3758/s13423-015-0903-7

Wernicke, C. (1969). *The symptom complex of aphasia* (pp. 34–97). Springer. https://doi.org/10.1007/978-94-010-3378-7_2

Wong, C., & Gallate, J. (2012). The function of the anterior temporal lobe: A review of the empirical evidence. *Brain Research, 1449*, 94–116. https://doi.org/10.1016/j.brainres.2012.02.017

9

MODELING THE ATTENTIONAL CONTROL OF VOCAL UTTERANCES:

From Wernicke to WEAVER++/ARC

Ardi Roelofs

Introduction

In *Die Sprache*, Wundt (1900) criticized the now classic model of normal and aphasic utterance production of Wernicke (1874) by arguing that producing verbal utterances is an active goal-driven process rather than a passive associative process proceeding from stimulus to vocal response, as held by the model. According to Wundt (1900, 1904), an attentional process located in the frontal lobes of the human brain actively controls an utterance perception and production network located in perisylvian brain areas, described by the Wernicke model (see Roelofs, 2021a, for discussion). Modern models of vocal utterance production, such as WEAVER++ (Levelt, Roelofs, & Meyer, 1999; Roelofs, 1992, 2018) and its more recent neurocognitive extension WEAVER++/ARC (Roelofs, 2014, 2022), build in many respects on the Wernicke model, but also address Wundt's critique by implementing assumptions on how the production-perception network is controlled. Characteristics of vocal utterance production, such as production onset latencies, errors, and corresponding brain activation, arise from the interplay of the production-perception network and the attentional control system. For example, patterns of speech errors by normal and aphasic speakers seem to be determined, at least in part, by self-monitoring, which is an important attentional control function (Roelofs, 2004, 2020). The extent to which presentation and recovery of language after stroke not only depend on the integrity of language systems but also on domain-general attentional control has become a topic of extensive investigation in recent years (Geranmayeh, Chau, Wise, Leech, & Hampshire, 2017; Kuzmina & Weekes, 2017; Pompon, McNeil, Spencer, & Kendall, 2015; Stefaniak, Alyahya, & Lambon Ralph, 2021; Wilson & Schneck, 2021). Models can benefit aphasia therapy. As Basso and Marangolo (2000) stated: "Clearly articulated and detailed hypotheses about representations and processing of cognitive functions allow rejection of all those strategies for treatment that are not theoretically justified. The more detailed the cognitive model, the narrower the spectrum of rationally motivated treatments" (p. 228).

The remainder of this chapter is organized as follows. I start by describing some of the key characteristics of the classic Wernicke model and outline Wundt's critique that the model lacks attentional control mechanisms. According to Wundt, understanding attentional control is important for aphasia therapy, because control processes may partly compensate the negative effects of lesions on language performance. Next, I describe vocal utterance production and perception

 DOI: 10.4324/9781003204213-11

in the WEAVER++/ARC model (Levelt et al., 1999; Roelofs, 1992, 2014, 2022) as well as the model's assumptions on attentional control. I then review brain imaging evidence on the attentional control of word production, which has confirmed Wundt's suggestion that control processes are localized in the frontal lobes. Controversy exists about the role of one of the frontal areas, the anterior cingulate cortex (ACC). Researchers generally agree that the ACC plays a role in the contextual regulation of nonverbal vocal utterances, including monkey calls and human crying, laughing, and pain shrieking (e.g., Scott, 2022). However, no agreement exists on the role of the ACC in spoken word production. Some researchers deny any role for the ACC in word production (e.g., Jürgens, 2009), while others assume involvement of the human ACC but disagree on whether the ACC plays a regulatory role (Cheney & Seyfarth, 2018; Posner & Raichle, 1994; Roelofs, 2020) or a role in detecting conflict and predicting error-likelihood (Miller & Cohen, 2001; Nozari, 2020; Nozari, Dell, & Schwartz, 2011). I review brain imaging evidence from my own laboratory for a regulatory role of the human ACC in attentional control. Finally, avenues for future research are indicated.

Wernicke's model and Wundt's critique

In a small monograph published in 1874, called *The aphasia symptom complex: A psychological study on an anatomical basis*, Wernicke presented a model for the functional neuroanatomy of vocal utterance production and comprehension. During the past century and a half, the model has been extremely influential in directing and organizing research results on aphasic and normal language performance. According to Wernicke (1874), verbal vocal utterances require both cortical and brainstem mechanisms, whereas nonverbal vocal utterances, such as crying, only need brainstem circuits. Figure 9.1 illustrates the structure of the model.

At the heart of the model, auditory images for words are linked to motor images for words. The auditory images were presumed to be stored in what is today called Wernicke's area, which includes the left posterior superior temporal gyrus. The motor images were assumed to be stored in Broca's area, which consists of the left posterior inferior frontal gyrus. The model assumes that when a word is heard (Wernicke used the example of hearing the word *bell*), auditory signals from sensory

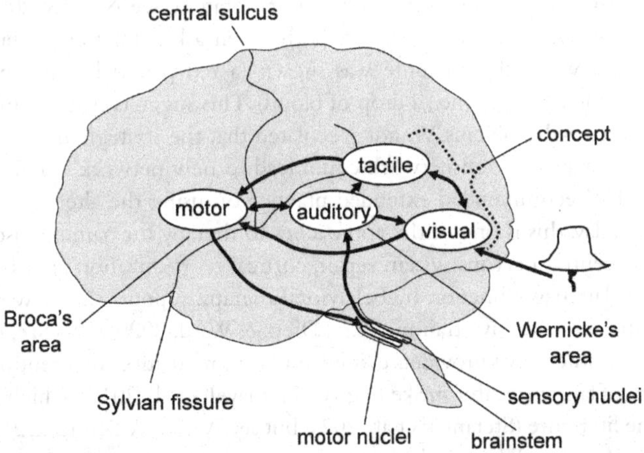

Figure 9.1 Illustration of the functional neuroanatomy for vocal utterance production and perception assumed by Wernicke's model. Auditory and motor images for words are located in a left-lateralized perisylvian network of brain areas, whereas concept images (representing, e.g., visual and tactile features) are represented in widely distributed areas.

brainstem nuclei travel to the primary auditory cortex and then activate the auditory images for words. The auditory images activate associated concept images, which include sensory images of the visual and tactile impressions of the corresponding object. This leads to comprehension of the word. In repeating a heard word, the auditory images activate the corresponding motor images in Broca's area, which then activate the motor nuclei in the brainstem via primary motor cortex. In naming a pictured bell, concept images corresponding to the bell are activated, which then activate the motor images. The motor image activates the auditory image for the word, which in turn activates the motor image. This reverberation of activation stabilizes the activation of the motor images, which serves a monitoring function.

Wernicke (1874) had developed the model to explain various types of poststroke aphasia, which were presumed to be the result of different loci of brain damage. For example, according to the model, damage to the auditory images gives rise to speech comprehension deficits (today called Wernicke's aphasia), whereas damage to the motor images gives rise to deficits in speech production (Broca's aphasia). The reverberation of activation between motor and auditory images in speech production explains why brain-damaged patients with speech recognition deficits (people with Wernicke's aphasia) often have fluent but phonemically disordered speech production. When the auditory word images are lesioned, activity of the motor images no longer sufficiently stabilizes, explaining the phonemic errors.

It is outside the scope of the present chapter to evaluate the scientific merits of Wernicke's model. A description of the early impact of the model can be found in Levelt (2013), and for an overview of key insights into aphasia obtained since Wernicke's seminal work, I refer to Kemmerer (2022). Relevant for the present chapter is the critique on the model advanced by Wundt (1900). According to Wundt, the retrieval of words from memory is an active goal-driven process rather than a passive associative process, as held by Wernicke's model. In particular, an attentional process located in the frontal lobes of the human brain controls the word perception and production network located in perisylvian brain areas, described by the Wernicke model. Consequently, characteristics of normal and impaired vocal performance arise from interactions between the production-perception network and the attentional control system.

Wundt (1900) maintained that such interactions may partly compensate the negative effects of lesions on language performance. In support of this claim, he referred to an anomic patient who tried to activate the spoken object name by making writing movements (today, first writing and then reading is recognized as a common compensatory strategy, see Nickels, 2002). Furthermore, the patient failed to name attributes of objects both when asked for the attribute ("what is the color of blood?") and when the attribute was shown (a red patch) but not when he saw the object together with the attribute (i.e., a drop of blood). This suggests that an enriched input may help remedy word retrieval problems. Wundt speculated that the strategic use of alternative routes through the perception-production network could lead to new network associations substituting the damaged ones. He recommended extended practice on using the alternative route as a form of aphasia therapy. Today, this is one of the approaches to therapy for naming disorders. Studies of phenomena such as central nervous system repair, cortical reorganization after brain damage, and the improvement of language function by behavioral therapy, support the view that patients may regain lost capabilities by extensive training (e.g., Dietz & Ward, 2020; Ping Sze, Hameau, Warren, & Best, 2021). Also, studies have provided evidence that upregulation of attentional control contributes to recovery of language after stroke (e.g., Geranmayeh et al., 2017), which is confirmed in a meta-analysis of the literature (Stefaniak et al., 2021; but see Wilson & Schneck, 2021). Surprisingly, although Wundt's critique on Wernicke's model seems fundamental, assumptions about attentional control have typically not been part of computational models of word production and perception that have been developed during the past century (e.g., Coltheart, Rastle, Perry, Langdon, & Ziegler, 2001; Dell, Schwartz, Nozari, Faseyitan, & Coslett, 2013; Ueno, Saito, Rogers, & Lambon Ralph, 2011).

In an early review of the literature on treatment for word-retrieval disorders, Nickels (2002) concluded:

> There can be no doubt that therapy for word-retrieval impairments can be highly successful, resulting in long-term improvements which can be of great communicative significance for the individual with aphasia. However, predicting the precise result of a specific treatment task with a specific individual with certainty is still not possible. (p. 935)

According to Nickels (2002), "[i]f one is ever to achieve (or even attempt) prediction in treatment, between task and impairment, a clearly articulated theory of the levels of processing that can be impaired is essential" (p. 955). However, according to her, "[o]ne of the limitations remains that while theories of language processing are becoming increasingly specified (e.g., Levelt, Roelofs & Meyer, 1999), how these models will function once damaged is not at all clear" (p. 955). Since then, this problem has been remedied. Assuming that brain damage leads to a loss of activation capacity in the lexical network, the theory of Levelt et al., implemented in the WEAVER++/ARC model, has been successfully applied to poststroke and progressive aphasias, at both patient group and individual patient levels (e.g., Roelofs, 2014, 2022). Moreover, it has been applied to remediation (Roelofs, 2021b). This theory is reviewed next.

The WEAVER++/ARC model

In a seminal article, Norman and Shallice (1986) made a distinction between "horizontal threads" and "vertical threads" in the control of perception and action. Horizontal threads are strands of processing that map perceptions onto actions and vertical threads are attentional influences on these mappings. Behavior arises from interactions between horizontal and vertical threads. WEAVER++/ARC is a model that computationally implements specific claims about how the horizontal and vertical threads are woven together in the planning and comprehending of spoken words (see Roelofs & Piai, 2011, for a review). Different from Wernicke's model, WEAVER++/ARC was originally designed to explain evidence from word production latencies (see Levelt et al., 1999, for an early review, and Roelofs & Ferreira, 2019, for a more recent one). In the past decade, the model has been extended to provide accounts of word production, comprehension, and repetition in poststroke and progressive aphasias (Roelofs, 2014, 2022). Also, the model has been applied to remediation of word production in poststroke aphasia (Roelofs, 2021). I first describe the functional claims of the model, and then the neuroanatomical basis, as assessed by functional brain imaging studies.

Functional aspects

Whereas the Wernicke model postulates an associative network of concept, auditory, and motor images for words, WEAVER++/ARC distinguishes concepts, lemmas, morphemes, phonemes, and syllable motor programs, as illustrated in Figure 9.2 (for reviews, see Kemmerer, 2019, 2022; Roelofs & Ferreira, 2019). This associative network is assumed to be part of a brain system for declarative knowledge, which is distinct from a brain system for procedural knowledge (e.g., Eichenbaum, 2012, for a review). Whereas the associative network instantiating declarative knowledge is thought to be represented in temporal and inferior frontal regions, condition-action (i.e., IF-THEN) rules instantiating procedural knowledge are thought to be represented in frontal regions, basal ganglia, and thalamus. In naming, the associative network is accessed by spreading activation while procedural rules select activated nodes that satisfy the task demands specified in working memory (here, to name a picture). The rules also exert top-down control in conceptually driven word production by selectively enhancing the activation of target lexical concept nodes in the network in order to achieve quick and accurate retrieval and encoding operations. For example, in naming a pictured

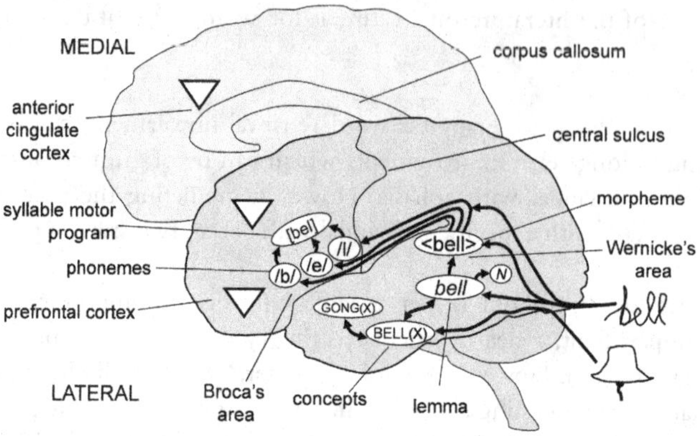

Figure 9.2 Illustration of the functional neuroanatomy for vocal utterance production and perception assumed by the WEAVER++/ARC model. Representations of concepts (e.g., BELL(X)), lemmas (e.g., *bell* specifying that the word is a noun), morphemes (e.g., <bell>), phonemes (e.g., /b/, /e/, and /l/), and syllable motor programs (e.g., [bel]) are located in a left-lateralized network of brain areas. An attentional control system located in anterior cingulate cortex and in ventrolateral and dorsolateral prefrontal cortex (indicated by triangles) exerts regulatory influences over the lexical network.

bell, activation spreads from the representation of the concept BELL(X) to the lemma of *bell* specifying that the word is a noun (for languages such as Dutch, lemmas also specify grammatical gender), the morpheme <bell>, the phonemes /b/, /e/, and /l/, and the syllable motor program [bel]. Each node sends a proportion of its activation to connected nodes. The activation flow from concepts to motor programs is limited unless attentional enhancements are involved to boost the activation (Roelofs, 1992, 2014). The rules select a lexical concept for the picture (i.e., BELL(X)), select a lemma for the selected lexical concept (i.e., *bell*), select a morpheme for the selected lemma (i.e., <bell>), select phonemes for the selected morpheme (i.e., /b/, /e/, and /l/) and syllabify them, and finally select a syllable motor program for the created phonological syllable (i.e., [bel]).

Following Wernicke's model, WEAVER++/ARC assumes that perceived objects have direct access to concepts (e.g., BELL(X)) and only indirect access to word forms (e.g., <bell> and /b/, /e/, /l/), whereas perceived spoken and written words have direct access to word forms and only indirect access to concepts (cf. Roelofs, 1992, 2014, 2022). Consequently, naming objects requires concept selection, whereas spoken words can be repeated without concept selection. The latter is achieved by mapping input word-forms (e.g., the input phonological or orthographic form of *bell*) directly onto output word-forms (e.g., <bell> and /b/, /e/, /l/), without engaging concepts and lemmas, as illustrated in Figure 9.2.

Whereas Wernicke's model lacks attentional control mechanisms, these are present in WEAVER++/ARC. In particular, goal-driven selection of information from the lexical network in the model is regulated by the rule system. When a goal is placed in working memory, word planning is controlled by those rules that include the goal among their conditions. For object naming, a rule would specify that

IF the goal is to say the name of the object,
and the concept corresponds to the object
THEN select the concept,
and enhance its activation.

The activation enhancements are required until appropriate syllable motor programs have been activated above an availability threshold. The attentional control system determines how strongly and for how long the enhancement occurs. A speaker may assess the required duration of the enhancement by monitoring the progress on word planning (Roelofs, 2004, 2020). The rules also allow for the specification of alternative naming routes. For example, the compensatory writing strategy discussed earlier may be specified as

IF the goal is to say the name of the object,
and naming fails
THEN set the goal to write the name of the object,
and read aloud the written name.

A compensatory strategy that has been studied in much detail is letter-by-letter reading in pure alexia (e.g., Dehaene, 2009), which is a frequent consequence of left occipitotemporal cortical damage. This area seems to implement the abstract identity of strings of letters. Pure alexic patients often retain single letter recognition abilities, and develop an effortful letter-by-letter strategy, which is the basis of most rehabilitation techniques. The strategy consists of silently sounding out the letters of the word from left to right. Consequently, word reading latency increases linearly with the number of letters of the word. Using brain imaging, Cohen et al. (2004) observed increased activation of the right occipitotemporal cortex in reading by a pure alexic patient compared to healthy controls, suggesting that letters were identified in the right rather than the left hemispheric area, as is normally the case. Moreover, the patient showed stronger than normal activation in left frontal and parietal areas that are implicated in phonological recoding and working memory, suggesting that the letter-by-letter strategy more strongly engages these functions. Examination of the patient eight months later revealed decreased word reading latencies and decreased activation in the right occipitotemporal cortex (Henry et al., 2005), suggesting that the area became better at identifying letters with practice. The work of Cohen et al. (2004) and Henry et al. (2005) demonstrates the utility of functional brain imaging in assessing the effect of strategy use. Moreover, it provides some evidence for Wundt's conjecture that compensatory strategies may establish new routes through the perception-production network.

Neuroanatomical aspects

Following Wernicke's model, WEAVER++/ARC assumes that the activation of representations underlying object naming proceeds from percepts in posterior cortical areas to articulatory programs in anterior areas, as illustrated in Figure 9.2. Indefrey and Levelt (2004) performed a meta-analysis of 82 neuroimaging studies on word production (updated by Indefrey, 2011), which suggested that the following cortical areas are involved. Information on the time course of word production in relation to these areas came from magnetoencephalographic studies. The meta-analysis included object naming (e.g., say "bell" to a pictured bell), word generation (producing a use for a noun, e.g., say "ring" to the spoken or written word *bell*), word repetition or reading (e.g., say "bell" to *bell*), and pseudoword repetition or reading (e.g., say "bez" to *bez*). Activation of percepts and concepts in object naming happens in occipital and inferotemporal regions of the brain. The middle part of the left middle temporal gyrus seems to be involved with lemma retrieval. When the total object naming time is about 600 ms, activity in these areas occurs within the first 275 ms after an object is presented. Next, activation spreads to Wernicke's area, where the morphological code (i.e., lexical phonological code) of the word seems to be retrieved. Activation is then transmitted to Broca's area for phoneme processing and syllabification, taking some 125 ms. During the next 200 ms, syllable motor programs are accessed. The sensorimotor areas control articulation. Word repetition and reading may be accomplished by activating the areas of Wernicke and Broca for aspects of form encoding, and motor areas for articulation.

The activation just described concerns learned declarative knowledge stored in cortical regions, while the hippocampus and surrounding regions underpin the learning and consolidation of new declarative knowledge. Analogous to this, several investigators (Ashby, Ennis, & Spiering, 2007; Hélie, Ell, & Ashby, 2015; Ullman, 2016) have proposed that cortical regions like frontal cortex store procedural knowledge, while the basal ganglia underpin the learning and consolidation of new procedural knowledge. Theoretical neuroscience work on the basal ganglia has shown how condition-action rules may be instantiated by networks of spiking neurons and how new rules may be learned (e.g., Eliasmith, 2013). This work suggests that input regions of the basal ganglia, like the caudate and putamen, represent the IF-part that is tested against information in cortex (e.g., in Broca's area), while output regions like the globus pallidus release the action specified in the THEN-part, via the thalamus, in cortex (again, in Broca's area). Over time, the IF-THEN link becomes directly established in cortex (via Hebbian learning), and the rule may operate without mediation by the basal ganglia.

Neuroimaging studies on word planning have confirmed Wundt's (1900, 1904) suggestion that the perisylvian production-perception network is controlled by attentional control mechanisms located in the frontal lobes. In particular, attentional control processes engage the lateral prefrontal cortex (LPFC) and the anterior cingulate cortex (ACC), as illustrated in Figure 9.2. The ACC and LPFC are more active in word generation (say "ring" to *bell*) when the attentional control demands are high than in word repetition (say "bell" to *bell*) when the demands are much lower (Petersen, Fox, Posner, Mintun, & Raichle, 1988; Thompson-Schill, D'Esposito, Aquirre, & Farah, 1997). The increased activity in the frontal areas disappears when word selection becomes easy after repeated generation of the same use to a word (Petersen, van Mier, Fiez, & Raichle, 1998). Moreover, activity in the frontal areas is higher in object naming when there are several good names for an object so that selection difficulties arise than when there is only a single appropriate name (Kan & Thompson-Schill, 2004). Also, the frontal areas are more active when retrieval fails and words are on the tip of the tongue than when words are readily available (Maril, Wagner, & Schacter, 2001). Frontal areas are also more active in naming objects with semantically related words superimposed (e.g., naming a pictured bell combined with the word *gong*) than without word distractors, as demonstrated by de Zubicaray, Wilson, McMahon, and Muthiah (2001). Thus, the neuroimaging evidence suggests that medial and lateral prefrontal areas exert attentional control over word planning. Along with the increased frontal activity, there is an elevation of activity in perisylvian areas (e.g., Piai, Roelofs, Jensen, Schoffelen, & Bonnefond, 2014; Raichle, Fiez, Videen, MacLeod, Pardo, Fox, & Petersen, 1994; Snyder, Abdullaev, Posner, & Raichle, 1995; de Zubicaray et al., 2001).

Evidence for the involvement of frontal areas in the attentional control of word production also comes from impaired performance. Semantic retrieval problems due to lesions of temporal areas of the human brain typically preserve the ability to generate category terms. For example, a patient may be able to say "instrument" to a bell, without being able to say "bell". Humphreys and Forde (2005) reported evidence on a patient with combined frontal-temporal damage, who had, instead, a specific impairment of generating category terms. According to Humphreys and Forde, the unusual impairment resulted because categorizing requires the attentional control provided by the frontal lobes.

Although both the ACC and LPFC are involved in the attentional control of word planning, the areas seem to play different roles. Evidence suggests that the dorsolateral prefrontal cortex (DLPFC) is involved in maintaining goals in working memory (for a review, see Kane & Engle, 2002). WEAVER++/ARC's assumption that abstract condition-action rules mediate goal-oriented retrieval and selection processes in prefrontal cortex is supported by evidence from single cell recordings and hemodynamic neuroimaging studies (e.g., Bunge, 2004; Bunge, Kahn, Wallis, Miller, & Wagner, 2003; Wallis, Anderson, & Miller, 2001). Moreover, evidence suggests that the ventrolateral prefrontal cortex plays a role in selection among competing response alternatives (Thompson-

Schill et al., 1997), the control of memory retrieval, or both (Badre, Poldrack, Paré-Blagoev, Insler, & Wagner, 2005). The ACC seems to exert regulatory influences over these processes.

In the light of Darwin's continuity hypothesis (i.e., new capabilities arise in evolution by modification and extension of existing ones), the involvement of the ACC in the attentional control of spoken word production seems plausible, because the area also controls nonverbal vocal utterances, considered by many to be the evolutionary forerunner of speech (e.g., Deacon, 1997; Jürgens, 2009; Ploog, 1992). Vocal utterances of nonhuman primates (monkeys and apes) consist of innate emotional vocalizations, such as fear, aggression, alarm, and contact calls. The two most stereotypical innate vocalizations in humans are crying and laughing (e.g., Newman, 2007). Evidence suggests that the ACC plays a critical role in the voluntary initiation and suppression of these nonverbal vocal utterances (e.g., Aitken, 1981; see Cheney & Seyfarth, 2018, for a review). The area does so by sending regulatory signals to the periaqueductal gray in the caudal midbrain. The periaqueductal area links emotional signals from the amygdala and other areas to the corresponding vocal responses. Also, the area gray links sensory stimuli, such as a heard vocal utterance, to corresponding vocal motor programs, thereby providing a low-level audio-vocal interface. Neighboring areas in the midbrain contain sensorimotor-orienting circuits underlying the automatic shift of gaze and attention and the turning of the head towards the sensory stimuli. The ACC signals the periaqueductal gray to initiate or withhold the motor program, depending on the context. The motor programs are embodied by premotor and motor nuclei in the lower brainstem and spinal cord (as assumed by Wernicke). The premotor nuclei coordinate the activity of the motor nuclei controlling the larynx, respiratory apparatus, and supralaryngeal tract. The three levels of vocal control (ACC, periaqueductal gray, lower brainstem nuclei) seem to be present in mammalian species as different as the cat and the bat (see Jürgens, 2009, for a review). For example, the ACC exerts control over the echolocation of bats (Duncan & Henson, 1994; Gooler & O'Neill, 1987), showing that the area also regulates noncommunicative use of the voice.

In the human speech system, the motor region of the posterior ventrolateral cortex directly projects onto the brainstem premotor and motor nuclei for the control of the oral, vocal, and respiratory muscles, bypassing the periaqueductal gray. Still, the ACC may exert regulatory influences over the speech system through its connections with ventrolateral prefrontal, premotor, and motor cortex (Deacon, 1997; Jürgens, 2009; Paus, 2001). The ACC seems implicated in enhancing the activation of target representations in the ventrolateral frontal areas until retrieval and selection processes have been accomplished in accordance with the goals maintained in DLPFC (Roelofs et al., 2006). According to this view, the ACC plays a role in the regulation of both verbal and nonverbal vocal utterances (cf. Deacon, 1997; Posner & Raichle, 1994), although through different neural pathways, as illustrated in Figure 9.3.

The activation enhancements provided by the ACC constitute a kind of driving force behind vocal utterance production. This fits with the idea that for action control, it is not enough to have goals in working memory, but one should be motivated to attain them. Anatomically, the ACC is in a good position to provide such a driving force (cf. Paus, 2001). The necessary arousal may be provided through the extensive projections from the thalamus and reticular brainstem nuclei to the ACC. The information on what goals to achieve may be provided through the extensive connections between the ACC and dorsolateral prefrontal cortex. Access to the motor system by the ACC is provided by the dense projections of the motor areas of the cingulate sulcus onto the brainstem and motor cortex. The idea that the ACC provides a kind of driving force behind vocal utterance production agrees with the effect of massive damage to the ACC.

Damage of the medial frontal cortex including the ACC typically results in transient akinetic mutism, which is characterized by reduced frequency of spontaneous speech with a preserved ability to repeat what is said (i.e., when externally triggered). The mutism arises with left or bilateral medial lesions, but damage to the right ACC may also result in transient speech aspontaneity (Chang, Lee, Lui, & Lai, 2007). Jürgens and Von Cramon (1982) reported a case study of a patient

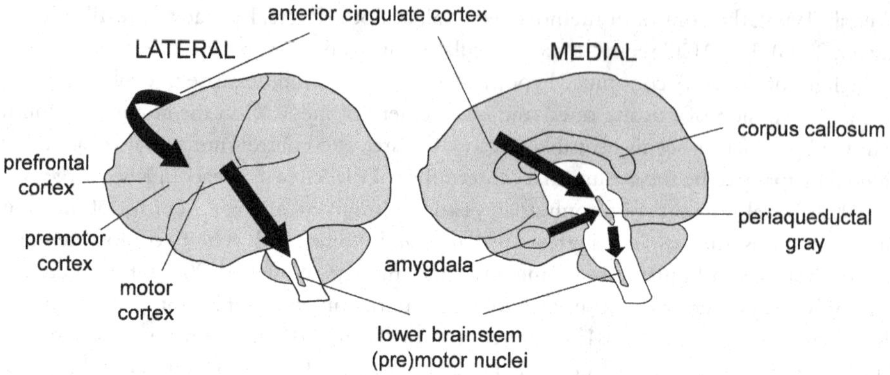

Figure 9.3 Illustration of the regulatory pathways of the anterior cingulate cortex in verbal (lateral view) and nonverbal vocal utterances (medial view). In verbal utterances, the ACC exerts control over lateral prefrontal, premotor, and motor cortex, which directly controls the pontine and medullary (pre)motor nuclei. In nonverbal utterances, the ACC exerts control over the periaqueductal gray.

with a lesion to the medial frontal cortex on the left side, which included damage to the ACC. The patient first exhibited a state of akinetic mutism during which no spontaneous vocal utterances were produced. After a few months, the patient could whisper but not produce voiced verbal utterances, which were restored only later. During the following months, the frequency of spontaneous utterances increased, but emotional intonation (e.g., an angry voice) remained impaired. A patient reported by Rubens (1975) presented with voiceless laughing and crying in the initial phase of mutism. Later, the ability to produce voiced verbal utterances was regained, but the intonation remained monotonous. According to Jürgens and Von Cramon (1982), these findings indicate a role for the ACC in the volitional control of the emotional aspect of spoken utterances, but not their verbal aspect.

Role of the ACC in attentional control

Although the role that I proposed for the ACC in the attentional control of both verbal and nonverbal vocal utterances seems plausible, this claim is controversial. Whereas researchers generally agree that the ACC plays a role in the attentional control of nonverbal vocal utterances, they have found no agreement on the role of the human ACC in the production of verbal vocal utterances. Some researchers deny any role for the ACC in spoken word production except for emotional aspects (e.g., Jürgens, 2009). Other researchers assume involvement of the human ACC in attentional control but disagree on whether the ACC plays a regulatory role (Cheney & Seyfarth, 2018; Posner & Raichle, 1994; Roelofs, 2020; Roelofs & Hagoort, 2002), as in call production, or a role in detecting conflict or predicting error-likelihood (Miller & Cohen, 2001; Nozari, 2020; Nozari et al., 2011). I discuss the different views on the role of the human ACC in attentional control, and review brain imaging evidence from my own laboratory supporting a regulatory role of the human ACC.

Emotional vocalization

Based on three decades of electrophysiological studies of monkey vocalization, Jürgens and colleagues developed a model of the role of the ACC in vocal utterances (see Jürgens, 2009, for a review), which has become a leading model in the literature on mammalian vocalization. This work has shown that the anterior cingulate is the only cortical area that is directly involved in call production by monkeys. Although extensive connectivity between the ACC and lateral prefrontal, premotor, and motor cortex is acknowledged, a role of the ACC in the control of speech is denied. The extensive connectivity between the ACC and lateral frontal cortex may serve functions unrelated to speech. For example, the ACC is implicated in the voluntary initiation of swallowing (Maeda, Takashi, Shinagawa, Honda, Kurabayashi, & Ohyama, 2006; Watanabe, Abe, Ishikawa, Yamada, & Yamane, 2004).

However, given the neuroimaging evidence on word production reviewed above, it seems difficult to maintain that the ACC plays no role in spoken word production. Vocalization, like swallowing, requires the coordinated activity of the oral, vocal, and respiratory muscles. Since swallowing and breathing are exclusive activities, the larynx plays a critical role in gating access to the respiratory tract. MacNeilage (1998) suggested that ingestion-related capabilities in lateral frontal cortex associated with chewing, sucking, and licking were modified in human evolution to serve a role in speaking. The extensive connectivity between the ACC and lateral frontal cortex, including Broca's area and the larynx motor cortex, may have become exploited in the control of speech production (cf. Ploog, 1992). Clearly, the ACC is involved in speech production only under certain circumstances, namely when utterance production requires attentional control. However, a circumscribed role of the ACC is also observed in call production, where the area plays a role only in the contextual regulation of vocalization, but not in its production per se.

Regulation versus conflict detection

Whereas Jürgens (2009) denies any role for the ACC in spoken word production, other researchers assume involvement of the human ACC but disagree on whether the area plays a regulatory role (Cheney & Seyfarth, 2018; Posner & Raichle, 1994; Roelofs, 2020; Roelofs & Hagoort, 2002) or a role in detecting conflict or predicting error-likelihood (e.g., Nozari, 2020; Nozari et al., 2011). According to the latter view, the ACC is involved in performance monitoring (Miller & Cohen, 2001). In particular, ACC activity reflects the detection of response conflict and acts as a signal that engages attentional control processes subserved by LPFC.

In a review of the monkey literature on the control of gaze by the frontal lobes, Schall and Boucher (2007) concluded that neurons in the supplementary eye field (part of the medial frontal cortex) exhibit activity specifically related to response conflict, but neurons in the ACC do not. ACC neurons only reflect the amount of control exerted. This conclusion was surprising given that the conflict detection hypothesis is the dominant view on ACC function in the literature on humans. According to Schall and Boucher, the difference between monkeys (control-related activity but no conflict-related activity in the ACC) and humans (ACC conflict detection) may reflect differences in species, tasks, or effectors. For example, monkey studies have typically employed saccadic stop-signal tasks, in which conflict is evoked by infrequently presenting a stop signal while preparation of a saccade is in progress. In contrast, human studies have typically employed Stroop-like tasks with vocal or manual responding. For example, in the color-word Stroop task, participants name the ink color of congruent or incongruent color words (e.g., the word *red* printed in green), whereby vocal responding is slower in the incongruent than the congruent condition. In the arrow-word version of this task, the stimuli consist of incongruent and congruent combinations of left or right pointing arrows and the words *left* or *right*, and the participants respond by pressing a left or right response button. According to Schall and Boucher, it is possible that the saccadic responses in monkey studies yielded less conflict than the vocal and manual responses in human studies, explaining the difference in results between monkeys and humans.

However, it is also possible that the difference in results between monkeys and humans has another ground, namely a confound between conflict and control in the human studies. Incongruent and congruent stimuli not only differ in the amount of conflict they evoke, but also in the amount of attentional control required by the corresponding responses. Thus, the conflict-related activity in Stroop-like tasks is compatible with both the regulative and conflict detection hypotheses on ACC function. It is possible to discriminate between the two hypotheses empirically by using neutral stimuli. A critical prediction made by the conflict hypothesis is that ACC activity should be increased only when conflicting response alternatives are present (e.g., in responding to the word *left* combined with a right-pointing arrow). ACC activity should not differ between congruent trials (e.g., the word *left* combined with a left-pointing arrow) and neutral trials (e.g., the word *left* only), because competing response alternatives are absent on both trial types. In contrast, the regulatory hypothesis (Posner & Raichle, 1994; Roelofs & Hagoort, 2002) not only predicts more ACC activity on incongruent than on neutral trials, but also less ACC activity on congruent than on neutral trials. Less ACC activity is predicted because the correct response (left) is already activated by the distractor (a left-pointing arrow) on congruent trials and therefore less enhancement of the target is required.

To test between the conflict detection and regulation hypotheses about ACC function, Roelofs et al. (2006) conducted a functional magnetic resonance imaging (fMRI) study. Participants were scanned while they were presented with arrow-word combinations. The participants were asked to communicate the direction denoted by the word by pressing a left or right button using the index and middle fingers of their left hand. A meta-analysis of the existing neuroimaging literature and the results from a new neuroimaging experiment by Barch, Braver, Akbudak, Conturo, Ollinger, and Snyder (2001) has shown that Stroop-like tasks activate the dorsal ACC regardless of whether the direction of the word is communicated through a spoken or manual response. On incongruent trials in the experiment of Roelofs et al. (2006), the word and the arrow designated opposite responses. On congruent trials, the word and arrow designated the same response. On neutral trials, a word was presented in combination with a straight line, so only one response was designated by the stimulus. Congruent, incongruent, and neutral trials were presented rapidly in a randomly intermixed order. The response time data showed that, consistent with earlier findings, responses to the words were much slower on incongruent than on neutral trials, and fastest on congruent trials. The neuroimaging data demonstrated that activity in the ACC was larger on incongruent than on congruent trials. The same held for activity in the LPFC. Importantly, ACC activity was larger for neutral than for congruent stimuli, in the absence of response conflict. This result demonstrates the engagement of the ACC in the regulation of communicative responses. This conclusion was corroborated by successful WEAVER++ simulations of the chronometric and neuroimaging findings (Roelofs et al., 2006).

Anticipatory adjustments

People are often faced with circumstances in which certain vocal behaviors are inappropriate, such as laughing at a funeral or talking aloud in a library. This raises the question whether the ACC is also involved in adjusting the control settings for responding (e.g., raising the response thresholds) depending on the communicative situation (cf. Cheney & Seyfarth, 2018). Sohn, Albert, Jung, Carter, and Anderson (2007) proposed that the ACC plays a role in signalling upcoming response conflict. Brown and Braver (2005) argued that the ACC signals upcoming error likelihood, independent of response conflict. More generally, environmental cues may provide information about which type of stimulus is coming and, as a consequence, about which control setting is most appropriate for responding to the stimulus. However, these contextual cues do not necessarily have to predict response conflict or error likelihood. This raises the question whether anticipatory activity in the ACC may be obtained independent of upcoming conflict or error likelihood. Aarts, Roelofs, and Van Turennout (2008) conducted an fMRI experiment that examined this issue.

As in the study of Roelofs et al. (2006), participants were scanned while they were presented with arrow-word combinations. Again, the index and middle fingers of the left hand were used for responding. On each trial, the participants were now informed about the arrow-word stimulus conditions by means of symbolic cues, which were presented well before the arrow-word stimulus. The cue was a colored square that indicated whether the upcoming arrow-word stimulus was congruent, incongruent, or neutral, or the cue provided no information about the upcoming condition. Green squares were always preceding congruent stimuli, red squares preceded incongruent stimuli, and yellow squares preceded neutral stimuli. The uninformative cues were grey squares, which could be followed by any of the stimulus types.

If the ACC plays a role in anticipatory adjustments in control, ACC activity should be higher in response to informative cues than to uninformative cues. If the adjustments are independent of response conflict or error likelihood, enhanced ACC activity should be obtained for cues preceding congruent stimuli. Adjustments are expected in premotor cortex, where response rules are implemented. An informative cue preceding an incongruent stimulus might encourage participants to weaken the connections between the arrows and their responses, because the arrows elicit the wrong response. However, an informative cue preceding a congruent target might encourage participants to strengthen the connections between the arrows and the corresponding responses, because the arrows now elicit the correct response. In WEAVER++, the adjustments may be achieved by condition-action rules specifying that

IF the goal is to indicate the direction denoted by the word,
and the cue is green
THEN strengthen the connection between arrows and responses.

If such advance adjustments are successful, ACC activity should exhibit smaller differences among target conditions in response to the arrow-word stimuli after informative cues (when control was adjusted in advance) than following uninformative cues (when control was not adjusted in advance).

Aarts et al. (2008) observed that participants responded faster to the arrow-word stimuli after informative than uninformative cues, indicating cue-based adjustments in control. Moreover, ACC activity was larger following informative than uninformative cues, as would be expected if the ACC is involved in anticipatory control. Importantly, this activation in the ACC was observed for informative cues even when the information conveyed by the cue was that the upcoming arrow-word stimulus evokes no response conflict and has low error likelihood. This finding demonstrates that the ACC is involved in anticipatory control processes independent of upcoming response conflict or error likelihood. Moreover, the response of the ACC to the target stimuli was critically dependent upon whether the cue was informative or not. ACC activity differed among target conditions after uninformative cues only, indicating ACC involvement in actual control adjustments. Taken together, these findings argue strongly for a role of the ACC in anticipatory control independent of anticipated conflict and error likelihood, and also show that such control can eliminate conflict-related ACC activity during target processing.

Premotor cortex activity should reflect the operation of control in response to informative cues. Therefore, we expected a positive correlation between cue-related ACC and premotor activity. The correlation should be confined to the right premotor cortex, contralateral to the response hand. Correlation analyses confirmed that cue-based activity in the ACC was positively correlated with activity in the dorsal premotor cortex and the supplementary motor area contralateral to the response hand. Although several other frontal areas were active in response to the cues, no correlations between cue-based ACC activity and the other regions were found. These results provide evidence for a direct influence of the ACC over premotor cortex (cf. Figure 9.3).

Summary and conclusions

This chapter outlined the classic model of Wernicke (1874) for the functional neuroanatomy of vocal utterance production and comprehension, and Wundt's (1900, 1904) critique that the model lacks attentional control mechanisms, which he localized in the frontal lobes. Next, the

WEAVER++/ARC model (Roelofs, 1992, 2014, 2022) was described, which builds in many respects on Wernicke's ideas but also addresses Wundt's critique by implementing assumptions on attentional control. Characteristics of utterance production by healthy and brain-damaged individuals arise from the interplay of a perisylvian production-perception network and the frontal attentional control system. I indicated that controversy exists about the role of one of the frontal areas, the ACC. Whereas some researchers deny any role for the ACC in spoken word production, other researchers assume involvement of the area but disagree on whether it plays a regulatory role, as in call production, or a role in detecting conflict or predicting error-likelihood. I reviewed evidence for a regulatory role of the ACC.

Aphasiologists agree that a good theoretical model is important for therapy (e.g., Basso & Marangolo, 2000). However, Nickels (2002) argued that it remained unclear how models like that of Levelt et al. (1999) will function once damaged. Over the past decade, this problem has been remedied. The theory of Levelt et al., implemented in the WEAVER++/ARC model, has been applied to poststroke and progressive aphasias, at both patient group and individual patient levels (e.g., Roelofs, 2014, 2022), and the model has been applied to remediation (Roelofs, 2021). Given the importance of modeling for therapy, future research should further theoretically analyze and model vocal utterance production and its attentional control, impairments, and their interactions. I hope this chapter has provided some helpful hints for this research and for clinical practice.

Further reading

Roelofs, A. (2020). Self-monitoring in speaking: In defense of a comprehension-based account. *Journal of Cognition, 3*(1), 1–13.

Roelofs, A. (2021a). How attention controls naming: Lessons from Wundt 2.0. *Journal of Experimental Psychology: General, 150*(10), 1927–1955.

Roelofs, A. (2022). A neurocognitive computational account of word production, comprehension, and repetition in primary progressive aphasia. *Brain and Language, 227*, 105094.

References

Aarts, E., Roelofs, A., & Van Turennout, M. (2008). Anticipatory activity in anterior cingulate cortex can be independent of conflict and error likelihood. *Journal of Neuroscience, 28*(18), 4671–4678.

Aitken, P. G. (1981). Cortical control of conditioned and spontaneous vocal behavior in rhesus monkeys. *Brain and Language, 13*(1), 171–184.

Ashby, F. G., Ennis, J. M., & Spiering, B. J. (2007). A neurobiological theory of automaticity in perceptual categorization. *Psychological Review, 114*(3), 632–656.

Badre, D., Poldrack, R. A., Paré-Blagoev, E., Insler, R. Z., & Wagner, A. D. (2005). Dissociable controlled retrieval and generalized selection mechanisms in ventrolateral prefrontal cortex. *Neuron, 47*(6), 907–918.

Barch, D. M., Braver, T. S., Akbudak, E., Conturo, T., Ollinger, J., & Snyder, A. (2001). Anterior cingulate cortex and response conflict: Effects of response modality and processing domain. *Cerebral Cortex, 11*(9), 837–848.

Basso, A., & Marangolo, P. (2000). Cognitive neuropsychological rehabilitation: The emperor's new clothes? *Neuropsychological Rehabilitation, 10*(3), 219–230.

Brown, J. W., & Braver, T. S. (2005). Learned predictions of error likelihood in the anterior cingulate cortex. *Science, 307*(5712), 1118–1121.

Bunge, S. A. (2004). How we use rules to select actions: A review of evidence from cognitive neuroscience. *Cognitive, Affective, and Behavioral Neuroscience, 4*(4), 564–579.

Bunge, S. A., Kahn, I., Wallis, J. D., Miller, E. K., & Wagner, A. D. (2003). Neural circuits subserving the retrieval and maintenance of abstract rules. *Journal of Neurophysiology, 90*(5), 3419–3428.

Chang, C.-C., Lee, Y. C., Lui, C.-C., & Lai, S.-L. (2007). Right anterior cingulate cortex infarction and transient speech aspontaneity. *Archives of Neurology, 64*(3), 442–446.

Cheney, D. L., & Seyfarth, R. M. (2018). Flexible usage and social function in primate vocalizations. *Proceedings of the National Academy of Sciences of the USA, 115*(9), 1974–1979.

Cohen, L., Henry, C., Dehaene, S., Martinaud, O., Lehéricy, S., Lemer, C., & Ferrieux, S. (2004). The pathophysiology of letter-by-letter reading. *Neuropsychologia, 42*(13), 1768–1780.

Coltheart, M., Rastle, K., Perry, C., Langdon, R., & Ziegler, J. (2001). DRC: A dual route cascaded model of visual word recognition and reading aloud. *Psychological Review, 108*(1), 204–256.

de Zubicaray, G. I., Wilson, S. J., McMahon, K. K., & Muthiah, S. (2001). The semantic interference effect in the picture-word paradigm: An event-related fMRI study employing overt responses. *Human Brain Mapping, 14*(4), 218–227.

Deacon, T. W. (1997). *The symbolic species: The co-evolution of language and the brain.* New York: Norton.

Dehaene, S. (2009). *Reading in the brain: The science and evolution of a human invention.* New York: Viking.

Dell, G. S., Schwartz, M. F., Nozari, N., Faseyitan, O., & Coslett, H. B. (2013). Voxel-based lesion-parameter mapping: Identifying the neural correlates of a computational model of word production. *Cognition, 128*(3), 380–396.

Dietz, V., & Ward, N. S. (Eds.). (2020). *Oxford textbook of neurorehabilitation* (2nd ed.). Oxford: Oxford University Press.

Duncan, G. E., & Henson, O. W. (1994). Brain activity patterns in flying, echolocating bats (*Pteronotus parnellii*): Assessed by high resolution autoradiographic imaging with [^{3}H]2-deoxyglucose. *Neuroscience, 59*(4), 1051–1070.

Eichenbaum, H. (2012). *The cognitive neuroscience of memory: An introduction* (2nd ed.). Oxford: Oxford University Press.

Eliasmith, C. (2013). *How to build a brain: A neural architecture for biological cognition.* Oxford: Oxford University Press.

Geranmayeh, F., Chau, T. W., Wise, R., Leech, R., & Hampshire, A. (2017). Domain-general subregions of the medial prefrontal cortex contribute to recovery of language after stroke. *Brain, 140*(7), 1947–1958.

Gooler, D. M., & O'Neill, W. E. (1987). Topographic representation of vocal frequency demonstrated by microstimulation of anterior cingulate cortex in the echolocating bat, *Pteronotus parnelli parnelli. Journal of Comparative Physiology, 161*(2), 283–294.

Hélie, S., Ell, S. W., & Ashby, F. G. (2015). Learning robust cortico-cortical associations with the basal ganglia: An integrative review. *Cortex, 64*, 123–135.

Henry, C., Gaillard, R., Volle, E., Chiras, J., Ferrieux, S., Dehaene, S., & Cohen, L. (2005). Brain activations during letter-by-letter reading: A follow-up study. *Neuropsychologia, 43*(14), 1983–1989.

Humphreys, G. W., & Forde, E. M. E. (2005). Naming a giraffe but not an animal: Basic-level but not superordinate naming in a patient with impaired semantics. *Cognitive Neuropsychology, 22*(5), 539–558.

Indefrey, P. (2011). The spatial and temporal signatures of word production components: A critical update. *Frontiers in Psychology, 2*, Article 255.

Indefrey, P., & Levelt, W. J. M. (2004). The spatial and temporal signatures of word production components. *Cognition, 92*(1–2), 101–144.

Jürgens, U. (2009). The neural control of vocalization in mammals: A review. *Journal of Voice, 23*(1), 1–10.

Jürgens, U., & von Cramon, D. (1982). On the role of the anterior cingulate cortex in phonation: A case report. *Brain and Language, 15*(2), 234–248.

Kan, I. P., & Thompson-Schill, S. L. (2004). Effect of name agreement on prefrontal activity during overt and covert picture naming. *Cognitive, Affective, and Behavioral Neuroscience, 4*(1), 43–57.

Kane, M. J., & Engle, R. W. (2002). The role of prefrontal cortex in working-memory capacity, executive attention, and general fluid intelligence: An individual-differences perspective. *Psychonomic Bulletin and Review, 9*(4), 637–671.

Kemmerer, D. (2019). From blueprints to brain maps: The status of the lemma model in cognitive neuroscience. *Language, Cognition and Neuroscience, 34*(9), 1085–1116.

Kemmerer, D. (2022). *Cognitive neuroscience of language* (2nd ed.). New York: Psychology Press.

Kuzmina, E., & Weekes, B. S. (2017). Role of cognitive control in language deficits in different types of aphasia. *Aphasiology, 31*(7), 765–792.

Levelt, W. J. M. (2013). *A history of psycholinguistics: The pre-chomskyan era.* Oxford: Oxford University Press.

Levelt, W. J. M., Roelofs, A., & Meyer, A. S. (1999). A theory of lexical access in speech production. *Behavioral and Brain Sciences, 22*(1), 1–38.

MacNeilage, P. F. (1998). The frame/content theory of evolution of speech production. *Behavioral and Brain Sciences, 21*(4), 499–511.

Maeda, K., Takashi, O., Shinagawa, H., Honda, E., Kurabayashi, T., & Ohyama, K. (2006). Role of the anterior cingulate cortex in volitional swallowing: An electromyographic and functional magnetic resonance imaging study. *Journal of Medical and Dental Sciences, 53*(3), 149–157.

Maril, A., Wagner, A. D., & Schacter, D. L. (2001). On the tip of the tongue: An event-related fMRI study of semantic retrieval failure and cognitive conflict. *Neuron, 31*(4), 653–660.

Miller, E. K., & Cohen, J. D. (2001). An integrative theory of prefrontal cortex function. *Annual Review of Neuroscience, 24*, 167–202.

Newman, J. D. (2007). Neural circuits underlying crying and cry responding in mammals. *Behavioural Brain Research, 182*(2), 155–165.

Nickels, L. (2002). Therapy for naming disorders: Revisiting, revising, and reviewing. *Aphasiology, 16*(10–11), 935–979.

Norman, D. A., & Shallice, T. (1986). Attention to action: Willed and automatic control of behavior. In R. J. Davidson, G. E. Schwarts, & D. Shapiro (Eds.), *Consciousness and self-regulation: Advances in research and theory* (pp. 1–18). New York: Plenum Press.

Nozari, N. (2020). A comprehension- or a production-based monitor? Response to Roelofs (2020). *Journal of Cognition, 3*(1), Article 19.

Nozari, N., Dell, G. S., & Schwartz, M. F. (2011). Is comprehension necessary for error detection? A conflict-based account of monitoring in speech production. *Cognitive Psychology, 63*(1), 1–33.

Paus, T. (2001). Primate anterior cingulate cortex: Where motor control, drive and cognition interface. *Nature Reviews Neuroscience, 2*(6), 417–424.

Petersen, S. E., Fox, P. T., Posner, M. I., Mintun, M., & Raichle, M. E. (1988). Positron emission tomographic studies of the cortical anatomy of single-word processing. *Nature, 331*(6157), 585–589.

Petersen, S. E., van Mier, H., Fiez, J. A., & Raichle, M. E. (1998). The effects of practice on the functional anatomy of task performance. *Proceedings of the National Academy of Sciences of the UnitedStates of America, 95*(3), 853–860.

Piai, V., Roelofs, A., Jensen, O., Schoffelen, J.-M., & Bonnefond, M. (2014). Distinct patterns of brain activity characterise lexical activation and competition in spoken word production. *PLOS ONE, 9*(2), e88674.

Ping Sze, W., Hameau, S., Warren, J., & Best, W. (2021). Identifying the components of a successful spoken naming therapy: A meta-analysis of word-finding interventions for adults with aphasia. *Aphasiology, 35*(1), 33–72.

Ploog, D. W. (1992). The evolution of vocal communication. In H. Papoušek, U. Jürgens, & M. Papoušek (Eds.), *Nonverbal vocal communication: Comparative and developmental approaches* (pp. 6–30). Cambridge: Cambridge University Press.

Pompon, R. H., McNeil, M. R., Spencer, K. A., & Kendall, D. L. (2015). Intentional and reactive inhibition during spoken-word Stroop task performance in people with aphasia. *Journal of Speech, Language, and Hearing Research, 58*(3), 767–780.

Posner, M. I., & Raichle, M. E. (1994). *Images of mind.* New York: W. H. Freeman.

Raichle, M. E., Fiez, J. A., Videen, T. O., MacLeod, A.-M. K., Pardo, J. V., Fox, P. T., & Petersen, S. E. (1994). Practice-related changes in human brain functional anatomy during nonmotor learning. *Cerebral Cortex, 4*(1), 8–26.

Roelofs, A. (1992). A spreading-activation theory of lemma retrieval in speaking. *Cognition, 42*(1–3), 107–142.

Roelofs, A. (2004). Error biases in spoken word planning and monitoring by aphasic and nonaphasic speakers: Comment on Rapp and Goldrick (2000). *Psychological Review, 111*(2), 561–572.

Roelofs, A. (2014). A dorsal-pathway account of aphasic language production: The WEAVER++/ARC model. *Cortex, 59*, 33–48.

Roelofs, A. (2018). A unified computational account of cumulative semantic, semantic blocking, and semantic distractor effects in picture naming. *Cognition, 172*, 59–72.

Roelofs, A. (2020). Self-monitoring in speaking: In defense of a comprehension-based account. *Journal of Cognition, 3*(1), Article 18.

Roelofs, A. (2021a). How attention controls naming: Lessons from Wundt 2.0. *Journal of Experimental Psychology: General, 150*(10), 1927–1955.

Roelofs, A. (2021b). Phonological cueing of word finding in aphasia: Insights from simulations of immediate and treatment effects. *Aphasiology, 35*(2), 169–185.

Roelofs, A. (2022). A neurocognitive computational account of word production, comprehension, and repetition in primary progressive aphasia. *Brain and Language, 227*, 105094.

Roelofs, A., & Ferreira, V. S. (2019). The architecture of speaking. In P. Hagoort (Ed.), *Human language: From genes and brains to behavior* (pp. 35–50). Cambridge, MA: MIT Press.

Roelofs, A., & Hagoort, P. (2002). Control of language use: Cognitive modeling of the hemodynamics of Stroop task performance. *Cognitive Brain Research, 15*(1), 85–97.

Roelofs, A., & Piai, V. (2011). Attention demands of spoken word planning: A review. *Frontiers in Psychology, 2*, Article 307.

Roelofs, A., van Turennout, M., & Coles, M. G. H. (2006). Anterior cingulate cortex activity can be independent of response conflict in Stroop-like tasks. *Proceedings of the National Academy of Sciences of the USA, 103*(37), 13884–13889.

Rubens, A. B. (1975). Aphasia with infarction in the territory of the anterior cerebral artery. *Cortex, 11*(3), 239–250.

Schall, J. D., & Boucher, L. (2007). Executive control of gaze by the frontal lobes. *Cognitive, Affective, and Behavioral Neuroscience, 7*(4), 396–412.

Scott, S. K. (2022). The neural control of volitional vocal production: From speech to identity, from social meaning to song. *Philosophical Transactions of the Royal Society of London: Series B, Biological Sciences, 377*(1841), 20200395.
Snyder, A. Z., Abdullaev, Y. G., Posner, M. I., & Raichle, M. E. (1995). Scalp electrical potentials reflect regional cerebral blood flow responses during processing of written words. *Proceedings of the National Academy of Sciences of the UnitedStates of America, 92*(5), 1689–1693.
Sohn, M.-H., Albert, M.V., Jung, K., Carter, C. S., & Anderson, J. R. (2007). Anticipation of conflict monitoring in the anterior cingulate cortex and the prefrontal cortex. *Proceedings of the National Academy of Sciences, 104*(25), 10330–10334.
Stefaniak, J. D., Alyahya, R., & Lambon Ralph, M. A. (2021). Language networks in aphasia and health: A 1000 participant activation likelihood estimation meta-analysis. *NeuroImage, 233*, 117960.
Thompson-Schill, S. L., D'Esposito, M., Aguirre, G. K., & Farah, M. J. (1997). Role of left inferior prefrontal cortex in retrieval of semantic knowledge: A reevaluation. *Proceedings of the National Academy of Sciences of the UnitedStates of America, 94*(26), 14792–14797.
Ueno, T., Saito, S., Rogers, T. T., & Lambon Ralph, M. A. (2011). Lichtheim 2: Synthesizing aphasia and the neural basis of language in a neurocomputational model of the dual dorsal-ventral language pathways. *Neuron, 72*(2), 385–396.
Ullman, M. T. (2016). The declarative/procedural model: A neurobiological model of language learning, knowledge and use. In G. Hickok & S. A. Small (Eds.), *The Neurobiology of language* (pp. 953–968). Boston, MA: Elsevier.
Wallis, J. D., Anderson, K. C., & Miller, E. (2001). Single neurons in prefrontal cortex encode abstract rules. *Nature, 411*(6840), 953–956.
Watanabe, Y., Abe, S., Ishikawa, T., Yamada, Y., & Yamane, G. (2004). Cortical regulation during the early stage of initiation of voluntary swallowing in humans. *Dysphagia, 19*(2), 100–108.
Wernicke, C. (1874). *Der aphasische Symptomencomplex. Eine psychologische Studie auf anatomischer Basis*. Breslau: Cohn & Weigert.
Wilson, S. M., & Schneck, S. M. (2021). Neuroplasticity in post-stroke aphasia: A systematic review and meta-analysis of functional imaging studies of reorganization of language processing. *Neurobiology of Language, 2*(1), 22–82.
Wundt, W. (1900). *Die Sprache*. Leipzig: Verlag von Wilhelm Engelmann.
Wundt, W. (1904). *Principles of physiological psychology*. London: Swan Sonnenschein.

10
THEORIES OF SEMANTIC PROCESSING

Elise Money-Nolan and John Shelley-Tremblay

Introduction

Semantics, broadly defined, refers to meaning. The study of semantics has been important in the fields of linguistics, rhetoric, law, philosophy, and political science as far back as the ancient Greeks. For the modern student of communication disorders, the study of semantics is critical for understanding the nature of any given language deficit. Why? It is because the intention of any communicative act ultimately is to convey meaning. The most common way that semantics impacts communication disorders is that in both developmental and acquired disorders of language, there can be observed some abnormality with either the structure of, or access to, concepts or their interconnections. The semantic system is one way that humans store information in memory, and as such semantic problems are memory problems. This chapter will review the most influential and widely researched theories of semantic representation, including distributed and local models, and the concept of spreading activation. Further reading (e.g., Chapters 6, 11, and 12) will show that problems with semantics have been implicated in many of the most common disorders encountered by speech pathologists or other communication disorders professionals, including the aphasias and Alzheimer's disease (AD).

Since the publication of the first edition of this text, much has changed in the study of semantics, but many concepts introduced in this chapter remain fundamental. For this reason, much of the initial work on definitions and theories of semantics remain in place, as they still form the basis for research in clinical and experimental linguistics today. However, we have expanded our discussion of semantics to include a review of theories that are "grounded," "embodied," and "perceptual." This work has dominated much of the thinking for the last two decades, and is important to understand if one wishes to work in semantics going forward. Additionally, we have updated work on the N400 Event-related Potential, and include classical psycholinguistics and simulation studies that reveal as much about the nature of semantics as they do about the N400 itself. Although this limited chapter is unable to cover the breadth of research associated with semantic processing, we hope that this brief survey engages your interest and leaves you asking more questions about this most important topic: the representation and processing of meaning.

Semantic memory has been conceptualized as a system for representing general world knowledge, linguistic skill, and aspects of vocabulary (Collins & Loftus, 1975; Moss et al., 1997; Zurif et al., 1974). This can be contrasted with episodic memory, which can be thought of as autobiographical memory for contextually specific events (Heilman & Valenstein, 1993; Tulving, 1984; Tulving & Thomson, 1973). Semantic memory is often thought of as the end result of a person's

DOI: 10.4324/9781003204213-12

abstracting the relevant information from multiple learning experiences. For example, as a young child encounters dogs for the first time, she may notice that all dogs have certain visual, structural, and functional features in common. She may also notice that dogs occur in certain contexts, emit specific noises, and may be associated with some of the goals of the child, such as throwing Frisbees or taking a walk. All of this information may become incorporated into different aspects of semantic memory, but the emphasis would not be on what specific dog could catch Frisbees or when this dog was first seen. Instead, the semantic system would specialize in storing the information about dogs, in general, and how they are related to the rest of the world.

In his introduction to a special issue of Brain and Language on the investigation of lexical semantic representation in AD, Henderson (1996) states that four general issues are of central importance to the current study of lexical semantic representation: (1) What are the processes by which semantic information comes to be stored in the lexicon? (2) How is meaning represented in the lexicon (what is its nature)? (3) How is this knowledge accessed and retrieved? (4) How do other cognitive operations affect these lexical semantic processes? It is the purpose of this chapter to address the state of the understanding of these issues, with a focus on issue number (2), as it bears most strongly on all others. Semantic priming is the most common technique for investigating issues number (2) and (3). This chapter will examine local, feature-based, and distributed models first and conclude with a discussion of the theories of grounded cognition and embodied semantics.

The lexicon versus the semantic system

Often times in published research the terms lexical and semantic are used interchangeably (Brown & Hagoort, 1993; Deacon et al., 2000; Holcomb, 1993), potentially due to an insufficient empirical basis upon which to discriminate between these closely related constructs. The lexicon refers specifically to a dictionary-like cognitive information structure that contains a person's vocabulary, including the morphology, argument structure, thematic role, and "meaning" of a vocabulary item. A conceptualization of the place of the lexicon in relationship to the rest of the language system is shown in Figure 10.1.

The difficulty with saying that any lexical item contains the meaning of a concept is that all meanings are dependent upon their relationships to other concepts. Thus, the lexical "definition" of any concept may best be thought of as an organized system of "pointers" to other concepts, or alternately, as the convergence of multiple concepts to form a unique reference. For example, one would not normally be said to know about the concept "dog" without an understanding of some of the critical components of a dog, including four legs, a tail, teeth, and so on. While "dog" is more than a collection of other concepts (a dog is not just a large cat with hair instead of fur, even though they are related and share many features), an understanding of "dog" rests on an understanding of its components. This notion is explored more below, in the section that critiques featural theories of meaning.

For the discussion that follows on local semantic systems, lexical and semantic may be interchangeable because any test of the semantic system must necessarily be carried out through access to the lexicon. As yet, I am unaware of any experimental manipulation that can achieve semantic access without lexical access first occurring. Even in the case of shapes or pictures serving as primes (Rock & Gutman, 1981), it is possible that the priming observed is a result of the pictorial codes activating the propositional codes stored in the lexical system. This is only a concern if one takes the "dual code" stance on the issue of multiple codes versus a unitary code for information storage in cortex (Kosslyn, 1981). If one takes the position that all information is represented in an elaborated propositional format (Paivio, 1991), then the idea of pictorial, auditory, and even somatosensory stimuli all converging on a single lexical system that serves to index semantic relationships is unproblematic.

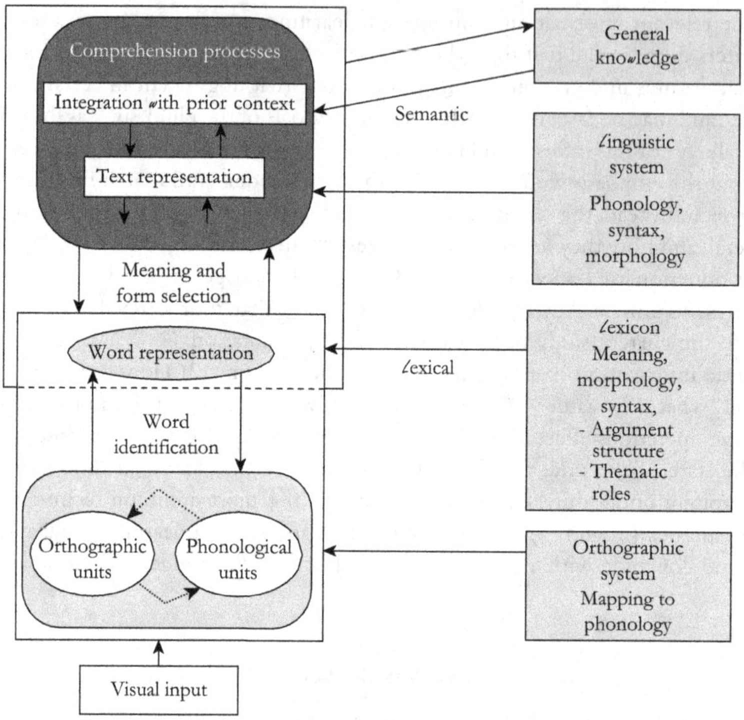

Figure 10.1 A schematic representation of the reader. The left column represents a sequential stream of hypothesized processing and representational stages as the language system processes a visually presented word. The right column refers to the general cognitive system that is subserved by the stages on the left. (Based on Perfetti, 2000, in Brown, C., and Hagoort, P., Eds., *The Neurocognition of Language*. Oxford.)

Models of semantic memory

The dominant models of semantic memory that have appeared over the last four decades can be roughly divided into one of two types: local or distributed. As these terms have been applied to a wide variety of models of semantic memory, it is possible to become confused about what stands as the defining features of these two types. At a basic level, local models are defined as those in which each "concept" in semantic memory has a unique location, or "node" in memory, while distributed systems posit that the same representational structures subserve multiple "concepts." Concepts, as defined in Collins & Loftus's (1975) local theory, are "particular senses of words or phrases." For example, "car," "driving a car," and "the particular car that I own" could all be thought of as concepts. Certainly, this is an extremely flexible and underspecified notion of a concept. At the core of both local and distributed models (which make few revisions to the construct of "concept") is a poor operational definition of a key aspect of the theory. This situation is similar, by analogy, to a theory of chemistry that makes no distinction between atoms and molecules, or acknowledges a distinction, but makes no attempt to look for functional differences between basic and conglomerated units.

A discussion of how this definitional deficiency may be addressed follows in the next section of the chapter. For now, setting aside this issue, an attempt to further delineate these classes of theory must be made. The whole notion of local versus distributed representation of information has a long history, and within the neurosciences can be traced back to the early aphasiologists. The heart of the difference between these types lies in the debate between the localizationists (Gaul &

Spurzheim, 1810–1819; Geschwind, 1965) and those who adhere to the doctrine of mass action (Lashley, 1938). Localizationists, in particular Barlow (1972), generally believe that individual neurons are capable of a high degree of coding specificity, such that a single neuron, or small group of neurons, would fire in response to a particular stimulus, and no other. The ubiquitous example of this doctrine is the notion of a "grandmother cell," which is sensitive only to the face of one's own grandmother. While this particular cell has not been found, similar instances of neuronal specificity have been discovered, such as a "monkey-hand cell," which responds most strongly to the image of a hand from its own species (Hinton & Anderson, 1989). This example may be instructive of the way that the brain can represent so many unique concepts. It seems that the cortex is structured to create fairly specific coding mechanisms for different basic stimuli that are encountered frequently, and that have a high survival value to the organism, such as the orientation sensitive cells described in cat visual cortex by Hubel and Wiesel (1979). This does not imply, however, that the majority of abstract semantic concepts would have their own neuron population assigned to them.

Local models

In discussing local semantic models, such as the most well-known version proposed by Collins and Quillian (1969) and Collins and Loftus (1975), the basic idea of a "node" may be somewhat incompatible with current conceptions of neuroanatomy/physiology. To the extent that Collins and Loftus (1975) is a Human Information Processing model (Neisser, 1967) that seeks only to provide a functional description of how the mind processes symbols, this discrepancy is unproblematic. However, if any modern theory wishes to employ models that can accommodate and integrate data from a wide range of sources, including the neurosciences, then the local models deserve a considerable revisiting. Such examination of the tenets of local theories has been attempted for the purposes of computational simulation (Fahlman et al., 1989), and word recognition (Rummelhart, 1986), but few authors have systematically attempted to create a local model that is both functionally descriptive of the vast body of experimental literature, as well as biologically plausible.

Perhaps the appeal of local models is their conceptual and diagrammatic simplicity. Shown in Figure 10.2 are concepts represented as circles, each depicting a unique informational location or node. These nodes are connected through links determining the strength and type of the relationship between nodes. The Collins and Quillian (1969) formulation of a semantic network allowed for five basic types of relationships, as well as for viewing links as a type of node, or concept, in themselves. Again, the advantage is flexibility, but the disadvantage is that it is difficult to conceive experiments that could disconfirm such a flexible theory such that it needed to be discarded. Perhaps the best candidates for such experiments are those semantic priming studies involving the interposition of an unrelated intervening item between the first and second stimuli. Such studies will be discussed in detail below, but unfortunately have yielded highly mixed results.

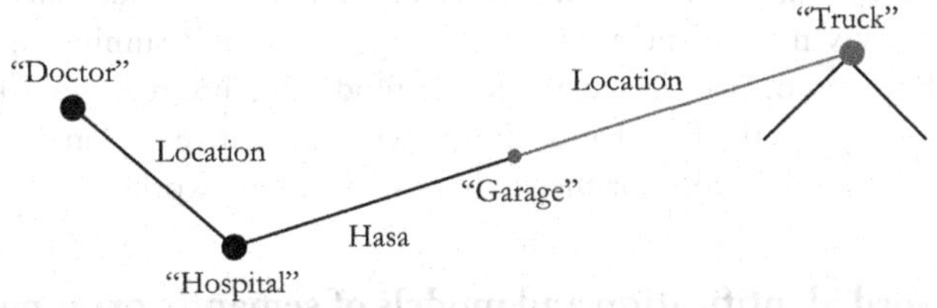

Figure 10.2 A portion of a local neural network. Words in parentheses indicate concepts that are represented in nodes (circles). The lines associate connections of the sort indicated by the labels, such as "DOCTOR" and "HOSPITAL" are related in that a doctor is found at the location, hospital. Strongly associated words are usually depicted as being closer together in the network. (Based on Collins, A. M. and Loftus, E. F., Psychol. Rev., 82, 407–428, 1975.).

In addition to the Collins and Loftus (1975) model and the Posner and Snyder (1975) model, which introduced the element of controlled processing into semantic network theory, the models of Anderson (1974, 1976, 1983; Anderson & Reder, 1999) were based on the assumption of spreading activation through a local network. Anderson's main finding was of a "fan effect," in which the ease of target recognition was inversely related to the number of concepts that it was associated to during a study phase. This effect, expressed most completely in the Adaptive Control of Thought (ACT) (Anderson, 1983) and ACT-R (Anderson, 1993) theories, supported the notion that when a word stimulus is presented, its corresponding representation becomes activated. This activation is finite, like an electrical charge, and then spreads out to all related concepts automatically. According to ACT, because the activation is of finite level and duration, the larger the number of related concepts, the smaller amount of activation for any single related concept. This proposition is expressed most basically as:

$$A_i = B_i + 3W_jS_{ji}.$$

Where latency to retrieve any piece of information from memory is determined by its current activation level, Ai, which is equal to the base level of activation Bi (determined by factors including recency and frequency of study), plus the sum of j concepts that make up the probe stimulus. Wj indicates the amount of attention given to any one source of information in the probe, and Sji equals the strength of association between source j and piece of information i. This equation is best illustrated in the simple propositional statements often used by Anderson, such as "A hippie is in the park." When hippie is paired with park, house, and bank (three pairs) during study, it takes longer to retrieve than if it was paired with park alone (one pair).

The utility of this mathematical formulation is that it has allowed Anderson and others (Anderson & Spellman, 1995; Radvansky et al., 1993) to test their reaction time and accuracy results against qualitative and quantitative predictions of the model. The results of such analyses over multiple experiments have generally confirmed the feasibility of spreading activation as a mechanism for explaining relationships between items in associative memory (Anderson & Reder, 1999). In a series of articles, Anderson and his associates proposed that the fan effect is equally well explained in terms of inhibitory processes (see Anderson & Spellman, 1995), rather than a simple dilution of facilitation across multiple items. In a paradigm similar to the typical study-and-test method of Anderson, these authors had participants practice particular associations to a category heading, for example, study "blood" and "tomato" for the category "red." One of the associates received more practice (here, blood), and subjects demonstrated an (unsurprising) boost in recall for that item. Interestingly, the less studied item (here, tomato) not only yielded poorer recall performance, but novel members of the same category as the less studied item also showed a recall decrement at test. For instance, the red food "strawberry" was more difficult to recall than another food (crackers) that did not fit into the category of red. While ACT-R did not predict such an effect, the presence of inhibition is in no way incompatible with spreading activation, assuming that the locus of the inhibition can be shown to operate in a manner that modulates, not replaces, automatic spreading of activation.[1] In recent years, the field has been ripe with alternative explanations for the priming effect that has been the primary tool for the study of semantic networks.

Word identification and models of semantic priming

Semantic information, simply, is just another type of data processed by the human brain on a regular basis. Thus, there is input of semantic information from the environment, most often in the form of written or spoken words, as well as the storage of semantic information, and the use of semantics by output systems to create meaningful writing and speech. It is to the first task of identifying words and extracting their meaning that we now turn our attention. Researchers have used a single experimental technique above all others in the past 35 years to investigate the process of word recognition: semantic priming.

Semantic priming refers to the processing advantage that occurs when a word (the target) is preceded by another word (the prime) when it is related in meaning to the target. The nature of the meaning relationship can be one or more of the following, but is not limited to, shared physical, functional, or visual features, membership in the same semantic category, or a simple associative relationship, such as ice cream scoop. An example of a typical semantic priming sequence is presented in Figure 10.3.

The phenomenon of priming has become ubiquitous with cognitive psychology, and the existence of positive semantic priming has been solidly established. However, the nature of the operations behind semantic priming is far from completely understood. What one believes about the process of semantic priming depends on one's view of the nature of semantic representation, and what operations are believed to be going on during the specific task required by the subject. This is because the strength and direction of priming effects vary greatly with the subject's task, as well as the stimulus and display parameters involved in task presentation. With that in mind, we can review some of the most influential theories of priming, and then discuss the most common parameters that have been found to influence priming in meaningful ways.

As mentioned above, perhaps the best known theory of semantic priming is that of Collins and Loftus (1975). Their explanation of semantic priming rested on (1) their proposal that semantic information is best described as being organized as a local network (see above), and (2) their notion of how the search of this network takes place. When a word is presented to a subject, for instance the prime "DOCTOR," the activation generated by the lexical identification of the stimulus begins to radiate out to all related concepts through the series of associative links described above. These authors proposed that, in addition to the nodes and links just described, a system of "tags" should be included to mark the path that spreading activation follows. As spreading activation travels, it leaves behind a trace (tag) that indicates not only its node of origin, but the last node that it had just passed through.

When the target is presented, the subject is supposed to initiate a search of their semantic memory to find the lexical entry of the word, in the case of a lexical decision task, or to find the

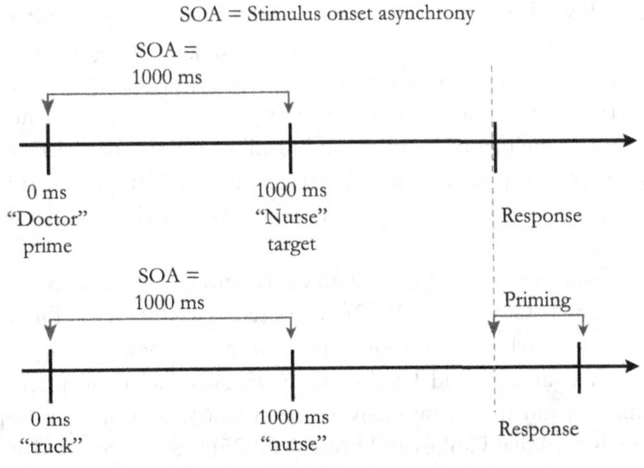

Figure 10.3 The target word, "NURSE," is preceded by a related prime, "DOCTOR," in the top time line. In the bottom time line, the target word is preceded by an unrelated prime, "TRUCK." The subject is asked to make a speeded response to the target word. A reduction in reaction time (RT) to the target is taken as an indication of the primes facilitative effect on the target.

word's semantic properties, such as its associates, in the case of a semantic relatedness judgment task. This theory was designed to account for data in semantic verification tasks of the sort, "All apples are fruit." In order to check for the truth of this proposition, the subject initiates a memory search to compare the information about these two items. If the word Macintosh had been presented prior to the to-be-verified proposition, then all its associatively related concepts, including "apple," will recently have had activation tags placed along their network. When the spreading activation from related tags "intersects," that is, tags from the two concepts are found in the same place, then an evaluation process occurs in which each path is traced back to its start. If the concepts link up, then they are judged to be related. If they do not link up, they are said to be unrelated.

In the case of the lexical decision task, targets that are merely letter strings are nonetheless still afforded some space in memory, albeit in an infrequently accessed portion of memory. This aspect of the theory at first seems untenable because of its notion that even nonsense strings would have representation in memory. However, the presence of priming effects, in both behavioral and event-related potential (ERP) studies for morphologically legal nonwords suggests that there may be some utility to this notion (Rugg, 1985). It may well be that every nonsense string is not uniquely represented, but is simply evaluated based on its physical proximity to the nearest real word; for instance, "BEEG," might elicit much the same pattern of activation as "BEEF." Essentially, the priming advantage for lexical decision tasks has been hypothesized to arise from a comparison process in which the memory search says, "Oh, BEEF has semantic associates, as indicated by this tag-related processing advantage, so if it has associates, it must be a word. Let's press the 'word' button more quickly."

It is important to note that the process thought to be operating during these tasks is word identification. A great deal of research has tried to isolate the nature of the processes underlying word identification, and the evidence tends to point to the notion that it can, but typically doesn't proceed without attention (Besner & Stolz, 1998). Posner and Snyder (1975) were the first authors to popularize the distinction between automatic and controlled processes in word identification. Their studies revealed that priming was greatly influenced by the length of delay between prime and target (see Posner & Snyder, 1975). At short delays, or stimulus onset asynchronies (SOAs) of less than 250 msec, only facilitatory effects were found, while both facilitation and inhibition were possible at long SOAs (greater than about 750 msec). It was theorized in addition to the automatic spreading activation already described, controlled processes would also be used when subjects were given ample time.

The two most often discussed types of controlled processes are expectancy generation, and various forms of post-lexical matching processes (de Groot, 1983; de Groot et al., 1982). These matching processes are referred to as post-lexical because they are thought to occur after the word form and meaning of a word stimulus have been accessed. The priming advantage is theorized to occur somewhere between meaning access and the motor response. This dichotomy is somewhat misleading, in that even in the original Collins and Quillian (1969) formulation of spreading activation in a local network, the priming effect produced by the system of activation tags was not realized until after activation had spread through the network and the paths were evaluated in a memory search process.

The matching mechanism was formulated as an explanation for the results obtained in studies by de Groot (de Groot, 1983; de Groot et al., 1982), who used a combination of masked and unmasked primes to test the limits to which activation spreads in a network. De Groot was interested in determining whether activation could be shown to spread to all concepts immediately related to a prime word, and beyond that, how many more distantly associated concepts would receive automatic facilitation. Recall that Collins and Loftus's (1975) theory predicted automatic spreading activation through all related nodes in a network, with this activation spreading first to all immediate associates (one-step pairs), followed by to more distant associates. Consider the pair Lion–Zebra (two-step pairs), which may not appear associatively related upon first inspection. Consider then the interposition of Tiger between Lion and Zebra, and the shared association of stripes becomes apparent. Thus, pairs like Lion–Tiger, as well as pairs like Lion–Zebra were tested under unmasked and masked conditions. Under unmasked conditions, only Lion–Tiger pairs received clear-cut facilitation in terms of decreased reaction time (RT) on a go/no-go lexical decision task.

De Groot speculated, however, that the failure to find reliable priming for second degree primes may have been due to a controlled checking strategy. Essentially, she suggested that subjects always look for a meaningful relationship between a prime and target after the recognition of both had occurred, and after a "Yes" response had been planned for the target in the case that it was a word. If subjects are presented with unrelated pairs, then somewhere between response planning and response execution they attempt to process the meaning of the pair until their discrepancy can be resolved. This is said to happen because readers are trained to expect that words in a normal text will be coherent, and contextually related as a rule. Violations of this rule lead to increased processing time. She proposed that such a process, if in operation, could preclude the detection of any automatic priming effects, as they would act to delay the decision process to a point where automatic facilitation would have dissipated. In further experiments, De Groot found that when her stimuli were masked, in an effort to limit conscious word identification and hence controlled meaning processing, no two-step priming was produced. Therefore, she concluded that no spreading activation occurred beyond the one-step associate.

Because of the lack of spreading activation beyond the first associate, she suggested a model in which the semantic network is composed of clusters of concepts, with a central concept (DOG) surrounded by its core associates (CAT). Activation may spread automatically between these concepts. However, she proposed that no direct associative links exist between central concepts and more peripheral ones, so that any priming that occurs between those concepts would be due to a post-lexical process involving a search of already active concepts. To date, this theory has received mixed support, but has not been conclusively disconfirmed.

The other mechanism that has been thought to be active at long SOAs is that of semantic expectancy. Here, when subjects have been exposed to an experimental situation in which the prime is somewhat predictive of the target, then it is thought that they begin to actively generate a set of possible targets after the appearance of the prime. This process is illustrated in Figure 10.4. Generally, when the proportion of primes and targets is relatively high (∃ .50), it would be reasonable to adopt such a strategy. If the subject happens to generate the target as part of his or her expectancy set, then the response to that target should be facilitated due to its prior activation by the expectancy mechanism.

While this strategy occurs after the prime has been processed, it does occur before the meaning of the target word has been processed, and so in that sense is a controlled process that is not post-lexical. In other words, it is distinct from expectancy generation because its effect is to change the level of activation of the target before it is encountered as a stimulus, not to facilitate a matching process after lexical activation. All of the mechanisms discussed in this section have been proposed to account for experimental data in local conceptions of a semantic network, but other possibilities for lexical–semantic organization exist.

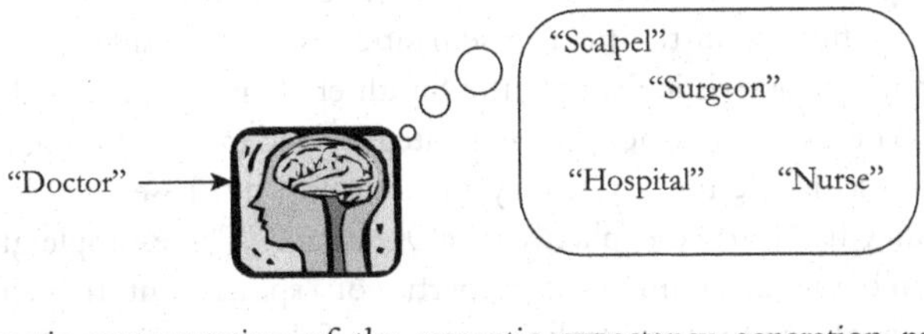

Figure 10.4 A schematic representation of the semantic expectancy generation process. After viewing "DOCTOR," the subject begins to produce candidate targets based on the expectation of semantic relatedness. If one of the generated possibilities is "NURSE," then response time will be shortened.

Feature-based semantic models

While the paradigms thus far have assumed that concepts are relatively unitary constructions linked together through some sort of associative connections, other proposed models view concepts as an aggregate of features. One of the best known models of this type is that of Smith et al. (1974), which theorizes that concepts are composed of both defining and characteristic features. The former are thought to be elements of a concept that are necessary and sufficient for the basic definition of the concept, while the latter may often be associated with, but not critical to, a concept's meaning. While not grouped by Smith et al., modern featural theory researchers have divided the majority of features into structural and functional features, with the structural features composed of both sensory aspects (square-shaped), and material qualities (made of clay; Moss et al., 1997). Functional features would permit the comparison of "spoon" and "shovel," because both can be used to scoop. Like Collins and Loftus's (1975) model, this model was designed to account for performance on a sentence verification task where subjects are asked to indicate the truth of a statement such as "All robins are birds." Memory access is accomplished through a two-stage search process in which (1) a set of category names are retrieved containing names of all categories that having members in common with the category of the predicate noun (bird in the previous example), and (2) a feature-by-feature comparison process occurs in which attributes of the subject and predicate of the sentence are checked for a match.

A major advantage of such a model is that it permits a detailed mapping of semantic space, such that the distances between concepts can be determined along empirically derived continua. This was accomplished by Smith et al. (1974) by the use of typicality ratings as the dependent measure in a factor analysis technique. Such a semantic space allows for the predictions to be made about the typicality of any new instance of a concept that is introduced to such a space. Network models must suppose the existence of a new node, not only for new concepts, but for even slightly different senses of an existing concept. For instance, the notion of a "Coke" and that of a "large Coke" would have separate representations in a local network, while a feature model would need only to change the weight on the dimension of size to encode this second concept. This seems to be a more precise and economical format for information storage.

Another advantage of such a conception of semantic representation is its ability to specify what elements are included in the definition of any concept. For instance, "dog" in a local network for one researcher may not be the same for another. In practice, however, this is enormously difficult due to several factors. In the first place, it may be impossible to determine what constitutes a necessary feature for any category. For example, the concept of "furniture" may typically include tables and chairs, which share four legs and the ability to hold other items on top of them. On the other hand, "furniture" may contain beanbag chairs, with no legs, and grandfather clocks that do not hold other objects. Second, there may be a great deal of difference between the featural composition of a concept between individuals. While two people may agree that the furry creature standing before them should be labeled "dog," this does not mean that they have the same set of key attributes in their representations of dog.

The model of Smith et al. (1974) was criticized so effectively by Collins and Loftus (1975) that it lost a good deal of influence in the field of semantic research. Besides the difficulty in distinguishing defining from characteristic features, the Smith et al. model proposed that people do not search the superordinate category when making category judgments. Often, as stated by Collins and Loftus, people must decide upon category membership not based on defining features, but simply on whether they had learned explicitly that "X was a Y." The example given by Collins and Loftus was of a person being uncertain of the properties of a sponge, but still being able to correctly categorize it as an animal due to their explicit learning of that fact. One way to view the critical difference between these types of theories is that featural theories permit a sort of calculation of the semantic status of each concept online, based on the evidence of its featural composition. Local network theories seem to propose that what gets stored and linked together are the outputs of processes. In other words, while features may be used to construct and judge instances of categories, local nodes are the output of such constructive or rote learning processes.

Distributed models

The doctrine of mass action stands somewhat at odds with local models. In this way of thinking, a relatively large proportion of all neurons are involved in the representation of every concept that is processed during one operation. Perhaps the most cogent formulation of such a model for use with semantic memory is that of Masson (1995; Masson & Borowsky, 1998). This model is truly "distributed" in that it postulates that every concept is represented over a large array of processing units that are generally the same within any one module of the system. Such an array is generally thought to consist of multiple layers, or levels, starting with an input unit, followed by some number of hidden layers, and finally an output layer. This arrangement is illustrated in Figure 10.5.

Masson's model proposed the division of the neural network into three main subnetworks based on their representational content: orthographic units, phono-logical units, and meaning units. These subsystems are completely interconnected though feed forward and feedback pathways, thus allowing the output of semantic and phonological analyses to influence the activity state of the orthographic units. This feature allows the network to account for such basic phenomenon as the word-superiority effect (Reicher, 1969), where word identification is faster than an equivalent nonword string. Here, lexical level information would bias orthographic processing units, causing a more rapid identification of previously encountered (legal) word forms.

If a word is presented visually, the orthographic system takes the word form as its input, which is then transduced into values that are passed to an unspecified number of intermediate units, and finally these values are passed as output to a higher-level subsystem. Orthographic output is proposed to pass either directly to the semantic unit, or by way of the phonological unit to the semantic unit. This architecture is necessary to account for evidence suggesting that while a phonological activation may be the default result of an orthographic analysis, meaning activation can take place in the absence of concomitant phonological analysis (Jared & Seidenberg, 1991). Whenever input enters one of the distributed processing subsystems, it is cycled through repeatedly, with output being fed back into the input channel until the most stable pattern of activation is found. In this sense, "identification" at any processing level means the point at which error between input and outpoint is minimized.

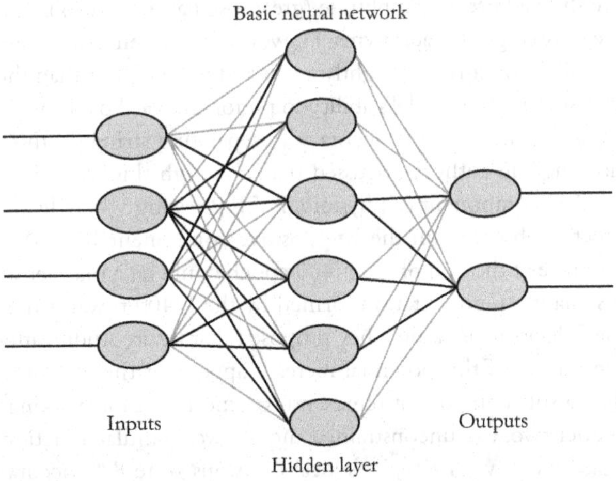

Figure 10.5 A basic three-level neural network model with parallel, distributed connections between each of the processing units. Activation levels of each node, on their own, represent no concepts. But when taken together the unique activity of the output level is suggested to be able to code for any unique concept. (Adapted from www.e-orthopaedics.com/sakura/images/neural.gif.)

The N400 event-related potential (ERP), which was introduced in Chapter 5 of this textbook, can be used to index semantic processing. Interestingly, some ERP studies have shown that semantic access as reflected by the N400 is engaged even in cases of illegal consonant strings. N400s to these nonwords were altered in response to manipulations such as changes in orthographic neighborhood size and orthographic neighbor frequency (Laszlo & Federmeier, 2009, 2011). Laszlo and Plaut (2012) attempted to test this "obligatory semantics" view using the Parallel Distributed Processing approach (PDP) in two simulations which varied the structure of the computational model. The PDP approach, first proposed by Seidenberg and McClelland (1989) "utilizes learned representations of a uniform set of principles." However, the initial PDP model, like localist models, has been criticized for not being neuro-biologically plausible (i.e., not truly representative of cognitive processes as they occur naturally in the brain during processing of words and meaning).

For simulation one of this study, Laszlo and Plaut (2012) modified the PDP model from its original format so that it was more representative of actual cognitive processes, separating excitatory and inhibitory inputs throughout the layers of the model, which they referred to as the "constrained model." Also, model one varied from the original PDP approach in that it did not examine the interaction of phonology with orthography and semantics. In simulation two, the model was not as neuro-biologically plausible, allowing excitatory and inhibitory outputs from single units, which was referred to as the "unconstrained model." In both simulations, the obligatory semantics view was tested, simulating N400 amplitudes in response to words, pseudowords, acronyms, and illegal strings.

Here, the models' autoencoders were trained to prefer CVC strings (such as words and pseudowords) and "disprefer" illegal strings and consonants. This training was based on the results of another study which found an "N effect," where individual lexical characteristics, (e.g., orthographic neighborhood size, neighbor frequency) were stronger predictors of N400 amplitude than lexical category (e.g., word, pseudoword) (Laszlo & Federmeier, 2011). For this study, Laszlo and Plaut (2012) also varied orthographic neighborhood size so that it was much larger for the words (N=6.83) than acronyms (N=0.8). Next, they trained the semantic access component of the model so that it had more exposure to words and acronyms, "preferring" their semantic features over those of pseudowords and illegal strings.

The results of simulation one showed that the accuracy for model one's autoencoder was 100%, and its semantic access accuracy was 93% (correct for all words and acronyms). The simulated amplitude results here showed greater amplitude (greater semantic access) for words and pseudowords compared to illegal strings and acronyms. However, by the end of the recording epoch, the amplitudes for words and acronyms rose slightly again and were higher than those of pseudowords and illegal strings, representing the model's ability to perform lexical decision-making. Also in support of this finding was the model's 90% accuracy in separating strings with semantic representations from those without. The authors discussed that, although this second amplitude increase is not observed in the N400 component of physiologic ERP testing where lexical decision tasks are required, such an effect is observed on the late positive component ERP (LPC). They proposed that this amplitude increase at the end of the N400 epoch could be a manner of feed-forward projection of the stable semantic representation formed by the N400 towards the LPC, which could form the basis of lexical decision-making. They proposed that future studies attempt to separate the LPC and N400 to determine if this potential increase appears at the end of the N400 recording epoch, which could be a sub-component representing lexical decision-making.

The results for model two, the unconstrained model, were similar functionally to model one, as the autoencoder's accuracy was 100%, its lexical decisions were 87% accurate, and its semantic access accuracy was 90% (though here, errors were distributed across all word categories). Although the two models were similar functionally, the manner in which semantic access was achieved differs, with model two being much less similar to physiologic N400 data. The simulated amplitude results for model two showed two peaks, with the initial peak occurring at stimulus onset (different from actual N400 data), having greater amplitudes than typical physiologic data, and equal amplitudes for all word categories. The second peak still showed greater amplitude for words and pseudowords, but here was followed closely by acronyms, and the amplitude for illegal strings was not as greatly reduced compared to model one.

Overall, the results showed that the separation of excitation and inhibition in model one was more successful in modelling the N400, with the constrained model being much more similar to actual N400 ERP data. Also, model one showed similar effects of orthographic neighborhood size compared to ERP data for words that had been trained (words and acronyms) vs. words that had not been trained (pseudowords and illegal strings). This was shown by the initial greater simulated N400 amplitude for words and pseudowords (higher Ns) vs. acronyms and illegal strings (lower Ns), providing additional support for the "obligatory semantics" view. However, the model successfully separated items with learned semantic representations (words and acronyms) by the end of the epoch, which differs from behavioral ERP results to date, but may be revealed in future ERP studies requiring lexical decision-making tasks. These results provide additional support for the PDP model of visual word recognition, and emphasize that separating excitation and inhibition is an important addition to the model.

Priming effects in distributed models

The basic explanation for semantic priming in a distributed model is that when a prime appears, it causes the processing units to take on the values associated with that word at each level of analysis. Because the processing units can only hold one value at a time, if a related target appears it will find the current pattern of semantic activation to be similar to its own. Thus, the time necessary for the target to reach a stable level of representation will be shortened. Unrelated words require a resetting of the units, while neutral stimuli would leave the network in a relatively unbiased state. Thus, RT for tasks requiring word identification should be slowest for unrelated, moderate for neutral, and quickest for related. In this way, distributed models can account for the same findings of inhibition for unrelated words at long SOAs that were discussed earlier in the work of Posner and Snyder (1975).

As alluded to above, distributed models can be viewed as having the advantage that they resemble, in function and somewhat in structure, the populations of neurons thought to be responsible for all cognition. However, as discussed in Masson (1995), the primary test of the utility of such models is in their ability to account for existing data parsimoniously, and to make unique predictions. The primary experimental evidence for the distributed model discussed by Masson concerns its ability to accurately predict the magnitude and direction of semantic priming effects in a situation in which an unrelated item is interposed between a related prime and target. Similar to the paradigm utilized by de Groot (above), the intervening item manipulation compares the RT results from two critical conditions: a prime followed by a related target (DOG–CAT), as opposed to a prime followed by an intervening item and then a target (DOG–ROCK–CAT).

The original formulation of local network models predicts that an intervening item should have no effect on the strength of priming effects because activation is thought to spread automatically to all nodes in the network. Presenting an intervening item should just serve to add another source of activation to the network, but not disrupt the initial activation. Because distributed networks can represent only one concept at a time in their processing units, the intervening item should disrupt priming to the extent that it is different from the activation pattern of the prime and target. Thus, unrelated intervening items should disrupt priming the most, and neutral stimuli (like "XXXX") should have a marginally disruptive influence.

Masson reports two studies designed to test these predictions. Study 1 presented subjects with a prime, intervening item on some trials, and target for 200 msec each, with an SOA of 400 msec. The subject's task was to name the target as quickly as possible. As predicted by his model, Masson found that the unrelated intervening item significantly disrupted priming when compared to the condition where the target followed the prime directly. Masson performed a second study in which priming across trials was assessed. In this experiment he lengthened both the duration and SOA of the stimuli and arranged the items so that the target of one pair would serve as a prime to the next pair. He predicted that under these conditions the disruption of priming seen in experiment 1 would diminish because the degree of disruption should be proportional to the amount of processing devoted to the intervening item, relative to the prime. In a sense, the pattern set up when processing the intervening item is more likely to disrupt priming if (1) the prime's pattern is less established, and (2) the intervening item's pattern is allowed to completely stabilize in the system. While the complexity of his results renders them prohibitively large to report in detail, he found that the intervening item disruption diminished as predicted.

Masson's paper aimed to provide support for the plausibility of an alternative representational scheme to the local network. In this endeavor he was initially successful. On the other hand, he pointed out that the model was incomplete in that it did not provide mechanisms to account for many of the common strategic processing factors encountered in priming research, including proportion of related to unrelated prime–target pairs (so-called relatedness proportion, or RP), proportion of nonwords, and semantic expectancy strategies. It also lacked an ability to account for a "learning effect" apparent in a comparison of the two studies. Briefly, when a legal word is used as the intervening item ("Ready"), subjects slowly become habituated to it, and the pattern of disruption changes.

Since the publication of the first edition of this chapter, a recent study by Cheyette and Plaut (2017) addressed many of these semantic priming factors in an N400 study which updated the previously mentioned modified PDP model developed by Laszlo and Plaut (2012). This model was applied to a paradigm used in another model developed by Rabovsky and McRae (2014), which was shown to be sensitive to many additional N400 effects including semantic priming, semantic richness, word frequency, repetition, and interactions of richness, frequency, and orthographic neighborhood (ON) size. Although successful in showing these effects, the original model by Rabovsky and McRae (2014) was limited in that it only focused on behavioral effects and the direction of N400 change, without actually simulating the N400's morphology and amplitude changes. Additionally, the neurological plausibility of the initial model is questionable, and the effect sizes of significant findings were small. The current study aimed to address the same phenomena as Rabovsky and McRae (2014), but using the neurologically constrained model from Laszlo and Plaut (2012), adding additional units representing separate excitatory and inhibitory influences along the pathway. The model was also altered to include a lexical decision-making system, and an activation-based decay function (Laszlo & Armstrong, 2014).

This study used the model for two simulations, the first of which studied N400 effects in response to several factors, modeling N400 amplitude using summed semantic activation. The second simulated behavioral effects, asking the model to perform lexical decisions and analyzing summed yes/no activations. Results of the first simulation (N400 effects) revealed decreased N400 amplitudes for words that were higher in frequency, lower in richness, repeated, and preceded by semantically or associatively related primes (vs. unrelated), and words with smaller ON sizes. Also, greater effects of repetition were found for words that were lower in frequency and higher in richness. Also, the model was reasonably successful in using semantic activation to approximate the shape of the N400 waveform. Results of the second simulation (behavioral effects) revealed that the model was successful in producing most of the relevant empirical effects, showing better performance for primed words, repeated words, and words with high frequency and richness. Overall, using the model of Laszlo and Plaut (2012) to address empirical findings related to semantic priming found in Rabovsky and McRae (2014) was successful in accounting for behavioral lexical decision-making and for effects of several priming factors on N400 amplitude.

Models of grounded cognition

Although distributed models have successfully provided an alternative explanation of semantic processing compared to local models, such distributed models have been criticized for being "disembodied," in that they only learn semantic information through textual information[2] (Silberer & Lapata, 2012). Models of grounded cognition reject the idea that knowledge is represented by amodal symbols, accounting for learning of semantic information and meaning through individuals' experiences and actions in their environment (Barsalou, 2008). This view is in opposition to standard views of cognition, which posit that the brain forms internal representations about information separately from the modality-specific areas of the brain associated with perception, action, and introspection. In the view of grounded cognition, the body acts as a source of external information about situations and actions experienced in the environment, which may be used to supplement internal representations driven by simulations within the brain's modal systems (Barsalou, 2008).

Simulations are an important aspect of the grounded cognition theories, proposing that the brain "re-enacts" multimodal representations of external experiences when attempting to draw meaning to some item or action. For example, as an individual performs an action such as eating a bite of a new food, the brain codes features of the experience across modalities, noting the look, feel and taste of the food, coding the action of eating, and any noting introspections such as like or dislike of the food. In later situations where the brain encounters the food again, or sees it written in text, these coded, modal representations may be drawn upon to give meaning to the word based upon past experiences. The idea that knowledge is learned from perceptual information, actions encountered in the environment, and simulations within the brain's modal systems is referred to as the theory of grounded cognition.

Theory of embodied semantics

One specific theory falling into the category of grounded cognition is the theory of embodied semantics, which states that information about an action or experience is coded within the brain in the same sensory-motor areas associated with performing the action. Recently, it has been suggested that the mirror neuron system may be involved in the process of embodied semantics (Aziz-Zadeh & Damasio, 2008). The mirror neuron system has been shown to be responsive to execution, observation, and mental simulation of an action in the F5 area in monkeys (di Pellegrino et al., 1992; Gallese et al., 1996; Umiltà et al., 2001). In humans, the mirror neuron system is within Broadman's Area 44 (BA 44), in dorsal areas of the premotor cortex, and within the inferior parietal lobule (IPL) (Aziz-Zadeh et al., 2004; Aziz-Zadeh et al., 2006; Geyer et al., 2000). Importantly, these neurons are sensitive to the goal of an action, no matter the manner of execution of the action.

It is proposed that as an individual learns about actions through environmental experiences, the primary and secondary sensory-motor areas may send information about the representation of such actions through "feed-forward" projections to the inferior frontal gyrus (IFG-contains BA 44 and 45) and the IPL. As these distributed signals converge, visual, somatosensory, and motor information are integrated, and mirror neurons code representations of the action within the brain. Findings of several fMRI studies have supported the theory of embodied semantics, revealing activation of the hand, foot, and mouth premotor regions in response to watching actions performed by each area (Aziz-Zadeh et al., 2006), and reading about actions performed by each area (Hauk et al., 2004). However, some studies have failed to localize the specific premotor regions associated with watching or reading of associated actions, with some studies indicating incorrect or overlapping areas.

In recent years, several perceptually grounded distributional models have arisen. These models are distributed in that they posit that a large amount of neurons throughout the cortex are activated to achieve semantic access, but oppose the idea that meaning is learned only through linguistic information. Silberer and Lapata (2012) aimed to examine how word meaning is derived from textual and perceptual (grounded) information encountered in the environment by comparing models representing word meaning based on perceptual data vs. linguistic information. The authors explained that there are two views of how perceptual and textual information may be integrated to form representations of meaning. Some researchers believe that textual and perceptual information is represented independently, and a grounded representation is formed by simply concatenating information from the two sources. Alternatively, some believe that the information from textual and perceptual sources is interpreted jointly, and that semantic knowledge is gained through shared representations from each of these sources. Researchers here aimed to determine whether models that integrate textual and perceptual information better capture the way individuals form representations of meaning, compared to models using only one source of information. Additionally, they wanted to determine the best mode of integration of textual and perceptual information, whether it be through simple concatenation of the two sources or joint integration of shared information.

Sibera and Lapata's (2012) experimental procedure involved comparing three models on three tasks, word association, word similarity, and the models' ability to infer perceptual information when none is provided. They adopted three models from previous experiments, firstly a "Feature-Topic Model" by Andrews et al. (2009). In this model, words in bodies of text are represented by their frequency of occurrence, and words within the text that also have feature information (from a database of features of common words derived behaviorally) are paired with their features and represented by the feature distribution of the word. Word meaning is represented by the distribution of joint, shared textual information and perceptual features over the learned words. The second model, called a "Global Similarity Model," was adopted from Johns and Jones (2012), which posits that perceptual representations of words are created through means of "global lexical similarity." The focus of this model is on creating perceptual representations when words have no perceptual correlates, based on the idea that "lexically similar words also share perceptual features and hence it should be possible to transfer perceptual information onto words that have none from their linguistically similar neighbors." Here, a word's meaning is represented by the concatenation of separate perceptual and textual information. The third model is called "Canonical Correlation Analysis," and was adopted from Hardoon et al. (2004). This statistical model jointly integrates perceptual and textual information in a way so that specific details of the representation (textual or perceptual) are removed from the analysis, leaving only the underlying common factors that generated a correlation.

The results of this study showed that across all models, the use of both textual and perceptual information more closely approximated behavioral data, rather than using only one source. Interestingly, though, for all models, when considering only perceptual or textual information, perceptual information yielded a higher correlation coefficient, speaking to the importance of perceptual information in forming representations of meaning. When comparing the three models on the word association task, it was clear that joint integration of perceptual and textual information was ideal over simple concatenation of the two information sources, which was shown by higher correlation coefficients for the Feature-Topic Model and the Canonical Correlation Analysis than the Global Similarity Model. The correlation coefficients between the two joint integration methods were not significantly different by a t-test. The word similarity task yielded similar results, with the two joint integration models performing better than the Global Similarity Model that concatenates the two information sources. For the inference task, the Global Similarity Model performed the best, as it is the only model with a built-in inference method. However, the authors noted that the concern of how to best integrate perceptual and textual information (concatenation or joint integration) seemed to have a larger impact on forming representations of meaning vs. the inference mechanism.

Summary and conclusion

We have reviewed the most common theories of semantic representation that have emerged in the last 35 years. The models consisted of local theories, feature-based theories, and distributed models. The advantage of local theories was that they were extremely flexible and powerful, and can model almost any experimental result. This was particularly true of Anderson's ACT models, which were so flexible that they may not be falsifiable. A theory that cannot be proven wrong is problematic for science, because it proves difficult to know when to discard it in favor of a better theory. Nonetheless, local models that operate using spreading activation have been the most influential and widely investigated since the 1970s.

Feature-based theories had the advantage of allowing the most precise and economical mapping of semantic knowledge, but suffered from the problem of finding good "critical" or defining features that would be necessary to differentiate one concept form from another. Powerful theories of semantic representation, like those of Anderson, include aspects both of local network and feature-based theories. Distributed models offered the distinct advantage of being more biologically plausible, especially when excitatory and inhibitory inputs are separated throughout layers of the model. Remember that our brains are composed of billions of highly flexible units (neurons) that may be reconfigured to complete many processing tasks, and that each neuron may be involved in the representation of many different pieces of semantic information. Distributed models were furthermore able to account for the intervening item phenomenon that was problematic for standard local spreading activation models. Grounded theories differ from both local and distributed theories suggesting that meaning is primarily derived from information from textual sources, and posit that meaning is derived from information encountered by the body within the environment.

In summary, the study of semantic representation has made great strides in accounting for the richness and complexity of human knowledge in the past 40 years. Elements of these theories still figure prominently in the 21st-century language studies, and they continue to provide a means to account for normal word recognition. Chapter 28 in this volume will examine how these models play a central role in understanding what breaks down in some common communication disorders.

Notes

1 Research revising early models of spreading activation suggests the operation of an attentional center-surround mechanism (CSM) which assists in coding weakly activated semantic representations, such as for newly learned words. The CSM assists in retrieving meaning from semantic memory by facilitating strongly related items in the "center" of the activation, and inhibiting weakly related items in the "surround" (Carr & Dagenbach, 1990; Dagenbach & Carr, 1994). Recent research on the CSM suggests that this process operates differentially in the left and right hemispheres, with only the left hemisphere supporting processes of spreading activation (Deacon et al., 2013).

2 However, in learning from textual information, perceptual information may be conveyed since information about features and experiences can be conveyed through text. Riordan and Jones (2011) argued that the amount of perceptual and semantic information accounted for in distributed computational models has been "underappreciated" in a review article comparing newer feature-based and distributed models.

Further reading

Evans, W. S., Cavanaugh, R., Gravier, M. L., Autenreith, A. M., Doyle, P. J., Hula, W. D., & Dickey, M. W. (2021). Effects of semantic feature type, diversity, and quantity on semantic feature analysis treatment outcomes in aphasia. *American Journal of Speech-Language Pathology, 30*(1S), 344–358.

Ding, J., Chen, K., Liu, H., Huang, L., Chen, Y., Lv, Y., & Lambon Ralph, M. (2020). A unified neurocognitive model of semantics language social behaviour and face recognition in semantic dementia. *Nature Communications, 11*(1), 1–14.

Gravier, M. L., Dickey, M. W., Hula, W. D., Evans, W. S., Owens, R. L., Winans-Mitrik, R. L., & Doyle, P. J. (2018). What matters in semantic feature analysis: Practice-related predictors of treatment response in aphasia. *American Journal of Speech-Language Pathology, 27*(1S), 438–453.

References

Anderson, J. R. (1974). Retrieval of propositional information from long-term memory. *Cognitive Psychology, 6*(4), 451–474.

Anderson, J. R. (1976). *Language, memory, and thought*. Potomac, MD: Lawrence Erlbaum.

Anderson, J. R. (1983). A spreading activation theory of memory. *Journal of Verbal Learning and Verbal Behavior, 22*(3), 261–295.

Anderson, J. R. (1993). Problem solving and learning. *American Psychologist, 48*(1), 35–44.

Anderson, J. R., & Reder, L. M. (1999). The fan effect: New results and new theories. *Journal of Experimental Psychology: General, 128*(2), 186–197.

Anderson, M. C., & Spellman, B. A. (1995). On the status of inhibitory mechanisms in cognition: Memory retrieval as a model case. *Psychological Review, 102*(1), 68–100.

Andrews, M., Vigliocco, G., & Vinson, D. (2009). Integrating experiential and distributional data to learn semantic representations. *Psychological Review, 116*(3), 463–498. https://doi.org/10.1037/a0016261.

Aziz-Zadeh, L., & Damasio, A. (2008). Embodied semantics for actions: Findings from functional brain imaging. *Journal of Physiology-Paris, 102*(1–3), 35–39.

Aziz-Zadeh, L., Iacoboni, M., Zaidel, E., Wilson, S., & Mazziotta, J. (2004). Left hemisphere motor facilitation in response to manual action sounds. *European Journal of Neuroscience, 19*(9), 2609–2612. https://doi.org/10.1111/j.0953-816X.2004.03348.x.

Aziz-Zadeh, L., Koski, L., Zaidel, E., Mazziotta, J., & Iacoboni, M. (2006). Lateralization of the human mirror neuron system. *Journal of Neuroscience: The Official Journal of the Society for Neuroscience, 26*(11), 2964–2970. https://doi.org/10.1523/JNEUROSCI.2921-05.2006.

Aziz-Zadeh, L., Wilson, S. M., Rizzolatti, G., & Iacoboni, M. (2006). Congruent embodied representations for visually presented actions and linguistic phrases describing actions. *Current Biology: CB, 16*(18), 1818–1823. https://doi.org/10.1016/j.cub.2006.07.060.

Barlow, H. B. (1972). Single units and sensation: A neuron doctrine for perceptual psychology? *Perception, 1*(4), 371–394.

Barsalou, L. W. (2008). Grounded cognition. *Annual Review of Psychology, 59*(1), 617–645. https://doi.org/10.1146/annurev.psych.59.103006.093639.

Besner, D., & Stolz, J. A. (1998). Unintentional reading: Can phonological computation be controlled? *Canadian Journal of Experimental Psychology, 52*(1), 35–42.

Brown, C., & Hagoort, P. (1993). The processing nature of the N400: Evidence from masked priming. *Journal of Cognitive Neuroscience, 5*(1), 10.

Carr, T. H., & Dagenbach, D. (1990). Semantic priming and repetition priming from masked words: Evidence for a center-surround attentional mechanism in perceptual recognition. *Journal of Experimental Psychology. Learning, Memory, and Cognition, 16*(2), 341–350.

Cheyette, S. J., & Plaut, D. C. (2017). Modeling the N400 ERP component as transient semantic over-activation within a neural network model of word comprehension. *Cognition, 162*, 153–166. https://doi.org/10.1016/j.cognition.2016.10.016.

Collins, A. M., & Loftus, E. F. (1975). A spreading activation theory of semantic processing. *Psychological Review, 82*(6), 407–428.

Collins, A. M., & Quillian, M. R. (1969). Retrieval time from semantic memory. *Journal of Verbal Learning and Verbal Behavior, 8*(2), 240–248.

Dagenbach, D., & Carr, T. H. (1994). Inhibitory processes in perceptual recognition: Evidence for a center-surround attentional mechanism. In D. Dagenbach & T. H. Carr (Eds.), *Inhibitory processes in attention, memory, and language* (pp. 327–357). Cambridge, MA: Academic Press.

de Groot, A. M. (1983). The range of automatic spreading activation in word priming. *Journal of Verbal Learning and Verbal Behavior, 22*(4), 417–436.

de Groot, A. M., Thomassen, A. J., & Hudson, P. T. (1982). Associative facilitation of word recognition as measured from a neutral prime. *Memory and Cognition, 10*(4), 358–370.

Deacon, D., Hewitt, S., Yang, C.-M., & Nagata, M. (2000). Event-related potential indices of semantic priming using masked and unmasked words: Evidence that the N400 does not reflect a post-lexical process. *Cognitive Brain Research, 9*(2), 137–146.

Deacon, D., Shelley-Tremblay, J. F., Ritter, W., & Dynowska, A. (2013). Electrophysiological evidence for the action of a center-surround mechanism on semantic processing in the left hemisphere. *Frontiers in Psychology, 4*, 936. https://doi.org/10.3389/fpsyg.2013.00936.

di Pellegrino, G., Fadiga, L., Fogassi, L., Gallese, V., & Rizzolatti, G. (1992). Understanding motor events: A neurophysiological study. *Experimental Brain Research*, *91*(1), 176–180. https://doi.org/10.1007/BF00230027.

Fahlman, S. E., Hinton, G. E., & Anderson, J. A. (1989). Representing implicit knowledge. In *Parallel models of associative memory (updated ed.)* (pp. 171–185). Lawrence Erlbaum Associates, Inc. Retrieved from http://search.ebscohost.com/login.aspx?direct=true&db=psyh&AN=1989-97439-005&loginpage=Login.asp&site=ehost-live&scope=site.

Gallese, V., Fadiga, L., Fogassi, L., & Rizzolatti, G. (1996). Action recognition in the premotor cortex. *Brain: A Journal of Neurology*, *119*(Pt 2), 593–609. https://doi.org/10.1093/brain/119.2.593.

Gaul, F., & Spurzheim, G. (1810). *The anatomy and physiology of the nervous system in general and the brain in particular* (Vols. 1–4). F. Schoell.

Geschwind, N. (1965). Disconnection syndromes in animals and man. *Brain*, *88*(2), 237–294.

Geyer, S., Matelli, M., Luppino, G., & Zilles, K. (2000). Functional neuroanatomy of the primate isocortical motor system. *Anatomy and Embryology*, *202*(6), 443–474. https://doi.org/10.1007/s004290000127.

Hardoon, D. R., Szedmak, S., & Shawe-Taylor, J. (2004). Canonical correlation analysis: An overview with application to learning methods. *Neural Computation*, *16*(12), 2639–2664. https://doi.org/10.1162/0899766042321814.

Hauk, O., Johnsrude, I., & Pulvermüller, F. (2004). Somatotopic representation of action words in human motor and premotor cortex. *Neuron*, *41*(2), 301–307. https://doi.org/10.1016/s0896-6273(03)00838-9.

Heilman, K., & Valenstein, E. (Eds.). (1993). *Clinical neuropsychology* (3rd ed.). Oxford: Oxford University Press.

Henderson, V. W. (1996). The investigation of lexical semantic representation in Alzheimer's disease. *Brain and Language*, *54*(2), 179–183.

Hinton, G. E., & Anderson, J. A. (1989). *Parallel models of associative memory (updated ed.)*. Lawrence Erlbaum Associates, Inc. Retrieved from http://search.ebscohost.com/login.aspx?direct=true&db=psyh&AN=1989-97439-000&loginpage=Login.asp&site=ehost-live&scope=site.

Holcomb, P. J. (1993). Semantic priming and stimulus degradation: Implications for the role of the N400 in language processing. *Psychophysiology*, *30*(1), 47–61.

Hubel, D. H., & Wiesel, T. N. (1979). Brain mechanisms of vision. *Scientific American*, *241*(3), 150–162.

Jared, D., & Seidenberg, M. S. (1991). Does word identification proceed from spelling to sound to meaning? *Journal of Experimental Psychology: General*, *120*(4), 358–394.

Johns, B. T., & Jones, M. N. (2012). Perceptual inference through global lexical similarity. *Topics in Cognitive Science*, *4*(1), 103–120. https://doi.org/10.1111/j.1756-8765.2011.01176.x.

Kosslyn, S. M. (1981). The medium and the message in mental imagery: A theory. *Psychological Review*, *88*(1), 46–66.

Lashley, K. S. (1938). Factors limiting reciovery after central nervous system lesions. *Journal of Mental and Nervous System Disorders*, *888*, 733–755.

Laszlo, S., & Armstrong, B. C. (2014). PSPs and ERPs: Applying the dynamics of post-synaptic potentials to individual units in simulation of temporally extended Event-Related potential reading data. *Brain and Language*, *132*, 22–27. https://doi.org/10.1016/j.bandl.2014.03.002.

Laszlo, S., & Federmeier, K. D. (2009). A beautiful day in the neighborhood: An event-related potential study of lexical relationships and prediction in context. *Journal of Memory and Language*, *61*(3), 326–338. https://doi.org/10.1016/j.jml.2009.06.004.

Laszlo, S., & Federmeier, K. D. (2011). The N400 as a snapshot of interactive processing: Evidence from regression analyses of orthographic neighbor and lexical associate effects. *Psychophysiology*, *48*(2), 176–186. https://doi.org/10.1111/j.1469-8986.2010.01058.x.

Laszlo, S., & Plaut, D. C. (2012). A neurally plausible parallel distributed processing model of event-related potential word reading data. *Brain and Language*, *120*(3), 271–281. https://doi.org/10.1016/j.bandl.2011.09.001.

Masson, M. E. J. (1995). A distributed model of semantic priming. *Journal of Experimental Psychology: Learning, Memory, and Cognition*, *21*, 3–23.

Masson, M. E. J., & Borowsky, R. (1998). More than meets the eye: Context effects in word identification. *Memory and Cognition*, *26*(6), 1245–1269.

Moss, H. E., Tyler, L. K., & Jennings, F. (1997). When leopards lose their spots: Knowledge of visual properties in category-specific deficits for living things. *Cognitive Neuropsychology*, *14*(6), 901–950.

Neisser, U. (1967). Cognitive psychology. Appleton-Century-Crofts. Retrieved from http://search.ebscohost.com/login.aspx?direct=true&db=psyh&AN=1967-35031-000&loginpage=Login.asp&site=ehost-live&scope=site.

Paivio, A. (1991). Images in mind: The evolution of a theory. Harvester Wheatsheaf. Retrieved from http://search.ebscohost.com/login.aspx?direct=true&db=psyh&AN=1991-98882-000&loginpage=Login.asp&site=ehost-live&scope=site.

Posner, M. I., & Snyder, R. R. (1975). Attention and cognitive control. In R. L. Solso (Ed.), *Information processing and cognition: The Loyola symposium* (pp. 55–85). Chichester: Wiley, John & Sons, Incorporated.
Posner, M., & Snyder, R. R. (1975). *Facilitation and inhibition in the processing of signals: Vol. V.* Cambridge, MA: Academic Press.
Rabovsky, M., & McRae, K. (2014). Simulating the N400 ERP component as semantic network error: Insights from a feature-based connectionist attractor model of word meaning. *Cognition, 132*(1), 68–89. https://doi.org/10.1016/j.cognition.2014.03.010.
Radvansky, G. A., Spieler, D. H., & Zacks, R. T. (1993). Mental model organization. *Journal of Experimental Psychology: Learning, Memory, and Cognition, 19*(1), 95–114.
Reicher, G. M. (1969). Perceptual recognition as a function of meaningfulness of stimulus material. *Journal of Experimental Psychology: General, 81*(2), 275–280.
Rock, I., & Gutman, D. (1981). The effect of inattention on form perception. *Journal of Experimental Psychology: Human Perception and Performance*, 7(2), 275–285.
Rugg, M. D. (1985). The effects of semantic priming and word repetition on event-related potentials. *Psychophysiology, 22*(6), 642–647.
Rummelhart, D. E., &. McClelland, J. E. (1986). *Parallel distributed processing: Explorations in the microstructure of cognition: Vol. 1. Foundations.* Cambridge, MA: MIT Press.
Seidenberg, M. S., & McClelland, J. L. (1989). A distributed, developmental model of word recognition and naming. *Psychological Review, 96*(4), 523–568. https://doi.org/10.1037/0033-295x.96.4.523.
Silberer, C., & Lapata, M. (2012). Grounded models of semantic representation. Retrieved from http://repositori.upf.edu/handle/10230/41868.
Smith, E. E., Shoben, E. J., & Rips, L. (1974). Structure and process in semantic memory: A featural model for semantic decisions. *Psychological Review, 81*(3), 214–241.
Tulving, E. (1984). Precis of Elements of episodic memory. *Behavioral and Brain Sciences*, 7(2), 223–268.
Tulving, E., & Thomson, D. M. (1973). Encoding specificity and retrieval processes in episodic memory. *Psychological Review, 80*(5), 359–380.
Umiltà, M. A., Kohler, E., Gallese, V., Fogassi, L., Fadiga, L., Keysers, C., & Rizzolatti, G. (2001). I know what you are doing. A neurophysiological study. *Neuron, 31*(1), 155–165. https://doi.org/10.1016/s0896-6273(01)00337-3.
Zurif, E. B., Caramazza, A., Myerson, R., & Galvin, J. (1974). Semantic feature representations for normal and aphasic language. *Brain and Language, 1*(2), 167–187.

11

LANGUAGE COMPREHENSION

A neurocognitive perspective

Catherine Longworth and William Marslen-Wilson

Introduction

Within milliseconds of perceiving speech or text, we recognize individual words from the tens of thousands we have learned, gain access to their linguistic properties, and integrate their meaning with that of the preceding words to compute an interpretation of the intended message. Language comprehension seems so rapid and effortless for most of us that the question hardly seems to arise of how this astonishing decoding operation is actually carried out. Nevertheless, common neurological conditions, such as strokes or forms of dementia, very often disrupt both general and specific aspects of the comprehension process, indicating the complexity of its cognitive and neural foundations. A complete understanding of language comprehension must therefore provide an account not only of the mental representations of language and the processes that operate upon them, but also of how these relate to the brain and to the breakdown of function following brain damage (i.e., a neurocognitive account). This chapter provides a historical overview of the ways in which the language comprehension system has been investigated and outlines the basis of our neurocognitive approach to language comprehension, illustrated by a clinical example.

Historical overview

The classic neurological account of language, the Wernicke–Lichtheim model, proposed that language depends upon a left lateralized network of discrete brain regions connected by white matter tracts. In this network the posterior left superior temporal gyrus (Wernicke's area) was thought to be critical for comprehension, whereas the anterior left inferior frontal gyrus (LIFG) (Broca's area) was critical for production and the arcuate fasciculus allowed information to flow between the two regions (see Figure 11.1). Thus, damage to Wernicke's area should result in comprehension failure, as opposed to damage to Broca's area, which should result in difficulties with language production. This model is often still used today to describe the aphasic syndromes associated with damage to these two regions (e.g., Broca's and Wernicke's aphasias). It relies on a methodology of lesion-deficit associations, by which observed language deficits were assumed to be related to brain lesions. At the time these lesions could only be identified at postmortem, but the methodology has been updated with the advent of structural brain scanning and today we can visualize brain lesions in vivo and pinpoint their location using voxel-based morphometry (VBM; Ashburner & Friston, 2000). It is risky, nonetheless, to assume a simple mapping between comprehension deficits and observable lesions, since deficits may reflect neural disruption that cannot be visualized in standard

DOI: 10.4324/9781003204213-13

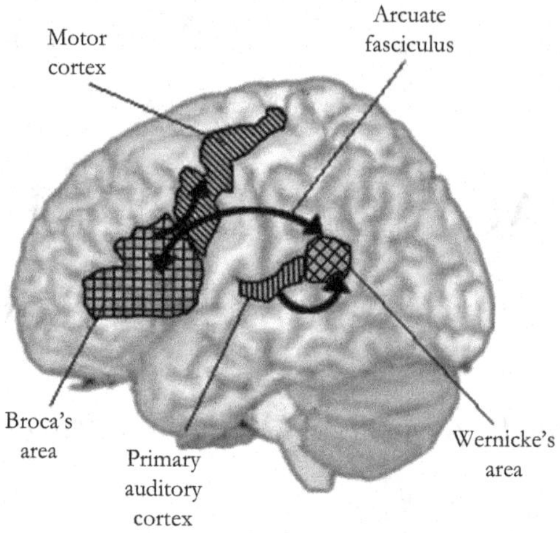

Figure 11.1 The classic Wernicke–Lichtheim model of language in the brain. (Adapted from Tyler, L. K. and Marslen-Wilson, W. D., Phil. Trans. R. Soc. B 363, 1493, 1037–1054, 2008 under CC BY 4.0 license.)

neuroimaging or in distant regions that rely on the damaged area. Lesion-deficit mapping must be combined with other methodologies to build up a full picture of how abilities such as language comprehension are instantiated in the brain. It is also necessary to specify those representations or processes that are associated with a particular lesion, rather than trying to localize comprehension as a whole.

The cognitive revolution of the 1960s onward addressed this omission by seeking to identify the mental processes and representations underlying human abilities, such as language comprehension, typically through the use of speeded experimental paradigms. Priming, for example, is an experimental paradigm in which responses to target words are facilitated by prior presentation of related words or primes. By manipulating the relationship between primes and targets it has been possible to investigate how words are represented in the mind (e.g., Marslen-Wilson, Tyler, Waksler, & Older, 1994) and the time course with which we access their meanings (e.g., Moss, McCormick, & Tyler, 1997; Tyler, Moss, Galpin, & Voice, 2002). The evidence gathered using methods such as these resulted in cognitive theories, such as the cohort theory of spoken word recognition, focusing on the critical early stages of relating sound to lexical form and meaning during language comprehension (Gaskell & Marslen-Wilson, 1997; Marslen-Wilson, 1987; Marslen-Wilson & Welsh, 1978).

In its classic formulation, the cohort theory suggests that spoken word recognition has three stages: lexical access, selection, and integration. The first two of these stages occur before a word can be identified, and the last stage occurs after word recognition, or postlexically. During the access stage, mental representations of all the lexical forms matching the speech input (the "cohort") are activated in parallel, together with their associated meanings. The extent to which these forms continue to match the incoming signal is mirrored in their level of activation. In the selection stage the form with the greatest level of activation (i.e., that which most closely matches the perceptual evidence) is identified as the best match to the speaker's intention and recognition occurs. Finally, during the integration stage the semantic and syntactic properties of the identified form are integrated with higher order representations of the message. The whole process occurs within a fraction of a second.

Cognitive science has helped to specify the representations and processes involved in language comprehension but does not tell us how these relate to their neural instantiation. For this reason many researchers have turned to cognitive neuroscience, which complements information about language pathology using lesion-deficit mapping, with information about the healthy language system using electrophysiological (EEG and MEG) methods (e.g., Hauk, Davis, Ford, Pulvermuller, & Marslen-Wilson, 2006) and functional neuroimaging (fMRI, PET) methods (e.g., Bozic, Marslen-Wilson, Stamatakis, Davis, & Tyler, 2007). For example, fMRI can be used to confirm that the brain-behavior associations implied by lesion-deficit mapping are present in the healthy brain. Two main methods of analysis are used. Subtractive analyses identify the brain regions in which activity increases during an experimental task, in contrast to a control condition. This identifies all the regions active for a given task, but does not establish those regions that are essential for this task or how the activity in different regions relates to each other. Connectivity analyses, on the other hand, allow us to identify how activity in a given region relates to activity elsewhere and thus can be used to develop maps of the neural systems underlying components of language comprehension. Electrophysiological techniques complement neuroimaging by providing a direct window onto the millisecond timecourse of language comprehension in the brain.

In addition to examining human abilities directly, cognitive neuroscience also makes use of primate research to investigate the nonhuman precursors for our major cognitive systems. In the case of language this has involved examining the extent to which knowledge of primate auditory processing informs our understanding of human speech processing. Research suggests that the differentiation of sensory processing into dorsal and ventral processing streams, previously established for primate visual processing (Ungerleider & Mishkin, 1982), also applies to primate auditory processing. Auditory information is initially processed in the auditory cortex and then travels either via a dorsal stream leaving the auditory cortex posteriorly and looping round to the inferior frontal cortex or via a ventral stream linking to the inferior frontal cortex anteriorly (Kaas & Hackett, 1999; Rauschecker & Tian, 2000). Research on macaques has proposed that the ventral route processes the identity of the sound (i.e., a "what" pathway) whereas the dorsal route processes the location of the sound (i.e., a "where" pathway; Kaas & Hackett, 1999; Rauschecker & Tian, 2000). This differentiation of the primate auditory system is echoed in suggestions that the language system in humans divides into multiple processing pathways (Hickok & Poeppel, 2004; Scott & Johnsrude, 2003; Figure 11.2). For example, in contrast to the simplified left hemisphere system proposed by the classic model of language, current neurocognitive models propose that language comprehension is instantiated in the brain through two neural pathways, each with distinct functions and with contributions made by both cerebral hemispheres.

A neurocognitive approach to language comprehension

Language conveys two types of information between sender and receiver: semantic information about meanings in the world and syntactic information about the grammatical properties of lexical forms (e.g., tense, number, aspect, etc.) and how they combine to form sentences. This information is associated with specific entries within a store of lexical representations known as the "mental lexicon." As we listen to speech or read text we match spoken or written inputs to lexical representations and access their meanings and grammatical properties.

Lexical representation and morphology

It is often assumed that the basic unit of language is the word. It is not clear, however, that this is the fundamental unit of representation in the mental lexicon, since linguistics recognizes an even smaller unit, the morpheme. This has been defined as "the smallest meaningful unit" of language (Bloomfield, 1933) or "the smallest unit of grammatical analysis" (Lyons, 1968). In English many morphemes occur as individual words, or monomorphemes, associated with specific semantic or syntactic information (e.g., the frog). However, there are also many morphologically complex words, formed by adding bound morphemes to word stems. Bound morphemes (e.g., pre-, -un,

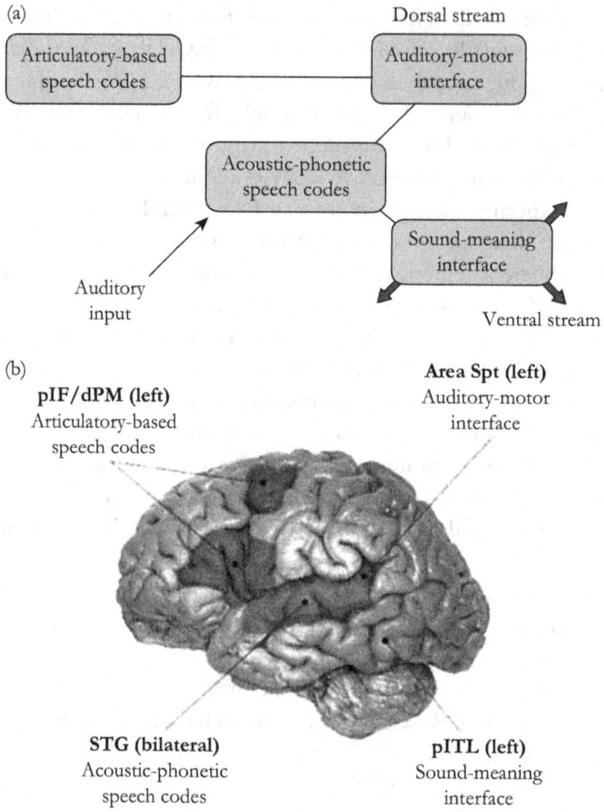

Figure 11.2 Hickok and Poeppel's model of language in the brain featuring dorsal and ventral processing streams. Panel (a) presents a schematic diagram of the two pathway model, with an auditory-motor dorsal stream and sound-meaning ventral stream. Panel (b) shows how these two streams map onto specific brain areas (pIF/dPM = posterior Inferior Frontal/dorsal Premotor cortex, STG = Superior Temporal Gyrus, Area Spt = Sylvian–parietal–temporal, an area of the Sylvian fissure at the boundary of the temporal and parietal lobes, pITL = posterior Inferior Temporal Lobe). (Reprinted from Hickok, G. and Poeppel, D., Cognition, 92, 67–99, 2004. With permission.)

-ing, -ness, -ed), or affixes, occur only in combination with stems. English has two means of generating these combinations: inflectional and derivational morphology. Inflectional affixes convey syntactic information that makes words appropriate for their role in a sentence, while maintaining their meaning and word class. Derivational affixes change the meaning or word class of a stem morpheme, generating new entries in the mental lexicon.

Inflectional morphology

A series of studies indicates that lexical access to words made up of stems and inflectional affixes differs from lexical access to words without an internal structure and relies on a different neurocognitive processing stream. In one such study (Marslen-Wilson & Tyler, 1997; Tyler et al., 2002a), we used auditory morphological priming to contrast lexical access to regular and irregular past tense forms. This allowed us to compare the processing of inflected forms with an internal structure divisible into component morphemes (e.g., jump-ed) and unstructured forms that must be processed as whole forms (e.g., taught). Both past tense conditions were compared to a semantic priming condition (e.g., swan/goose) and a phonological control condition (e.g., tinsel/tin).

A group of healthy volunteers showed a pattern of response facilitation to target words that were preceded by morphologically related prime words (e.g., jumped/jump, taught/teach) relative to unrelated control words (e.g., played/jump, bought/teach) for both regular and irregular verbs. They also showed response facilitation to targets preceded by semantically related words (semantic priming, e.g., swan/goose) but no facilitation of words related only by form (e.g., gravy/grave). Nonfluent (or Broca's) aphasics, in contrast, showed normal priming for irregular verbs and semantically related words, but no priming from the regular past tense (Figure 11.3). Neuroimaging indicated that their brain damage was confined to left perisylvian regions (e.g., LIFG and superior temporal gyrus). Two further patients showed a converse pattern, with priming from regular verbs and semantically related words, but no facilitation for irregular past tense forms (Marslen-Wilson & Tyler, 1997, 1998). One of these patients was a nonfluent aphasic with bilateral lesions, including damage to the right temporal lobe and the other suffered from semantic dementia, which is associated with temporal lobe atrophy. This double dissociation between regular and irregular past tense priming suggests the existence of two language processing routes through the brain: a dorsal route decomposing the words into stems and affixes and a ventral route recognizing unstructured words (and processing whole forms and stems).

A second study strengthens the evidence for a decompositional dorsal route (Longworth, Marslen-Wilson, Randall, & Tyler, 2005). This compared auditory semantic priming from regular and irregular verb stems and their past tense forms (e.g., blame/accuse, blamed/accuse, teach/learn, taught/learn). Nonfluent aphasic patients showed preserved semantic priming from verb stems and irregular forms, as did healthy volunteers, indicating an intact ability to map unstructured forms onto meaning. In contrast, however, they showed an absence of normal semantic priming following

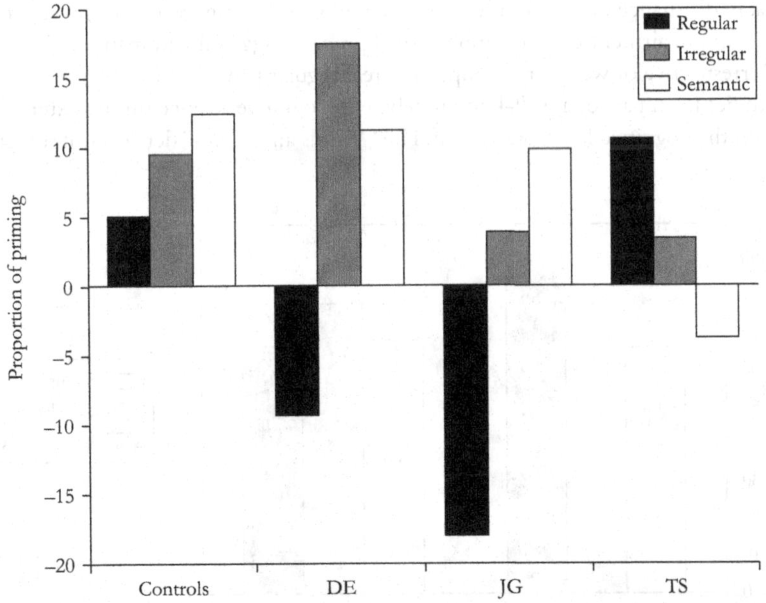

Figure 11.3 The double dissociation between regular and irregular past tense priming across patients. The labels DE and JG are the initials of two non-fluent left hemisphere patients; TS is a third patient with bilateral damage. The Controls are healthy individuals matched for age and education. (Reprinted from Marslen-Wilson, W. D. and Tyler, L. K., Trends in Cognitive Science, 2, 428–436, 1998. With permission.)

regular past tense forms (Figure 11.4). The mapping of form onto meaning appears to be disrupted by their impairment in processing words with a complex internal structure. This indicates that rather than being stored in the mental lexicon in their own right, in the same way as stems and irregular past tenses, regular past tense forms must be decomposed into their component parts in order to identify the stem and access its meaning and to process the syntactic implications of the past tense affix.

A third study indicates that the decomposition of inflected forms into stems and affixes is an early, obligatory stage of processing. This study used an auditory same–different task to contrast the processing of regular and irregular past tense forms and words and nonwords matched to their phonology. Nonfluent aphasics and a group of age-matched healthy volunteers were asked whether the second of two spoken stimuli, either two words or two nonwords spoken in a male and a female voice, was the same as the first (Tyler et al., 2002b). For healthy volunteers this is an easy task, yet the patients not only had difficulties with regularly inflected word pairs (e.g., played/play) but also, crucially, with any word or nonword pair that ended in the phonetic hallmark of the regular past tense (e.g., trade/tray, snade/snay), which we have termed the English inflectional rhyme pattern (IRP). The IRP, characteristic not only of the regular past tense but also of the English "s" inflection, consists of a final coronal consonant (d, t, s, z) that agrees in voicing with the preceding consonant. The experiment compared performance on regular verbs (played/play) with other stimuli with the IRP: pseudoregular pairs (trade/tray), where the first word has the IRP and could potentially be a past tense of the second word; and nonwords matched to real and pseudoregular pairs (snayed/snay). These conditions were contrasted with performance in "additional phoneme" conditions, in which the stimuli were matched to the consonant vowel structure of the other conditions, so that the final consonant was dropped in the second of each pair, but this consonant was not a potential English inflection (e.g., claim/clay, blane/blay). The patients performed worst on regular verb pairs, confirming their impairment in decomposing inflected forms into morphemes. However, they also performed very poorly on pseudoregular and nonword regular pairs, despite near normal performance on the additional phoneme pairs (see Figure 11.5). This suggests that the patients have an impairment of a decompositional process triggered automatically by the presence of the IRP, irrespective of whether the input is a real regular past tense or not.

These studies form part of a well-known debate in cognitive science on the extent of differentiation within the cognitive language system. The "Words and Rules" debate contrasts single route

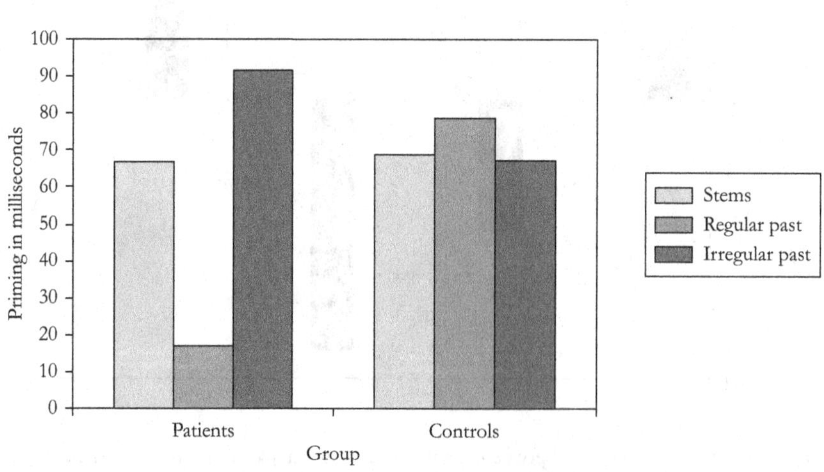

Figure 11.4 The failure of semantic priming from the regular past tense in patients with Broca's aphasia. (Adapted from Longworth, C. E., Marslen-Wilson, W. D., Randall, B., and Tyler, L. K. Journal of Cognitive Neuroscience, 17, 7, 1087–1097, 2005.)

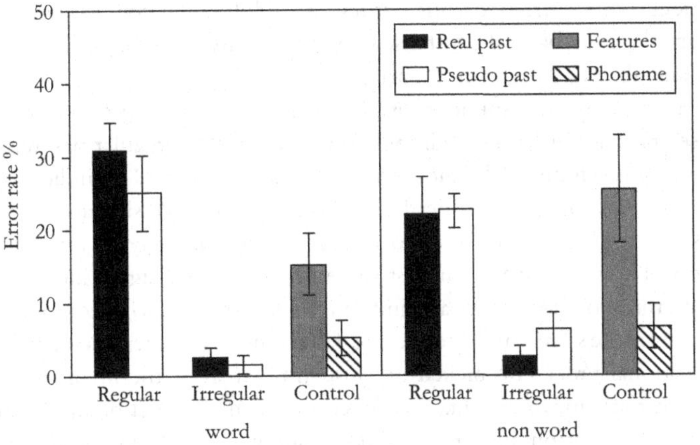

Figure 11.5 Patient error rates for words and nonwords in the same-different task. (Reprinted from Tyler, L. K. et al. Neuropsychologia, 40(8), 1154–1166, 2002. With permission.)

accounts, which argue that all words are accessed as whole forms in terms of learned associations between sensory inputs and representations of form and meaning (McClelland & Patterson, 2002; Rumelhart & McClelland, 1986) with dual route accounts, which claim that there is differentiation within the language processing system, with the form and meaning of some inputs computed from their component parts (Pinker & Prince, 1988; Pinker & Ullman, 2002). The studies summarized above provide evidence for differentiation within the language system in that regular inflectional morphology appears to engage a separate processing system than uninflected stems or irregular forms that are not analyzable into a stem and a regular inflectional affix.

In response to studies such as these, single route theorists argued that regular and irregular past tense deficits in language comprehension do not reflect impairments of decompositional and whole word access procedures, but difficulties with phonology or semantics, respectively (Joanisse & Seidenberg, 1999). Processing regular verbs was argued to depend on general phonological processing since the regular past tense differs from its verb stems by a single phoneme, which might be difficult to perceive. Processing irregular verbs was argued to depend on semantic processing due to the absence of a reliable phonological relationship between irregular past tense forms and their stems. It was argued that both phonological and semantic information are processed by an undifferentiated associative memory system. Such an account, however, makes the wrong predictions about patients with past tense deficits. As shown in the third study described, although nonfluent patients may have difficulties with words and nonwords matched to past tense phonology, their difficulties are greatest for regular past tense forms. In addition, dissociations have been reported between difficulties with the irregular past tense and semantic impairments (Miozzo, 2003; Tyler et al., 2004). Although these two types of deficit may co-occur, this is not necessarily the case, as demonstrated by patients with irregular past tense deficits but intact semantic processing (Miozzo, 2003).

However, perhaps the strongest evidence against the single route interpretation of past tense deficits comes from combining behavioral evidence with structural brain imaging. Tyler and colleagues (2005) correlated variations in behavioral performance with variations in MRI signal intensity to identify areas where abnormal performance is linked to neuroimaging evidence of damaged tissue. On MRI scans, differences in neural tissue integrity are reflected in characteristic variations in signal intensity, which can be visualized on a black–white scale. Relative to normative scan data, damaged areas of the brain often have lower signal intensity and appear darker on MRI scans. The Tyler et al. (2005) study correlated these variations in MRI signal intensity, across the whole brain, with variations in performance on the auditory morphological priming task for 22 neurological patients with a variety of different lesions and different cognitive deficits. The patients were not preselected on the basis of past tense deficits, but simply on the inclusion criteria of suitability for MRI and ability to perform the priming task.

Contrary to a single mechanism account, the results show double dissociations between the regular past tense and phonological conditions and between the irregular past tense and semantic conditions, in the regions found to be most critical for performance. This indicates that processing regular inflectional morphology is distinct from phonological processing and processing irregular past tense forms is distinct from semantic processing, because they rely on different brain regions.

The correlation between the regular past tense condition and signal intensity peaked in the LIFG at a standard threshold for statistical significance and extended to encompass the left superior temporal gyrus, Wernicke's area, and the arcuate fasciculus at a more lenient threshold. In other words, the correlational procedure picked out just those areas of the brain thought to be critical for core grammatical (morpho-syntactic) functions in the normal brain. Performance on the phonological control condition, in contrast, did not show a statistically significant correlation in this area, and the two correlations were significantly different from one another. Instead, the phonological condition correlated with signal intensity in a more medial brain area called the insula, with increased damage being associated with more disrupted performance. The insula is a region previously associated with phonological processing (Noesselt, Shah, & Jancke, 2003), and therefore likely to be involved in the phonological comparison processes on which performance here presumably depends. The regular past tense condition, however, did not correlate significantly with intensity in this region, consistent with the view that what drives performance here are factors to do with combinatorial linguistic analysis (elicited by the presence of an inflectional morpheme).

The correlation between the irregular past tense condition and signal intensity peaked at the left superior parietal lobule and extended to encompass surrounding areas at a more lenient threshold. These areas, which have been implicated in lexical access processes in other studies, are not only quite different from those seen in the regular past tense condition, but also quite different from those that correlate with performance in the semantic condition. This condition showed no significant correlation in the areas linked to irregular past tense performance, and instead correlated with signal intensity in the left medial fusiform gyrus (BA 37, hippocampus, and surrounding parahippocampal regions), extending to the left middle temporal gyrus (LMTG). These are areas found in other studies to play a role in linking phonological inputs to lexical semantic representations, and showed no correlation in this study with performance on the irregulars.

In subsequent investigations, we confirmed that the brain behavior relationships that had been implied by language pathology extended to the normal language system. To do this we used event-related fMRI to identify those brain regions that were active when healthy volunteers performed the same–different task described above (Tyler, Stamatakis, Post, Randall, & Marslen-Wilson, 2005). We also used connectivity analysis to investigate how activity in key regions correlated with activity elsewhere in the brain for the different conditions (Tyler & Marslen-Wilson, 2008). Healthy volunteers were asked to judge whether word pairs were the same or different while fMRI scans were conducted. The conditions allowed us to contrast the brain regions activated by regular verb pairs with those activated by pseudoregulars, irregular verbs, pseudoirregulars, pairs with an additional phoneme (e.g., claim/clay), and matching nonword conditions.

The results showed that the regular past tense condition, and all other conditions, containing the IRP (e.g., pseudo and non-word regulars) engaged significantly more activity in the LIFG and bilateral superior and middle temporal gyri, than either irregular past tense forms and stimuli matched to these (e.g., pseudo and nonword irregulars), or the additional phoneme conditions (e.g., real and nonword pairs with an additional phoneme). The increased temporal lobe activation may reflect processes operating on embedded lexical content (e.g., the jump in jumped and embedded tray in trade), since nonwords with or without the IRP, which by definition have no lexical content, did not differ in activation in these regions. In contrast, nonwords with the IRP (e.g., pairs like snayed/snay) activated the LIFG more strongly than nonwords without the IRP (e.g., blane/blay). Since neither condition has lexical content and they differ only in the presence of the IRP, the increased activation of the LIFG appears to reflect processes specific to the IRP. Finally, there was an interaction between regularity (regular versus irregular past tense) and word type (real versus pseudo) such that the real regular past tense condition, but not the pseudo or nonword regular past tense conditions, activated the left anterior cingulate more than real, pseudo, and nonword irregulars. This suggests that the left anterior cingulate is involved when, in addition to featuring embedded lexical content and the IRP, words can be genuinely segmented into stems and inflectional affixes.

A connectivity analysis (reported in Stamatakis, Marslen-Wilson, Tyler, & Fletcher, 2005) showed that activity in the LIFG and left anterior cingulate indeed covaried with activity in a third region, the left posterior middle temporal gyrus, to a greater extent for stimuli with the IRP, than they did for irregular past tense forms and words and nonwords matched to these. However, the covariance was stronger for real regular past tense forms than for pseudoregulars and nonwords matched to regular past tense forms (Stamatakis et al., 2005). Neuroimaging research suggests that the anterior cingulate may play a role in integrating information from different processing streams in frontal and temporal regions (Braver, Barch, Gray, Molfese, & Snyder, 2001; Fletcher, McKenna, Friston, Frith, & Dolan, 1999). It is possible that in the context of language comprehension, the anterior cingulate is differentially activated by real regular past tense forms due to the greater processing demands of integrating frontal systems supporting morpho-phonological segmentation with temporal processes involved in the access of the lexical content of their stems.

Derivational morphology

The meaning and syntactic properties of regularly inflected words can be computed from the combination of their stems and affixes, making them fully compositional, and uniformly analyzed, as argued above, by cooperating left hemisphere fronto-temporal systems (Marslen-Wilson & Tyler, 2007).

Research on derived words, on the other hand, shows a more complex pattern of findings (Marslen-Wilson, 2007). This reflects the fact that derivational morphology creates new lexical entries, with their own meanings and syntactic properties, which vary in compositionality. In addition, responses to derived words are influenced by many properties of stems and affixes, such as the frequency with which stems are encountered in the language; the number of words sharing a stem morpheme (morphological family size); affix homonymy, or whether or not the form of the affix is associated with one meaning or several; the degree of semantic transparency in the relationship between the stem and derivational variants; allomorphy, or the phonetic or orthographic similarity between stem and derived form; and productivity, the extent to which an affix is used to create new words in the language. Many of these variables influence behavioral responses to derived words simultaneously, necessitating the use of multivariate approaches (for review, see Ford, Davis, & Marslen-Wilson, in press).

Despite the differences between inflectional and derivational morphology, research suggests that derived words engage an early, obligatory segmentation process, triggered by the presence of potential derivational affixes, in a similar manner to regularly inflected words. This research uses a paradigm known as visual masked priming, which involves presenting a written prime word so briefly that the reader is only aware of the subsequent target word, allowing us to investigate the earliest stages of visual word processing. Using this paradigm it has been found that derived words prime their stems in many different languages (e.g., Boudelaa & Marslen-Wilson, 2005; Deutsch, Frost, & Forster, 1998; Dominguez, Segui, & Cuetos, 2002; Marslen-Wilson, Bozic, & Randall 2008). Moreover, pseudoderived pairs that feature a potential derivational affix (e.g., corner/corn), but which are not themselves morphologically related also show priming (Rastle, Davis, Marslen-

Wilson, & Tyler, 2000; Rastle, Davis, & New, 2005). Even non-words composed of nonoccurring combinations of real stems and derivational affixes (e.g., tallness) have been found to prime their pseudostems (e.g., tall) as well as existing legal combinations (e.g., taller), suggesting that the priming reflects a prelexical segmentation process, blind to lexical status (Longtin, Segui, & Halle, 2003; Longtin & Meunier, 2005). An area of the left fusiform gyrus known as the visual word form area may be involved in this prelexical segmentation. An event-related fMRI study comparing masked priming effects in behavioral and neural responses to morphologically transparent (teacher/teach), semantically opaque (department/depart), and pseudoderived word pairs (slipper/slip) found that the visual word form area showed stronger priming for opaque and pseudoderived pairs than morphologically transparent pairs (Devlin, Jamison, Matthews, & Gonnerman, 2004).

In contrast to masked priming, however, overt priming—when the prime is presented for a long enough period for participants to become aware of its presence—is influenced by lexical properties and compositionality, and suggests that some derived words are stored as morphemes in a similar manner to regularly inflected words. For example, using cross-modal priming it has been found that spoken derived words facilitate responses to their visually presented stems when the relationship between the two is semantically transparent (darkness/dark) but not when it is opaque (department/depart) (Marslen-Wilson et al., 1994). This finding was interpreted as indicating that the same underlying lexical representation of the stem (e.g., dark) is accessed by both prime (darkness) and target (dark) (Marslen-Wilson et al., 1994). Similarly, semantically transparent words sharing a derivational suffix (e.g., darkness/toughness) facilitate responses to each other in cross-modal priming, suggesting that the same lexical representation of the suffix (e.g., -ness) is accessed by both prime and target (Marslen-Wilson, Ford, Older, & Zhou, 1996). Moreover, related derived words with different suffixes (e.g., darkness/darkly) produce a phenomenon called suffix–suffix interference, argued to reflect interference between suffixes competing to link with the same representation of the stem (Marslen-Wilson et al., 1994). As with regular inflectional morphology, the LIFG appears to be involved in segmenting derived words to identify potential compositional representations in the mental lexicon. An event-related fMRI study using delayed priming found that both semantically transparent (bravely/brave) and opaque (archer/arch) pairs showed priming in the LIFG, whereas words with the same degree of semantic or orthographic relatedness showed no priming (Bozic et al., 2007).

Sentence-level syntactic and semantic information

So far, we have considered how the language system in the brain is modulated by the nature of individual lexical representations. We have argued that accessing the lexical content of morphologically unstructured words (e.g., monomorphemic, irregularly inflected, or semantically opaque derived words) engages a ventral processing stream in the temporal lobes. Forms that are potentially compositional—in particular stimuli bearing the phonetic signature of the regular past tense form (the IRP)—engage a dorsal system that attempts to segment them into component morphemes, so that the syntactic properties of inflectional suffixes can be analyzed and the semantic content of stems or derivational affixes can be accessed by the ventral system. In addition, written stimuli with potential derivational affixes engage an obligatory prelexical process of segmentation that may involve a region of the brain known as the visual word form area.

We now turn briefly to the issue of how the language system is modulated by combinatorial processes operating at the level of the sentence (for a more detailed review see Tyler & Marslen-Wilson, 2008). In one recent study, this was investigated using an fMRI study contrasting responses to syntactic and semantic ambiguities (Rodd, Longe, Randall, & Tyler, 2004; Tyler & Marslen-Wilson, 2008). Healthy volunteers were presented with spoken sentences containing either a semantic or a syntactic ambiguity that was subsequently resolved (e.g., "She quickly learned that injured calves ... moo loudly" or "Out in the open, flying kites ... are liable to get tangled"). To make the task as naturalistic as possible volunteers listened passively to each sentence and were only then required to judge whether a visually presented word was related in meaning to the sentence. The degree of ambiguity was quantified by collecting ratings of the extent to which one reading of each ambiguous phrase was preferred over the other. Processing syntactic ambiguities engaged the LIFG, the LMTG extending forward into the anterior portion and backward into the inferior parietal lobule and the right superior temporal gyrus. Activity in these regions increased with increasing dominance, such that they were most strongly activated when the preferred reading was overturned by the continuation. This suggests that listeners developed a strong preference for a particular interpretation, which might then have to be overturned by subsequent information. Processing semantic ambiguities also engaged the LIFG and the LMTG. However, the LMTG activation was significantly less than that elicited by syntactic ambiguities and confined to the middle portion of the gyrus. The activation elicited by semantic ambiguities showed no effect of dominance, suggesting that both meanings of the ambiguous word were initially activated in parallel and only disambiguated later. A connectivity analysis showed further differences between the two conditions. Activation of the LIFG predicted activity in the left temporal pole, but in the case of the syntactic ambiguity condition the LIFG predicted temporal pole activation in the right hemisphere as well. In the syntactic ambiguity condition, the LIFG also predicted activation in posterior regions, such as the posterior LMTG, inferior parietal gyrus, angular gyrus, and supramarginal gyrus of the left hemisphere. The posterior LMTG region identified was adjacent to that previously identified as covarying with activity in the LIFG and the left anterior cingulate for regular past tenses (Stamatakis et al., 2005). Thus, it is possible that different types of combinatorial processes engage adjacent portions of the posterior LMTG.

A clinical example

A clinical example exemplifies the consequences of damage to dorsal language processing pathways in the left hemisphere. Patient DE is a right-handed man who suffered a middle cerebral artery infarct following a road traffic accident at age 16, damaging the posterior inferior frontal gyrus and superior and middle temporal gyri of his left cerebral hemisphere. His language abilities have been investigated in depth in psycholinguistic research (Patterson & Marcel, 1977; Tyler, 1985, 1992; Tyler et al., 2002a, 2002b; Tyler, Moss, & Jennings, 1995; Tyler & Ostrin, 1994) and he participated in many of the studies that informed the neurocognitive model of language comprehension outlined in this chapter (Tyler et al., 2002a, 2002b, 2005). His acquired brain injury resulted in dysfluent speech and a number of selective deficits in combinatorial linguistic processing. For example, he has deep dyslexia, which is typified by morphological errors in reading aloud. Recent research confirms that these errors reflect the morphological status of words (Rastle, Tyler, & Marslen-Wilson, 2006) rather than other confounding linguistic features, such as word imageability or frequency as previously suggested (Funnell, 1987). DE also has impaired speech comprehension for morphologically complex words, as shown in his lack of morphological and semantic priming from regularly inflected words (Longworth et al., 2005; Tyler et al., 2002a) and high error rate in the regular past tense condition of the same-different task (Tyler et al., 2002b). At the sentence level, DE also shows agrammatic speech comprehension, again indicating impairment in the ability to combine linguistic units (Tyler et al., 2002a).

Connectivity analyses of fMRI data from DE reveal the unilateral nature of combinatorial linguistic processes. To examine his pattern of connectivity in the morphological domain, DE participated in the fMRI version of the same-different task (Tyler & Marslen-Wilson, 2008). For healthy age-matched volunteers, activity in the left inferior frontal cortex and anterior cingulate cortex predicted activity in the left posterior middle temporal gyrus. In contrast, DE showed a more right hemisphere pattern of connectivity, with increased activity in the inferior and middle temporal gyrus of the right hemisphere and bilateral anterior temporal lobes. His comprehension deficits for regularly inflected words suggest that this reorganization of function to the right hemisphere is insufficient to support combinatorial processes operating at the level of the word. He also participated in the fMRI study of semantic and syntactic ambiguity, allowing us to examine his pattern of connectivity in the syntactic domain. Syntactic ambiguities activated his left middle frontal gyrus and pre- and postcentral gyri and right inferior parietal lobule. A connectivity analysis showed that the peak of this left hemisphere activity predicted activation of posterior regions of the right hemisphere, in contrast to the left hemisphere posterior regions found in connectivity analyses of healthy volunteers. Again, despite this reorganization of function to the right hemisphere, his syntactic processing remains impaired, suggesting that a left hemisphere language processing stream is critical, not only for combinatorial processes at the level of lexical representation, but also at the level of the sentence. This contrasts with semantic processing, which remains seemingly intact in DE (Longworth et al., 2005) suggesting that comprehension of word meaning relied on primarily ventral pathways that function bihemispherically.

Questions and answers

Why do we need a neurocognitive model of language comprehension?

Cognitive and neurological approaches to understanding language comprehension gain from the theoretical constraints provided by each other. Well-specified cognitive models of the mental representations and processes involved in language comprehension are necessary precursors to understanding how comprehension is instantiated in the brain. Equally, however, knowledge of the neural bases for language comprehension can be useful in distinguishing between competing cognitive models. Both domains of knowledge are required to understand how language comprehension occurs normally and breaks down after brain damage.

How does the current model differ from the classic Wernicke–Lichtheim model of language in the brain?

The classic model proposed a single, dorsal language processing pathway in the left hemisphere. In contrast, the current neurocognitive model posits at least two processing pathways: a unilateral dorsal pathway in the left hemisphere, required for combinatorial processes at the level of lexical representation and at the sentence level; and a bilateral ventral pathway required for processing unstructured lexical representations and semantic information.

How does the current model fit into broader theoretical debates?

The current model forms part of the "Words and Rules" debate in cognitive science, which asks whether language processing and by extension human cognition in general, shows evidence of differentiation or can be handled by an undifferentiated associative memory system. The neurocognitive model posits the existence of two distinct pathways for language comprehension, along the lines of dual route models of other primate systems.

What outstanding questions remain?

The neurocognitive model has implications for speech pathology. It suggests that combinatorial linguistic processes will be more vulnerable to brain damage than the processing of unstructured lexical representations and semantic information. Further research is required to assess the practical implications of this model for the assessment and rehabilitation of acquired language comprehension deficits.

Further reading

Fonteneau, E., Bozic, M., & Marslen-Wilson, W. D. (2015). Brain network connectivity during language comprehension: Interacting linguistic and perceptual subsystems. *Cerebral Cortex*, *25*(10), 3962–3976.

Marslen-Wilson, W. D., Bozic, M., & Tyler, L. K. (2014). Morphological systems in their neurobiological contexts. In M. S. Gazzaniga & G. R. Mangun (Eds.), *The cognitive neurosciences* (5th ed.). Cambridge, MA: MIT Press.

Nili, H., Wingfield, C., Walther, A., Su, L., Marslen-Wilson, W., & Kriegeskorte, N. (2014). A toolbox for representational similarity analysis. *PLOS Computational Biology, 10*(4), e1003553.

Shafto, M. A., Tyler, L. K., Dixon, M., Taylor, J. R., Rowe, J. B., Cusack, R., ... Cam, C. A. N. (2014). The Cambridge centre for ageing and neuroscience (Cam-CAN) study protocol: A cross-sectional, lifespan, multidisciplinary examination of healthy cognitive ageing. *BMC Neurology, 14*, 204.

Su, L., Zulfiqar, I., Jamshed, F., Fonteneau, E., & Marslen-Wilson, W. (2014). Mapping tonotopic organization in human temporal cortex: Representational similarity analysis in EMEG source space. *Frontiers in Neuroscience, 8*, 368.

References

Ashburner, J., & Friston, K. J. (2000). Voxel-based morphometry: The methods. *Neuroimage, 11*(6/1), 805–821.

Bloomfield, L. (1933). *Language*. New York: Holt.

Boudelaa, S., & Marslen-Wilson, W. D. (2005). Discontinuous morphology in time: Incremental masked priming in Arabic. *Language and Cognitive Processes, 20*(1–2), 207–260.

Bozic, M., Marslen-Wilson, W. D., Stamatakis, E., Davis, M. H., & Tyler, L. K. (2007). Differentiating morphology, form, and meaning: Neural correlates of morphological complexity. *Journal of Cognitive Neuroscience, 19*(9), 1464–1475.

Braver, T. S., Barch, D. M., Gray, J. R., Molfese, D. L., & Snyder, A. (2001). Anterior cingulate cortex and response conflict: Effects of frequency, inhibition and errors. *Cerebral Cortex, 11*(9), 825–836.

Deutsch, A., Frost, R., & Forster, K. I. (1998). Verbs and nouns are organized and accessed differently in the mental lexicon: Evidence from Hebrew. *Journal of Experimental Psychology: Learning, Memory, and Cognition, 24*(5), 1238–1255.

Devlin, J. T., Jamison, H. L., Matthews, P. M., & Gonnerman, L. (2004). Morphology and the internal structure of words. *Proceedings of the National Academy of Sciences, 101*(41), 14984–14988.

Dominguez, A., Segui, J., & Cuetos, F. (2002). The time-course of inflexional morphological priming. *Linguistics, 40*(2), 235–259.

Fletcher, P., McKenna, P. J., Friston, K. J., Frith, C. D., & Dolan, R. J. (1999). Abnormal cingulate modulation of fronto-temporal connectivity in schizophrenia. *Neuroimage, 9*(3), 337–342.

Ford, M. A., Davis, M. H., & Marslen-Wilson, W. D. (2010). Affix productivity promotes decomposition of derived words: Evidence from effects of base morpheme frequency. *Journal of Memory and Language, 63*(1), 117–130.

Funnell, E. (1987). Morphological errors in acquired dyslexia: A case of mistaken identity. *Quarterly Journal of Experimental Psychology, 39A*(3), 497–539.

Gaskell, M. G., & Marslen-Wilson, W. D. (1997). Integrating form and meaning: A distributed model of speech perception. *Language and Cognitive Processes, 12*(5–6), 613–656.

Hauk, O., Davis, M. H., Ford, M., Pulvermuller, F., & Marslen-Wilson, W. D. (2006). The time course of visual word-recognition as revealed by linear regression analysis of ERP data. *Neuroimage, 30*(4), 1383–1400.

Hickok, G., & Poeppel, D. (2004). Dorsal and ventral streams: A framework for understanding aspects of the functional anatomy of language. *Cognition, 92*(1–2), 67–99.

Joanisse, M. F., & Seidenberg, M. S. (1999). Impairments in verb morphology after brain injury: A connectionist model. *Proceedings of the National Academy of Sciences of the United States of America, 96*(13), 7592–7597.

Kaas, J. H., & Hackett, T. A. (1999). "What" and "where" processing in auditory cortex. *Nature Neuroscience, 2*(12), 1045–1047.

Longtin, C.-M., & Meunier, F. (2005). Morphological decomposition in early visual word processing. *Journal of Memory and Language, 53*(1), 26–41.

Longtin, C.-M., Segui, J., & Halle, P. A. (2003). Morphological priming without morphological relationship. *Language and Cognitive Processes, 18*(3), 313–334.

Longworth, C. E., Marslen-Wilson, W. D., Randall, B., & Tyler, L. K. (2005). Getting to the meaning of the regular past tense: Evidence from neuropsychology. *Journal of Cognitive Neuroscience, 17*(7), 1087–1097.

Lyons, J. (1968). *Introduction to theoretical linguistics*. Cambridge: Cambridge University Press.

Marslen-Wilson, W. D. (1987). Functional parallelism in spoken word-recognition. *Cognition, 25*(1–2), 71–102.

Marslen-Wilson, W. D. (2007). Morphological processes in language comprehension. In G. Gaskell (Ed.), *Oxford handbook of psycholinguistics* (pp. 175–193). Oxford: OUP.

Marslen-Wilson, W. D., Bozic, M., & Randall, B. (2008). Early decomposition in visual word recognition: Dissociating morphology, form, and meaning. *Language and Cognitive Processes, 23*(3), 394–421.

Marslen-Wilson, W. D., Ford, M., Older, L., & Zhou, X. (1996). The combinatorial lexicon: Priming derivational affixes. In G. Cottrell (Ed.). *Proceedings of the 18th annual conference of the cognitive science society* (pp. 223–227). Mahwah, NJ: LEA.

Marslen-Wilson, W. D., & Tyler, L. K. (1997). Dissociating types of mental computation. *Nature, 387*(6633), 592–594.

Marslen-Wilson, W. D., & Tyler, L. K. (1998). Rules, representations and the English past tense. *Trends in Cognitive Science, 2*(11), 428–436.

Marslen-Wilson, W. D., & Tyler, L. K. (2007). Morphology, language and the brain: The decompositional substrate for language comprehension. *Philosophical Transactions of the Royal Society of London Series B, 362*(1481), 823–836.

Marslen-Wilson, W. D., Tyler, L. K., Waksler, R., & Older, L. (1994). Morphology and meaning in the English mental lexicon. *Psychological Review, 101*(1), 3–33.

Marslen-Wilson, W. D., & Welsh, A. (1978). Processing interactions during word recognition in continuous speech. *Cognition, 10*, 29–63.

McClelland, J., & Patterson, K. (2002). Rules or connections in past-tense inflections: What does the evidence rule out? *Trends in Cognitive Sciences, 6*(11), 465–472.

Miozzo, M. (2003). On the processing of regular and irregular forms of verbs and nouns: Evidence from neuropsychology. *Cognition, 87*(2), 101–127.

Moss, H. E., McCormick, S., & Tyler, L. K. (1997). The time course of activation of semantic information during spoken word recognition. *Language and Cognitive Processes, 12*(5/6), 695–731.

Noesselt, T., Shah, N., & Jancke, L. (2003). Top-down and bottom-up modulation of language related areas—An fMRI study. *BMC Neuroscience, 4*, 13.

Patterson, K., & Marcel, A. (1977). Aphasia, dyslexia and the phonological coding of written words. *Quarterly Journal of Experimental Psychology, 29*(2), 307–318.

Pinker, S., & Prince, A. (1988). On language and connectionism: Analysis of a parallel distributed-processing model of language-acquisition. *Cognition, 28*(1–2), 73–193.

Pinker, S., & Ullman, M. (2002). The past and future of the past tense. *Trends in Cognitive Sciences, 6*(11), 456–463.

Post, B., Marslen-Wilson, W. D., Randall, B., & Tyler, L. K. (2008). The processing of English regular inflections: Phonological cues to morphological structure. *Cognition, 109*(1), 1–17.

Rastle, K., Davis, M. H., Marslen-Wilson, W. D., & Tyler, L. K. (2000). Morphological and semantic effects in visual word recognition: A time-course study. *Language and Cognitive Processes, 15*(4–5), 507–537.

Rastle, K., Davis, M. H., & New, B. (2005). The broth in my brother's brothel: Morphoorthographic segmentation in visual word recognition. *Psychonomic Bulletin, 11*(6), 1090–1098.

Rastle, K., Tyler, L. K., & Marslen-Wilson, W. D. (2006). New evidence for morphological errors in deep dyslexia. *Brain and Language, 97*(2), 189–199.

Rauschecker, J. P., & Tian, B. (2000). Mechanisms and streams for processing of 'what' and 'where' in auditory cortex. *Proceedings of the National Academy of Sciences, 97*(22), 11800–11806.

Rodd, J. M., Longe, O. A., Randall, B., & Tyler, L. K. (2004). Syntactic and semantic processing of spoken sentences: An fMRI study of ambiguity. *Journal of Cognitive Neuroscience, 16*(Suppl. C), 89.

Rumelhart, D. E., & McClelland, J. L. (1986). On learning the past tenses of English verbs. In D. E. Rumelhart, J. L. McClelland, & P. R. Group (Eds.), *Parallel distributed processing: Explorations in the microstructure of cognition: Foundations* (Vol. 2). Cambridge, MA: MIT Press.

Scott, S. K., & Johnsrude, I. S. (2003). The neuroanatomical and functional organization of speech perception. *Trends in Neuroscience, 26*(2), 100–107.

Stamatakis, E. A., Marslen-Wilson, W. D., Tyler, L. K., & Fletcher, P. C. (2005). Cingulate control of fronto-temporal integration reflects linguistic demands: A three-way interaction in functional connectivity. *NeuroImage, 28*(1), 115–121.

Tyler, L. K. (1985). Real-time comprehension processes in agrammatism: A case-study. *Brain and Language, 26*(2), 259–275.

Tyler, L. K. (1992). *Spoken language comprehension: An experimental approach to disordered and normal processing.* Cambridge, MA: MIT Press.

Tyler, L. K., de Mornay-Davies, P., Anokhina, R., Longworth, C. E., Randall, B., & Marslen-Wilson, W. D. (2002a). Dissociations in processing past tense morphology: Neuropathology and behavioral studies. *Journal of Cognitive Neuroscience, 14*(1), 79–94.

Tyler, L. K., & Marslen-Wilson, W. D. (2008). Frontotemporal brain systems supporting spoken language comprehension. *Philosophical Transactions of the Royal Society of London Series B, 363*(1493), 1037–1054.

Tyler, L. K., Marslen-Wilson, W. D., & Stamatakis, E. A. (2005). Dissociating neuro-cognitive component processes: Voxel-based correlational methodology. *Neuropsychologia, 43*(5), 771–778.

Tyler, L. K., Moss, H. E., Galpin, A., & Voice, J. K. (2002). Activating meaning in time: The role of imageability and form-class. *Language and Cognitive Processes, 17*(5), 471–502.

Tyler, L. K., Moss, H. E., & Jennings, F. (1995). Abstract word deficits in aphasia: Evidence from semantic priming. *Neuropsychology*, *9*(3), 354–363.
Tyler, L. K., & Ostrin, R. K. (1994). The processing of simple and complex words in an agrammatic patient: Evidence from priming. *Neuropsychologia*, *32*(8), 1001–1013.
Tyler, L. K., Randall, B., & Marslen-Wilson, W. D. (2002b). Phonology and neuropsychology of the English past tense. *Neuropsychologia*, *40*(8), 1154–1166.
Tyler, L. K., Stamatakis, E. A., Jones, R., Bright, P., Acres, K., & Marslen-Wilson, W. D. (2004). Deficits for semantics and the irregular past tense: A causal relationship? *Journal of Cognitive Neuroscience*, *16*(7), 1159–1172.
Tyler, L. K., Stamatakis, E. A., Post, B., Randall, B., & Marslen-Wilson, W. D. (2005). Temporal and frontal systems in speech comprehension: An fMRI study of past tense processing. *Neuropsychologia*, *43*(13), 1963–1974.
Ungerleider, L. G., & Mishkin, M. (1982). Two visual pathways. In D. J. Ingle, M. A. Goodale, & R. J. W. Mansfield (Eds.), *Analysis of visual behavior* (pp. 549–586). Cambridge, MA: MIT Press.

12

FAMILIAR LANGUAGE

Formulaic expressions, lexical bundles, and collocations in mind and brain

Diana Sidtis

Background and purpose

Familiar language—referring to formulaic expressions, lexical bundles, and collocations—has come into its own. These utterances have been named "nonpropositional," precisely because they are not generated anew by the application of grammatical rules on the lexicon. Attempts to treat familiar expressions using generative linguistic approaches resembled, in the opinion of many today, forcing a square peg into a round hole. Fixed, familiar expressions constitute a very vibrant sector of language competence, worthy of examination on their own terms. Observations of familiar language in diverse discourse contexts have greatly increased our perspective in the past decade, and theories have begun to mature (Pawley, 2007; Conklin & Schmitt, 2012; Coulmas, 1994). Much of this growth is attributable to the burgeoning interest in pragmatics—language use in everyday settings, and to the embracing of spoken discourse as staunchly undertaken by sociolinguists. A further impetus to delve into the world of fixed expressions arises from second language interests, where the phenomenon brings unique challenges to learner and teacher alike (Edmonds, 2014; Ellis, 2008).

This chapter reviews progress in our understanding of fixed, familiar expressions, beginning with a background discussion and continuing with an overview of representative studies of normal use and incidence. A new schema for classifying these individualized, variegated, and often controversial expressions is offered. Many types of familiar expressions flourish in spontaneous language use. It is therefore useful to focus on spoken texts, corpus studies, and discourse analyses. It is also important to supplement these observations by formal studies that quantify findings derived from measures of spoken language.

The overview in this chapter then proceeds from normal to disordered speech. A "dual process" model that accommodates both familiar (other terms: overlearned, fixed, routinized, holistic, configurational, unitary) and novel (newly created, grammatical) language has been proposed (Heine, Kuteva, & Kaltenböck, 2014; Erman & Warren, 2000). From a neurolinguistic perspective, accountable brain structures may differ for these two modes of language competence (Van Lancker Sidtis, 2004). Given more recent in-depth descriptions of lexical bundles (Biber, Conrad, & Cortes, 2004; Biber & Barbieri, 2007) and collocations (Vilkaitė, 2016), which have distinctive linguistic, psychological, and distributional characteristics that differ from those for conversational speech formulas, expletives, idioms, and proverbs (which form the class of formulaic expressions), a more modern proposal looks to a multi-process model of language competence in mind and brain.

 DOI: 10.4324/9781003204213-14

Definitions and theory

A first satisfying definition of familiar expressions is an exclusionary one, with the descriptor "non-novel" as the selection criterion; that is, these expressions have in common that they are *not* newly created from the operation of grammatical rules on lexical items. They all have this in common: the expressions are *cohesive*, and they are *familiar* to a language community. They are holistically acquired and produced, and they are stored as memory traces and recognized in unitary form (Rammell, Pisoni, & Van Lancker Sidtis, 2018). Fixed expressions have a major place in a language community; talkers manifest shared knowledge of the canonical forms, the conventionalized meanings, and the appropriate linguistic and social contexts as conditions of use. The characteristics, cohesion, and stereotyped form entail that familiar expressions, in their canonical form, contain precisely specified words in a certain word order, usually spoken on a set intonation contour (Hallin & Van Lancker Sidtis, 2017). Secondly, meanings are conventionalized, which means the semantic aspects are idiosyncratic in various ways; many familiar expressions carry nonliteral meanings, some serve mainly as social signals, and all can be said to communicate a meaning that is greater than the sum of their parts (Wray, 2002). And third, as fixed expressions live in the realm of pragmatics, conditions of use, or context, constitute the third defining characteristic. The appropriate contexts of use are stored in the language user with the expressions.

This treatment of familiar language proposes three distinct classes, based on linguistic and psychological characteristics: formulaic expressions, lexical bundles, and collocations. Fuzzy edges in categorizing these phenomena are to be expected, and many exemplars may belong to more than one class, depending on use. Much attention has been paid to formulaic expressions: the major subsets of this class are idioms, proverbs, conversational speech formulas, and expletives (Wray, 2002). These are mostly nonliteral in meaning and they are high in nuance—affective and attitudinal connotations. Analysis of repetition behaviors in conversation revealed a significantly higher rate of repetition for formulaic than novel expressions (Wolf, Van Lancker Sidtis, & Sidtis, 2014).

More recently, speech scientists have described the second class, lexical bundles (Biber & Barbieri, 2007; Biber, Conrad, & Cortes, 2003; Chen, & Baker, 2010); these are sequences of two or more words that co-occur frequently in corpora. They function to express stance and qualify the speaker's intention (Kaltenböck, Mihatsch, & Schneider, 2010), enhance verbal fluency, and organize the discourse (Biber, Conrad, & Cortes, 2004; Vilkaitė, 2016; Heng, Kashiha, & Tan, 2014). Like all the others, they are unitary in structure, and they are recognized in holistic form (Jeong & Jiang, 2019), but they differ from formulaic expressions in being mostly literal in meaning and in conveying little or no nuance.

A third class has arisen as prominent among holistic expressions: collocations (Mackin, 1978). Collocations can be identified by the "tendency of two or more words to co-occur in discourse" (González Fernández, & Schmitt, 2015, p. 95) but care should be taken to distinguish collocations from lexical bundles, which are also identified using these same procedures. Members of the collocation class differ in being mostly literal in meaning process (e.g., *salt and pepper, absolutely ridiculous*) and having variable nuance, depending on the meanings of the constituent words. These three classes have in common that they are cohesive in structure, nonnovel and not newly created, and familiar to a language community.

The three classes are presented in Table 12.1. From the examples, it can be seen that the exemplars are distinguished by linguistic and psychological characteristics: the degree of nuance (affective and attitudinal load), whether their meanings are primarily nonliteral or literal, and their relationship to social and verbal context. It is proposed that the role of text frequency in acquisition varies for three classes of utterances.

The examples in Table 12.1 reveal that formulaic expressions have the most nuance—attitudinal and affective connotations—of the three classes. Idioms, such as *she has him eating out of her hand*, transmit a more or less punchy affective load. The same is true for proverbs, conversational speech

Table 12.1 Three classes of fixed, familiar expressions, with examples

A cold day in hell	All that sort of stuff	A cautionary tale
A cut above the rest	All things being equal	A hop, skip, and a jump
Birds of a feather	But wait, there's more	Better late than never
Bite my head off	By the way	Better safe than sorry
Cat got your tongue?	Correct me if I'm wrong	Breathe a sigh of relief
Cheek to jowl	Did it occur to you	Cast of characters
Down in the dumps	Due to the fact that	He has a lot of gall
Down the tubes	First and foremost	He'll never learn
Fast on the draw	For some reason	He's learned his lesson
Fat chance	From the perspective of	He's troubled with the gout

formulas, and expletives, all classic members of the formulaic expression class. It is also apparent that these expressions typically carry nonliteral meanings. Analyses of the incidence of formulaic expressions in written and spoken discourse suggest that many occur relatively infrequently (Moon, 1998), so that mechanisms other than frequent exposure must be operative in achieving some subsets of this repertory. It will be proposed below that familiarity with fixed expressions can occur, under certain circumstances, rapidly and from only one or a few exposures.

As can be seen in the examples in the second box ofTable 12.1, lexical bundles rank very low on the nuance (attitudinal and affective connotation) parameter. It follows that they are less subject to the attentional and arousal mechanisms that are proposed to be active in recognizing and acquiring exemplars in the other two classes, formulaic expressions and collocations. As such, their acquisition is tied to frequent exposure in talk and text.

The third class, collocations, is also made up of phrases that are cohesive, unitary, and known to a language community, but these differ from the others in that they do not usually cavort in nonliteral meanings, and they typically convey more propositional meaning than the other two classes. Collocations are based on constructions, the building blocks of language (Michaelis, 2017). Facts about discourse frequency for collocations in comparison with other classes of familiar language are coming to light (Vilkaitė, 2016; Durrant, 2014), but the role of frequency in their acquisition is not well established.

Members of the classes differ in their relations to social and linguistic context. Social and verbal context plays a major role, as has been described for discourse in dementia (Müller & Guendouzi, 2002). Formulaic expressions are especially sensitive to context, while lexical bundles and collocations permit more contextual flexibility. Greetings and leave taking, classic exemplars of the formulaic expression class, are tightly tied to context. People in a language community know not to say *see you later* on first entering a room; they do not give a *good morning* greeting twice in a row, when passing in the hall, to the same person. Members of the other two classes, although less afflicted by contextual constraints, may also find that social and linguistic contingencies impinge on appropriate use. Some such "rules" are very subtle, falling on a continuum of formality, so that using a light-hearted, casual expression in a serious situation can land as inappropriate. A lexical bundle such as *I need you to focus* probably should not be said to one's boss or professor. The collocation *here today, gone tomorrow* might ring a sour note if uttered at a funeral. Considering the important role of social context, one perspective says that the acquisition of fixed familiar expressions allows for socialization in the first and second language (Burdelski & Cook, 2012).

Flexibility of form

A property of fixed expressions that has wreaked havoc in linguistic circles is, paradoxically, their flexibility: many variants can and do appear. The canonical form can be, and usually is, altered in actual usage. Alterations referencing the canonical form are acceptable as long as the underlying form remains recognizable (Kuiper, 2009); this is Kuiper's Law (Sidtis, 2021). To alter fixed expressions is to engage in theme and variation (Kecskés, 2017), one of the oldest and most pervasive practices in art and culture. The creative potential of fixed, familiar expressions (Pagán Cánovas & Antović, 2016; Kecskés, 2017) as well as the colorful practice (Kuiper, 2007; Sidtis, 2021) have been given detailed treatment.

Syntactic, lexical, phonetic, phonological, and semantic operations can be performed on any fixed expression (Sidtis, 2021; Kuiper, 2007), providing that the canonical form remains recognizable. Alternations, then, will not affect the features of fixed expressions: familiarity, stereotyped form, cohesion, conventional meanings, and specific conditions of use. Knowledge of these features is revealed in surveys, sentence completion studies, and association studies (Van Lancker Sidtis & Rallon, 2004; Clark, 1970); such knowledge appears to continue over two generations of speakers (Van Lancker Sidtis, Cameron, Bridges, & Sidtis, 2015).

Fixed expressions, depending on the intent and verbal creativity of the speaker and context, can be altered using a range of standard grammatical and lexical choices. This is particularly true of formulaic expressions and collocations; lexical bundles appear to be relatively intransigent to such manipulation. Because of flexibility and context dependency, in formal studies of fixed expressions, it is likely that task demands in psycholinguistic approaches exert an overriding influence on the results. When subjects are involved in metalinguistic decisions about the interplay between fixed and novel expressions, their performance will be highly influenced by contingencies of the experimental setting. The idiom studies do not lead to the conclusion that fixed expressions and novel language are processed in the same way, but rather show that grammar can operate on any legitimate utterance, and that standard lexical meanings can be discerned in any phrase. Again, the interesting point is not that fixed, familiar expressions can be semantically transparent and composed and are therefore alterable, but that there is a *known entity to analyze and to alter.*

An analysis of article titles and advertisements from newspapers and magazines reveals frequent use of fixed expressions, often with minor changes to reference or advocate the purpose and content of the ad or article. A comprehensive study of these allusions to fixed expressions over two years of publications revealed no instances of the application of generative rules on an expression. Instead, alterations consisted of replacing a word or words (e.g., *The Politburo loves a parade*, from *I love a parade*; *Boston Sea Party* from *Boston Tea Party*); adding text to recast the fixed expression to fit the purpose (*People lie through their teeth, but their teeth can't lie* in an article about forensic dentistry); or redirection of the conventional meaning of the fixed expressions (*Why don't you go away*, in an ad for a travel agency). For further examples of alterations of fixed expressions in the media for special purposes, see Sidtis (2021, Appendix X). Cartoons also manipulate and deform fixed expressions in various ways. For a full display of fixed expression "deformations" as documented from a cartoon series, see Kuiper (2007).

Regarding flexibility: the stereotyped, cohesive form, its conventional meaning, and its conditions of usage are known to the language community. Grammatical, lexical, morphological, phonetic, and phonological alterations (and all do occur)—are "permitted" in the communicative context, provided that enough of the underlying canonical form remains identifiable and the context allows for the intended interpretation. The key feature of fixed, familiar expressions is their personal familiarity: people know them. Their status as common knowledge in a linguistic community forms the major portion of their *raison d'être*. People easily endorse knowledge of fixed expressions, but it is not only a matter of native speakers' intuitions, which stand as valid linguistic evidence (Devitt, 2006); stored knowledge of fixed expressions has been demonstrated in formal studies.

People are free to apply linguistic alterations on familiar expressions for any purpose: communication, verbal playfulness, performing a new twist on a conventionalized meaning, allusion to a previous instance of a formula, conflation of two formulas, even pure fun, and so on. The speaker's meaning under these situations will be determined by linguistic and social context, as has been found in earlier studies (Gibbs, 1981). From anecdotal observation, it appears that "acceptability" parameters for formulaic expressions, lexical bundles, and collocations work from particularly soft constraints, meaning that acceptability judgments are highly subject to local linguistic and contextual effects (Sorace & Keller, 2005).

Familiarity

Familiarity, as a psychological state, evokes a change in consciousness (Titchener, 1916, p. 407). It is a unique sentiment, a "warm glow," eliciting sensations of well-being, security, and belonging (Monin, 2003). The experience of familiarity is by and large a positive one (Garcia-Marques, Mackie, Claypool, & Garcia-Marques, 2004) and it is often accompanied by smiling (Stephens, 1988; Baudouin, Gilibert, Sansone, & Tiberghien, 2000; Moreland & Zajonc, 1982; Claypool, Hall, & Mackie, 2008; Carr, Brady, & Winkielman, 2017). Familiar stimuli are preferred "presumably because familiarity signals safety" (De Vries, Holland, Chenier, Starr, & Winkielman, 2010, p. 321). According to Bartlett (1967), the familiarity sensation is

> an attitude, or orientation, which we cannot ascribe to any localized physiological apparatus, but which has to be treated as belonging to 'the whole' subject, or organism, reacting
>
> *(p. 191).*

As stated by Jackendoff (1995), a very large number of a broad range of formulaic expressions "are familiar to American speakers of English; that is, an American speaker must have them stored in memory" (p. 135). Fixed, familiar expressions are "familiar" in the sense that a native speaker will recognize them as having this special status. For example, the sentence *He knew already a few days ago about the anniversary of the first actual moon landing* has probably not been said or heard before; this sentence has none of the properties of familiarity, cohesion, and predictability mentioned above (Pinker, 1995). On the other hand, the expressions *David spilled the beans* or *It's a wrap* or *The early bird catches the worm* (formulaic expressions) are all "familiar," in that native speakers recognize these utterances—they say that they do, and they demonstrate knowledge of their specialized meanings and appropriate contexts. A great number of lexical bundles, such as *At this point in time*, and *Any way, shape, or form* are similarly known to speakers in a language community. The third class, collocations, also take their place in the stored repertory of language users: *First come, first served*; *he doesn't meet my needs*; *hermetically sealed* (see Sidtis, 2021). Studies have begun to examine knowledge of lexical bundles (Vilkaitė, 2016) and collocations, especially in the field of second language learning (Durrant, 2014; González Fernández, & Schmitt, 2015; Edmonds, 2014).

Saying that fixed expressions are familiar is another way of affirming that they are known, stored as traces in the brain (Rammell, Pisoni, & Van Lancker Sidtis, 2018). This knowledge is demonstrated in myriad ways. Some notable signs are ubiquitous allusions to fixed expressions in the public media (see comments on newspaper and magazine usage below). Humorous treatments of fixed expressions are common, using playful alterations of form and meaning (Kuiper, 2007; Sidtis, 2021). Other sources are counts of transcribed conversations, other corpora of all kinds, field and survey studies, and studies of word association. As an operational test, native speakers of a language accurately fill in blanks in such utterances, when key words are omitted in a range of fixed expressions (Van Lancker Sidtis, & Rallon, 2004) and in schemata (i.e., *down with …*) (Van Lancker Sidtis, Kougentakis, Cameron, Falconer, & Sidtis, 2012). Approximately a third of word association results are attributable to the "idiom effect," which means that given a target word, subjects produce the word from a known fixed expression (Clark, 1970).

How are familiar expressions acquired?

Revealing to the contrasts between familiar and novel language competence are findings from developmental language studies, including first and second language acquisition. Researchers in child language document acquisition of holistic "chunks" of speech (Ambridge & Lieven, 2015; Bannard & Lieven, 2012; Grimm, Cassani, Gillis, & Daelemans, 2019) which evolve into compositional structures (Peters, 1977, 1983; Lieven, Salomo, & Tomasello, 2009; Tomasello, 2003; Locke, 1993, 1997; MacWhinney, 2004). Selected formulaic expressions are taught by parents (Gleason & Weintraub, 1976). While unitary utterances are utilized by children early on, acquisition of the larger set of the three classes of familiar language at adult levels lags behind acquisition of grammatical competence (Kempler, Van Lancker, Marchman, & Bates, 1999; Prinz, 1983). This suggests that the two processes, holistic and analytic, perform different roles at different stages of language acquisition, and, further, that different maturational schedules are in play for novel versus holistic language knowledge.

Similarly, in adult second language acquisition, the difficulty posed by all three classes of familiar expressions is well known. It is likely that critical periods for native-like acquisition exist for various types of language competences, including for acquisition of formulaic expressions. Using a broad set of comprehensive measures, the use and comprehension of familiar expression in English and Russian was measured, targeting Russian bilingual speakers who arrived in the USA at two different ages, the early and the later arriving groups (Vaynshteyn & Van Lancker Sidtis, 2019). The early group arrived at about age 12, and later group at 30 years old or older. The result was clear: the early arriving group did not perform better than the later group on tasks probing competence with fixed expressions, suggesting that the maturational age for acquiring native-like knowledge of fixed expression occurs at some time before puberty.

Grammatical and holistically processed language may be acquired according to two or more disparate modes. It is possible that the three classes, formulaic expressions, lexical bundles, and collocations engage brain structures in different ways and in different times in cerebral maturation. Clinical studies of over a century establish with certainty that grammatical language is processed in the left hemisphere. Clinical and experimental studies point to the right hemisphere and a strong involvement of the basal ganglia for acquisition and production of some kinds of fixed expressions. These processes may be based in different brain maturational schedules (Thatcher, Walker, & Giudice, 1987), accounting for the discrepancy in early consolidation of grammatical knowledge contrasting with later acquisition of familiar language.

The question of acquisition of familiar language in the native speaker generally assumes that a major force in acquisition of formulaic expressions is frequency of exposure, such that many repetitions (one prominent speech scientist has proposed a minimum requirement of 50 exposures) eventually make a lasting impression in the developing child's or adult's memory. A companion assumption is that, because our brains are finite, novel language is learned primarily by abstract rules. The emphasis on the finiteness of our brains arises from the postulate that memory capacity is severely limited, when considering the very large set of phrases and sentences we command, and that therefore an entirely generative process must be in play. More recent viewpoints indicate that both of these assumptions—frequency of exposure and limited memory capacity—are questionable and fail to provide a basis for either a viable model or for empirical observations in familiar language competence (Kecskés, 2014).

The "slow exposure" assumption is most likely limited as an explanation, because, as mentioned above, the number of known expressions is very high. Native speakers acquire precise forms and complex semantic and pragmatic meanings of these expressions; unlike newly created sentences, they are all learned "by heart." If memory is poor for exact verbal replicas, then very many exposures of each expression are required. It is not a logical possibility that a sufficient number of repetitions of each of 100,000 (or, as some researchers say, 500,000) exact forms and contexts are provided for each language user, adequate to satisfy the requirements of the incremental learning process, leading to the huge repertory of pristinely stored canonical forms.

The role of frequency seems to vary for formulaic expressions, lexical bundles, and collocations. The "colorful" and high nuance characteristics of formulaic expressions assist in the uploading process, as arousal mechanisms are more obviously in play for these expressions. For example, idioms appear infrequently or not at all in analyzed corpora. In contrast, lexical bundles, the low-nuance class, manifest high counts in discourse samples, such that frequent exposure likely contributes to their being acquired in language users (Hassanzadeh & Tamleh, 2022). As mentioned previously, frequency counts of collocations are limited and scarce and do not yet permit the role of frequency in speakers' knowledge.

It follows from this point, then, that the "highly limited memory" assumption is also misguided. As the first bit of evidence, people know tens of thousands of multiword expressions. Of interest here are recent findings by Gurevich, Johnson, and Goldberg (2010) showing a successful verbatim memory for language, as well as a study by Reuterskiöld and Van Lancker Sidtis (2013), revealing that one-time exposure to an unfamiliar idiom, during a casual crafts session, sufficed for children to retain the idiom, a holistic form, better than a matched novel expression (exposed in a similar manner). Children ages 9 to 13 recognized the target idioms better than the novel expressions, also presented in the session, and target, one-time exposed idioms were better comprehended than non-exposed idioms.

In these studies, participants reliably recognized and recalled full sentences and idioms that they were exposed to only once. This view is amply represented by the episodic theory of speech perception (Goldinger, 1996; Nygaard, Sommers, & Pisoni, 1994; Pisoni, 1993; Geiselman & Crawley, 1976) revealing that listeners retain "surface" material from speech, such as unique pronunciation and voice quality (Lachs, McMichael, & Pisoni, 2012). It is likely that this fundamental ability to capture verbal material exactly is greatly heightened by the properties of formulaic expressions, and possibly of collocations, and that this ability follows a unique maturational schedule.

It appears from many observations that a specialized form of knowledge acquisition may be operative for familiar, fixed language, especially formulaic expression (idioms, swearwords, proverbs, conversational speech formulas) and collocations (e.g., *fast and furious*; *red, white, and blue*; *land of fire and ice*). For example, something comparable to one-trial learning, a special case in classic learning theory, should be considered. In this type of learning, rather than acquiring a piece of information through repeated exposure or trials, organisms "learn" (acquire a conditioned response) immediately or very quickly as the result of a "strong contingency"[1] reinforcement (Lattal, 1995). Another kind of instantaneous "learning" that is well studied is imprinting. Brain biochemistry and localization for imprinting have been extensively investigated in birds (Horn, 1985; Knudson, 1987). It is known that forebrain hemispheres with strong connections to striatal (subcortical) and brainstem structures are operative in imprinting, and these structures are also involved in visceral and endocrine functions as well as emotional expression (Horn, 1985, p. 243). Genetic determinants control the basic neuronal circuitry in some species studied, but flexibility allows for experience to shape the perceptual system (Knudsen, 1987).

There are critical time windows, but these sensitive periods are often labile and flexible (Marler, 1987). Also, worth mentioning as a rapid memory process are "flash bulb memories," in which an unusual amount of experiential detail is retained in memory in association with receiving surprising information (Brown & Kulik, 1977). Features of the processes include arousal, surprise, and personal relevance in addition to affect, attention, distinctiveness, and poststimulus elaboration (Christianson, 1992). It has been suggested that this function is part of an automatically preattentive mechanism (Neisser, 1976). Arousal levels may arise from hormonal influences (Gold, 1992), leading to a "Now Print" command in the nervous system, which results in immediate and detailed acquiring of a stimulus.

One plausible perspective is that the acquisition of familiar, fixed expressions occurs according to a unique learning process comparable to the three relatively instantaneous types described above. It is a fair assumption that throughout the early lifespan, formulaic expressions are acquired in a manner quite different from processes involved in learning the rules and lexicon that underlie the generation of novel expressions. In view of the difficulties encountered by adult second language learners, it is likely that the rapid acquisition ability diminishes with age. This fact is commonly observed in second language teaching and studies and was formally demonstrated by examining English familiar language competence in native speakers of Russian (Vaynshteyn & Van Lancker Sidtis, 2019).

These three examples of extraordinary learning and memory functions are offered to provoke new ways of looking at acquisition of formulaic expressions. These examples of near-instantaneous acquisition of information all demonstrate the coordinated roles of procedural, episodic, and declarative memory, as well as arousal and attention, rendering a special status to some kinds of knowledge acquisition. An alerting mechanism may be engaged by the fact that many kinds of fixed expressions pattern differently in the conversational setting, are tightly bound to social context, or utilize unconventional semantic processes. In summary, it is here proposed that many kinds of fixed expressions, under specialized circumstances not yet understood, ascend quickly and suddenly into a native speaker's language competence.

Functions of formulaic language in everyday discourse

The pervasive nature of these types of expressions in our daily repertoire of communication has been examined in studies documenting the function and frequency of familiar language in conversations and in literary texts and films (Van Lancker Sidtis, 2004; Van Lancker Sidtis & Rallon, 2004). High nuance appears in formulaic expressions, and, to a lesser and more variable extent, collocations. Certain function-based divisions of formulaic expressions reflect these features; for example, thanking, apologies, requests, and offers (Aijmer, 1996; Wray & Perkins, 2000; Tannen & Öztek, 1981). Others, falling under the heading of social interactions, include conversational maintenance and purpose (e.g., *How've you been? No kidding!*) These appear in negotiating complaints (Drew & Holt, 1988) and signaling partnership solidarity (Bell & Healey, 1992; Bruess & Pearson, 1993). Lexical bundles, much lower in nuance, also serve special purposes in communication (Oktavianti & Prayogi, 2022), including structuring talk (Fox Tree, 2006; Jucker, 1993), maintaining fluency in various contexts such as sport, weather forecasting, horse races, and auctions (Kuiper, 1991, 1992, 1996, 2004, Kuiper & Haggo, 1985), and generally sounding like a native speaker of the language (Fillmore, 1979; Pawley & Syder, 1983). Collocations carry more information in the discourse than the other two classes, as they typically utilize the literal or propositional meanings of their constituent lexical items.

Because fixed expressions are not newly formed, they free up resources in the speaker to look ahead to the next part of the encoding process. Production of ready-made phrases allows for a more consistent rate of speech and greater fluency (Fillmore, 1979; Guz, 2014; McGuire, 2017; Uchihara, Eguchi, Clenton, Kyle, & Saito, 2022) also giving the advantage of "buying time" during speech production for novel verbal material to be accessed and generated (Tremblay, Derwing, Libben, & Westbury, 2011). Their properties of stereotyped form and cohesion, conventionalized, often idiosyncratic meanings, and restricted pragmatic conditions are easily apprehended. Native speakers recognize them as familiar and know implicitly how they function in discourse.

Quantity of fixed expressions in everyday discourse

The actual number of these expressions is debated. Persons accumulating lists have not seen an upper limit. While experts toiling in the fields of fixed expressions differ somewhat in how widely to throw the net to catch the candidates, all agree that the number making up a typical speaker's repertory exceeds many tens of thousands, and some say the totals are upwards of hundreds of thousands (Kuiper, personal communication). All kinds of fixed expressions occur in daily speech a great deal of the time, but a compiled sum remains difficult to come by at the present time, in part because analytic efforts examining incidence of exemplars have been fragmented and piecemeal.

Naturalistic speech is a notoriously difficult beast and establishing word counts of any kind is challenging (Brysbaert, Stevens, Mandera, & Keuleers, 2016). Difficult questions arise regarding the kinds of expressions and how many of them, in what social and linguistic contexts do they appear, by whom are they spoken and how frequently do they appear, and with which themes and discourse styles are they associated. This requires qualitative and quantitative examination of natural speech. Some local, limited field studies of incidence have appeared. Jay (1980) tabulated use of cursing in specific populations (e.g., college students) and Gallahorn (1971) kept records of expletives emitted during team meetings of health care professionals on a psychiatric ward.

A singular contribution utilizing the fieldwork method came from Hain (1951), who recorded over 350 proverbs in actual use among people who lived in a small German village, Ulfa, between the years of 1938 and 1943. Hain, a folklorist using sociolinguistic, field study methods, was interested in documenting veridical, spontaneous production of proverbs, and in simultaneously recording the linguistic and social contexts of these specialized utterances. In this way, she could concern herself with quantity—how many different proverbial utterances appeared in the years that she lived in the village performing field work, and quality—how was each utterance used to communicate in the unique context. She examined the time of appearance of a proverb in the conversational setting (early, late, toward the end) and how the utterance was dealt with by the speaker and the listener (Hain, 1951). She set about to record the function of proverbs in everyday life as well as their position in a discussion. Here are some speech situations from the Ulfa village life recorded by Hain (1951). In the second example, the same proverb appeared in two settings:

1. The baptism of an infant with about 30 guests … Two older farmer women talk about the local young teacher, his performance in school and his meager salary. Especially Mrs. X. has a lot of information, she knows him and his modest means. X.: *Er ess hoard gscheit!* (er ist sehr klug) (Engl: he is very smart). At first K. listens pensively, then she responds slowly: *Aich saan als, wer de Hoawwern vedint hot, kritt en näid* (I always say, those who deserve the \ oats don't get them). Mrs. X. energetically agrees: *Joa, so ess!* (That's for sure!). And so, this topic has ended; the individual case has become part of the general.
2. The old dirt farmer Ch., in his late 70s, always has a joke at hand tells an acquaintance from the city about his daughter in law's long illness. How long they tried to heal her and how much money they spent! It would not have been necessary if she would have gone for x-rays in Giessen right away. B.: "One only knows in hindsight." As he is getting ready to leave Ch. replies loudly, so that you can even hear it across the street: *Joa, wann's Kend gehowe ess, gitts Gevadderleut* (ja, wenn das Kind aus der Taufe gehoben ist, gibt's Gevatterleute) (Engl: yes, when the child is baptized there will be godparents)!

   I heard the same proverb in other situations. A dirt-farmer of about 50 years told me about her misfortune with her cows. When another one was infected with brucellosis the year before, she bought insurance for all animals. She ended her story calmly, almost wearily: *Wann's Kend gehouwe ess, gitt's Gevadderleut!* (translated above). In both situations the proverb offered a way out into a consoling generic situation.

This labor-intensive study provides a rare record of ordinary usage of one particular category of formulaic expressions, proverbs. From the examples provided throughout her field work record, it is clear that each time a proverb is used, the speaker has an expectation that its stereotyped form and conventionalized meaning will be recognized by the listener(s) as part of their linguistic knowledge. Never was the meaning glossed or explained. Three main facts about personal familiarity that must not be lost or ignored in any treatment: people know fixed expressions in a language; speakers using them expect listeners to know them and to appreciate the meaning conveyed; and, indeed, mutual familiarity with the specialized expressions forms an essential part of the reason for using them: establishing solidarity and common foundations of understanding.

In the past few decades, discourse samples, or corpora, have been examined, using spoken samples and written texts (Biber & Conrad, 1999). With the benefit of computerized searching, various texts have been analyzed using different algorithms to count incidence of fixed expressions, including lexical bundles and collocations (Biber, Conrad, & Reppen, 1994; Durrant, 2014). Many others have not separated fixed expressions into categories, or the classification system has been unique to each study. Using a mathematical standard only, Altenberg (1998) listed three-word combinations that occurred ten times or more in the London-Lund Corpus (Greenbaum & Svartvik, 1990). Other studies have utilized a human interface to classify utterance types. Some analyses have focused on a particular type of formula, such as proverbs. Cowie (1992) performed a study on "multiword lexical units" in newspaper language, differentiating idioms from collocations of various kinds. In an extensive treatment, Moon (1998) performed a descriptive study of formulaic expressions and idioms in an 18-million-word corpus of contemporary English, the Oxford Hector Pilot Corpus (Glassman et al., 1992), augmenting her analysis from other text sources. Norrick (1985) reports only one complete proverb, plus a few proverbial allusions, in the 43,165-line corpus transcribed conversation published by Svartvik and Quirk (1980). A comparative frequency count of proverbs in French and English conversational corpora is described by Arnaud and Moon (1993).

Some quantitative and qualitative data on fixed expressions come from studies of literary texts, especially in oral literature (Kiparsky, 1976; Kuiper, 2000). Tilley counted proverbs in the plays of Shakespeare (Tilley, 1950; see Mieder, 1993). Schweizer (1978) listed 194 idioms in 2,876 pages of six novels of Günter Grass, yielding an average of 14.8 idioms per page. For the qualitative contribution, she describes numerous literary devices throughout Grass's writings that involve idiomatic forms and meanings. The plays of Ionesco utilize an abundance of speech formulas to artistic effect as discussed by Klaver (1989). Familiar phrases play a major role in the works of Homer (Lord, 1960). In his study of Homer's *Iliad*, Page (1959) estimates that about one-fifth of the poem is "*composed of lines wholly repeated from one place to another*" (p. 223), and that within the *Iliad*'s 28,000 lines, there are approximately 25,000 repeated phrases. In the screen play "Some Like it Hot" idioms, proverbs, and conversational speech formulas constituted 25% of the total number of phrases in the text (Van Lancker & Rallon, 2004).

Psycholinguistic studies

Comprehension studies of one subset of formulaic expressions, idioms, offer some understanding of what makes these expressions special and the questions that have been asked. Using idioms, speakers convey ideas and emotions using words that do not refer to their usual lexical meanings. *She's skating in thin ice* can be said without directly referring to skating, but to convey the idea of risky behavior. How the listener apprehends idiomatic meaning remains entirely mysterious. Three models proposed to explain this process are literal-first (serial) processing, literal and idiomatic (parallel) processing, and direct access of idiomatic meaning (depending on the context). These models differ in their use of the notion of compositionality, as some are based on the assumption that idioms not "composed," but are processed as cohesive unitary items (Titone & Libben,

2014). The foundation for this idea comes from studies showing that people remember idioms as chunks rather than composite forms (Osgood & Hoosain, 1974; Pickens & Pollio, 1979; Horowitz & Manelis, 1973; Simon, 1974; Jacobs, Dell, Benjamin, & Bannard, 2016), a result also shown for Chinese idioms (Simon, Zhang, Zang, & Peng, 1989).

The two models of noncompositionality are The Idiom List Hypothesis and The Lexical Representation Model. The Idiom List Hypothesis (Bobrow & Bell, 1973) proposes that idioms are lexical items stored in memory and that upon encountering an idiom, the comprehension device first attempts a literal interpretation. After failing, the idiom retrieval mode kicks in and the idiom is selected from the look-up list. Thus, serial processing predicts greater response time latencies for idioms than for literal utterances because literal interpretation is the first step in any language task. A number of later studies refuted these findings by showing that visual classification of idioms is faster than literal phrases, forming the basis for the Lexical Representation model. Originally formulated by Swinney and Cutler (1979), the Lexical Representation model suggests that idiomatic meaning is processed in parallel with literal meaning, and that idioms are stored and retrieved whole, accounting for the faster reaction times.

The question remains as to how idioms can undergo syntactic and semantic modifications and maintain their pragmatic identity. Different studies have addressed these two separate underlying issues: are idioms stored and accessed as whole units, and/or are their individual words and syntactic form taken into account during the retrieval process? Experimental approaches to these questions involve measuring production errors, response time, accuracy in recall and recognition memory tasks, and various kinds of rating surveys. Fixed expressions that can undergo syntactic modifications yet maintain their conventional meaning are said to have syntactic flexibility (or productivity). For example, one could say *For years, she had been skating on really thin ice,* and listeners, depending on context, could assume the nonliteral meaning.

The notion "degree of compositionality," established using native speakers' ratings, has been proposed to determine the flexibility of an idiom's comprehension (Gibbs et al, 1989; Gibbs & Gonzales, 1985). This finding is interesting although the reliability of the approach has been questioned (Titone & Connine, 1999; Cacciari & Tabossi, 1988). An idiom's "degree of compositionality" is likely not an all or none property, but instead viewed as a falling along a continuum, highly influenced by context. In addition, ratings in these surveys depend greatly on task instructions. Further, linguistic and situational contexts facilitate several aspects of nonliteral language comprehension, including how rapidly formulaic expressions (e.g., indirect requests and idioms) are processed, how they are interpreted (literally or figuratively), and how accurately and quickly they are retrieved from memory (Gibbs, 1980; Gibbs, 1981). Context plays a major role in judgments or perceptions of lexical transparency and syntactic flexibility.

The various findings of syntactic and lexical flexibility have led to hybrid psycholinguistic models. The earliest example is the Configurational Model (Cacciari & Tabossi, 1988), which integrates literal-first and idiomatic-only approaches. This states that initially the idiom's potential literal meaning is activated until a key word is encountered which unlocks the idiom's figurative meaning. The idiom meaning is encoded within a specific word configuration that has weighted connections between its lexical nodes. Idioms are considered to have either high or low predictability, depending on how early the key occurs in the string.

Several creative approaches to the production mode have been designed. From studies using speech-error elicitation experiments (Cutting & Bock, 1997), the authors conclude that idioms are not frozen or devoid of information about their syntactic and semantic structure. Interference in the form of blending errors was more likely to occur between idioms sharing the same syntactic form, and resultant word substitutions were in the same grammatical class. This is a highly sensible finding, as any object can be deconstructed into compositional parts; this is especially true of linguistic objects. Another experiment showed that idiom production can result in activation of corresponding literal meaning. The authors put forth the argument that what is special about idioms is their relationship to a conceptual representation, which is a nonlinguistic entity, and that in normal language production, idioms are not special. Another study using a priming technique, in which a probe word is used to influence later online processing of a test word, also concluded that words in idioms stimulate word association networks as readily as words in literal sentences (Smolka, Rabanus, & Rösler, 2007).ab

A series of idiom production experiments by Sprenger and colleagues (Sprenger, 2003; Kuiper, van Egmond, Kempen, & Sprenger, 2007) using a priming paradigm with response time measurement addressed this question, yielded the notion of superlemma, which corresponds to the idea proposed in this article of canonical form underlying fixed expressions. Similarly, analysis of speech errors involving idioms suggest that "idioms are both compositional and noncompositional at the same time, at different levels of processing" (Kuiper, van Egmond, Kempen, & Sprenger, 2007, p. 324). This superlemma or canonical form is stored and processed as a whole, but because it contains syntactic and semantic information of various kinds (as does any linguistic entity in the speaker's repertory), it can link to other parts of the lexicon and grammar, and it can be manipulated in any number of ways.

Auditory contrasts of idiomatic and literal meanings

Another set of studies highlights speakers' knowledge of differences between literal and idiomatic utterances. Using American English ditropic sentences, those having both idiomatic and literal meanings, such as *He was at the end of his rope*, it was seen that listeners can distinguish between these kinds of meanings from the acoustic signal alone. Listening studies confirmed the discriminability of these utterance types, and acoustic measures of rate, pitch mean and variability, and terminal pitch revealed significantly contributory auditory cues. These observations implied that native speakers articulate literal and idiomatic utterances differently, formulating consistent and stable auditory-acoustic cues that listeners use to distinguish between the two meanings (Van Lancker, Canter, & Terbeek, 1981).

Later studies examined utterances in French and Korean, revealing differences and similarities in the use of acoustic-phonetic cues to successfully convey contrastively idiomatic and literal interpretations of ditropic sentences (Abdelli-Baruh, Yang, Ahn, & Van Lancker Sidtis, 2007). It was found that Parisian French and American English speakers utilized the same cues to distinguish the sentences, but in an opposite manner: French idioms were significantly longer, while for English, the literal versions were longer. Pitch was also differently utilized to signal the meaning differences. When Korean ditropic sentences were analyzed, it was seen that native speakers of Korean used duration, amplitude variations, and contrasting fundamental frequency in the last two words to mark utterances as either literal or idiomatic in Korean (Yang, Ahn, & Van Lancker Sidtis, 2015). Literal utterances have longer durations than idiomatic utterances, whereas idiomatic utterances are more varied in amplitude than literal utterances. Intonation contours differ for the two types of meanings: literal utterances end more often with falling pitch whereas idiomatic utterances end with rising pitch. Thus, formulaic and literal meaning contrasts, in utterances where the words and grammar do not differ, are successfully signaled by various acoustic-auditory cues known to the native speaker community.

Disordered language

Psychiatric disturbance

Fixed expressions play a special role in psychiatric diagnoses, including autism (Paul, 2004), Gilles de la Tourette syndrome (Shapiro, Shapiro, Bruun, & Sweet, 1983), treatment-resistant depression (Holtzheimer & Mayberg, 2011), and schizophrenia (Carlsson & Carlsson, 1990). Persons on the autistic spectrum "echo" holistic expressions spoken by themselves and others (Prizant, 1983; Lord & Paul, 1997), and they "pick up" sayings and jingles heard on radio and television (Dobbinson, Perkins, & Boucher, 2003). In Gilles de la Tourette disease, expletives and other unitary taboo utterances are emitted in a semi-compulsive manner. Speech in severe depression was observed to have a preponderance of low-nuance expressions (Bridges, Sidtis, Mayberg, & Van Lancker Sidtis, 2023). An examination of connected speech by persons diagnosed with schizophrenia, accompanied by formal testing, revealed a pathological diminution of fixed, familiar expressions (Garidis, Van Lancker Sidtis, Tartter, Rogers, Sidtis, & Javitt, 2009). This condition, along with the signature thought disorder, likely contributes to the impression of abnormal speaking profiles.

Neurological disturbance

A neurological account of familiar phrase processing as an independent mode in language use can be found in clinical observations of aphasia (impairment of language due to neurological injury). Speech and language behaviors are represented in the left cerebral hemisphere (Espir & Rose, 1970; Geschwind, 1970). In clinical domains, the notion of familiar language traces back to the concept of "automatic speech"[2] in aphasia, first identified and described by Jackson (1874). Automatic speech includes "overlearned" utterances such as counting, formulaic expressions (salutations and conversational formulae), swearing, nursery rhymes, familiar song lyrics (Bartlett & Snelus, 1980), and other routinized, overlearned, conventional expressions (Van Lancker, 1988; Code, 1989; Van Lancker & Cummings, 1999). Preservation of certain kinds of speech is dramatic when experienced in the context of severe cases of language disturbance following left hemisphere stroke: the afflicted person cannot articulate a novel word, propositional phrase, or grammatical sentence, or can do so only with extreme effort and limited articulatory success. In contrast, he or she can fluently swear, count to ten, recite nursery rhymes and song lyrics, and produce a set of fixed expressions such as *how are you, goodbye, I don't know, wait and see.* This well-known fact remained anecdotally transmitted among neurologists and speech pathologists until survey studies by Code (1982) and Blanken and his colleagues (Blanken & Marini, 1997), which systematically documented preserved expressions in severe aphasia in English and in Cantonese Chinese (Chung, Code, & Ball, 2004).

Group studies of production abilities in aphasia, applying formal measures, support impressions about preservation of formulaic expressions. Using three paired tasks, Lum and Ellis (1994) compared speech production in formulaic versus propositional contexts. First, counting was compared to naming Arabic numbers in nonconsecutive order; second, naming pictures with cues from formulaic expressions (e.g., *Don't beat around the BUSH*) was compared to naming pictures depicting novel phrases (*Don't dig behind the BUSH*); and third, formulaic and novel expressions were compared in a repetition task. Subjects performed better on automatic speech and formulaic subtests for number production and picture naming, with a slight advantage also for phrase repetition. A similar finding (Van Lancker Sidtis & Yang, 2016) arose from comparing matched propositional and formulaic expressions in aphasic speakers also in the repetition and sentence completion tasks, again with the result of weaker differences in the repetition task.

The three classes of familiar language have their most authentic presence in spontaneous speech, but the written language more properly exhibits an abundance of lexical bundles and collocations. Formulaic expressions are rampant in conversation; lexical bundles appear extensively in extended spoken and written discourse; and collocations are present in all forms of talk (Schmitt, Sonbul, Vilkaitė-Lozdienė, & Macis, 2019). Questions arise about the neurological foundations of the production and comprehension of fixed, familiar expressions. In our laboratory, we have examined the naturalistic speech of persons with left or right hemisphere damage due to stroke to determine the effect of localized damage on use of fixed expressions.

Natural speech of right and left hemisphere damaged persons compared to normal controls was examined by Van Lancker and Postman (2006). Persons with left hemisphere damage suffer from aphasia, or disordered speech and language. The incidence of fixed expressions was significantly higher in left hemisphere damage resulting in aphasia than in matched normal control speakers, while in right hemisphere damage, such expressions were significantly diminished in comparison to normal speech. Similar differing abilities to produce fixed expressions, corresponding to left or right hemisphere damage, were reported also for the Korean language (Yang, & Van Lancker Sidtis, 2016; Yang, Sidtis, & Yang, 2016). Similarly, a case studied revealed that aphasic speaker utilized a much greater proportion than all other groups (Sidtis, Canterucci, & Katsnelson, 2009). These studies were performed before categorization into three classes had been undertaken. For left hemisphere damaged persons, these results suggest that fixed expressions become a vehicle for communication in aphasia, and for right hemisphere damaged persons, who do not have phonological, syntactic, or linguistic-semantic deficits, these results may help clarify the clinical impression of abnormal pragmatics of communication.

Case studies and other observations in neurologically impaired speech have implicated subcortical structures in the brain; these regions are responsible for effective production of motor gestures. In one case report, a loss of formulaic speech production abilities, targeting prayers and sayings, occurred following damage in the basal ganglia, namely a right caudate stroke (Speedie, Wertman, T'air, & Heilman, 1993). Another examination of two individuals with damage confined to subcortical nuclei, utilizing discourse obtained from structured interviews, revealed a significantly smaller proportion of fixed expressions when compared to similar interview settings obtained from normal control speakers matched for education and age (Sidtis, Canterucci, & Katsnelson, 2009). In another instance, which involved a motor speech disorder likely due to a subcortical stroke, a pathologically intrusive syllable (*sis*) occurred with greater frequency during recitation, counting, and other formulaic expressions than in novel speech (Van Lancker, Bogen, & Canter, 1983).

Still other differences between fixed and novel language production have been seen in analyses of speech samples from Parkinson's patients, who have diminished basal ganglia function, revealing reduced familiar expressions when speaking (Illes, Metter, Hanson, & Iritani, 1988). A later study documented dysfunction in recited speech, whereby the impairment in subcortical (basal ganglia) nuclei resulted in faulty retention of overlearned nursery rhymes and culturally familiar song lyrics (Bridges, Van Lancker Sidtis, & Sidtis, 2013). This group study of persons diagnosed with Parkinson's disease provided support to the single case study of a person who suffered a subcortical stroke, who lost his ability to recite well-established prayers (Speedie, Wertman, T'air, & Heilman, 1993). In Parkinson's speakers, preliminary acoustic measures of voice and articulation, as well as listeners' ratings, differed significantly for novel and fixed expressions (Sidtis, Rogers, Katsnelson, & Sidtis, 2008). These analyses merit further examination.

Incidence of fixed expressions in Parkinson's disease, in comparison with the Alzheimer diagnosis, was further investigated by Van Lancker Sidtis, Choi, Alken, and Sidtis (2016), who reported a complementary profile for persons with Alzheimer's disease (who have intact basal ganglia and impaired cortical function): greatly increased incidence of familiar expressions compared to normal or Parkinsonian speakers. The proportion of fixed, familiar expressions in continuous speech was found to be greatly increased in persons with moderately severe Alzheimer's disease, compared to normal and Parkinsonian speakers (Bridges & Van Lancker Sidtis, 2013). This finding reveals an important role of subcortical structures in producing fixed, familiar expressions, where impairment results in loss or diminution, while intactness, even in the face of cognitive, cortical decline, as seen in dementia, is associated with their abundance in fluent speech.

Examining naturalistic language of persons with dementia reveals insights about the structure of everyday conversation and discourse (Kindell, Keady, Sage, & Wilkinson, 2017; Müller & Guendouzi, 2005). Using different approaches, strategies of chunking and repetition were described in narratives (Guendouzi, Davis, & Maclagan, 2015a, 2015b), and careful consideration of the influence of social context, including use of politeness and formulaic expressions, has been also examined in persons diagnosed with dementia (Guendouzi & Pate, 2014).

Verbal completion phenomena in brain damage yield compelling evidence of a privileged status for fixed expressions. A case study a person with the diagnosis of "presenile dementia" was one of the first to suggest the intact presence of fixed expressions in the context of full cognitive loss. The relative preservation was observed in a severely aphasic 59-year-old woman, who was never observed to produce a meaningful utterance, but could complete idioms and other familiar conventional expressions spoken to her with the last word missing (Whitaker, 1976). Similarly, an aphasic individual with a severe comprehension deficit and a diagnosis of transcortical sensory aphasia was unable to produce meaningful speech, but correctly completed 50% of idiomatic and other formulaic expressions presented verbally (Van Lancker Sidtis, 2001); analysis of his connected speech revealed a proportion of over 50% of fixed expressions, well over the average of 24% seen in normal talkers. Idiom completion in another case of transcortical sensory aphasia was also reported by Nakagawa et al. (1993).

As mentioned above, observations in Alzheimer speech corroborate a role of the basal ganglia in production of fixed expressions (Bridges & Van Lancker Sidtis, 2013). It is commonly observed in the clinical setting that persons with considerable progression in the disease, with MiniMental State Examination scores as low as 7 (on a scale of 0–30), who have lost most cognitive capacity, continue to produce formulaic expressions, such as *Nice seeing you again*, *Excuse me*, and *Good-bye*. Informal observations of conversational speech in Alzheimer's disease reveal a large proportion of formulaic expressions (Davis & Maclagan, 2010). These clinical presentations have been substantiated by formal studies (Bridges & Van Lancker Sidtis, 2013; Van Lancker Sidtis, Choi, Alken, & Sidtis, 2016), documenting an abnormally high proportion of fixed, familiar expressions in Alzheimer speech.

While group studies yield general results, in the clinical setting, it can be seen that the conventional expressions are sometimes used inappropriately. An Alzheimer patient said *I haven't seen you for a while* to a stranger in the hallway, while the two were waiting together for the elevator. In some speech samples, distortions of a fixed expressions appear, such as *But they were very good down there by me for*, or a blend of two or more expressions, such as *put down my mind to it*. In considering a brain model underlying the use of fixed and novel expressions, the relative preservation of fixed in comparison to novel expressions is likely attributable to the fact that Alzheimer's disease attacks the cortical layers, leaving the subcortical nuclei intact until very late in the disease, by which time the patient is mute.

Functional imaging

The few functional brain imaging studies examining familiar language have been inconsistent, and findings are not always in agreement with well-established information derived from clinical observations and lesion studies. Earlier studies of cerebral blood flow using SPECT methodology associated bilateral hemisphere activation with automatic speech (Larsen, Skinhoj, & Lassen, 1978; Ryding, Bradvik, & Ingvar, 1987), but with the proliferation of functional imaging of language studies, bilateral signal is reported for most language tasks, and the early SPECT results are no longer interpretable. Published studies of language processing in general typically report bilateral hemispheric blood flow responses, for reasons that are not yet well understood (Van Lancker Sidtis, 2006). More recently, Blank et al. (2002) reported bilateral activation for both propositional and automatic speech, which does not reveal an interpretable contrast between the two language modes. Another study using PET imaging employed two automatic speech tasks: the months of the year and the Pledge of Allegiance (Bookheimer, Zeffiro, Blaxton, Gaillard, & Theodore, 2000), compared to tongue movements and consonant–vowel syllable production. Continuous production of the Pledge of Allegiance showed activation in traditional language areas; reciting the months of the year selectively engaged language areas Brodmann areas 44 and 22. These studies did not examine counting, which has been the most widely used task in cortical mapping and is the most frequent type of preserved aphasic speech.

Van Lancker, McIntosh, and Grafton (2003) reported that counting and word generation differed in brain activity, with only word generation showing activation in Broca's area, or the left anterior frontal area, and counting associated with more diffuse brain activity, including some subcortical sites. This finding has clinical corroboration, given that nearly all persons with nonfluent aphasia (all having left hemisphere damage) retain the ability to count from one to ten, presumably drawing for this performance on structures other than those in the left anterior area of the brain.

Approaches to functional imaging generally utilized a subtraction measure, whereby activation data for one task was subtracted from activation data obtained in a contrasting task or from the rest state. It has been suggested that one reason for the inconsistent functional brain imaging results is that that cerebral blood flow is influenced by multiple factors and is not a direct surrogate of behavior (Sidtis, 2022). Rather the relationship between cerebral blood flow and behavior requires modeling a relationship between a specific behavior and a network of multiple brain areas. This is called Performance Based Behavior, which quantifies the performance of persons in the scanner in association with brain regions (Sidtis et al., 2003; Sidtis, 2007; 2012a, 2012b; Sidtis et al., 2018). In the PET environment, where ongoing behavior can be examined, participants spoke on a topic of their choice for 60 seconds (Sidtis, Van Lancker Sidtis, Dhawan, & Eidelberg, 2018). Performance based analysis was utilized on these data. From transcriptions of these speech samples, formulaic expressions and lexical bundles, including conversational speech formulas, idioms, proverbs, expletives, sentence initials (*I think*), discourse elements (*well, then*), and pause fillers (*um, uh*) were identified and expressed as proportions of total word counts obtained for the monologues. Spoken samples of syllables, words, and phrases—the propositional condition, obtained in separate PET sessions, were also analyzed.

Multiple linear regression analyses examined the production rates of propositional elements and the proportion of words in fixed expressions (Van Lancker Sidtis, & Sidtis, 2018a, b). As the rate of spoken syllables and words increased, blood flow increased in the *left* inferior frontal region of the cerebral cortex (an area known to modulate speech production) and decreased in a key structure in the basal ganglia (*right* caudate nucleus). In contrast, the proportion of fixed expressions in the monologues yielded a complementary pattern: blood flow increased in the *right* inferior frontal region and decreased in the *left* caudate. This cerebral profile resonates with the known effects of right hemisphere and subcortical damage on the production of fixed expressions, as seen in clinical studies. An exception was seen for the pause fillers *uh* and *um*, which patterned like propositional, lexical items. These findings lend support to a classification of these pause fillers as lexical items (Clark & FoxTree, 2002).

Relationship of fixed, familiar expressions to animal vocalization and role in evolution

The notion that a right hemisphere-subcortical circuit plays a role in formulaic verbal behavior in humans is especially interesting when considering the relationship of human phonatory behaviors to animal vocalization. We defined one class of familiar language, formulaic (or automatic) expressions, as routinized, holistic, emotional, and attitudinal utterances of various kinds; these kinds of speech bear a certain similarity to animal calls. In humans, such vocalizations have occurred when subcortical sites are electrically stimulated during stereotaxic surgical techniques, usually for treatment of epilepsy (Schaltenbrand, 1965; Petrovici, 1980). As mentioned above, subcortical dysfunction is associated with diminution of formulaic expressions. On the other side of the coin, hyperfunction of the basal ganglia/limbic system, as in persons with Tourette's syndrome, gives rise to semi-compulsive emotive utterances (called coprolalia or "foul speaking").

Animal vocalization is almost exclusively social[3] in nature, with some vocalizations indicating anger and warning and others facilitating social interactions (Marler, 1998). Similarly, many formulaic expressions in humans (e.g., expletives, warnings) represent vocalizations mediated by limbic system structures and originally intended to perform the social functions of repulsing intruders, bonding, and expressing anger and dissatisfaction. As such, formulaic expressions have been proposed as antecedent to the evolution of human language (Jespersen, 1933; Patel, 2008; Wray, 2002; Code, 2005). In this view, the evolutionarily older system also continues to perform in emotional and routinized vocal behaviors. Use of lexical bundles and collocations, the other two classes of familiar language, appears to differ from these contingencies, having different linguistic characteristics. Further understanding of brain function underlying the three classes is needed.

Ploog (1975) proposed a hierarchical system of neuronal organization in the central nervous system, corresponding with evolutionary development, with brainstem control of vocal gestures, with higher level control in anterior limbic cortex in primates, and with cortical representation occurring only in humans. This resembles the notion of two levels of nervous system control for vocalization in humans: an older system, which terminates in the cingulate gyrus (part of the limbic, or emotional, circuit) at the bilateral, rostral (rear) end of the limbic system, and which is capable of emotive and formulaic speech behavior; and a newer system that is cortical, unilateral, and involved in voluntary, novel, and planned speech (Robinson, 1987; Ploog, 1975). As mentioned above, the relationship of lexical bundles and collocations, also manifesting many characteristics of fixed, familiar language, to these theoretical positions has not been investigated or considered. Disparate neurological circuits have been seen for control of "innate" vocal reactions (such as cries in response to pain) and "voluntary" vocalization, which appear to be differentially distributed in human and nonhuman brain organization (Jürgens, 2002). Thus, studies in primates and humans lend credence to the notion that one important class of familiar language, formulaic expressions, emerged in humans from an evolutionary history different from that proposed for novel language, and is differently structured and controlled in the brain, and possibly different from the emergence of lexical bundles and collocations.

It is possible that further studies, examining the three classes of familiar language in psycholinguistic studies and neurological conditions will lead to a multi-process model of language competence in the brain.

Dual or multi-processing model of language competence

The "dual model" of language competence, which has been advanced by several writers (Koestler, 1967; Wray & Perkins, 2000; Heine, Kuteva, & Kaltenböck, 2014; Erman & Warren, 2000; Lounsbury, 1963; Ullman, Corkin, Coppola, Hickok, Growdon, Koroshetz, & Pinker, 1997), accommodates many of the clinical observations described above. Some of these proposals, when brain structures are considered, identify overlearned, routinized, grammatical, and holistic speech material with right hemisphere and subcortical (basal ganglia) modulation (Lieberman, 2000; Zanini, Tavano, & Fabbro, 2010; Lee & Van Lancker Sidtis, 2020; Bridges, Van Lancker Sidtis, & Sidtis, 2013), and associate newly created linguistic processing with left sided cortical structures. The inconsistencies arising from some of the idiom studies might be explained by the interplay of holistic and novel processing.

The dual process model proposes that fixed expressions, which by definition are cohesive, have stereotyped form and conventionalized meanings, are familiar to speakers of a language community (Kitzinger, 2000), and exist in harmony with the grammar, which consists of rules and a lexicon. A dual process model of language processing, accommodating two modes of language use, familiar and novel, has several advocates (some referenced above). Neurological damage can disturb, diminish, or enhance various subsets of familiar language. Novel and many kinds of fixed, known expressions are affected differently by different types of brain damage: left hemisphere damage leads to selective impairment of novel language and relative preservation of many types of fixed, unitary expressions, while right hemisphere and/or subcortical damage lead to selective impairment of, primarily, formulaic expressions (especially conversational speech formulas, recited speech) sparing novel language. Enhancements or selective presentation are seen in aphasia (conversational speech formulas, swearing), Tourette's syndrome (expletives and taboo utterances), and Alzheimer's disease (conventional expressions of all kinds), while diminution of many kinds of fixed expressions is observed in right hemisphere and subcortical disease. It is likely that more such differences will be documented as information about the three classes, and all the various subsets, of familiar language is gleaned from research studies and disseminated into clinical practice. Recognition of the important role of these expressions in evaluation and recovery in aphasia (Stahl & Van Lancker Sidtis, 2015; Stahl, Gawron, Regenbrecht, Flöel, & Kotz, 2020) and other neurological disorders has barely begun, despite the "automatic speech" tradition extending more than a hundred years into the past.

The notion of more than one processing mode has emerged from studies of learning and memory, comparing, for example, procedural and declarative knowledge (Mishkin, Malamut, & Bachevalier, 1984). Subcortical structures have been associated with "chunking of action repertoires" (Greybiel, 1998) or "habit learning" (Knowlton, Mangels, & Squire, 1996). These perspectives have been aligned with hierarchical levels of the central nervous system, such that automated motor gestures are accommodated by subcortical structures, which developed phylogenetically earlier in human evolution (Koestler, 1967). Correspondingly, it has been suggested that the origin of human language might be located in initial use of formulaic expressions (Jaynes, 1976; Code, 2005; Wray, 1998, 2000; Wray & Grace, 2007).

Summary

The fixed, familiar expression has unique properties: it is cohesive and unitary in structure (sometimes with aberrant grammatical form), while easily subject to variation. It features conventionalized meaning and sensitivity to social and linguistic context. Most important, as reflected in its name, the expression is familiar, which means that it is known in a special way to members of a speech community. Three classes are proposed, distinguished by important linguistic, social, and psychological characteristics. Unitary utterances may or may not be nonliteral and deviant in meaning properties; some carry more or less strongly nuanced meanings or transmit meanings transcend the sum of their (lexical) parts. Some conform essentially to a pragmatic dimension of language, being intimately tied to social context and having subtle specifications of usage (Kuiper & Flindall, 2000). This is especially true of formulaic expressions. Others, particularly lexical bundles, serve primarily to organize discourse and underpin fluency, carrying little propositional meaning. The third class, collocations, vary the most in nuance, depending on their lexical constituents, which tend to convey the most propositional meaning.

The special properties that differentiate the three classes of fixed expressions might be reflected in differing underlying neurological processes. The dual process model proposes that novel, grammatical language is modulated by the left hemisphere, which features categorization, material detail, and sequential processing modes, while familiar language relies more heavily on the right hemisphere, where holistic, affective, contextual, and personally familiar phenomena preside (Van Lancker, 1991; McGilchrist, 2009). The motor systems of the basal ganglia modulate routinized motor gestures (Marsden, 1982). As such they play varied roles in the production of novel versus familiar expressions: grammatical morphemes and syntactic structures appear to require intact basal ganglia (Zanini, Tavano, & Fabbro, 2010), as do holistically produced, fixed expressions (Lee & Van Lancker Sidtis, 2020); these observations pertain for the first language only. Most studies of speech production following left or right hemisphere or subcortical damage have examined an array of fixed expressions, with little attention to subtyping. Given the differing features inhering in the three classes proposed here, further research may reveal varying and stronger associations within the large body of familiar language. It is with this perspective in mind that the notion of a multi-process model of language processing in the brain is proposed (Table 12.2).

Table 12.2 Behavioral properties of three major structures in the brain that process speech and language. The **left hemisphere** excels at linguistic meanings, sequential processing, and grammar. The **right hemisphere** manages affect and nuanced meanings, patterns and configurations, and personally familiar phenomena. The **basal ganglia** modulate routinized, overlearned vocal motor patterns.

Left Hemisphere	*Basal Ganglia*	*Right Hemisphere*
linguistic meanings	routinized motor gestures	nuanced meanings
sequences		configurations
grammar		familiarity

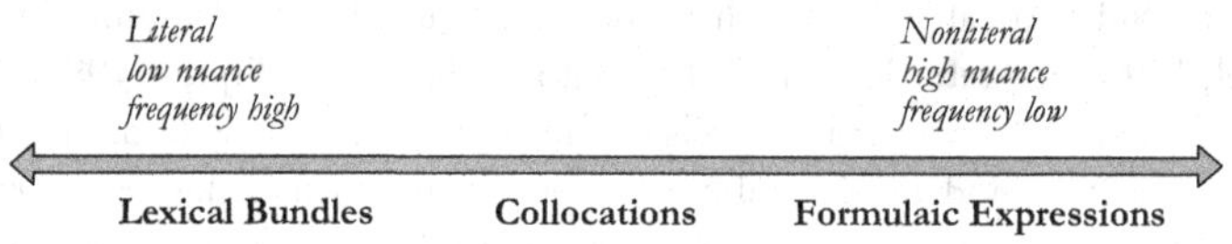

Figure 12.1 Characteristics of the three classes of familiar language on a proposed continuum.

Traditionally, left and right hemispheres are said to perform using generally different behavioral modes, as outlined in Table 12.2 (Bever, 1975; Bryden, 1982; Hellige, 1993; Ley & Bryden, 1982; Martin, 1979; Springer & Deutsch, 2001). Given the association of affective processing with the right hemisphere, the finding that formulaic expressions, the high nuanced class, are favored there is not surprising. The right hemisphere modulates familiarity in the environment (Van Lancker, 1991) and excels at the pragmatic requirements of language use, such as recognizing context (Baldo, Kacinik, Moncrief, Beghin & Dronkers, 2016), humor, and inferences (Brownell & Martino, 2013). The right hemisphere is also the pattern recognizer, processing configurations and holistic stimuli more aptly than elsewhere in the brain. This property would appear also to draw lexical bundles, despite their low load on nuance, as well as collocations. The basal ganglia formulate and manage the output of complex motor gestures of all kinds, including vocalization and speech, so that the overlearned, routinized feature of fixed expressions naturally finds a home here. Some of these proposals and speculations are backed by clinical data, but, as mentioned previously, careful examination of how and where different classes and subtypes of fixed, familiar expressions are stored and processed in the mind and brain is still in its infancy.

Most importantly, the canonical form of the typical fixed expression is known to native speakers. The expressions are acquired and transmitted because they "sound right" (Van Lancker Sidtis, 2019). All these expressions function differently in form, meaning, and use from the literal, novel, newly created, propositional, grammatical expressions (Lounsbury, 1963).

Fixed, familiar, unitary expressions are informed by principles and properties that cause them to be essentially different from newly created sentences. They cannot usefully be handled by the same analytic apparatus. Familiar and novel language are disparate modes of language competence. Further examination of the various classes and subtypes will reveal more about how to establish a model of language competence, and how to line these behaviors up with brain function. Creative linguistic processes of all sorts can and do operate on any canonical form, which can be varied providing it remains identifiable. Unitary expressions are learned according to a distinctive maturational schedule in ways that are different from those operative for learning grammar, and, in many cases, they may draw on instantaneous rather than incremental learning. These perspectives have relevance for models of language competence, language learning, and language loss in psychiatric and neurological disorders.

Notes

1 "Contingency" of reinforcement is a relation between environmental events (i.e., stimuli) and responses (Lattal, 1995).

2 The terms "automatic and voluntary," "automatic and propositional," and "nonpropositional and propositional" have been both useful and troublesome. The terms were introduced by Jackson (1874) to characterize preserved vocalizations in severe aphasia, including emotional outbursts, swearing, clichés, greetings, yes, no. The terms "voluntary" and "propositional" speech were used for novel or newly created speech. However, preserved vocalizations are used voluntarily to communicate, and much of motor speech production, including the inclusion of grammatical morphemes and grammatical structure, can be called "automatic."

3 Vervet monkeys and other nonhuman primates have a small set of vocalizations that refer to a predator or to an action to take in the response to the predator (Cheney & Seyfarth, 1980).

Further reading

Lee, B., & Van Lancker Sidtis, D. (2020). Subcortical involvement in formulaic language: Studies on bilingual individuals with Parkinson's disease. *Journal of Speech, Language, and Hearing Research, 63*(12), 4029–4045.

Sidtis, D. (2022). *Foundations of familiar language.* NJ: Wiley-Blackwell.

Wray, A. (2013). Formulaic language. *Language Teaching, 46*(3), 316–334.

References

Abdelli-Baruh, N., Yang, S.-Y., Ahn, J.-S., & Van Lancker Sidtis, D. (2007). *Acoustic cues differentiating idiomatic from literal expressions across languages.* American Speech-Language Hearing Association, Boston, MA, November 15–17.

Aijmer, K. (1996). *Conversational routines in English.* London and New York: Longman.

Altenberg, B. (1998). On the phraseology of spoken English: The evidence of recurrent word-combinations. In A. P. Cowie (Ed.), *Phraseology: Theory, analysis and application* (pp. 101–124). Oxford: Clarendon Press.

Ambridge, G., & Lieven, E. (2015). A constructive account of child language acquisition. In B. MacWhinney & W. O'Grady (Eds.), *The handbook of language emergence* (pp. 478–510). London: John Wiley and Sons.

Arnaud, P., & Moon, R. E. (1993). Fréquence et emploi des proverbes anglais et français. In C. Plantin (Ed.), *Lieux communs: Topoï, stéréotypes, clichés* (pp. 323–341). Paris: Kime.

Baldo, J. V., Kacinik, N. A., Moncrief, A., Beghin, F., & Dronkers, N. F. (2016). You may now kiss the bride: Interpretation of social situations by individuals with right or left hemisphere injury. *Neuropsychologia, 80*, 133–141.

Bannard, C., & Lieven, E. (2012). Formulaic language in L1 acquisition. *Annual Review of Applied Linguistics, 32*, 3–16.

Bartlett, F. C. (1967). *Remembering: A study in experimental and social psychology.* London: Cambridge University Press.

Bartlett, J. C., & Snelus, P. (1980). Lifespan memory for popular songs. *American Journal of Psychology*, 551–560.

Baudouin, J. Y., Gilibert, D., Sansone, S., & Tiberghien, G. (2000). When the smile is a cue to familiarity. *Memory, 8*(5), 285–292.

Bell, R. A., & Healey, J. G. (1992). Idiomatic communication and interpersonal solidarity in friends' relational cultures. *Human Communication Research, 3*(3), 307–335.

Bever, T. G. (1975). Cerebral asymmetries in humans are due to the differentiation of two incompatible processes: Holistic and analytic. *Annals of the New York Academy of Science, 263*, 251–262.

Biber, D., & Barbieri, F. (2007). Lexical bundles in university spoken and written registers. *English for Specific Purposes, 26*(3), 263–286.

Biber, D., & Conrad, S. (1999). Lexical bundles in conversation and academic prose. *Language and Computers, 26*, 181–190.

Biber, D., Conrad, S., & Cortes, V. (2003). Lexical bundles in speech and writing: An initial taxonomy. In A. Wilson, P. Rayson, & T. McEnery (Eds.), *Corpus linguistics by the Lune: A festschrift for Geoffrey Leech* (pp. 71–92). Frankfurt: Peter Lang.

Biber, D., Conrad, S., & Cortes, V. (2004). If you look at …: Lexical bundles in university teaching and textbooks. *Applied Linguistics, 25*(3), 371–405. http://doi.org/10.1093/applin/25.3.371.

Biber, D., Conrad, S., & Reppen, R. (1994). Corpus-based approaches to issues in applied linguistics. *Applied Linguistics, 15*(2), 169–189. http://doi.org/10.1093/applin/15.2.169.

Blank, S. C., Scott, S., Murphy, K., Warburton, E., & Wise, R. (2002). Speech production: Wernicke, Broca and beyond. *Brain, 125*(8), 1829–1838.
Blanken, G., & Marini, V. (1997). Where do lexical speech automatisms come from? *Journal of Neurolinguistics, 10*(1), 19–31.
Bobrow, S., & Bell, S. (1973). On catching on to idiomatic expressions. *Memory and Cognition, 1*(3), 343–346.
Bookheimer, S.Y., Zeffiro, T. A., Blaxton, T. A., Gaillard, P. W., & Theodore, W. H. (2000). Activation of language cortex with automatic speech tasks. *Neurology, 55*(8), 1151–1157.
Bridges, K., & Van Lancker Sidtis, D. (2013). Formulaic language in Alzheimer's disease. *Aphasiology, 27*(7), 799–810.
Bridges, K., Van Lancker Sidtis, D., & Sidtis, J. J. (2013). The role of subcortical structures in recited speech: Studies in Parkinson's disease. *Journal of Neurolinguistics, 26*(6), 591–601.
Bridges, K. A., Mayberg, H., Van Lancker Sidtis, D., & Sidtis, J. J. (2023). Familiar language in treatment-resistant depression: Effects of deep brain stimulation of the subcallosal cingulate. *Journal of Neurolinguistics, 65*, 101110.
Brown, R., & Kulik, J. (1977). Flashbulb memories. *Cognition, 5*(1), 73–93.
Brownell, H., & Martino, G. (2013). In Beeman, M., & Chiarello, C. (Eds.), *Getting it right: The cognitive neuroscience of right hemisphere language comprehension*. Hillsdale, NJ: Lawrence Erlbaum Associates.
Bruess, C. J., & Pearson, J. C. (1993). 'Sweet pea' and 'pussy cat': An examination of idiom use and marital satisfaction over the life cycle. *Journal of Social and Personal Relationships, 10*(4), 609–615.
Bryden, M. P. (1982). *Laterality: Hemispheric specialization in the intact brain*. New York: Academic Press.
Brysbaert, M., Stevens, M., Mandera, P., & Keuleers, E. (2016). How many words do we know? Practical estimates of vocabulary size depending on word definition, the degree of language input, and the participant's age. *Frontiers in Psychology*, 7, 1116.
Burdelski, M., & Cook, H. M. (2012). Formulaic language in language socialization. *Annual Review of Applied Linguistics, 32*, 173–188. https://doi.org/10.1017/S0256190512000049.
Cacciari, C., & Tabossi, P. (1988). The comprehension of idioms. *Journal of Memory and Language, 27*(6), 668–683.
Carlsson, M., & Carlsson, A. (1990). Schizophrenia: A subcortical neurotransmitter imbalance syndrome? *Schizophrenia Bulletin, 16*(3), 425–432.
Carr, E. W., Brady, T. F., & Winkielman, P. (2017). Are you smiling, or have I seen you before? Familiarity makes faces look happier. *Psychological Science, 28*(8). https://doi.org/10.1177/0956797617702003.
Chen, Y.-H., & Baker, P. (2010). Lexical bundles in L1 and L2 academic writing. *Language Learning and Technology, 14*(2), 30–49.
Cheney, D. L., & Seyfarth, R. M. (1980). Vocal recognition in free-ranging vervet monkeys. *Animal Behaviour, 28*(2), 362–367.
Christianson, S.-Å. (1992). Do flashbulb memories differ from other types of emotional memories? In E. Winograd & U. Neisser (Eds.), *Affect and accuracy in recall: Studies of "flashbulb memories"* (pp. 191–211). Cambridge: Cambridge University Press.
Chung, K. K. H., Code, C., & Ball, M. J. (2004). Lexical and non-lexical speech automatisms in aphasic Cantonese speakers. *Journal of Multilingual Communication Disorders, 2*(1), 32–42.
Clark, H. H. (1970). Word associations and linguistic theory. In J. Lyons (Ed.), *New horizons in linguistics* (pp. 271–286). Baltimore, MD: Penguin Books.
Clark, H. H., & Fox Tree, J. E. (2002). Using uh and um in spontaneous speaking. *Cognition, 84*(1), 73–111.
Claypool, H. M., Hall, C. E., Mackie, D. M., & Garcia-Marques, T. (2008). Positive mood, attribution, and the illusion of familiarity. *Journal of Experimental Social Psychology, 44*(3), 721–728. https://doi.org/10.1016/j.jesp.2007.05.001.
Code, C. (1982). Neurolinguistic analysis of recurrent utterance in aphasia. *Cortex, 18*(1), 141–152.
Code, C. (1989). Speech automatisms and recurring utterances. In C. Code (Ed.), *The characteristics of aphasia* (pp. 155–177). London: Taylor and Francis.
Code, C. (2005). First in, last out? The evolution of aphasic lexical speech automatisms to agrammatism and the evolution of human communication. *Interaction Studies, 6*(2), 311–334.
Conklin, K., & Schmitt, N. (2012). The processing of formulaic language. *Annual Review of Applied Linguistics, 32*, 45–61.
Coulmas, F. (1994). Formulaic language. In R. E. Asher (Ed.), *Encyclopedia of language and linguistics* (pp. 1292–1293). Oxford: Pergamon.
Cowie, A. P. (1992). Multiword lexical units and communicative language teaching. In P. Arnaud & H. Bejoint (Eds.), *Vocabulary and applied linguistics* (pp. 1–12). London: Macmillan.
Cutting, J. C., & Bock, K. (1997). That's the way the cookie bounces: Syntactic and semantic components of experimentally elicited idiom blends. *Memory and- Cognition, 25*(1), 57–71.

Davis, B. H., & Maclagan, M. (2010). Pauses, fillers, placeholder, and formulaicity in Alzheimer's discourse: Gluing relationships as impairment increases. In N. Amiridze, B. H. Davis, & M. Maclagan (Eds.), *Fillers, pauses, and placeholders* (pp. 189–216). Amsterdam: John Benjamins.

de Vries, M., Holland, R. W., Chenier, T., Starr, M. J., & Winkielman, P. (2010). Happiness cools the warm glow of familiarity: Psychophysiological evidence that mood modulates the familiarity-affect link. *Psychological Science, 21*(3), 321–328. https://doi.org/10.1177/0956797609359878.

Devitt, M. (2006). Intuitions in linguistics. *British Journal for the Philosophy of Science, 57*(3), 481–513.

Dobbinson, S., Perkins, M. R., & Boucher, J. (2003). The interactional significance of formulas in autistic language. *Clinical Linguistics and Phonetics, 17*(4), 299–307.

Drew, P., & Holt, E. (1988). Complainable matters: The use of idiomatic expressions in making complaints. *Social Problems, 35*, 398–417.

Durrant, P. (2014). Corpus frequency and second language learners' knowledge of collocations: A meta-analysis. *International Journal of Corpus Linguistics, 19*(4), 443–477. https://doi.org/10.1075/ijcl.19.4.01dur.

Edmonds, A. (2014). Conventional expressions: Investigating pragmatics and processing. *Studies in Second Language Acquisition, 36*(1), 69–99.

Ellis, N. C. (2008). Constructions, chunking, and connectionism: The emergence of second language structure. Revised chapter for C. J. Doughty & M. H. Long (Eds.), *Handbook of second language acquisition* (pp. 63–103). Oxford: Blackwell. https://doi.org/10.1002/9780470756492.ch4.

Erman, B., & Warren, B. (2000). The idiom principle and the open choice principle. *Text-International Journal for the Study of Discourse, 20*(1), 29–62.

Espir, L., & Rose, F. (1970). *The basic neurology of speech*. Oxford: Blackwell Scientific Publications.

Fillmore, C. (1979). On fluency. In C. J. Fillmore, D. Kempler, & W. S.-Y. Wang (Eds.), *Individual differences in language ability and language behavior* (pp. 85–102). London: Academic Press.

Fox Tree, J. E. (2006). Placing like in telling stories. *Discourse Studies, 8*(6), 723–743.

Gallahorn, G. E. (1971). The use of taboo words by psychiatric ward personnel. *Psychiatry, 34*(3), 309–321.

Garcia-Marques, T., Mackie, D. M., Claypool, H. M., & Garcia-Marques, L. (2004). Positivity can cue familiarity. *Personality and Social Psychology Bulletin, 30*(5), 585–593.

Garidis, C., Van Lancker Sidtis, D., Tartter, V. C., Rogers, T., Sidtis, J. J., & Javitt, D. C. (2009). The use of formulaic expressions in schizophrenia: A basis for identifying neural substrates. Presentation at the International Congress on Schizophrenia Research, March 28-April 1. San Diego, CA.

Geiselman, R. E., & Crawley, J. M. (1976). Long-term memory for speaker's voice and source location. *Memory and Cognition, 4*(15), 483–489.

Geschwind, N. (1970). The organization of language in the brain. *Science, 170*(3961), 940–944.

Gibbs, R. W. (1980). Spilling the beans on understanding and memory for idioms in conversation. *Memory and Cognition, 8*(2), 149–156.

Gibbs, R. W. (1981). Your wish is my command: Convention and context in interpreting indirect requests. *Journal of Verbal Learning and Verbal Behavior, 20*(4), 431–444.

Gibbs, R. W., Jr., & Gonzales, G. P. (1985). Syntactic frozenness in processing and remembering idioms. *Cognition, 20*(3), 243–259.

Gibbs, R. W., Jr., Nayak, N. P., Bolton, J. L., & Keppel, M. E. (1989). Speaker's assumptions about the lexical flexibility of idioms. *Memory and Cognition, 17*(1), 58–68.

Glassman, L., Grinberg, D., Hibbard, C., Meehan, J., Reid, L. G., & van Leunen, M.-C. (1992). *Hector: Connecting words with definitions. SRC Report 92a*; Digital Equipment Corporation Systems Research Center, Palo Alto, CA.

Gleason, J. B., & Weintraub, S. (1976). The acquisition of routines in child language. *Language in Society, 5*(2), 129–139.

Gold, P. E. (1992). A proposed neurobiological basis for regulating memory storage for significant events. In E. Winograd & U. Neisser (Eds.), *Affect and accuracy in recall: Studies of "flashbulb memories"* (pp. 141–161). Cambridge: Cambridge University Press.

Goldinger, S. D. (1996). Words and voices: Episodic trace in spoken work identification and recognition memory. *Journal of Experimental Psychology: Learning, Memory, and Cognition, 22*(5), 1166–1183.

González Fernández, B., & Schmitt, N. (2015). How much collocation knowledge do L2 learners have?: The effects of frequency and amount of exposure. *ITL-International Journal of Applied Linguistics, 166*(1), 94–126. https://doi.org/10.1075/itl.166.1.03fer.

Graybiel, A. M. (1998). The basal ganglia and chunking of action repertoires. *Neurobiology of Learning and Memory, 70*(1–2), 119–136.

Greenbaum, S., & Svartik, J. (1990). The London-Lund corpus of spoken English. In J. Svartik (Ed.), *The London-Lund corpus of spoken English: Description and research* (pp. 11–45). Lund: Lund University Press.

Grimm, R., Cassani, G., Gillis, S., & Daelemans, W. (2019). Children probably store short rather than frequent or predictable chunks: Quantitative evidence from a corpus study. *Frontiers in Psychology, 10* (Jan), art. no. 80.
Guendouzi, J., Davis, B. H., & Maclagan, M. (2015a). Expanding expectations for narrative styles in the context of dementia. *Topics in Language Disorders, 35*(3), 237–257.
Guendouzi, J., Davis, B. H., & Maclagan, M. (2015b). Listening to narratives from people recently diagnosed with dementia. *Transactions in Language Disorders, 35*(3), 237–257.
Guendouzi, J., & Pate, A. (2014). Interactional and cognitive resources in dementia: A perspective from politeness theory. In R. Schrauf & N. Müller (Eds.), *Dialogue and dementia: Cognitive and communicative resources for engagement* (pp. 121–146). London: Blackwell.
Gurevich, O., Johnson, M. A., & Goldberg, A. E. (2010). Incidental verbatim memory for language. *Language and Cognition, 2–1*(1), 45–78.
Guz, E. (2014). Formulaic sequences as fluency devices in the oral production of native speakers of Polish. *Research in Language, 12*(2), 113–129.
Hain, M. (1951). *Sprichwort und Volkssprache*. Giessen: Wilhelm Schmitz Verlag. English trans., in D. Sidtis & S. Mohr (Eds.), *Formulaic language in the field*, Anja Tachler, translator. Copyright.
Hallin, A., & Van Lancker Sidtis, D. (2017). A closer look at formulaic language: Prosodic characteristics of Swedish proverbs. *Applied Linguistics, 38*(1), 68–89. https://doi.org/10.1093/applin/amu078.
Hassanzadeh, M., & Tamleh, H. (2022). The use of lexical bundles by native English authors in applied linguistics: A corpus-driven study. *Language Related Research, 13*, in press.
Heine, B., Kuteva, T., & Kaltenböck, K. (2014). Discourse grammar, the dual process model, and brain lateralization: Some correlations. *Language and Cognition, 6*(1), 146–180.
Hellige, J. B. (1993). *Hemispheric asymmetry: What's right and what's left*. Cambridge, MA: Harvard University Press.
Heng, C. S., Kashiha, H., & Tan, H. (2014). Lexical bundles: Facilitating university "talk" in group discussions. *English Language Teaching*, 7(4), 1–10.
Holtzheimer, P. E., & Mayberg, H. (2011). Stuck in a rut: Rethinking depression and its treatment. *Trends in Neuroscience, 34*(1), 1–9.
Horn, G. (1985). *Memory, imprinting and the brain*. Oxford Psychology Series No. 10. Oxford: Clarendon Press.
Horowitz, L. M., & Manelis, L. (1973). Recognition and cued recall of idioms and phrases. *Journal of Experimental Psychology, 100*(2), 291–296.
Hughlings Jackson, J. (1874). On the nature of the duality of the brain. In J. Taylor (Ed.), *Selected writings of John Hughlings Jackson* (Vol. 2, pp. 129–145). London: Hodder & Stoughton.
Illes, J., Metter, E. J., Hanson, W. R., & Iritani, S. (1988). Language production in Parkinson's disease: Acoustic and linguistic considerations. *Brain and Language, 33*(1), 146–160.
Jackendoff, R. (1995). The boundaries of the lexicon. In M. Everaert, E. van der Linden, A. Schenk, & R. Schreuder (Eds.), *Idioms: Structural and psychological perspectives* (pp. 133–166). Hillsdale, NJ: Lawrence Erlbaum Associates.
Jacobs, C. L., Dell, G. S., Benjamin, A. S., & Bannard, C. (2016). Part and whole linguistic experience affect recognition memory for multiword sequences. *Journal of Memory and Language, 87*, 38–58.
Jay, T. B. (1980). Sex roles and dirty word usage: A review of the literature and a reply to Haas. *Psychological Bulletin, 88*(3), 614–621.
Jaynes, J. (1976). *The origin of consciousness in the breakdown of the bicameral mind*. Boston, MA: Houghton Mifflin.
Jeong, H., & Jiang, N. (2019). Representation and processing of lexical bundles: Evidence from word monitoring. *System, 80*, 188–198.
Jespersen, O. (1933). *Essentials of English grammar*. London: George Allen and Unwin, Ltd.
Jucker, A. H. (1993). The discourse marker 'well': A relevance-theoretical account. *Journal of Pragmatics, 19*(5), 435–452.
Jürgens, U. (2002). Neural pathways underlying vocal control. *Neuroscience and Biobehavioral Reviews, 26*(2), 235–258.
Kaltenböck, G., Mihatsch, G., & Schneider, S. (Eds.). (2010). *New approaches to hedging*. Emerald Publishers.
Kecskés, I. (2014). *Intercultural pragmatics*. Oxford: Oxford University Press.
Kecskés, I. (2017). Deliberate creativity and formulaic language use. In K. Allan, A. Capone, & I. Kecskés (Eds.), *Pragmemes and theories of language use* (pp. 3–20). *Perspectives in Pragmatics, Philosophy & Psychology, 9*. Springer International Publishing, Switzerland. https://doi.org/10.1007/978-3-319-43491-9.
Kempler, D., Van Lancker, D., Marchman, V., & Bates, E. (1999). Idiom comprehension in children and adults with unilateral brain damage. *Developmental Neuropsychology, 15*(3), 327–349.
Kindell, J., Keady, J., Sage, K., & Wilkinson, R. (2017). Everyday conversation in dementia: A review of the literature to inform research and practice. *International Journal of Language and Communication Disorders, 52*(4), 392–406.

Kiparsky, P. (1976). Oral poetry: Some linguistic and typological considerations. In B. A. Stolz & R. S. Shannon (Eds.), *Oral literature and the formula*. Michigan University, Center for Coordination of Ancient and Modern Studies: Trillium Pr.

Kitzinger, C. (2000). How to resist an idiom. *Research on Language and Social Interaction, 33*(2), 121–154.

Klaver, E. (1989). The play of language in Ionesco's play of chairs. *Modern Drama, 32*(4), 521–531.

Knowlton, B., Mangels, J., & Squire, L. (1996). A neostriatal habit learning system in humans. *Science, 273*(5280), 1399–1402.

Knudsen, E. I. (1987). Early experience shapes auditory localization behavior and the spatial tuning of auditory units in the barn owl. In J. P. Rauschecker & P. Marler (Eds.), *Imprinting and cortical plasticity* (pp. 3–7). New York: John Wiley & Sons.

Koestler, A. (1967). *The ghost in the machine*. Chicago, IL: Henry Regnery Company.

Kuiper, K. (1991). The evolution of an oral tradition: Race-calling in Canterbury, New Zealand. *Oral Tradition, 6*, 19–34.

Kuiper, K. (1992). The English oral tradition in auction speech. *American Speech, 67*(3), 279–289.

Kuiper, K. (1996). *Smooth Talkers: The linguistic performance of auctioneers and sportscasters*. Mahwah, NJ: Erlbaum Association Publishers.

Kuiper, K. (2000). On the linguistic properties of formulaic speech. *Oral Tradition, 15*(2), 279–305.

Kuiper, K. (2004). Formulaic performance in conventionalised varieties of speech. In N. Schmitt (Ed.), *Formulaic sequences: Acquisition, processing, and use* (pp. 37–54). Amsterdam: John Benjamins.

Kuiper, K. (2007). Cathy Wilcox meets the phrasal lexicon. In J. Munat (Ed.), *Lexical creativity, texts and contexts* (Vol. 58, pp. 93–112). John Benjamins Publishing.

Kuiper, K. (2009). *Formulaic genres*. Basingstoke: Palgrave Macmillan.

Kuiper, K., & Flindall, M. (2000). Social rituals, formulaic speech and small talk at the supermarket checkout. In J. Coupland (Ed.), *Small talk* (pp. 183–207). London: Longman.

Kuiper, K., & Haggo, D. (1985). The nature of ice hockey commentaries. In R. Berry & J. Acheson (Eds.), *Regionalism and national identity: Multidisciplinary essays on Canada* (pp. 189–197). Christchurch: Association for Canadian Studies in Australia and New Zealand.

Kuiper, K., van Egmond, M., Kempen, G., & Sprenger, S. (2007). Slipping on superlemmas: Multi-word lexical items in speech production. *Mental Lexicon, 2*(3), 313–357.

Lachs, L., McMichael, K., & Pisoni, D. B. (2012). Speech perception and implicit memory: Evidence for detailed episodic encoding of phonetic events. In J. S. Bowers & C. J. Marsolek (Eds.), *Rethinking implicit memory* (pp. 215 –238). Oxford: Oxford University Press.

Larsen, B., Skinhoj, E., & Lassen, H. A. (1978). Variations in regional cortical blood flow in the right and left hemispheres during automatic speech. *Brain, 10*, 193–200.

Lattal, K. A. (1995). Contingency and behavior analysis. *Behavior Analyst, 24*, 147–161.

Lee, B., & Van Lancker Sidtis, D. (2020). Subcortical involvement in formulaic language: Studies on bilingual individuals with Parkinson's disease. *Journal of Speech, Language, and Hearing Research, 63*(12), 4029–4045.

Ley, R. G., & Bryden, M. P. (1982). A dissociation of right and left hemispheric effects for recognizing emotional tone and verbal content. *Brain and Cognition, 1*(1), 3–9.

Lieberman, P. (2000). *Human language and our reptilian brain: The subcortical bases of speech, syntax, and thought*. Cambridge, MA: Harvard University Press.

Lieven, E., Salomo, D., & Tomasello, M. (2009). Two-year-old children's production of multiword utterances: A usage-based analysis. *Cognitive Linguistics, 20*(3), 481–507.

Locke, J. L. (1993). *The child's path to spoken language*. Cambridge, MA: Harvard University Press.

Locke, J. L. (1995). Development of the capacity for spoken language. In P. Fletcher & B. MacWhinney (Eds.), *The handbook of child language* (pp. 278–302). Oxford: Blackwell.

Locke, J. L. (1997). A theory of neurolinguistic development. *Brain and Language, 58*(2), 568–576.

Lord, A. (1960). *The singer of tales*. Cambridge, MA: Harvard University Press.

Lord, C., & Paul, R. (1997). Language and communication in autism. In D. J. Cohen & F. R. Volkmar (Eds.), *Handbook of autism and pervasive developmental disorders* (pp. 195–225). New York: John Wiley & Sons.

Lounsbury, F. G. (1963). Linguistics and psychology. In S. Koch (Ed.), *Psychology: Study of a science* (pp. 553–582). New York: McGraw-Hill.

Lum, C. C., & Ellis, A. W. (1994). Is nonpropositional speech preserved in aphasia? *Brain and language, 46*(3), 368–391.

Mackin, R. (1978). On collocations: 'Words shall be known by the company they keep'. In P. Strevens (Ed.), *Papers in honour of A. S. Hornby* (pp. 149–165). Oxford: Oxford University Press.

MacWhinney, B. (2004). A multiple process solution to the logical problem of language acquisition. *Journal of Child Language, 31*(4), 883–914.

Marler, P. (1987). Sensitive periods and the role of specific and general sensory stimulation in birdsong learning. In J. P. Rauschecker & P. Marler (Eds.), *Imprinting and cortical plasticity* (pp. 99–135). New York: John Wiley & Sons.

Marler, P. (1998). Animal communication and human language. In G. Jablonski & L. C. Aiello (Eds.), *The origin and diversification of language*. Wattis Symposium Series in Anthropology (pp. 1–19). Memoirs of the California Academy of Sciences, No. 24, San Francisco, CA: California Academy of Sciences.

Marsden, C. D. (1982). The mysterious motor function of the basal ganglia: The Robert Wartenberg lecture. *Neurology, 32*(5), 514–539.

Martin, M. (1979). Hemispheric specialization for local and global processing. *Neuropsychologia, 17*(1), 33–40.

McGilchrist, I. (2009). *The master and his emissary: The divided brain and the making of the Western World.* New Haven, CT and London: Yale University Press.

McGuire, M., & Larson-Hall, J. (2017). Teaching formulaic sequences in the classroom: Effects on spoken fluency. *TESL Canada Journal, 34*(3), 1–25.

Michaelis, L. A. (2017). Constructions are patterns and so are fixed expressions. In B. Busse & R. Moehlig (Eds.), *Patterns in language and linguistics*. Berlin: Mouton de Gruyter.

Mieder, W. (1993). *Proverbs are never out of season: Popular wisdom in the modern age.* New York: Oxford University Press.

Mishkin, M., Malamut, B., & Bachevalier, J. (1984). Memories and habits: Two neural systems. In G. Lynch, J. L. McGaugh, & N. M. Weinberger (Eds.), *Neurobiology of learning and memory* (pp. 65–67). New York: The Guilford Press.

Monin, B. (2003). The warm glow heuristic: When liking leads to familiarity. *Journal of Personality and Social Psychology, 85*(6), 1035–1048.

Moon, R. E. (1998). *Fixed expressions and text: A study of the distribution and textual behaviour of fixed expressions in English.* Oxford studies in lexicology and lexicography. Oxford: Clarendon Press.

Moreland, R. L., & Zajonc, R. B. (1982). Exposure effects in person perception: Familiarity, similarity, and attraction. *Journal of Experimental Social Psychology, 18*(5), 395–415.

Müller, N., & Guendouzi, J. A. (2002). Transcribing discourse: Interactions with Alzheimer's disease. *Clinical Linguistics and Phonetics, 16*(5), 345–359.

Müller, N., & Guendouzi, J. A. (2005). Order and disorder in conversation: Encounters with dementia of the Alzheimer's type. *Clinical Linguistics and Phonetics, 19*(5), 393–404.

Nakagawa, Y., Tanabe, H., Ikeda, M., Kazui, H., Ito, K., Inoue, N., … Shiraishi, J. (1993). Completion phenomenon in transcortical sensory aphasia. *Behavioural Neurology, 6*(3), 135–142.

Neisser, U. (1976). *Cognition and reality: Principles and implications of cognitive psychology*. San Francisco, CA: W. H. Freeman & Co.

Norrick, N. R. (1985) *How proverbs mean: Semantic studies in English proverbs*. Mouton.

Nygaard, L. C., Sommers, M. S., & Pisoni, D. B. (1994). Speech perception as a talker-contingent process. *Psychological Science, 5*(1), 42–46.

Oktavianti, I. N., & Prayogi, I. (2022). Discourse functions of lexical bundles in Indonesian EFL learners argumentative essays: A corpus study. *Studies in English Language and Education, 9*(2), 61–83.

Osgood, C., & Hoosain, R. (1974). Salience of the word as a unit in the perception of language. *Perception and Psychophysics, 15*(1), 168–192.

Pagán Cánovas, C., & Antović, M. (2016). Formulaic creativity: Oral poetics and cognitive grammar. *Language and Communication, 47*, 66–74.

Page, D. L. (1959). *History and the Homeric Iliad*. Berkeley, CA: University of California Press.

Patel, A. D. (2008). *Music, language, and the brain.* Oxford: Oxford University Press.

Paul, R. (2004). Autism. In R. D. Kent (Ed.), *The MIT handbook of communication disorders*. Cambridge, MA: MIT Press.

Pawley, A. (2007). Developments in the study of formulaic language since 1970: A personal view. In P. Skandera (Ed.), *Phraseology and culture in English* (pp. 3–45). Berlin: Mouton de Gruyter.

Pawley, A., & Syder, F. H. (1983). Two puzzles for linguistic theory: Nativelike selection and nativelike fluency. In J. C. Richards & R. Schmidt (Eds.), *Language and communication* (pp. 191–225). London: Longman.

Peters, A. (1977). Language-learning strategies: Does the whole equal the sum of the parts? *Language, 53*(3), 560–573.

Peters, A. M. (1983). *The units of language acquisition*. Cambridge: Cambridge University Press.

Petrovici, J.-N. (1980). Speech disturbances following stereotaxic surgery in ventrolateral thalamus. *Neurosurgical Review, 3*(3), 189–195.

Pickens, J. D., & Pollio, H. R. (1979). Patterns of figurative language competence in adult speakers. *Psychological Research, 40*(3), 299–313.

Pinker, S. (1995). *The language instinct.* New York: Harper Collins.

Pisoni, D. B. (1993). Long-term memory in speech perception: Some new findings on talker variability, speaking rate and perceptual learning. *Speech Communication, 13*(1–2), 109–125.
Ploog, D. (1975). Vocal behavior and its 'localization' as prerequisite for speech. In K. J. Zülch, O. Creutzfeldt, & G. C. Galbraith (Eds.), *Cerebral localization*. Pp. 239-238. Berlin: Springer-Verlag.
Poljac, E., de-Wit, L., & Wagemans, J. (2012). Perceptual wholes can reduce the conscious accessibility of their parts. *Cognition, 123*(2), 308–312.
Prinz, P. M. (1983). The development of idiomatic meaning in children. *Language and Speech, 26*(3), 263–271.
Prizant, B. M. (1983). Language acquisition and communicative behavior in autism: Toward an understanding of the 'whole' of it. *Journal of Speech and Hearing Disorders, 48*(3), 296–307.
Rammell, C. S., Pisoni, D., & Van Lancker Sidtis, D. (2018). Perception of formulaic and novel expressions under acoustic degradation: Evidence for a unitary memory. *Mental Lexicon, 12*(2), 234–262.
Reuterskiöld, C., & Van Lancker Sidtis, D. (2013). Incidental learning of formulaic expressions. *Child Language Teaching and Therapy, 29*(2), 216–228.
Robinson, B. W. (1987). Limbic influences on human speech. *Annals of the New York Academy of Sciences, 280*, 761–771.
Ryding, E., Bradvik, B., & Ingvar, D. (1987). Changes of regional cerebral blood flow measured simultaneously in the right and left hemisphere during automatic speech and humming. *Brain, 110*(5), 1345–1358.
Schaltenbrand, G. (1965). The effects of stereotactic electrical stimulation in the depth of the brain. *Brain, 88*(4), 835–840.
Schmitt, N., Sonbul, S., Vilkaite-Lozdienė, L., & Macis, M. (2019). Formulaic language and collocation. In *The concise encyclopedia of applied linguistics*. Wiley-Blackwell.
Schweizer, B.-M. (1978). *Sprachspiel mit Idiomen: Eine Untersuchung am Prosawerk von Günter Grass*. Zürich: Juris Druk Verlag.
Shapiro, A., Shapiro, E., Bruun, R. D., & Sweet, K. D. (Eds.). (1983). *Gilles de la Tourette syndrome*. New York: Raven Press.
Sidtis, D., Canterucci, G., & Katsnelson, D. (2009). Effects of neurological damage on production of formulaic language. *Clinical Linguistics and Phonetics, 23*(15), 270–284. PMID: 19382014
Sidtis, J. J., Van Lancker Sidtis, D., Dhawan, V., & Eidelberg, D. (2018). Switching language modes: Complementary brain patterns for formulaic and propositional language. *Brain Connectivity, 8*(3), 189–196. Published online: April 1, 2018. https://doi.org/10.1089/brain.2017.0573.
Sidtis, D. (2021). *Foundations of familiar language: Formulaic expressions, lexical bundles, and collocations at work and play*. London: Wiley-Blackwell.
Sidtis, D., Canterucci, G., & Katsnelson, D. (2009). Effects of neurological damage on production of formulaic language. *Clinical Linguistics and Phonetics, 23*(15), 270–284.
Sidtis, D., Rogers, T., Katsnelson, D., & Sidtis, J. J. (2008). Effects in Parkinson's subjects ON vs OFF deep brain stimulation on overlearned and serial speech. Motor Speech Conference, March 6–9, Monterey, CA.
Sidtis, J. J. (2007). Some problems for representations of brain organization based on activation in functional imaging. *Brain and Language, 102*(2), 130–140.
Sidtis, J. J. (2012a). Performance-based connectivity analysis: A path to convergence with clinical studies. *NeuroImage, 59*(3), 2316–2321.
Sidtis, J. J. (2012b). What the speaking brain tells us about functional imaging. In M. Faust (Ed.), *Handbook of the neuropsychology of language* (Vol. 2, pp. 565–618). Malden, MA: Blackwell.
Sidtis, J. J. (2022). Cerebral blood flow is not a direct surrogate of behavior: Performance models suggest a role for functional meta-networks. *Frontiers in Neuroscience, 16*, 771594. https://doi.org/10.3389/fnins.2022.771594.
Sidtis, J. J., Strother, S. C., & Rottenberg, D. A. (2003). Predicting performance from functional imaging data: Methods matter. *NeuroImage, 20*(2), 615–624.
Sidtis, J. J., Van Lancker Sidtis, D., Dhawan, V., & Eidelberg, D. (2018). Switching language modes: Complementary brain patterns for formulaic and propositional language. *Brain Connectivity, 8*(3), 189–196. https://doi.org/10.1089/brain.2017.0573.
Simon, H. A. (1974). How big is a chunk? *Science, 183*(4124), 482–448.
Simon, H. A., Zhang, W., Zang, W., & Peng, R. (1989). STM capacity for Chinese words and idioms with visual and auditory presentations. In H. A. Simon (Ed.), *Models of thought, II* (pp. 68–75). New Haven, CT and London: Yale University Press.
Smolka, E., Rabanus, S., & Rösler, F. (2007). Processing verbs in German idioms: Evidence against the configuration hypothesis. *Metaphor and Symbol, 22*(3), 213–231.
Sorace, A., & Keller, F. (2005). Gradience in linguistic data. *Lingua, 115*(11), 1497–1524.
Speedie, L. J., Wertman, E., Tair, J., & Heilman, K. M. (1993). Disruption of automatic speech following a right basal ganglia lesion. *Neurology, 43*(9), 1768–1774.

Springer, S., & Deutsch, G. (2001). *Left brain, right brain* (5th ed.). W. H. Freeman and Company/Worth Publishers.
Sprenger, S. A. (2003). Fixed expressions and the production of idioms. Doctoral dissertation, University of Nijmegen.
Stahl, B., Gawron, B., Regenbrecht, F., Flöel, A., & Kotz, S. A. (2020). Formulaic language resources may help overcome difficulties in speech-motor planning after stroke. *PLOS One*.
Stahl, B., & Van Lancker Sidtis, D. (2015). Tapping into neural resources of communication: Formulaic language in aphasia therapy. *Frontiers in Psychology*, *6*, 1526.
Stephens, L. L. (1988). The role of memory in the relationship between affect and familiarity. *Cognition and Emotion*, *2*(4), 333–349.
Svartvik, J., & Quirk, R. (1980). *A corpus of English conversation*. Lund studies in English. Lund: CWK Gleerup.
Swinney, D. A., & Cutler, A. (1979). The access and processing of idiomatic expressions. *Journal of Verbal Learning and Verbal Behavior*, *18*(5), 523–534.
Tannen, D., & Öztek, P. C. (1981). Health to our mouths: Formulaic expressions in Turkish and Greek. In F. Coulmas (Ed.), *Conversational routine: Explorations in standardized communication situations and prepatterned speech* (pp. 37–57). The Hague: Mouton.
Thatcher, R. W., Walker, R. A., & Giudice, S. (1987). Human cerebral hemispheres develop at different rates and ages. *Science*, *236*(4805), 1110–1113. https://doi.org/10.1126/science.3576224.
Tilley, M. P. (1950). *A dictionary of proverbs in England in the 16th and 17th centuries*. Ann Arbor, MI: University of Michigan Press.
Titchener, E. G. (1916). *A textbook of psychology*. New York: MacMillan.
Titone, D. A., & Connine, C. M. (1999). On the compositional and noncompositional nature of idiomatic expressions. *Journal of Pragmatics*, *31*(12), 1655–1674.
Titone, D. A., & Libben, M. (2014). Time-dependent effects of decomposability, familiarity, and literal plausibility on idiom meaning activation: A cross-modal priming investigation. *Mental Lexicon*, *9*(3), 473–496.
Tomasello, M. (2003). *Constructing a language: A usage-based theory of language acquisition*. Cambridge, MA and London: Harvard University Press.
Tremblay, A., Derwing, B., Libben, G., & Westbury, C. (2011). Processing advantages of lexical bundles: Evidence from self-paced reading and sentence recall tasks. *Language Learning*, *61*(2), 569–613.
Uchihara, T., Eguchi, M., Clenton, J., Kyle, K., & Saito, K. (2022). To what extent is collocation knowledge associated with oral proficiency? A corpus-based approach to word association. *Language and Speech*, *65*(2), 311–336.
Ullman, M. T., Corkin, S., Coppola, M., Hickok, M., Growdon, J. H., Koroshetz, W. J., & Pinker, S. (1997). A neural dissociation within language: Evidence that the mental dictionary is part of declarative memory, and that grammatical rules are processed by the procedural system. *Journal of Cognitive Neuroscience*, *9*(2), 266–276.
Van Lancker, D. (1988). Nonpropositional speech: Neurolinguistic studies. In A. Ellis (Ed.), *Progress in the psychology of language* (pp. 49–118). Hillsdale, NJ: Lawrence Erlbaum.
Van Lancker, D. (1991). Personal relevance and the human right hemisphere. *Brain and Cognition*, *17*(1), 64–92.
Van Lancker, D., Bogen, J. E., & Canter, G. J. (1983). A case report of pathological rule- governed syllable intrusion. *Brain and Language*, *20*(1), 12–20.
Van Lancker, D., Canter, J., & Terbeek, D. (1981). Disambiguation of ditropic sentences: Acoustic and phonetic cues. *Journal of Speech and Hearing Research*, *24*(3), 330–335.
Van Lancker, D., & Cummings, J. (1999). Expletives: Neurolinguistic and neurobehavioral perspectives on swearing. *Brain Research Reviews*, *31*(1), 83–104.
Van Lancker, D., McIntosh, R., & Grafton, R. (2003). PET activation studies comparing two speech tasks widely used in surgical mapping. *Brain and Language*, *85*(2), 245–261.
Van Lancker Sidtis, D. (2001). Preserved formulaic expressions in a case of transcortical sensory aphasia compared to incidence in normal everyday speech. *Brain and Language*, *79*(1), 38–41.
Van Lancker Sidtis, D. (2004). When novel sentences spoken or heard for the first time in the history of the universe are not enough: Toward a dual-process model of language. *International Journal of Language and Communication Disorders*, *39*(1), 1–44.
Van Lancker Sidtis, D. (2006). Has neuroimaging solved the problems of neurolinguistics? *Brain and Language*, *98*(3), 276–290.
Van Lancker Sidtis, D. (2009). Formulaic and novel language in a 'dual process' model of language competence: Evidence from surveys, speech samples, and schemata. In R. L. Corrigan, E. A. Moravcsik, H. Ouali, & K. M. Wheatley (Eds.), *Formulaic language: Volume 2. Acquisition, loss, psychological reality, functional applications* (pp. 151–176). Amsterdam: Benjamins Publishing Co.

Van Lancker Sidtis, D. (2019). "Because it sounds right": A guiding light to speaker knowledge. *Studies in English Language Teaching*, 7(3).

Van Lancker Sidtis, D., Cameron, K., Bridges, K., & Sidtis, J. J. (2015). The formulaic schema in the minds of two generations of native speakers. *Ampersand*, *2*, 39–48.

Van Lancker Sidtis, D., Choi, J.-H., Alken, A., & Sidtis, J. J. (2016). Formulaic language in Parkinson's and Alzheimer's disease: Complementary effects of subcortical and cortical dysfunction. *Journal of Speech, Language, and Hearing Research*, *58*(5), 1493–1507.

Van Lancker Sidtis, D., Kougentakis, K., Cameron, K., Falconer, C., & Sidtis, J. J. (2012). "Down with ____": The schema as intermediary between formulaic and novel expressions. *International Journal of Phraseology*, *3*, 87–108. https://doi.org/10.1515/phras-2012-0005.

Van Lancker Sidtis, D., & Postman, W. A. (2006). Formulaic expressions in spontaneous speech of left- and right-hemisphere damaged subjects. *Aphasiology*, *20*(5), 411–426.

Van Lancker Sidtis, D., & Rallon, G. (2004). Tracking the incidence of formulaic expressions in everyday speech: Methods for classification and verification. *Language and Communication*, *24*(3), 207–240.

Van Lancker Sidtis, D., & Sidtis, J. J. (2018a). Cortical-subcortical production of formulaic language: A review of linguistic, brain disorder, and functional imaging studies leading to a production model. *Brain and Cognition*, *126*, 53–64.

Van Lancker Sidtis, D., & Sidtis, J. J. (2018b). The affective nature of formulaic language: A right-hemisphere subcortical process. *Frontiers in Neurology*. Published online July 14.

Van Lancker Sidtis, D., & Yang, S.-Y. (2016). Formulaic language performance in left- and right-hemisphere damaged patients: Structured testing. *Aphasiology*, *31*, 82–99.

Vaynshteyn, I., & Van Lancker Sidtis, D. (2019). Effects of age of arrival on acquisition of formulaic expressions in the second language. *Studies in English Language Teaching*, 7(4).

Vilkaitė, L. (2016). Formulaic language is not all the same: Comparing the frequency of idiomatic phrases, collocations, lexical bundles, and phrasal verbs. *Taikomoji kalbotyra* (8). www.taikomojikalbotyra.lt.

Whitaker, H. (1976). A case of the isolation of the language function. In H. Whitaker & H. A. Whitaker (Eds.), *Studies in neurolinguistics* (Vol. 2, pp. 1–58). London: Academic Press.

Wolf, R., Van Lancker Sidtis, D., & Sidtis, J. J. (2014). The ear craves the familiar: Pragmatic repetition in left and right cerebral damage. *Aphasiology*, *28*(5), 596–615.

Wray, A. (1998). Protolanguage as a holistic system for social interaction. *Language and Communication*, *18*(1), 47–67.

Wray, A. (2000). Holistic utterances in protolanguage: The link from primates to humans. In C. Knight, J. R. Hurford, & M. Studdert-Kennedy (Eds.), *The evolutionary emergence of language: Social function and the origins of linguistic form* (pp. 285–302). Cambridge: Cambridge University Press.

Wray, A. (2002). *Formulaic language and the lexicon*. Cambridge: Cambridge University Press.

Wray, A., & Grace, G. W. (2007). The consequences of talking to strangers: Evolutionary corollaries of socio-cultural influences on linguistic form. *Lingua*, *117*(3), 543–578.

Wray, A., & Perkins, M. (2000). The functions of formulaic language: An integrated model. *Language and Communication*, *20*(1), 1–28.

Yang, S. Y., Ahn, J.-S., & Van Lancker Sidtis, D. (2015). The perceptual and acoustic characteristics of Korean idiomatic and literal sentences. *Speech Language and Hearing*, *18*(3), 166–178. https://doi.org/10.1179/2050572814Y.0000000061.

Yang, S.-Y., Sidtis, D., & Yang, S.-N. (2016). Listeners' identification and evaluation of Korean idiomatic utterances produced by persons with left- or right-hemisphere damage. *Clinical Linguistics and Phonetics*, *31*(2), 155–173.

Yang, S.-Y., & Van Lancker Sidtis, D. (2016). Production of Korean idiomatic utterances following left- and right-hemisphere damage: Acoustic studies. *Journal of Speech, Language, and Hearing Research*, *59*(2).

Zanini, S., Tavano, A., & Fabbro, F. (2010). Spontaneous language production in bilingual Parkinson's disease patients: Evidence of greater phonological, morphological and syntactic impairments in native language. *Brain and Language*, *113*(2), 84–89.

13

RELEVANCE THEORY AND LANGUAGE INTERPRETATION

Nuala Ryder and Eeva Leinonen

Introduction

For many years now, there have been reports of children and adults with difficulties with how to use language in communication. The utterances produced are generally grammatically and semantically well-formed but do not always seem to fit the conversational context. Often the listener is unable to infer what the given utterance means in a particular conversational context because of the unusual and disconnected nature of the utterance. They can be described as not always having the necessary degree of relevance with regard to the ongoing topic. Speech and language therapists have been providing therapy for individuals whose difficulties seem to lie with the understanding and/or production of connected discourse rather than linguistic structures but it was not until the 1980s that researchers (McTear & Conti-Ramsden, 1992; Rapin & Allen, 1983) began to investigate such difficulties. First referred to as "semantic-pragmatic disorders" (Bishop & Rosenbloom, 1987; Rapin & Allen, 1998; Vance & Wells, 1994), they came to be known as "pragmatic language impairments," or "pragmatic impairment" (Bishop, 2000) to reflect the primary difficulties of using language in context. It is now recognized that pragmatic impairments are a likely reflection of some underlying cognitive and social impairments (Bishop, 2000; Brook & Bowler, 1992; Hays, Niven, Godfrey, & Linscott, 2004; Linscott, 2005) and exist across a range of diagnostic boundaries such as autistic spectrum disorder (ASD) and pervasive developmental disorder not otherwise specified (PPDNOS). The relationship of such impairments experienced by children and adults on the autistic continuum has been subject to much debate (Bishop, 2000; Botting & Conti-Ramsden, 1999; Brook & Bowler, 1992; Gagnon, Mottron, & Joanette, 1997) with the outcome that the term "pragmatic impairment" is best considered a descriptive tool rather than a diagnostic entity. However, there is general agreement that, especially in children, the identification of pragmatic language impairment is important in the consideration of appropriate therapeutic and educational needs (Bishop, 2002). The remediation of children with pragmatic language impairment (PLI) continues to form a significant part of the caseload of speech and language therapists (Adams, Lloyd, Aldred, & Baxendale, 2006).

Early investigations of pragmatic difficulties were based on conversational analysis approaches where conversations involving individuals with such difficulties were analyzed for various characteristics such as turn-taking, degree of coherence, and use of cohesive devices (Bishop, Chan, Adams, Hartley, & Weir, 2000). The common communicative behaviors were identified as strategies the children used to handle a failure to understand, and focused on language production rather than comprehension. These analyses provided a useful starting point but carried with them

DOI: 10.4324/9781003204213-15

problems associated with a lack of a rigorous theoretical framework that would generate testable predictions. Though expressive language was characterized by coherence and turn-taking, the comprehension abilities were undefined. It became clear that the cognitive nature of pragmatic understanding in relation to the social difficulties associated with inadequate pragmatic skills and weaknesses in communicative competence was needed (Shields, Varley, Broks, & Simpson, 1996). One cognitive pragmatic approach focused on speech acts defined these as simple (direct) versus complex (indirect) according to the number or chain of inferences necessary for understanding (Airenti, Bara, & Colombetti, 1993; Bara, Bosco, & Bucciarelli, 1999). Around this time, Sperber and Wilson's (1995) Relevance Theory (RT) was being recognized as a theory of communication that defined the processes necessary for language interpretation, and went some way to explaining the dynamic nature of the generation of inferences (based on context) and how linguistic and nonlinguistic meaning were interactively achieved.

Happé (1993, 1995) found the framework of RT useful in the investigation of pragmatic language understanding and theory of mind abilities in children with autism. Leinonen and Kerbel (1999) later explored children's impairment of pragmatic comprehension within an RT paradigm. Leinonen and Ryder furthered this research (Leinonen & Ryder, 2003; Ryder & Leinonen, 2003) and found the framework useful and robust for investigating both typical development and disorders of pragmatic functioning in both English-speaking and Finnish-speaking children (Loukusa et al., 2007). The use of a framework developed on the basis of this theory has enabled rigorous and testable hypotheses to be generated that in turn has advanced our ability to study pragmatic language functioning in both normal and disordered children in a solid and systematic way.

Relevance theory

Relevance theory (Sperber & Wilson, 1995) is a psychological theory of communication. It details the processes of meaning interpretation in communicative situations and lends itself to empirical investigation of language impairment, especially the use of language in communication. Relevance theory supports Grice's (1989) assertion that looking at language structure alone ignores the reality of the communicative situation, where the interpretation of meaning by the hearer often involves understanding more than the meaning of the words and inferences alone. Meaning in communication is said to be derived from the context in which the communication takes place. Utterances such as "He was late again" can be produced in different contexts with different meanings. The words themselves (linguistic form and syntax) are frequently underdetermined and much of the meaning intended by the speaker is derived from intonation, gesture, eye gaze, the physical environment, and the knowledge/experience of the hearer including that of similar communicative situations. This cognitive view suggests that often, in order to interpret intended meaning, the ability to integrate relevant information is necessary and RT details the processes facilitating this. Based on the assumptions of cognition, RT argues that humans have an inborn inferential ability and a cognitive system is geared toward the processing of relevant information (governed by a principle of relevance and logical operations). They develop the ability to draw implicated conclusions from this information often necessary in communicative situations. In communication, the speakers want to be understood and therefore make their utterances as easy as possible for the hearer to understand. This results in the hearer being able to recover the intended meaning with minimum processing effort and the most accessible interpretation is therefore the most relevant one.

Pragmatic processes

In RT's view, the processes of reference assignment, enrichment, disambiguation, and implicature facilitate successful interpretation. The first three of these processes are argued to require inferences based on context. Reference assignment is the assignment of the relevant referent intended by the speaker in a communicative exchange, such as the person or thing a pronoun is used to refer to. Disambiguation refers to the meaning derived from context via inference when the expressed word has multiple meanings. For example, "rich" can mean wealthy, fertile, or calorific depending on the context. Similarly, enrichment relates to the relevant semantic meaning based on the context. When a hearer comprehends the meaning of words uttered in communication, enrichment of the linguistic meaning with other aspects of meaning are needed to form a coherent conceptualization. Inferring the meaning of words such as "enough" or "nothing" vary according to the context in which they are used. In the context of going to a party, the words in the phrase "nothing to wear" are enriched together to mean "nothing suitable or that I want to wear" rather than "nothing at all to wear." The conceptual information in memory about having "nothing to wear" to events such as parties are accessed on hearing the utterance. To constrain the possibilities of all the possible inferences from the conceptual information overloading our interpretation process, an unconscious logical operator guides access to conceptual information and a principle of relevance constrains interpretation such that the first relevant interpretation is taken as the one meant. In utterances with ambiguous words and ambiguous contexts the wrong interpretation can be reached as can and does happen in normal communication. RT suggests that in addition to these inferential processes, a process of implicature is necessary. Implicatures are not inferred but are the result of a process of integrating previously generated inferences with perceptual information and knowledge as is necessary for interpreting the intended meaning. This process facilitates the understanding of meaning that is not inferable from the linguistic form and conceptual information alone. Implicatures are then the result of the combination of the inferences following from the linguistic form of an utterance and relevant contextual information. What determines whether some or all of these processes are necessary for a successful interpretation is the specificity of the utterance being interpreted (akin to how literally they can be interpreted). Utterances intended to be interpreted literally are relatively infrequent and do not necessitate recovering implicature(s). Most often in communication, the words uttered and their meanings have to be enriched and relevant contextual information integrated to understand the intended meaning. RT suggests that the result of integrating or combining information (implicated premises) leads to an implicated conclusion (an implicature). The interpretation of intended meaning reached via the process of implicature is therefore contextually based. Context in this sense refers to the information available to the hearer at the time of the interpretation including perceptual information (e.g., facial expression, gesture, nodding in the direction of something or someone), intonation, the words uttered, and knowledge and experiences in memory. Examples of meaning that depend on the generation of implicatures include the understanding of indirect answers to questions, of figurative language such as metaphor, irony, lies, sarcasm, and of understanding vague expressions.

It can be seen then that the more underdetermined a language expression, the more contextual information has to be processed (increasing cognitive effort) for comprehension. Increased cognitive effort is incurred when implicatures are recovered (unless they are very frequent or routinely processed in everyday communication). Therefore, this theory allows predictions in terms of complexity of a language expression. In RT, cognitive effort positively correlates with increased assumptions or contextual effects derived from the context necessary for successful understanding. For example, if the answer to the question "Do you know where the dog is?" is indirect as in "The back gate's open" then increased cognitive effort is incurred as the interpretation gives rise to the implication that the dog may have gone out of the gate. Whereas, a direct answer such as "It's behind the shed" does not give rise to these implications and therefore cognitive effort in interpretation is decreased. Therefore, understanding a language expression that requires inferencing (reference assignment, enrichment, disambiguation) is less demanding in terms of cognitive effort than language expressions that necessitate recovery of implicature(s). However, it is important to note that these processes are not suggested to be linear.

RT therefore lends itself to empirical investigation of the processes involved in the comprehension of language, the validity of the notion of cognitive effort (the path of least effort to successfully process the utterance) or of communicative competence and the nature of the development of pragmatic language comprehension. It provides a comprehensive account of how underdetermined language expressions can be interpreted in context. The theory has been utilized in the investigation of the notion of complexity of pragmatic language understanding in autism (Happé, 1995; Loukusa et al., 2007), in patients with right hemisphere lesions and TBI (Dipper, Bryan, & Tyson, 1997; McDonald, 1999), in young typically developing children (Papafragou & Tantalou, 2004; Ryder & Leinonen, 2003), in children with specific language impairment (SLI), and in children with PLI (Leinonen & Ryder, 2003; Ryder, Leinonen, & Schulz, 2008).

Pragmatic language comprehension

Bridging inferences and right hemisphere brain injury

Research into communicative disorders of patients with right hemisphere damage (RHD) suggests that they can have impaired pragmatic language abilities. Dipper et al. (1997) investigated the reduced ability of patients with RHD to draw correct inferences from texts using an RT approach. Dipper and colleagues noted that when answering questions based on a story, patients with RHD did not use the context of the story in their answers, but were able to justify their answers. The justifications revealed that the RHD participants did not appear to be aware of the contextual information but were relying on world knowledge (from memory) generating semantically related inferences rather than utilizing the story context. Dipper et al. (1997) proposed that RT provided a way of investigating the reasons for these incorrect answers. Six stroke patients with a single neurological episode resulting in unilateral RHD participated (aged 31–74 years) and there were 12 age-matched controls. The experimenters based the study on RT's predictions regarding an unconscious logical deductive system said to operate on linguistic input and the notion that concepts consist of addresses in memory that give rise to logical (e.g., or, either), encyclopedic (cutting your finger makes it bleed, etc.), and lexical information (syntactical and grammatical information). When words are heard or seen, an automatic process of meaning retrieval accesses the appropriate concept address. The participants listened and read two sentence scenarios and answered three question types that targeted three types of bridging inference. The first (textual inference) required utilizing linguistic input in order to answer correctly. The second (textually reinforced inference) targeted information generated by discourse connectives where the contextually generated inference does not require accessing encyclopedic information (RT suggests that discourse connectives are procedural and do not have encyclopedic entries). The third inference required encyclopedic information to answer correctly.

Findings revealed that RHD participants performed less well than controls on all inference types. This group relied on encyclopedic information and questions targeting linguistic deduction were problematic for this group, particularly discourse connectives. Dipper et al. (1997) suggest that if RT's view of the procedural and nonencyclopedic nature of discourse connective concepts is correct, then the brain damage suffered by RHD patients affects the deductive device. Utilizing linguistic context to infer intended meaning is therefore affected. They suggest that this inability to use linguistic information from the text in the deductive system, was coupled with an over-reliance on encyclopedic information (not a preferential use of encyclopedic information). It is interesting to note that in typically developing four- and five-year-old children a tendency to use their own experiential knowledge of events (rather than the information in the story) was found when answering questions requiring semantic inferencing (enrichment) in context (Ryder & Leinonen, 2003). In a similar way to the answers given by RHD patients, the ability to utilize the relevant given context was implicated.

Sarcasm and traumatic brain injury

As mentioned, complexity in pragmatic language understanding is dependent on the cognitive effort involved in combining relevant information from context. The interpretation of irony and sarcasm, for example, is effortful in the sense that an additional recognition of the speaker's emotion or intentions is required for interpretation. In patients with traumatic brain injury (TBI) difficulties in understanding sarcasm are well-documented (McDonald, 1999). Often these patients interpret sarcastic utterances literally (where a literal interpretation is possible). McDonald (1999, p. 489) investigated the understanding of sarcasm in patients with TBI using RT to examine more closely the nature of the difficulty. In utterances such as "A lovely day for a picnic indeed" the interpretation depends on the hearer recognizing the echoed proposition from previously shared knowledge. That is, if previously it was suggested that it was a lovely day for a picnic and it was now cold or raining, the speaker's utterance echoes the previous utterance. Relevance theory suggests the understanding of sarcasm requires inferences about both the facts of the situation and of the mental state of the speaker (attitudes, knowledge, and intentions). In the same way that other linguistic expressions are interpreted, linguistic and contextual features are integrated but RT suggests that sarcastic comments additionally echo a prior assertion, and this echo communicates the speaker's derogatory attitude. Patients with TBI have been shown to be better able to interpret literal sarcastic utterances than when the sarcastic utterances were intended to mean the opposite of what was said (McDonald & Pearce, 1996). Patients watched videotapes of the interaction between two people and conversations included utterances that were sincerely meant or were sarcastic. In some cases, understanding the emotion of the speaker was necessary to understand that the literal utterance was not intended (the speaker does not mean what they say) but if this was not recognized a literal meaning could be comprehended. For example, patients were asked whether the speaker in saying "Sorry I made you come" was pleased that he made his addressee come. In another variation, the speaker's utterance could not be understood literally; that is, the speaker asked the hearer if they remembered their passport and the hearer replied saying they had torn it up and thrown it away. Patients were also asked questions about the emotions of the speaker. Findings suggested that the patients had no appreciable difficulty in understanding literal utterances or the emotional tone of the speaker. They performed poorly (failed to understand sarcasm) in these verbal exchanges, particularly when no literal interpretation was possible. McDonald suggests the patients' ability to understand sarcasm was independent of their ability to comprehend emotional tone and the difficulty lay in inferential reasoning of verbal information. In his review of studies of patients with TBI, McDonald notes that patients with TBI performed better when interpreting physically presented counterfactual sarcastic comments than verbally presented counterfactual comments. This suggests that these patients can utilize relevant visual information from context, but have particular difficulty when this information is verbal. According to McDonald (1999), RT's account of interpretation is well-founded with the exception of the notion of comprehending scornful echo. The patients with TBI were able to understand the literal meaning suggesting that they comprehended the previous assumption (and they were able to understand the speaker's emotion), but still they were unable to interpret the sarcastic intent. McDonald points out that studies (Kaplan, Brownell, Jacobs, & Gardner, 1990; McDonald & Pearce, 1996) have shown that even when the speaker's attitude is explicit (rather than inferred) patients with TBI still did not recognize the sarcastic intent. Therefore, a mentalizing ability is suggested to be crucial.

Mentalizing and autism

In a study by Happé (1993), RT's predictions of complexity of processing and notion of attributing mental states to others (understanding communicative intention) were used to examine the communicative competence of children and adults with autism (aged 9–28 years old) and children and adults with mild learning disabilities (aged 12–38 years). The participants answered questions targeting similes, metaphors, and irony. Based on RT, similes were suggested to require less processing than metaphors whereas irony was the most complex to process because of the necessity of attributing mental states to others. The ability to understand figurative language (sarcasm, metaphor, irony) develops gradually from the age of five in typically developing children (Laval & Bert-Erboul, 2005). However, in children and adults with autism this development is not seen and in addition the ability to understand other's intentions (suggested to be key in communication) and to integrate contextual information such as knowledge of the hearer during communication, appears either delayed or deviant. Happé (1993, 1995) found that in children with autism, the ability to understand the intentions of others was directly associated with the comprehension of pragmatically demanding figurative language such as metaphor and irony. There were underlying differences in the mentalizing ability of the two groups with autism, which mediated false-belief performance and utterance comprehension. Findings supported relevance theory's predictions regarding the increasing degree of mind necessary for understanding simile, metaphor, and irony.

The development of pragmatic language comprehension

Dipper et al. (1997) focused on the inferential and conceptual claims of RT whereas McDonald (1999) and Happé (1995) focused on the notion of increased cognitive effort or more pragmatically demanding language expressions in relation to communication difficulties. Another approach used to investigate the use of context in pragmatic language understanding (and hence the notion of pragmatic complexity) focuses on the processes suggested to be involved in pragmatic language comprehension. These have been used to investigate the pragmatic language abilities of children with high functioning autism (HFA), Asperger syndrome (AS), SLI, and PLI. Children with autism and AS have difficulties in social interaction suggested to be linked to problems in attributing mental states to others or recognizing others' intentions. They often interpret language expressions literally. Relevance theory's outline of pragmatic language understanding suggests that understanding the intention of the speaker is linked to an inherent ability to infer, to attend to relevant information, and to process implicatures. Children with SLI have been suggested to have some problems with inferencing (Botting & Adams, 2005) and a subgroup of children with PLI have similar but more marked difficulties. Relevance theory suggests that inferencing is only one process in language understanding and this ability is necessary to assign referents (e.g., assigning meaning to pronouns) and to enrich semantic meaning in context (as in disambiguation). These processes, particularly pronoun resolution, are common in everyday communication. RT suggests that frequency can lead to automaticity of processing, which is facilitated by a logical deductive device (see Sperber & Wilson, 1995 for details). Thus, the development of pronoun resolution or reference assignment occurs early in language development (around the age of three) and is suggested to be a relatively automatic process compared to inferring semantic meaning or enriching meaning in context (loosening, broadening, or disambiguating meaning), which continues to develop between the ages of three and five. Examples of reference assignment and enrichment can be seen in the following example.

Speaker A: Jane worked hard in her aerobic class.
Speaker B: The wedding's in six weeks.

In this example "Jane" is assigned to the person known as Jane to both speakers (reference assignment) and "worked hard" is enriched to mean exercising most energetically and not other meanings of "work" and "hard" that are not relevant in this context. The understanding of Speaker A's utterance is not dependent on the recovery of an implicature. Comprehension of the intended meaning of Speaker B's utterance is not achieved by inferring referents and enriching meaning alone. For speaker A to recover the meaning of "Jane is working hard at aerobics because she wants to look good at the forthcoming wedding," further processing is necessary. When the intended meaning is not recoverable from inferencing alone as in this example, previous relevant inferences, knowledge from memory, and perceptual information combine to yield implicatures. Intonation, facial expression, and world knowledge (including knowledge of these kinds of exchanges) are part of the contextual information the hearer uses to recover the intended meaning. RT suggests that this process incurs increased cognitive effort compared to the solely inferential processes of reference assignment and enrichment. Therefore, increased pragmatic demands may be associated with each of these processes (reference assignment < enrichment < implicature).

Leinonen and Kerbel (1999) explored data from three children with language impairment. The characteristic features of pragmatic impairment were examined within the RT framework. The processes detailed in RT were found to be useful in interpreting the difficulties. Communication breakdown could be attributed to difficulties in enriching meaning and in understanding implicatures. In production, the children's use of pronouns instead of naming the referent was suggested to reflect difficulty with relevance in relation to reference assignment. The seemingly irrelevant answers of the children in different communicative situations revealed that the children sometimes answered when they did not know what a word meant and on explanation of the word could then answer correctly. The children sometimes knew the meaning of a word but had difficulty in disambiguating or enriching the meaning in context. For example, interpreting "hole" (in the context of planting trees) to mean a place where you put a treasure rather than a hole to plant a tree in. This interpretation was arrived at despite having discussed the context of the picture beforehand (workmen in the park using spades to dig holes, the trees ready for planting). Interpreting the children's utterance within RT's framework was suggested to be clinically useful and shows the importance of understanding the language abilities of the child in order to decide on how best to communicate meaning.

In line with RT's view of cognitive processes and cognitive effort, studies using questions targeting reference assignment, enrichment, and implicatures have supported the notion of increased pragmatic language demands of the question types, in particular those targeting implicature. A developmental trend was evident in young children when answering the three question types (based on stories or scenarios) in both English and Finnish children (Loukusa et al., 2007; Ryder & Leinonen, 2003; Ryder, Leinonen, & Schulz, 2008). Three-year-old English children were unable to answer questions targeting implicatures, a finding that was also found in Finnish three-year-olds except when answering implicature questions based on very familiar daily routines, for example, interpreting "it's dinner time" to mean a request to go inside and get ready to have dinner. At the age of four both English and Finnish children were competent at enriching semantic meaning. Although this ability is still developing and by the age of five, children were found to be still developing the ability to recover implicatures (competence is evident by the age of seven). The wrong answers of the four-year-olds suggest that these children tend to rely on their world knowledge when they did not recover the intended implicature. For example, they would use their own knowledge of going to a birthday party rather than the information about the birthday party given in the story context. Three-year-olds also used world knowledge but most frequently produced answers that were irrelevant in the given context (Ryder & Leinonen, 2003).

Comparing the typically developing children (Ryder & Leinonen, 2003) to children with SLI, a further study by Leinonen and Ryder (2003) found the children with SLI performed less well than their peers. Children with SLI are a heterogeneous group presenting with various structural language deficits. Bates (2004, p. 249) suggests the deficits in SLI manifest themselves as a result of problems in the cognitive domain during development. In this study the children with SLI performed similarly to the typically developing four-year-olds when enriching semantic meaning and generating implicatures suggesting delayed language development.

The pragmatic comprehension of a subgroup of children with SLI who had difficulties with pragmatic language understanding (whose primary difficulties are with pragmatic language meaning in the absence of autistic spectrum symptoms) was recently investigated (Ryder et al., 2008). The children, aged 7–11 years, perform significantly below their peers and children with SLI without pragmatic impairment, when answering questions targeting implicature(s) based on verbal scenarios and stories. The children with PLI could be identified from the rest of the SLI group on their performance on questions targeting implicatures. These children had particular difficulty in using the given verbal context (scenario or story). All groups were competent at reference assignment and had no appreciable difficulties on the whole with enriching semantic meaning, but wrong answers revealed that the children tended to use world knowledge in preference to the context when incorrectly answering. The tasks in the study included verbal input with and without pictures. In the with-picture task where the answer was available in the picture, the children with SLI performed similarly to their peers when answering questions targeting implicatures. However, when pictures were not available and the input was verbal only, these children appear significantly delayed in understanding implicatures. The children with PLI performed worst of all on this task, a finding that was not explained by their structural language or auditory memory abilities. RT's framework was useful in examining the role of context in interpretation and highlights the interactive nature of meaning in interpretation.

Loukusa et al. (2007) carried out a similar study of Finnish children. Typically developing Finnish children were compared with children with AS and HFA. The reference assignment, enrichment, and implicature questions in this study were asked on the basis of verbal scenarios. The youngest children with AS/HFA (seven- to nine-year-olds) had some difficulties in answering questions targeting enrichment but this was not evident in the older (10 to 12-year-old) group. However, both groups were found to have significant difficulties with questions targeting implicatures (Loukusa et al., 2007) compared to typically developing children. This finding, taken with Happé's findings (1993, 1995) indicates the difficulty in understanding implicatures as being a core deficit in children and adults in autism affecting the ability to interpret metaphor and other language expressions requiring the generation of implicatures.

The studies discussed, taken together, show that the clinical groups were competent at reference assignment (resolution of pronouns, assigning referents), a process that develops relatively early in language development as seen in the typically developing children (English and Finnish) who were competent at the age of three to four years and by the age of six were competent at enriching semantic meaning.

Summary and conclusions

There had been comparatively little progress in the understanding of the nature of pragmatic language abilities compared to structural language abilities largely because of a need for a theoretical framework. RT has provided a framework with which to investigate the nature of language comprehension in disordered populations including details of the processes that may be impaired and the prediction of cognitive effort involved in communicative utterances. The studies discussed have supported RT's notion of pragmatic complexity and language development. It has also shown that instances of pragmatic language breakdown can be explained and predicted by this theory.

Relevance theory has provided testable predictions about language impairment and the kinds of language behavior that children and adults with communication difficulties may exhibit. It has enabled us to move away from a description of the communication behaviors to a better understanding of pragmatic language difficulties including why they result in difficulties in communication and their effects on the quality of conversational interactions. RT may provide a useful tool for addressing the issue of the assessment of PLI, given that the interpretation of implicature was found to be problematic in children and adults with pragmatic language difficulties. The findings that individuals with PLI often produce irrelevant utterances/answers as do very young children (three-year-olds) suggests that the processing involved in integrating contextual information or utilizing relevant context is implicated. RT maintains that humans cannot help but interpret the relevant meaning. However, in development children may stop processing at the first relevant interpretation because they have not yet developed the ability (or do not have the knowledge) to fully interpret the speaker's perspective. It is not clear how children develop this ability, though it may be the experience of interacting and conversing that provides the knowledge that they can then use in interpretation. On this view, children with PLI might lack this knowledge because of different experiences with language use during development. However, there is currently little data to support this and more research is needed. The data from typically developing children suggests that the development of the ability to recover implicatures occurs between the ages of four and seven years and therefore early intervention would be recommended. We have found that using this theoretical framework is useful in suggesting ways of facilitating interactions with pragmatically impaired individuals for example, consideration of the conceptual properties of words in relation to the context, and the context itself. The consequences of both the specificity of the verbal information used in tasks and the perceptual information/materials have consequences that ought to be considered in the assessment process.

The research has largely supported the psychological validity of the theory, but further research is necessary to validate the notion of relevance. Some also refute RT's view of an unconscious deductive device operating on linguistic input and consequent automatic conceptual access said to occur during enrichment (Cummings, 1998). Similarly, McDonald (1999) casts doubt on RT's notion of scornful echo as an explanation for the comprehension of sarcasm.

The data from the studies of patients with TBI was not consistent with this explanation. However, these theoretical considerations do not alter the contribution of the theory in focusing attention on other factors besides language structure that are important in the assessment of language and communication disorders.

RT's view of communication demonstrates both the responsibilities of the speaker and the limitations of the hearer in the interactional process. The studies have shown how individuals are responsible for communicative success or breakdown and how interaction in communication is facilitated. When breakdown occurs in communication, repair depends on knowledge of the hearer's language difficulties and their developmental level. These observations have important implications for therapy in the clinical setting. Difficulties with utilizing relevant context or integrating information from both the context and memory may be addressed in the clinical setting by encouraging our understanding of how the context is relevant to the interpretation. Within this framework, it is possible to explore the language of those engaging with language-impaired children and consider what kinds of contributions may be most facilitative.

"The influence of relevance theory has spread … contributing to cognitive sciences … the emergent domain of experimental pragmatics … it was, after all, originally conceived as a model of communication and cognition" (Wharton, Jagoe, & Wilson, 2022, p.1)

Further reading

Gabbatore, I., Bosco, F. M., Mäkinen, L., Leinonen, E., & Loukusa, S. (2021). Social-pragmatic contextual comprehension in Italian preschool and school-aged children: A study using the Pragma test. *Intercultural Pragmatics*, *18*(2), 131–162.

Kotila, A., Hyvärinen, A., Mäkinen, L., Leinonen, E., Hurtig, T., Ebeling, H., … Loukusa, S. (2020). Processing of pragmatic communication in ASD: A video-based brain imaging study. *Scientific Reports*, *10*(1), Art. 21739.

Loukusa, S., Mäkinen, L., Gabbatore, I., Laukkanen-Nevala, P., & Leinonen, E. (2017). Understanding contextual and social meaning in typically developing Finnish-speaking four- to eight-year-old children. *Psychology of Language and Communication*, *21*(1), 408–428.

Loukusa, S., Mäkinen, L., Kuusikko-Gauffin, S., Ebeling, H., & Leinonen, E. (2018). Assessing social-pragmatic inferencing skills in children with autism spectrum disorder. *Journal of Communication Disorders, 73*, 91–105.

References

Adams, C., Lloyd, J., Aldred, C., & Baxendale, T. (2006). Exploring the effects of communication intervention for developmental pragmatic language impairments: A signal-generation study. *International Journal of Language and Communication Disorders, 41*(1), 41–65.

Airenti, G., Bara, B. G., & Colombetti, M. (1993). Failures, exploitations and deceits in communication. *Journal of Pragmatics, 20*(4), 303–326.

Bara, B. G., Bosco, F. M., & Bucciarelli, M. (1999). Developmental pragmatics in normal and abnormal children. *Brain and Language, 68*(3), 507–528.

Bates, E. A. (2004). Explaining and interpreting deficits in language development across clinical groups: Where do we go from here? *Brain and Language, 88*(2), 248–253.

Bishop, D.V. M. (2000). Pragmatic language impairment: A correlate of SLI, a distinct subgroup, or part of the autistic continuum? In D.V. M. Bishop & L. B. Leonard (Eds.), *Speech and language impairments in children: Causes, characteristics, intervention and outcome* (pp. 99–114). Hove: Psychology Press.

Bishop, D.V. M. (2002). Speech and language difficulties. In M. Rutter & E. A. Taylor (Eds.), *Child and adolescent psychiatry* (pp. 782–802). London: Blackwell.

Bishop, D.V. M., Chan, J., Adams, C., Hartley, J., & Weir, F. (2000). Conversational responsiveness in specific language impairment: Evidence of disproportionate pragmatic difficulties in a subset of children. *Development and Psychopathology, 12*(2), 177–199.

Bishop, D. V. M., & Rosenbloom, L. (1987). Classification of childhood language disorders. In W. Yule & M. Rutter (Eds.), *Language development and disorders* (pp. 61–81). London: Mac Keith Press.

Botting, N., & Adams, C. (2005). Semantic and inferencing abilities in children with communication disorders. *International Journal of Language and Communication Disorders, 4*(1), 49–66.

Botting, N., & Conti-Ramsden, G. (1999). Pragmatic language impairment without autism: The children in question. *Autism, 3*(4), 371–396.

Brook, S. L., & Bowler, D. (1992). "Autism by another name?" Semantic and pragmatic impairments in children. *Journal of Autism and Developmental Disorders, 22*(1), 61–81.

Cummings, L. (1998). The scientific reductionism of relevance theory: The lesson from logical positivism. *Journal of Pragmatics, 29*(1), 1–12.

Dipper, L. T., Bryan, K. L., & Tyson, J. (1997). Bridging inference and relevance theory: An account of right hemisphere inference. *Clinical Linguistics and Phonetics, 11*(3), 213–228.

Gagnon, L., Mottron, L., & Joanette, Y. (1997). Questioning the validity of the semantic-pragmatic syndrome diagnosis. *Autism, 1*(1), 37–55.

Grice, H. P. (1989). *Studies in the way of words*. Cambridge, MA: Harvard University Press.

Happé, F. G. E. (1993). Communicative competence and theory of mind in autism: A test of relevance theory. *Cognition, 48*(2), 101–119.

Happé, F. G. E. (1995). Understanding minds and metaphors: Insights from the study of figurative language in autism. *Metaphor and Symbol, 10*(4), 275–295.

Hays, S. J., Niven, B. E., Godfrey, H. P. D., & Linscott, R. J. (2004). Clinical assessment of pragmatic language impairment: A generalizability study of older people with Alzheimer's disease. *Aphasiology, 18*(8), 693–714.

Kaplan, J. A., Brownell, H. H., Jacobs, J. R., & Gardner, H. (1990). The effects of right hemisphere brain damage on the pragmatic interpretation of conversational remarks. *Brain and Language, 38*(2), 315–333.

Laval, V., & Bert-Erboul, A. (2005). French-speaking children's understanding of sarcasm: The role of intonation and context. *Journal of Speech, Language, and Hearing Research, 48*(3), 610–620.

Leinonen, E., & Kerbel, D. (1999). Relevance theory and pragmatic impairment. *International Journal of Language and Communication Disorders, 34*(4), 367–390.

Leinonen, E., & Ryder, N. (2003). The use of context in pragmatic comprehension by specifically language-impaired and control children. *Linguistics, 41*(2), 407–423.

Linscott, R. J. (2005). Thought disorder, pragmatic language impairment, and generalized cognitive decline in schizophrenia. *Schizophrenia Research, 75*(2–3), 225–232.

Loukusa, S., Leinonen, E., Kuusikko, S., Jussila, K., Mattila, M. L., Ryder, N., … Moilanen, I. (2007). Use of context in pragmatic language comprehension by children with Asperger syndrome or high-functioning autism. *Journal of Autism and Developmental Disorders, 37*(6), 1049–1059.

McDonald, S. (1999). Exploring the process of inference generation in sarcasm: A review of normal and clinical studies. *Brain and Language, 68*(3), 486–506.

McDonald, S., & Pearce, S. (1996). Clinical insights into pragmatic language theory: The case of sarcasm. *Brain and Language, 53*(1), 81–104.

McTear, M., & Conti-Ramsden, G. (1992). *Pragmatic disability in children.* London: Whurr.

Papafragou, A., & Tantalou, N. (2004). Children's computation of implicatures. *Language Acquisition, 12*(1), 71–82.

Rapin, I., & Allen, D. (1983). Developmental language disorders: Nosologic considerations. In U. Kirk (Ed.), *Neuropsychology of language, reading, and spelling* (pp. 155–184). New York: Academic Press.

Rapin, I., & Allen, D. A. (1998). The semantic-pragmatic deficit disorder: Classification issues. *International Journal of Language and Communication Disorders, 33*(1), 82–87.

Ryder, N., & Leinonen, E. (2003). Use of context in question answering by 3-, 4- and 5-year-old children. *Journal of Psycholinguistic Research, 32*(4), 397–415.

Ryder, N., Leinonen, E., & Schulz, J. (2008). A cognitive approach to assessing pragmatic language comprehension in children with specific language impairment. *International Journal of Language and Communication Disorders, 43*(4), 427–447.

Shields, J., Varley, R., Broks, P., & Simpson, A. (1996). Social cognition in developmental language disorders and high level autism. *Developmental Medicine and Child Neurology, 38*(6), 487–495.

Sperber, D., & Wilson, D. (1995). *Relevance: Communication and cognition* (2nd ed.). Oxford: Blackwell.

Vance, M., & Wells, B. (1994). The wrong end of the stick: Language-impaired children's understanding of non-literal language. *Child Language Teaching and Therapy, 10*(1), 23–46.

Wharton, T., Jagoe, C., & Wilson, D. (2022). Relevance theory: New horizons Foreword by Tim Wharton, Caroline Jagoe and Deirdre Wilson. *Journal of Pragmatics, 194*, 1–5.

14

HOW SIMILARITY INFLUENCES WORD RECOGNITION

The effect of neighbors

Mark Yates and Devin Dickinson

Introduction

One of the most researched topics in cognitive psychology has been the study of single-word recognition (Balota, Cortese, Sergent-Marshall, Spieler, & Yap, 2004). Of this research, one issue that has received considerable attention is how word processing is affected by orthographic and phonological similarity. The impetus for much of this research has been the predictions made by models of word recognition as to how similarity should influence word processing. A particular class of models that has been extremely influential along these lines are models that are characterized by *interactive activation and competition* (IAC). Models that embody the assumptions of IAC are among some of the oldest models in psycholinguistics (e.g., McClelland & Elman, 1986; McClelland & Rumelhart, 1981; Rumelhart & McClelland, 1982). IAC models consist of multiple hierarchical levels that are interconnected with excitatory and/or inhibitory connections. Within each level are nodes denoting the representation that is processed at that level (e.g., whole words or letters).

The seminal interactive activation model of McClelland and Rumelhart (1981) provides a good example of an IAC model. The interactive activation model was designed to explain letter perception and to provide an account of the word superiority effect (Reicher, 1969; Wheeler, 1970). The model consists of a visual feature level, letter level, and word level. The feature level feeds excitatory and inhibitory activation to the letter level. Likewise, the letter level passes both types of activation to the word level. For instance, if the node for the letter *L* occurring in the first position becomes active, it will increase the activation of any words beginning with the letter *L* (e.g., *LOVE*), and at the same time, it will inhibit the activation of any words *not* containing the letter *L* in the first position (e.g., *MAST*). Additionally, the word level feeds back activation, both excitatory and inhibitory, to the letter level. This means that as the word *LOVE* becomes active it will increase the activation of the *L* node and inhibit the other letter nodes. Finally, there are within level inhibitory connections in both the letter and word levels, meaning as a word or letter becomes active it tries to inhibit all other letters or words.

Given the current interest in IAC models and their predictions regarding the influence of similarity on word recognition, there are two goals of this chapter. The first is to review how orthographic and phonological similarity have been used to better understand both written and spoken word recognition. Specifically, we will focus on the effect of *neighbors*. There are various ways of determining whether two words are neighbors, but in general, a neighbor is simply a word that is like the target word in terms of spelling (i.e., an orthographic neighbor) or sound (i.e., a phono-

DOI: 10.4324/9781003204213-16

logical neighbor). The second goal of this chapter is to explain the effects of neighbors within the context of models that have an IAC architecture. Although this chapter will concentrate on IAC models, this should not be taken as an indication that other types of models could not account for these effects. Another class of model that is common in word recognition are those that employ some type of learning algorithm (e.g., Harm & Seidenberg, 2004; Plaut, McClelland, Seidenberg, & Patterson, 1996; Seidenberg & McClelland, 1989), and some researchers have argued that these models can account for effects of similarity better than IAC models (Sears, Hino, & Lupker, 1995). Nevertheless, the reason for concentrating this chapter on IAC models is because these models have been studied extensively in relation to similarity effects.

Orthographic neighborhood

Orthographic neighbors were initially studied in relation to visual word recognition. As detailed below, exactly how orthographic neighbors influence processing has been a matter of some debate. Interestingly, in recent research, orthographic neighbors have been shown to influence auditory word recognition as well. In this section, we will cover the research dealing with orthographic neighborhood effects on both visual and auditory word recognition and relate this research to IAC models.

Orthographic neighborhood effects on visual word recognition

The origins of orthographic neighborhood research can be traced to the work of Landauer and Streeter (1973) who reported that frequent words tended to have more orthographic neighbors than infrequent words. Two words are defined as neighbors if they have the same number of letters and differ by one letter substitution. For example, *gate* and *game* are orthographic neighbors. Although Landauer and Streeter were the first to discuss orthographic neighbors, it was the work of Coltheart and colleagues (Coltheart, Davelaar, Jonasson, & Besner, 1977) that really sparked interest in the idea and led to a flurry of orthographic neighborhood studies. In fact, orthographic neighborhood is commonly referred to as Coltheart's N. Interestingly, Coltheart et al. (1977) failed to find an effect of orthographic neighborhood on lexical decisions to words. While Coltheart et al. (1977) failed to find an effect, subsequent research has shown that the size of the orthographic neighborhood is an important determinant of word recognition. The first researcher to do so was Andrews (1989) who demonstrated that words with a dense orthographic neighborhood (i.e., words having many neighbors) were verified more rapidly in a lexical decision task than were words having a sparse neighborhood (i.e., words with few neighbors). However, Andrew's results were quickly called into question by Grainger and Segui (1990) who noted that Andrew's stimuli were confounded with bigram frequency. To counter this criticism, Andrews (1992) showed that orthographic neighborhood facilitated lexical decisions even when bigram frequency was controlled. Later research in the area produced inconsistent results. Some researchers reported a facilitative effect of orthographic neighborhood density on lexical decisions (Balota et al., 2004; Forster & Shen, 1996; Huntsman & Lima, 2002; Sears et al., 1995), whereas others reported an inhibitory effect (Johnson & Pugh, 1994). It is worth noting that Johnson and Pugh's research differed from the other studies because their stimuli were blocked by orthographic neighborhood size. This means that participants saw all the high neighborhood words together in one block of trials and all small neighborhood words together in another block. As this experiment is the only one showing an inhibitory effect of orthographic neighborhood size, it seems likely that the inhibitory effect of orthographic neighborhood can be attributed to strategic factors that are employed when the words are blocked according to neighborhood size (Andrews, 1997).

An even more contentious issue is the nature of orthographic neighborhood frequency on lexical decisions. Grainger, O'Regan, Jacobs, and Segui (1989) demonstrated that words having at least one higher frequency neighbor were responded to more slowly than words without any higher frequency neighbors. Subsequent research also showed an inhibitory effect (Carreiras, Perea, & Grainger, 1997; Grainger, 1990; Grainger, O'Regan, Jacobs, & Segui, 1992; Huntsman & Lima, 1996; Perea & Pollatsek, 1998). Complicating matters, however, was additional research showing that orthographic neighborhood frequency facilitated lexical decisions, rather than inhibiting them (Sears et al., 1995). Unfortunately, it is not entirely clear why there is this discrepancy between the results generated from different labs, though at least two explanations have been suggested. One has to do with the different languages used in the various studies. Experiments demonstrating facilitation have been conducted with English words, whereas those reporting inhibition have typically used other languages (Andrews, 1997). One interesting hypothesis for this discrepancy is that English word recognition is more influenced by body neighbors (i.e., the vowel plus remaining consonants) and that body neighbors have a facilitative effect on processing (Ziegler & Perry, 1998). However, for other languages, body neighbors do not affect processing to the same degree as in English, and as such, inhibitory effects emerge in these languages. The second potential reason for the equivocal pattern of orthographic neighborhood results has to do with the confounding of orthographic neighborhood and phonological neighborhood (Yates, Locker, & Simpson, 2004). In visual word recognition, phonological neighbors are defined as two words that differ by one *phoneme* substitution. For example, *gate* has *bait* and *game* as two of its neighbors. Because a one letter change is often the same as a one phoneme change (cf. *gate* and *game*), many neighbors that are orthographic neighbors will also be phonological neighbors. Yates et al. (2004) showed that past studies investigating orthographic neighborhood have been significantly confounded with phonological neighborhood, making it difficult to tell exactly what the effect of orthographic neighborhood really is. In fact, there is some evidence that when phonological neighborhood is controlled there is no effect of orthographic neighborhood on visual word recognition (Mulatti, Reynolds, & Besner, 2006).

In contrast to the debate regarding the influence of orthographic neighbors on lexical decisions, their influence in the naming task appears to be relatively straightforward. In the naming task, participants are shown a word on the screen and are asked to name the word as rapidly as possible. The primary measure from this task is the latency between the onset of the stimulus and the onset of acoustic energy. Using the naming task, researchers have shown that orthographic neighborhood density facilitates responding (Andrews, 1989, 1992; Balota et al., 2004; Carreiras et al., 1997; Grainger, 1990; Peereman & Content, 1995; Sears et al., 1995). Likewise, the research seems to indicate that orthographic neighborhood frequency also facilitates naming (Grainger, 1990; Sears et al., 1995, but see Carreiras et al., 1997).

To be sure, much of the orthographic neighborhood research has been conducted using the lexical decision and naming tasks. However, some have argued that these tasks are not ideal because they do not necessarily require word identification before giving a response, and it would be more appropriate to use a task that requires lexical selection before a response is given (Forster & Shen, 1996). Two such tasks are perceptual identification and semantic categorization. There are several different perceptual identification tasks that have been used in orthographic neighborhood research. The common aspect to all of them is that they require the participant to identity the word when it is shown in a degraded form (e.g., masked). In the semantic categorization task, participants are asked to decide if a word belongs to some semantic category (e.g., is it an animal). The results from these tasks are mixed. Using the perceptual identification task, some researchers have reported inhibitory effects of neighborhood density and frequency (Carreiras et al., 1997; Grainger, 1990; Grainger & Jacobs, 1996; Snodgrass & Mintzer, 1993), whereas others have reported facilitation (Sears, Lupker, & Hino, 1999; Snodgrass & Mintzer, 1993). For the semantic categorization task, there have been reports of inhibitory (Carreiras et al., 1997), facilitative (Sears et al., 1999), and null (Forster & Shen, 1996) effects of orthographic neighbors. As was the case for lexical decision, it is not clear why the results from these studies are so divergent, but the explanations given above in relation to the lexical decision data may also be relevant in explaining the discrepancy in the perceptual identification and semantic categorization data.

An extension of the original interactive activation model known as the Multiple Read-Out Model (MROM) (Grainger & Jacobs, 1996) has been applied extensively to the study of orthographic neighborhood effects. In the MROM there are multiple ways that a response can be produced. In terms of lexical decisions, one way the model can make a response is when the activation level of an orthographic whole word node reaches a criterion value referred to as the *M* criterion (Grainger & Jacobs, 1996). The second way that a lexical decision can be made is determined by the Σ criterion. Using this criterion, a response is made based on the total summed orthographic activation. Finally, a nonword response is given if neither the *M* nor Σ has occurred before a given amount of time has transpired. The amount of time that must elapse before a nonword response is referred to as the *T* criterion.

In the MROM as the letter nodes receive activation from the feature level they will increase the activation for the whole word orthographic nodes with which they are consistent. The result of this is that the target word's activation at the lexical level will increase. In addition, the target word's orthographic neighbors' nodes will also receive activation due to the shared overlap at the letter level. To give an example, consider the word *drop* that has as one of its neighbors the word *prop*. When the letter nodes for *d*, *r*, *o*, and *p* become active they will all increase the activation of the *drop* node at the lexical level. The nodes corresponding to the letters *r*, *o*, and *p* will also increase the activation for the orthographic neighbor *prop*, but the *d* node will provide inhibition to the *prop* node. An interesting aspect of the MROM model is that it makes specific predictions about how orthographic neighbors should affect processing. If the Σ criterion is used, the orthographic neighbors should facilitate lexical decisions as the orthographic neighbors would help to increase the amount of summed orthographic activation. On the other hand, if the lexical decision is made based on the *M* criterion, then orthographic neighbors, particularly those higher in frequency, would slow responding because they would slow the accumulation of activation for the target word through lateral inhibition.

In the MROM, the *M* criterion is fixed and cannot be adjusted. Conversely, the Σ and *T* criteria are under strategic control. If Σ is set low, then responses will be made based on the summed orthographic activation, but if Σ is set high, responses will be based on the *M* criterion. This means unique word identification must occur before a response is given. In the lexical decision task, one factor that determines the value of the Σ criterion is the nonword environment. When the nonwords are easy (i.e., they are low in wordlikeness), then the Σ criterion can be set low and unique word identification need not occur to give a response. The reason the Σ criterion can be set low is because nonwords low in wordlikeness will create minimal activation within the orthographic lexicon. Consequently, summed orthographic activation is sufficient for the model to distinguish words and nonwords. On the other hand, if the nonwords are hard (i.e., they are high in wordlikeness), then the Σ criterion will need to be adjusted upward and lexical decisions will rely on the *M* criterion. In support of these predictions, Grainger and Jacobs (1996) showed that the facilitative effect of orthographic neighborhood size was only evident in the presence of easy nonwords. Interestingly, a similar conclusion was reached by Andrews (1989) who found a significant facilitative effect of orthographic neighborhood density by items only in the presence of easy nonwords. In terms of neighborhood frequency, Grainger and Jacobs (1996) showed that the MROM model could successfully simulate both the inhibitory effect reported by Grainger and Segui (1990) and the facilitative effect reported by Sears et al. (1995). This lead Grainger and Jacobs to conclude that the neighborhood frequency effect can range from inhibition to facilitation and what determines the nature of the effect is how low the Σ criterion is set.

The MROM has been fairly successful in explaining orthographic neighborhood effects in the lexical decision task, and it is clear that the ability to adjust the Σ criterion is responsible for the model's success. However, in other tasks where only the *M* criterion can be used, the model has had difficulty. For instance, in perceptual identification and semantic categorization tasks it is assumed that unique word identification must occur. For the MROM, this means a response can only be given once an orthographic word node exceeds the *M* criterion. The prediction from the MROM in this case is straightforward. Orthographic neighbors should slow responding because they will inhibit the accumulation of activation for the target word. Unfortunately, this has not always been the case. As mentioned above, there have been reports of facilitative effects of orthographic neighborhood density and orthographic neighborhood frequency in both perceptual identification and semantic categorization tasks, and this has led some to claim that the MROM overestimates the impact of inhibition on visual word recognition (Sears, Campbell, & Lupker, 2006; Siakaluk, Sears, & Lupker, 2002). Others have noted that it is possible for models with an interactive activation framework, such as the MROM, to simulate facilitative effects of orthographic neighbors by increasing the facilitation between the letter and word levels to offset the lateral inhibition within the word level (Andrews, 1997). Increasing the facilitation between the two levels means that as the neighbors became active they also increase the activation of their constituent letters through feedback activation to the letter level. As these letters are also shared with the target word, the letters in the target word increase in activation. This leads to an increase in activation at the word level for the target word node, allowing it to be identified more rapidly. Thus, it is possible to simulate either inhibitory or facilitative effects of orthographic neighbors as a function of the tradeoff between within level inhibition and between level excitation, and as result, it can be argued that these types of models are too powerful (Andrews, 1992).

Another model that should be discussed in relation to orthographic neighborhood effects on visual word recognition is the dual-route cascaded (DRC) model of Coltheart and colleagues (Coltheart, Rastle, Perry, Langdon, & Ziegler, 2001). The DRC model has primarily been applied to simulating data from the naming task. According to the model, there are two ways that a word can be named. One way is through a sublexical pathway that involves mapping letters to phonemes according to a set of rules. The other pathway is a lexical pathway that incorporates the assumptions of IAC. Both pathways pass activation to a shared phoneme system that consists of a series of phoneme units. A word is said to have been named once a phoneme unit within each of the positions in the phoneme system have reached some criterion.

In relation to orthographic neighborhoods, the lexical pathway of the DRC model has received the most attention, so it is worth describing in more detail. As in the original interactive activation model (McClelland & Rumelhart, 1981), the first part of the lexical pathway of the DRC model consists of a set of visual feature units that are connected to a letter level which in turn is connected to an orthographic whole word lexicon. Additionally, the orthographic lexicon is attached to a phonological lexicon that consists of whole word phonological units. Finally, the phonological lexicon passes activation to the shared phoneme system. Thus, as a node in the orthographic lexicon becomes activated, it increases the activation of its corresponding phonological node in the phonological lexicon, which in turn increases the activation level of its constituent phonemes. Using the standard parameter set from Coltheart et al. (2001), the DRC model was unable to simulate the facilitative effect of orthographic neighbors on naming, but Coltheart et al. did show that the DRC model could simulate the effect when the within level inhibition was turned off in the orthographic and phonological lexicons and the letter to word inhibition was reduced. Unfortunately, using this modified parameter set, the model failed to simulate effects that it had previously been able to simulate, such as nonword reading (Coltheart et al., 2001). Clearly more work is needed to provide a satisfactory account of how orthographic neighborhood affects visual word naming.

Orthographic neighborhood effects on spoken word recognition

Research demonstrating an effect of orthography on spoken word processing is not new. Early work by Seidenberg and Tanenhaus (1979) showed that participants were slower in a rhyme detection task when two words had different orthographic bodies (e.g., *rye* and *tie*) than when they had the same orthographic bodies (e.g., *pie* and *tie*). However, the interest in the role of orthography on spoken word recognition has increased dramatically. Leading this surge was a study by Ziegler and Ferrand (1998) showing that feedback consistency affects auditory lexical decisions. Feedback consistency refers to the reliability with which a word's phonological rime maps on its orthographic body. A word is considered feedback consistent if its rime can only be spelled one way (e.g., /-ɪmp/ is only spelled *–imp*). If a word's rime can be spelled more than one way, then it is said to be feedback inconsistent (e.g., /-eɪt/ can be spelled *–ate* and *–ait*.) There have now been numerous studies showing that words that are feedback inconsistent are responded to more slowly than are words that are feedback consistent (Pattamadilok, Morais, Ventura, & Kolinsky, 2007; Ventura, Morais, & Kolinsky, 2007; Ziegler, Ferrand, & Montant, 2004; Ziegler, Petrova, & Ferrand, 2008). Furthermore, it has been shown that the feedback consistency effect on auditory word recognition is not present for those without sufficient reading experience (Ventura et al., 2007; Ziegler & Muneaux, 2007), suggesting that the effect is truly orthographic in nature.

In terms of orthographic neighbors, the consensus of the few studies that have examined this variable in relation to auditory word recognition indicate that words with large orthographic neighborhoods are responded to more rapidly than are words with small orthographic neighborhoods (Ziegler & Muneaux, 2007; Ziegler, Muneaux, & Grainger, 2003). Using the bimodal interactive activation model (Grainger & Ferrand, 1994, 1996), Ziegler et al. (2003) showed that this effect can be explained as a consistency effect. The bimodal interactive activation model is based on the work of the original interactive activation model (McClelland & Rumelhart, 1981). The model contains two sublexical (one orthographic and one phonological) and two lexical (one orthographic and one phonological) levels. These levels are connected with excitatory connections, and the lexical levels contain lateral inhibitory connections. In more recent forms of the model, there is a central interface that converts orthography to phonology (e.g., letters to phonemes) and phonology to orthography (e.g., phonemes to letters). By having both phonological and orthographic processing systems, the model has the desirable property of making predictions about both spoken and written word recognition, as well as being able to account for cross modality neighborhood effects.

In the bimodal interactive activation model, when a spoken word is presented to the model it will first activate the phonological sublexical units. Next, it will pass activation to the phonological lexicon. Additionally, activation from the sublexical phonological units will activate their corresponding orthographic sublexical units, leading to an increase in activation within the orthographic lexicon for the target word even though the input is phonological. Importantly, not only will the target word's node become active within the orthographic lexicon, but the word's orthographic neighbors will also receive activation as they share all but one letter with the target word. Thus, in the bimodal interactive activation model, when the input is auditory, both the orthographic and phonological neighbors receive activation. The same is true when the input is visual.

On the face of it, it would seem that the bimodal interactive activation would have trouble explaining a facilitative effect of orthographic neighborhood as the within level inhibition in the orthographic lexicon would lead to inhibition for the target word from its orthographic neighbors. However, Ziegler et al. (2003) state that the effect is being driven by sublexical consistency and not lexical processing. They argue that words with few orthographic neighbors have an atypical orthographic pattern, and as a result, the link between phonology and orthography is weak for these words. For words with many orthographic neighbors, the link between phonology and orthography is stronger. Consequently, words with few orthographic neighbors will take longer to process due to the increased phonological-orthographic inconsistency. There are two findings that lend credence to this account. First, as previously mentioned, there have been numerous studies indicating that feedback consistency affects auditory word recognition. Second, when consistency was regressed out, the effect of orthographic neighborhood was no longer significant (Ziegler et al.,

2003). This indicates that it is not the neighborhood size that matters, but rather feedback consistency is what is important.

Regardless of whether the orthographic neighborhood effect arises from neighbors or feedback consistency, the critical point is that the effect provides strong support for the assertion that orthography influences auditory word recognition. As virtually all models of auditory word recognition do not include orthographic representations, the finding of orthographic effects on auditory word recognition represents one of the most difficult challenges for these models (Ziegler et al., 2008). Exactly how these models will answer this challenge is unclear at this time.

Phonological neighborhood

Phonological neighborhood research began in the area of auditory word recognition and later was extended to visual word recognition. As will be discussed below, the effect of phonological neighborhood is relatively consistent within the two modalities, although the direction of the effect reverses as a function of input modality. It should be noted that there have been different ways of defining phonological neighbors. In auditory word recognition research, neighbors are typically defined as words differing by one phoneme substitution, deletion, or addition, whereas in visual word recognition research, neighbors are defined as words that differ by one phoneme substitution. The reason for defining phonological neighbors this way in visual word recognition is to make the measure congruent with past research on orthographic neighborhood. The two ways of defining neighbors are obviously highly correlated and should lead to similar measures of neighborhood structure.

Phonological neighborhood effects on auditory word recognition

There have been many studies of how phonological neighbors influence spoken word recognition and the data clearly indicate that phonological neighborhood density and phonological neighborhood frequency inhibit auditory word recognition (Goldinger, 1989; Goldinger, Luce, & Pisoni, 1989; Luce, 1986; Luce & Pisoni, 1998; Luce, Pisoni, & Goldinger, 1990; Vitevitch & Luce, 1998, 1999). Furthermore, this inhibitory effect has been found using a number of different tasks including lexical decision, perceptual identification, and auditory naming. In line with the finding that phonological neighbors slow auditory word processing, essentially all models of spoken word recognition assume that neighbors compete for activation in some manner.

One of the first IAC models of spoken word recognition was the TRACE model (McClelland, 1991; McClelland & Elman, 1986). In similar fashion to the interactive activation model of visual word recognition, the TRACE model contains three hierarchical levels. The first is a phonetic feature level that is directly connected to a phoneme level that is in turn connected to a level containing whole word phonological nodes. There are excitatory connections between levels, and within the phoneme and word level there are inhibitory connections. In addition, as auditory word recognition naturally has a temporal component, each unit at the three levels is repeated across multiple time slices. This temporal component means that the between level excitatory connections only extend to units that are in the same or neighboring time slices. Likewise, the inhibitory connections between units will be strongest when they overlap closely in time and nonexistent if there is no temporal overlap.

When a word is first presented to the model, the feature detectors in the first time slice will become active and propagate activation to the phoneme level and then to the word level. As more of the utterance becomes available, activation for subsequent time slices will be computed based on the input pattern at that point in time as well as activation resulting from previous time slices. Word recognition is assumed to occur based on readout from the word level (McClelland & Elman, 1986).

In terms of phonological neighborhood, it is the within level inhibitory connections that account for the effect. As the model is presented with a word, the initial phoneme of the target word will become active via bottom-up activation from the feature level. This phoneme will likewise begin to pass activation to every word with which it is congruent. This means that every word beginning with this phoneme will receive activation early in processing. As more of the utterance becomes available, words that do not match the input will be inhibited by words that do. For words that have many phonological neighbors, there will be increased inhibition from the neighborhood, resulting in slower processing for these words.

The account given by TRACE is not the only account for the neighborhood effect. Indeed, virtually all models of spoken word recognition hold that similar sounding words interfere with recognition, although in quite different ways. Therefore, it is worth considering another way of explaining the neighborhood effect. One model that is particularly relevant to neighborhood effects is the neighborhood activation model (NAM; Luce & Pisoni, 1998).

According to NAM, when a word is encountered it will activate a pattern of acoustic-phonetic information. This acoustic-phonetic information then activates a set of word decision units that are congruent with the acoustic-phonetic activation. Once activated, a word decision unit monitors not only the acoustic-phonetic information with which it corresponds but also higher-level lexical information (e.g., frequency) that pertains to the particular word it represents. Furthermore, the word decision units monitor the overall level of activation in the word decision system. Word recognition occurs when one of the word decision units reaches a recognition criterion. During word processing, the word decision units compute decision values based on a decision rule where decision values decrease as neighborhood size increases. Because of this, NAM correctly predicts that phonological neighbors should hinder target word processing. It is important to note that both TRACE and NAM predict inhibitory effects of phonological neighbors, but for different reasons. In TRACE, the inhibitory effect exists because neighbors actively inhibit one another. In NAM, on the other hand, the inhibitory effect arises because neighbors raise the overall level of activity within the decision system, and this has the result of lowering the decision values, which slows responding.

One related effect that has proven difficult for NAM to explain is the effect of phonotactic probability. Phonotactic probability refers to the frequency of the phonetic segments in a word and is positively correlated with neighborhood density. Research has shown that *nonwords* that are high density/high phonotactic probability are processed more rapidly than are nonwords than are low density/low phonotactic probability. The opposite is true for words (Vitevitch & Luce, 1998, 1999). Vitevitch and Luce (1998) argue that when nonwords are processed there is no lexical representation for the stimuli, and as a result, sublexical processing dominates, leading to a facilitative effect. However, when the stimuli are words any sublexical facilitation is squelched by the competition at the lexical level, leading to an inhibitory effect. It is the facilitative effect for nonwords that is problematic for NAM as it predicts that stimuli with large neighborhoods should be processed more slowly (Vitevitch & Luce, 1999). Additionally, NAM suffers from the fact that it does not include a sublexical level, and therefore, cannot accommodate the effect of phonotactic probability. The architecture of the TRACE model is more in agreement with the data in that it contains lexical and sublexical levels. However, there have been no formal simulations of the effect, and it is not clear that the model could simulate the data given that Vitevitch and Luce (1999) have argued that sublexical and lexical processing need to be independent to explain the effects.

Because of the limitations with models such as NAM and TRACE, Vitevitch and Luce (1999) chose to discuss their results in terms of Grossberg's adaptive resonance theory (ART) of speech perception (Grossberg, 1986; Grossberg, Boardman, & Cohen, 1997; Grossberg & Myers, 2000). Within the ART framework, there are two levels of processing. In the first level, the incoming phonetic signal is mapped onto phoneme items in working memory. The second level is a short-term memory that consists of list chunks of different sizes (e.g., phonemes, syllables, whole word, etc.) representing different combinations of the items in working memory. The items in working memory are connected with bidirectional excitatory links to the list chunks in short-term memory. Within short-term memory, list chunks equal in size are connected with inhibitory connections (i.e., all words are connected, all syllables are connected, etc.). Also, larger list chunks in short-term memory can inhibit smaller list chunks (a process referred to as masking). For example, words mask syllables and syllables mask phonemes. When presented with a word, the items in working memory excite the list chunks that contain them. In turn, the active list chunks then send feedback to the items in working memory. As processing continues a resonance emerges between the list chunks and the items that support them. It is this resonance that gives rise to perception.

In terms of phonological neighborhood density, when a word chunk gets activated, it will receive inhibition from its phonological neighbors. It will take longer for the chunks of words with many neighbors to overcome this inhibition and establish a resonance with the items in working memory. Furthermore, for word processing, the largest chunks that will be activated are the word chunks, and these will mask all smaller chunks, removing any effect of phonotactic probability. However, when nonwords are processed, the largest chunks that will be become active are smaller than the word chunks. Consequently, the resonance between the chunks in short-term memory and the items in working memory will be driven by phonotactic probability and not density (Vitevitch & Luce, 1999). Thus, the ART framework seems capable of explaining the opposite effects of phonological neighborhood density and phonotactic probability, and the key to its ability to do so is that processing is driven by the properties of the longest chunks that become strongly activated. Although Vitevitch and Luce (1999) only discuss their effects in terms of a verbal description of ART, recent work has shown that ARTphone, a computational model based on the ART framework, can simulate the Vitevitch and Luce data (Pitt, Myung, & Altteri, 2007).

Phonological neighborhood effects on visual word recognition

As detailed in the preceding section, there is a rich history on the effect of phonological neighborhood on auditory word recognition, but in terms of visual word recognition, phonological neighborhood has only recently begun to receive attention. Interestingly, one of the first studies failed to find an effect of phonological neighborhood density on nonword naming (Peereman & Content, 1997). However, later research has shown that phonological neighborhood density facilitates visual word recognition in the lexical decision, naming, and semantic categorization tasks (Mulatti et al., 2006; Yates, 2005; Yates et al., 2004). There has been one report indicating that phonological neighbors may inhibit processing. Grainger, Muneaux, Farioli, and Ziegler (2005) crossed orthographic and phonological neighborhood density in a factorial design. Their results indicated that for words with few orthographic neighbors, phonological neighborhood had an inhibitory effect, but for words with large orthographic neighborhoods, the effect of phonological neighborhood was facilitative. They explained this interaction in terms of cross-code consistency within the bimodal interactive activation model. Cross-code consistency refers to whether activation within the phonological and orthographic systems is consistent. Any inconsistency between these systems will slow processing. For example, the word *bait* has some phonological neighbors that are not orthographic neighbors (e.g., *gate*, *hate*, and *bake*). Thus, the activation of these words within the phonological system will be inconsistent with activation in the orthographic system. Grainger et al. argued that words with orthographic and phonological neighborhoods that are similar in size (e.g., both large or both small) should be more cross-code consistent while words where one neighborhood is large and the other small should be more cross-code inconsistent. This means for words with small orthographic neighborhoods as the phonological neighborhood size *increases* so does the cross-code inconsistency. The result is slower responses to words with many phonological neighbors. For words with large orthographic neighborhoods, increasing the number of phonological neighbors *decreases* the cross-code inconsistency, leading to faster responses to words with many phonological neighbors.

The cross-code consistency account is intriguing, but it does not seem capable of explaining some of the facilitative effects seen in other studies. For example, using words controlled on measures of cross-code consistency (i.e., feedback and feedforward consistency), both Yates (2005) and Mulatti et al. (2006) found that phonological neighbors facilitated word recognition. One potential difference between these studies is that Grainger et al. (2005) used French words, and Yates and Mulatti et al. used English words. It is also worth noting that Peereman and Content's (1997) study that failed to find an effect of phonological neighborhood on word naming consisted of French stimuli. It is not clear why (or if) language is a determining factor in the nature of the phonological neighborhood effect.

In terms of the facilitative effect of phonological neighborhood density on English word naming, Yates (2005) argued that phonological neighbors increase the activation levels of the target word's phonemes through interactive activation between the lexical and sublexical levels. More recently it has been shown that what is important is not the number of neighbors per se but instead it is the number of neighbors for the least supported phoneme (LSP) that matters (Yates, Friend, & Ploetz, 2008; Yates, 2010). The LSP is defined as the phoneme within a word that receives the least amount of support from the word's phonological neighbors. For example, the word *geese* has the following words as neighbors: *cease, lease, niece, piece, gas, goose*, and *guess*. For the word *geese* the first phoneme /g/ is the LSP as it overlaps with the fewest phonological neighbors. As the LSP receives the least support, it should take longer to reach threshold than the other phonemes in the word that benefit from additional neighbor overlap. In word naming, it is assumed that the pronunciation for a word cannot be initiated until the complete phonological code has been determined (Rastle, Harrington, Coltheart, & Palethorpe, 2000). This means that the pronunciation of a word can only be as fast as the amount of time it takes the slowest phoneme (i.e., the LSP) to reach threshold. Yates et al. showed that words with large phonological neighborhoods tended to have more neighbors for their LSP than did words with small phonological neighborhoods. Moreover, they showed that the data from the naming experiments of Yates (2005) and Mulatti et al. (2006) could be explained in terms of the LSP and argued that the important variable was not the overall neighborhood density but was instead the number of neighbors for the LSP. Words with many neighbors overlapping with their LSP are named more rapidly than are words with few neighbors overlapping with their LSP. This claim was subsequently verified with simulations using a modification of the DRC model (Yates, 2010).

Individual differences

There have been numerous studies that have looked at how individual differences influence visual and auditory word recognition from a developmental perspective. However, more recently, there has been an interest in how individual differences in skilled readers influences visual word recognition. It is this work that we turn to now as it relates to the influence of similarity on word recognition.

Perfetti's Lexical Quality Hypothesis (LQH) argues that readers differ in terms of the quality of their lexical representations (Perfetti & Hart, 2002). As such, the LQH makes the prediction that individual differences will influence the word recognition process. In a reader with well specified lexical representations, the orthographic, phonological, and semantic constituents of words are fully specified and tightly coupled. As a result, the visual input to the reading system will be able to activate the correct representation with little competition from other representations. The net result is that readers with high quality lexical representations can more easily and quickly decode lexical stimuli.

Work by Sally Andrews and colleagues (Andrews & Hersch, 2010; Andrews & Lo, 2012) has found clear support for the predictions of the LQH. Their initial work using the masked priming paradigm showed that better spellers showed inhibitory priming from orthographic neighbors while poorer spellers showed facilitative priming (Andrews & Hersch, 2010). Readers with well specified orthographic representations (i.e., better spellers) can activate the prime to a level that it provides competition to the target. Readers with less well specified orthographic representations (i.e., poorer spellers) do not activate the prime sufficiently to provide competition. Instead, they benefit from sublexical activation provided from the prime as seen by the facilitative priming effect.

Subsequent research investigated the influence of lexicality (i.e., word vs. nonword) of orthographically similar primes (Andrews & Lo, 2012). They used both orthographic neighbors and transposed letter primes (i.e., *calm* as a prime for *clam*) as orthographically similar primes. The results show that participants scoring high on a factor that captured reading, vocabulary, and spelling ability (i.e., a proficiency factor) showed larger inhibitory priming when primes were words, but facilitation when the primes were nonwords. This indicates that participants with well specified representations can rapidly process the prime and benefit from the prime/target orthographic overlap, provided the prime is nonword. If, however, the prime is an orthographically similar word this rapid prime processing results in competition with the target word manifesting as an inhibitory priming effect, particularly for transposed letter primes. Finally, they found that participants who were better spellers than would be expected based on their reading/vocabulary scores were particularly likely to show inhibitory word priming effects. Whereas participants who had higher reading/vocabulary scores than would be expected based on their spelling scores were more likely to show stronger faciliatory priming by nonwords.

To investigate whether the influence of phonological similarity on visual word recognition is moderated by spelling ability, Yates and Slattery (2019) compared lexical decisions to words varying on phonological neighborhood spread. Phonological spread refers to how many phoneme positions in a word can be changed to form a neighbor and is denoted by the letter P. An example of a P = 3 word is *dish* as all three phoneme positions can be changed to form a word (e.g., *fish*, *dash*, and *dill*). On the other hand, *chill* is a P = 2 word as there is no neighbor that can be formed by changing the /ɪ/ phoneme. Previous research has shown that P = 3 words are responded to more rapidly in a lexical decision task than are P = 2 words (Yates, 2009). Research from Yates and Slattery (2019) showed larger phonological spread effects when spelling recognition (i.e., being able to recognize if a letter string correctly spells a word) was high and spelling production (i.e., ability to correctly spell a word presented auditorily) was low. To explain these opposing effects, we argued for a model in which there are separate orthographic systems for reading (measured by spelling recognition) and spelling (measured by spelling production) that communicate through a shared response buffer (Jones & Rawson, 2016). Our results showed that the quality of the orthographic connections in both systems influences phonological processing, albeit in different ways.

Taken together, the results of the research on individual differences indicates that the assumption skilled readers read alike is more myth than fact. These findings are also problematic for many computational models that employ IAC as they assume the quality of the representations is identical for all readers. The research on individual differences indicates that this assumption is incorrect, and these models need to be modified to account for effects of individual differences.

Summary and conclusions

As detailed throughout this chapter there is a rich history of studying how similarity among representations stored in memory affects word recognition. One of the most common ways of explaining these effects is in terms of IAC models. However, from the beginning, some of the research on similarity has proven difficult for these models to handle. Most notably are the facilitative effects of neighbors as most IAC models would, on the surface, seem to predict inhibition due to lateral inhibition from their neighbors. Nevertheless, researchers have shown that it is possible for models that employ interactive activation to produce facilitative effects by either reducing the influence of inhibitory connections and/or increasing the influence of facilitatory connections (Andrews, 1997; Mulatti et al., 2006; Yates et al., 2008; Yates, 2010). Unfortunately, when the models are modified in this manner, they lose the ability to explain other word recognition effects such as nonword naming (Coltheart et al., 2001). Also from a model standpoint, the study of neighborhoods has also brought to light a fundamental problem that is present in nearly all models of spoken word recognition. Specifically, they do not contain orthographic representations. The finding that orthographic neighbors, or more specifically feedback consistency, affect auditory word recognition poses a serious challenge for these models (Ziegler et al., 2008). Any model that claims to be a complete account of spoken word processing will need to include orthographic representations, just as models of visual word recognition include phonological representations.

Finally, throughout this chapter we have defined similarity in terms of neighbors. Historically this has been the most common way of defining similarity. Nevertheless, this is not the only or necessarily the best way to do so. For instance, research has shown that visual word recognition is influenced by words that share transposed letters (e.g., salt/slat, Andrews, 1996) and neighbors that are formed by deleting a letter (e.g., tablet/table, Davis & Taft, 2005). Although these words are clearly similar, they would not be considered neighbors using the conventions of Coltheart et al (1977). Additionally, others have argued that defining orthographic similarity in terms of Levenshtein distance (i.e., the minimum number of substitutions, insertions, or deletions needed to change one letter string to another) provides a better account of the lexical decision and naming data (Yarkoni, Balota, & Yap, 2008). Clearly there is still much work to be done in determining the best way(s) to define similarity, and as this research progresses, it should prove invaluable in helping to further refine our understanding of the role of orthography and phonology on word recognition.

Further reading

Caselli, N. K., Emmorey, K., & Cohen-Goldberg, A. M. (2021). The signed mental lexicon: Effects of phonological neighborhood density, iconicity, and childhood language experience. *Journal of Memory and Language, 121*, 104282.

Karimi, H., & Diaz, M. (2020). When phonological neighborhood density both facilitates and impedes: Age of acquisition and name agreement interact with phonological neighborhood during word production. *Memory and Cognition, 48*(6), 1061–1072.

Yates, M., Shelley-Tremblay, J., & Knapp, D. L. (2020). Measuring the influence of phonological neighborhood on visual word recognition with the N400: Evidence for semantic scaffolding. *Brain and Language, 211*, 104866.

References

Andrews, S. (1989). Frequency and neighborhood effects on lexical access: Activation or search? *Journal of Experimental Psychology: Learning, Memory, and Cognition, 15*(5), 802–814.

Andrews, S. (1992). Frequency and neighborhood effects on lexical access: Lexical similarity or orthographic redundancy? *Journal of Experimental Psychology: Learning, Memory, and Cognition, 18*(2), 234–254.

Andrews, S. (1996). Lexical retrieval and selection processes: Effects of transposed-letter confusability. *Journal of Memory and Language, 35*(6), 775–800.

Andrews, S. (1997). The effect of orthographic similarity on lexical retrieval: Resolving neighborhood conflicts. *Psychonomic Bulletin and Review, 4*(4), 439–461.

Andrews, S., & Hersch, J. (2010). Lexical precision in skilled readers: Individual differences in masked neighbor priming. *Journal of Experimental Psychology: General, 139*(2), 299.

Andrews, S., & Lo, S. (2012). Not all skilled readers have cracked the code: Individual differences in masked form priming. *Journal of Experimental Psychology: Learning, Memory, and Cognition, 38*(1), 152.

Balota, D. A., Cortese, M. J., Sergent-Marshall, S. D., Spieler, D. H., & Yap, M. (2004). Visual word recognition of single-syllable words. *Journal of Experimental Psychology: General, 133*(2), 283–316.

Carreiras, M., Perea, M., & Grainger, J. (1997). Effects of the orthographic neighborhood in visual word recognition: Cross-task comparisons. *Journal of Experimental Psychology: Learning, Memory, and Cognition, 23*(4), 857–871.

Coltheart, M., Davelaar, E., Jonasson, J., & Besner, D. (1977). Access to the internal lexicon. In S. Dornic (Ed.), *Attention and performance VI* (pp. 535–555). Hillsdale, NJ: Erlbaum.

Coltheart, M., Rastle, K., Perry, C., Langdon, R., & Ziegler, J. (2001). DRC: A dual route cascaded model of visual word recognition and reading aloud. *Psychological Review, 108*(1), 204–256.

Davis, C. J., & Taft, M. (2005). More words in the neighborhood: Interference in lexical decision due to deletion neighbors. *Psychonomic Bulletin and Review, 12*(5), 904–910.

Forster, K. I., & Shen, D. (1996). No enemies in the neighborhood: Absence of inhibitory neighborhood effects in lexical decision and semantic categorization. *Journal of Experimental Psychology: Learning, Memory, and Cognition, 22*(3), 696–713.

Goldinger, S. D. (1989). Neighborhood density effect for high frequency words: Evidence for activation-based models of word recognition. *Research on Speech Perception Progress Report, 16*, 163–186.

Goldinger, S. D., Luce, P. A., & Pisoni, D. B. (1989). Priming lexical neighbors of spoken words: Effects of competition and inhibition. *Journal of Memory and Language, 28*(5), 501–518.

Grainger, J. (1990). Word frequency and neighborhood frequency effects in lexical decision and naming. *Journal of Memory and Language, 29*(2), 228–244.

Grainger, J., & Ferrand, L. (1994). Phonology and orthography in visual word recognition: Effects of masked homophone primes. *Journal of Memory and Language, 33*(2), 218–233.

Grainger, J., & Ferrand, L. (1996). Masked orthographic and phonological priming in visual word recognition and naming: Cross-task comparisons. *Journal of Memory and Language, 35*(5), 623–647.

Grainger, J., & Jacobs, A. M. (1996). Orthographic processing in visual word recognition: A multiple read-out model. *Psychological Review, 103*(3), 518–565.

Grainger, J., Muneaux, M., Farioli, F., & Ziegler, J. C. (2005). Effects of phonological and orthographic neighbourhood density interact in visual word recognition. *Quarterly Journal of Experimental Psychology Section A, 58*(6), 981–998.

Grainger, J., O'Regan, J. K., Jacobs, A. M., & Segui, J. (1989). On the role of competing word units in visual word recognition: The neighborhood frequency effect. *Perception and Psychophysics, 45*(3), 189–195.

Grainger, J., O'Regan, J. K., Jacobs, A. M., & Segui, J. (1992). Neighborhood frequency effects and letter visibility in visual word recognition. *Perception and Psychophysics, 51*(1), 49–56.

Grainger, J., & Segui, J. (1990). Neighborhood frequency effects in visual word recognition: A comparison of lexical decision and masked identification latencies. *Perception and Psychophysics, 47*(2), 191–198.

Grossberg, S. (1986). The adaptive self-organization of serial order in behavior: Speech, language, and motor control. In E. C. Schwab & H. C. Nusbaum (Eds.), *Pattern recognition by humans and machines: Vol. 1 speech perception* (pp. 187–294). New York: Academic Press.

Grossberg, S., Boardman, I., & Cohen, M. (1997). Neural dynamics of variable-rate speech categorization. *Journal of Experimental Psychology: Human Perception and Performance, 23*(2), 481–503.

Grossberg, S., & Myers, C. W. (2000). The resonant dynamics of speech perception: Interword integration and duration-dependent backward effects. *Psychological Review, 107*(4), 735–767.

Harm, M. W., & Seidenberg, M. S. (2004). Computing the meanings of words in reading: Cooperative division of labor between visual and phonological processes. *Psychological Review, 111*(3), 662–720.

Huntsman, L. A., & Lima, S. D. (1996). Orthographic neighborhood structure and lexical access. *Journal of Psycholinguistic Research, 25*(3), 417–429.

Huntsman, L. A., & Lima, S. D. (2002). Orthographic neighbors and visual word recognition. *Journal of Psycholinguistic Research, 31*(3), 289–306.

Johnson, N. F., & Pugh, K. R. (1994). A cohort model of visual word recognition. *Cognitive Psychology, 26*(3), 240–346.

Jones, A. C., & Rawson, K. A. (2016). Do reading and spelling share a lexicon. *Cognitive Psychology, 86*, 152–184.

Landauer, T. K., & Streeter, L. A. (1973). Structural differences between common and rare words: Failure of equivalence assumptions for theories of word recognition. *Journal of Verbal Learning and Verbal Behavior, 12*(2), 119–131.

Luce, P. A. (1986). *Neighborhoods of words in the mental lexicon. Research on speech perception technical report* (No. 6). Bloomington, IN: Speech Research Laboratory, Psychology Department, Indiana University.

Luce, P. A., & Pisoni, D. B. (1998). Recognizing spoken words: The neighborhood activation model. *Ear and Hearing, 19*(1), 1–36.

Luce, P. A., Pisoni, D. B., & Goldinger, S. D. (1990). Similarity neighborhoods of spoken words. In G. T. M. Altmann (Ed.), *Cognitive models of speech processing: Psycholinguistic and computational perspectives* (pp. 122–147). Cambridge, MA: The MIT Press.

McClelland, J. L. (1991). Stochastic interactive processes and the effect of context on perception. *Cognitive Psychology, 23*(1), 1–44.

McClelland, J. L., & Elman, J. L. (1986). The TRACE model of speech perception. *Cognitive Psychology, 18*(1), 1–86.

McClelland, J. L., & Rumelhart, D. E. (1981). An interactive activation model of context effects in letter perception: I. An account of basic findings. *Psychological Review, 88*(5), 375–407.

Mulatti, C., Reynolds, M. G., & Besner, D. (2006). Neighborhood effects in reading aloud: New findings and new challenges for computational models. *Journal of Experimental Psychology: Human Perception and Performance, 32*(4), 799–810.

Pattamadilok, C., Morais, J., Ventura, P., & Kolinsky, R. (2007). The locus of the orthographic consistency effect in auditory word recognition: Further evidence from French. *Language and Cognitive Processes, 22*(5), 700–726.

Peereman, R., & Content, A. (1995). Neighborhood size effect in naming: Lexical activation or sublexical correspondences? *Journal of Experimental Psychology: Learning, Memory, and Cognition, 21*(2), 409–421.

Peereman, R., & Content, A. (1997). Orthographic and phonological neighborhoods in naming: Not all neighbors are equally influential in orthographic space. *Journal of Memory and Language, 37*(3), 382–410.

Perea, M., & Pollatsek, A. (1998). The effects of neighborhood frequency in reading and lexical decision. *Journal of Experimental Psychology: Human Perception and Performance, 24*(3), 767–779.

Perfetti, C. A., & Hart, L. (2002). The lexical quality hypothesis. In L. Verhoeven, C. Elbro, & P. Reitsma (Eds.), *Precursors of functional literacy* (pp. 189–213). Amsterdam: John Benjamins.

Pitt, M. A., Myung, J. I., & Altteri, N. (2007). Modeling the word recognition data ofVitevitch and Luce (1998): Is it ARTful? *Psychonomic Bulletin and Review, 14*(3), 442–448.

Plaut, D. C., McClelland, J. L., Seidenberg, M. S., & Patterson, K. (1996). Understanding normal and impaired word reading: Computational principles in quasi-regular domains. *Psychological Review, 103*(1), 56–115.

Rastle, K., Harrington, J., Coltheart, M., & Palethorpe, S. (2000). Reading aloud begins when the computation of phonology is complete. *Journal of Experimental Psychology: Human Perception and Performance, 26*(3), 1178–1191.

Reicher, G. M. (1969). Perceptual recognition as a function of meaningfulness of stimulus material. *Journal of Experimental Psychology, 81*(2), 275–280.

Rumelhart, D. E., & McClelland, J. L. (1982). An interactive activation model of context effects in letter perception: II. The contextual enhancement effect and some tests and extensions of the model. *Psychological Review, 89*(1), 60–94.

Sears, C. R., Campbell, C. R., & Lupker, S. J. (2006). Is there a neighborhood frequency effect in English? Evidence from reading and lexical decision. *Journal of Experimental Psychology: Human Perception and Performance, 32*(4), 1040–1062.

Sears, C., Hino, Y., & Lupker, S. J. (1995). Neighborhood size and neighborhood frequency effects in word recognition. *Journal of Experimental Psychology: Human Perception and Performance, 21*(4), 876–900.

Sears, C., Lupker, S. J., & Hino, Y. (1999). Orthographic neighborhood effects in perceptual identification and semantic categorization tasks: A test of the multiple read-out model. *Perception and Psychophysics, 61*(8), 1537–1554.

Seidenberg, M. S., & McClelland, J. L. (1989). A distributed, developmental model of word recognition and naming. *Psychological Review, 96*(4), 523–568.

Seidenberg, M. S., & Tanenhaus, M. K. (1979). Orthographic effects on rhyme monitoring. *Journal of Experimental Psychology: Human Learning and Memory, 5*(6), 546–554.

Siakaluk, P. D., Sears, C. R., & Lupker, S. J. (2002). Orthographic neighborhood effects in lexical decision: The effects of nonword orthographic neighborhood size. *Journal of Experimental Psychology: Human Perception and Performance, 28*(3), 661–681.

Snodgrass, J. G., & Mintzer, M. (1993). Neighborhood effects in visual word recognition: Facilitatory or inhibitory? *Memory and Cognition, 21*(2), 247–266.

Ventura, P., Morais, J., & Kolinsky, R. (2007). The development of the orthographic consistency effect in speech recognition: From sublexical to lexical involvement. *Cognition, 105*(3), 547–576.

Vitevitch, M. S., & Luce, P. A. (1998). When words compete: Levels of processing in perception of spoken words. *Psychological Science, 9*(4), 325–329.

Vitevitch, M. S., & Luce, P. A. (1999). Probabilistic phonotactics and neighborhood activation in spoken word recognition. *Journal of Memory and Language, 40*(3), 374–408.

Wheeler, D. D. (1970). Processes in word recognition. *Cognitive Psychology, 1*(1), 59–85.

Yarkoni, T., Balota, D., & Yap, M. (2008). Moving beyond Coltheart's N: A new measure of orthographic similarity. *Psychonomic Bulletin and Review, 15*(5), 971–979.

Yates, M. (2005). Phonological neighbors speed visual word processing: Evidence from multiple tasks. *Journal of Experimental Psychology: Learning, Memory, and Cognition, 31*(6), 1385–1397.

Yates, M. (2009). Phonological neighbourhood spread facilitates lexical decisions. *Quarterly Journal of Experimental Psychology (2006), 62*(7), 1304–1314.

Yates, M. (2010). Investigating the importance of the least supported phoneme on visual word naming. *Cognition, 11*(1), 197–201.

Yates, M., Friend, J., & Ploetz, D. M. (2008). Phonological neighbors influence word naming through the least supported phoneme. *Journal of Experimental Psychology: Human Perception and Performance, 34*(6), 1599–1608.

Yates, M., Locker, L. J., & Simpson, G. B. (2004). The influence of phonological neighborhood on visual word perception. *Psychonomic Bulletin and Review, 11*(3), 452–457.

Yates, M., & Slattery, T. J. (2019). Individual differences in spelling ability influence phonological processing during visual word recognition. *Cognition, 187*, 139–149.

Ziegler, J. C., & Ferrand, L. (1998). Orthography shapes the perception of speech: The consistency effect in auditory word recognition. *Psychonomic Bulletin and Review, 5*(4), 683–689.

Ziegler, J. C., Ferrand, L., & Montant, M. (2004). Visual phonology: The effects of orthographic consistency on different auditory word recognition tasks. *Memory and Cognition, 32*(5), 732–741.

Ziegler, J. C., & Muneaux, M. (2007). Orthographic facilitation and phonological inhibition in spoken word recognition: A developmental study. *Psychonomic Bulletin and Review, 14*(1), 75–80.

Ziegler, J. C., Muneaux, M., & Grainger, J. (2003). Neighborhood effects in auditory word recognition: Phonological competition and orthographic facilitation. *Journal of Memory and Language, 48*(4), 779–793.

Ziegler, J. C., & Perry, C. (1998). No more problems in Coltheart's neighborhood: Resolving neighborhood conflicts in the lexical decision task. *Cognition, 68*, B53–B62.

Ziegler, J. C., Petrova, A., & Ferrand, L. (2008). Feedback consistency effects in visual and auditory word recognition: Where do we stand after more than a decade? *Journal of Experimental Psychology: Learning, Memory, and Cognition, 34*(3), 643–661.

15
TWO THEORIES OF SPEECH PRODUCTION AND PERCEPTION

Mark Tatham and Katherine Morton

Introduction

In this chapter, we focus on two speech theories: Classical Phonetics and Cognitive Phonetics. Classical phonetics forms the basis of all modern research in speech, whereas cognitive phonetics is contemporary.

Classical phonetics (Abercrombie, 1967; Cruttenden, 2001) gave to mental representations of speech a central position in the theory, making it a cognitively based model. Relatively informal inspection of articulation enabled phoneticians to correlate the mental representation with vocal tract shapes for various speech sounds. Together with a symbol system—the International Phonetic Alphabet—the approach often enabled large scale comparisons between representations in many different languages.

There were two key problems with classical phonetics: it failed to tackle the difference between cognitive representation and physical instantiation, believing that because cognitively we tend to proceed in a symbolic categorical way the same must be true of the physical instantiation. In the 1960s, when it was pointed out that the cognitive representations are all about discrete segments and that the physical signals are all about continuousness, the model was restated by Coarticulation Theory (MacNeilage & De Clerk, 1969), which attempted to explain how discrete segments "become" continuous.

The inherent confusions in classical phonetics and its failure to explain more and more empirical observations as instrumentation developed from the 1950s onward led to several developments. Description of the data as the goal of the theory gave way to the more usual scientific goal of explanation of the data. Linear representations of speech gave way to nonlinear hierarchical representations. Researchers began to look behind the simple configurations of the vocal tract observed by eye and the audio signal registered by ear. Suggestions for integrated models of speech production and perception began to appear. Action Theory (Fowler, 1980) led the way, suggesting a layered model linking cognitively based speech processing (in linguistics: phonology) and physically based speech processing (phonetics), considerably downgrading the role of mental representation and processing that had been the central consideration of classical phonetics and linguistics.

Cognitive phonetics (Tatham, 1984, 1990) rested on the same basic ideas as action theory, but focused on developing ideas about cognition in speech, particularly concentrating on computationally adequate dynamic modeling of utterances from their phonological representations and on to the perceived soundwave (Tatham & Morton, 2002). Cognitive phonetics embodied a model of the perceiver in the speaker and a model of the speaker in the perceiver. Speech production

 DOI: 10.4324/9781003204213-17

and perception became essentially relatively simple processes compared with the earlier complex extensions to classical phonetics made by coarticulation theory. In the new model the surface complexity was explained by using the principle of supervision continuously controlling and therefore varying a basic and relatively uncomplicated articulation (Tatham, 1995). The simple categorical suggestions of classical phonetics gave way to explanation of the continuousness of speech production, but more importantly to a systematic explanation of the continuously varying nature of speech.

Classical phonetics (1900+)

Developed from the late 19th century onward, classical phonetics was the first true attempt at a scientific theory of speech. The focus of the theory is the segmental object, strings of which form speech. Experimental techniques as we know them today were not available to early phoneticians who relied on strict training in listening to give them the ability to perceive nuances in the acoustic signal and to introspect on how vocal tract shapes were set up to produce individual sounds. Classical phonetics developed symbolic representations for speech sounds and for some prosodic effects spanning groups of individual sounds.

Classical phonetics is a descriptive theory that does not extend to an explanatory level. Its subjective methodology for investigating speech asserted that speech is a concatenation of individually manipulable sounds. It relied on perception and limited observation of how the articulators produce speech to assign segment labels. Questions such as the shape of the vocal tract and neuromuscular control had to wait until the 1960s when techniques were developed such as electromyography, air pressure measurement, and video x-ray, allowing correlations between shapes and the acoustic wave. The new techniques generated many new questions:

(a) What aerodynamic properties of the general vocal tract are used in speaking? In general, speech is carried by an egressive air stream; that is, air flows out from the lungs, through the vocal tract, and exits via the mouth and/or nose. Some languages employ ingressive sounds, and it is possible to create localized aerodynamic effects (and hence sounds) within the vocal tract, such as clicks, and so on. Researchers have noted that airflow and the dynamic response to its impedance contribute to certain coarticulatory effects such as aspiration.

(b) How are the vocal shapes specified? Various proposals (Baer, Gore, Gracco, & Nye, 1991; Rubin & Vatikiotis-Bateson, 1998) are made in terms of
   1. The overall shape (the projected final shape within which the aerodynamics takes place).
   2. The configuration of the individual organs (a parametric representation).
   3. Parametrically in terms of the individual muscles.
   4. Parametrically in terms of muscle groupings (coordinative structures).

(c) What are the constraints (particularly temporal) on the mechanics of the vocal tract in a dynamic mode, rather than static single segment mode? We need to distinguish between constraints in moving in zero time from one static position to another and those constraints associated with dynamic movement (where the emphasis is on the movement rather than the underlying vocal tract shapes).

(d) Are these constraints fixed or can they deliberately be manipulated to the limits of the physical system? For example, manipulation can potentially have a considerable influence on constraints governed by time: it is possible to decide to speak fast or slow, but the constraint, even in slow speech, remains at the "boundaries," though with more time during the segment to render the target specification more accurately.

In general, classical phonetics made no attempt to address such questions, which by the 1970s were becoming center stage in speech production research.

Coarticulation theory (from around 1965)

From the 1940s onward, developments in instrumentation enabled researchers to examine directly the nature of the speech soundwave. It became obvious that it is rarely possible to find separate speech sounds within the signal. Work began to investigate how the discontinuity of the cognitive representation of speech (classical phonetics' segments) becomes continuous in the soundwave, and how the perceiver reconstructs the discontinuity when listening to the soundwave. We would not today consider that discrete objects become continuous, or that discrete objects are reconstructed from the soundwave. The kinds of questions being addressed at that time included:

(a) What is the precise nature of the acoustic signal of speech? The acoustic signal of speech has been studied extensively since the 1950s (Fant, 1960). The signal is modeled as the result of a filtered source, where the source can be either periodic, aperiodic, or mixed, originating with vocal cord vibration or due to some constriction-based impedance at some point(s) within the vocal tract. The vocal tract forms a resonance cavity responsible for the filtering of the source signal; the nasal cavity constitutes an additional resonance cavity that can be shunted into the system at will. The size and shape of the vocal tract cavities determine some aspects of the resultant waveform's spectral properties, with the resonance energized by characteristically shaped source signals. Recognition of unclear boundaries and so-called blurred effects across approximate boundaries led to coarticulation theory. A range of summarizing articles can be found in the collection edited by Hardcastle and Hewlett (1999). This model proposed that although a string of speech segments is intended by the speaker, the inertial properties of the various stages of production (in the motor control system, mechanics of muscle and articulator movement and the aerodynamics) introduce a smoothing, or overlap effect producing the observed continuousness of the final signal (MacNeilage, 1970). This smoothing is time dependent: a landmark change in speech production theory, since for the first time we have a truly dynamic and explanatory perspective on speech, which contrasted strikingly with the static and atemporal descriptive perspective of classical phonetics.

(b) What is encoded in the signal? Initially it was thought that the temporal rendering of the intended speech plan for a sequence of words directly encoded the basic meaning of the string of syntactic objects, and it was then up to phonological processing and phonetic rendering to determine what acoustic features can be assigned to prosody (intonation, stress, rhythm). There was no clear correlation in the sense that it is still unclear, for example, how the prosody of a particular sentence on a particular occasion will turn out in terms of the timing, frequency, and amplitude parameters of the acoustic signal (Matthies, Perrier, Perkell, & Zandipour, 2001).

(c) Are there specific aerodynamic coarticulatory constraints? Observations were made, for example, on vocal cord movement.

1. Intended vocal cord vibration from the start of the rendering of a vowel nucleus segment following a syllable initial voiceless plosive (as in a word like pat, /pæ.../, for example), is delayed because of instability in the air pressure and flow above the larynx following the release of the built-up air pressure. There is an oscillatory settling of the pressure, but until the necessary ratio between supra- and subglottal pressures and vocal cord tension is reestablished vibration will not begin. This delay is called voice onset time (VOT) (Lisker & Abramson, 1964) and varies across languages.
2. Vocal cord vibration for a phonologically voiced stop cannot be continued indefinitely if the air flow is stopped above the larynx. Again the build up of supraglottal air pressure behind the stop eventually destroys the required ratio—as in a sequence like /ada/ in English (Higgins, Netsell, & Schulte, 1998).

The general case of coarticulation resulting from a pressure ratio disturbance during stops specified as [+ voice] phonologically involves curtailment of vibration if the air flow is impeded above the larynx. Specific cases are progressive vocal cord vibration attenuation with partial impedance (in, say, a voiced fricative in a word like measure in English) and vibration failure with full impedance (in, say, a voiced stop in a word like adder) to air flow through the vocal tract. Deliberate curtailment of vocal cord vibration occurs when tension in the vocal cords (the third parameter in the equation) is too great or the vocal cords are held too stiffly, as in whispered vowels.

Cognitive phonetics (from around 1980)

The basic theory

Although coarticulation theory (MacNeilage & De Clerk, 1969) appeared to explain time governed dynamic effects in speech production and was able to use these to throw light on the mismatch between the segmentally oriented focus of classical phonetics and the more recent detailed observations of the acoustic signal, there remained some unexplained phenomena. Cognitive phonetics (Tatham, 1984) was devised to explain a class of observations that coarticulation theory failed to explain.

The idea that the continuousness of the soundwave results from the inertial properties of the production system implies that coarticulation is universal. Closer inspection reveals however that coarticulatory effects vary from language to language, even from accent to accent within a language and even within the speech of a single person on different occasions. Two explanations are possible: either there are no truly universal properties of coarticulation or the concept needs refining to account for these apparent discrepancies.

Cognitive phonetics took the second view, proposing that coarticulation is indeed a truly universal phenomenon since it is determined by the way nonlinguistic universal physical factors that are mechanical or aerodynamic in origin constrain the linguistic use of speech production processes. But at the same time linguistically (and therefore cognitively) sourced considerations determine the extent of coarticulatory phenomena. In other words, coarticulation is a two-stage process.

1. There are universal physically determined constraints.
2. These constraints are manipulable (Tatham, 1971).

The concept of cognitive intervention in somatic behavior here is different from usage of the term in education and therapy. Here intervention means disturbance or modification of an otherwise automatic or universal process. The source of the intervention is cognitive and relies on tacit knowledge of the coarticulatory process and knowledge of the speaker's phonological intentions. Intervention is rarely a consciously aware process and is performed by the Cognitive Phonetic Agent (CPA; Tatham, 1995). The concept of the agent is adapted from Artificial Intelligence (Garland & Alterman, 2004).

In phonetics, it is impossible to isolate cognitive considerations from physical considerations. In fact, much of the theorizing in phonetics over the past half century has explicitly addressed the relationship between the cognitive processes of phonology and the physical processes of speech production. We feel there must be a relationship, but what that relationship is still defeats theorists: at the most, we are able to characterize a rather loose correlative association between the two.

Speech production models usually propose that the cognitive processing underlying speech is handled along with all of language as a symbolic system that ultimately terminates in an output: a symbolic representation that specifies the linguistically significant properties of what is to be spoken. We have called this the utterance plan (Figure 15.1).

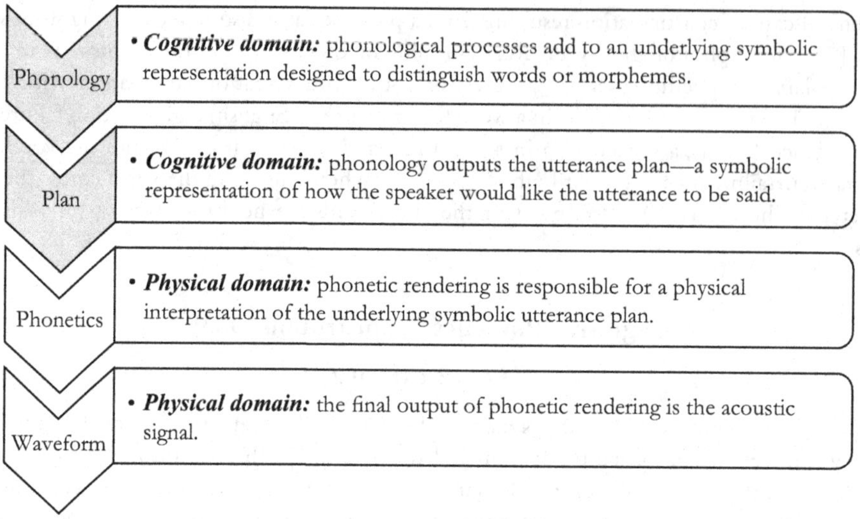

Figure 15.1 The relationship between cognitive phonology and physical phonetics.

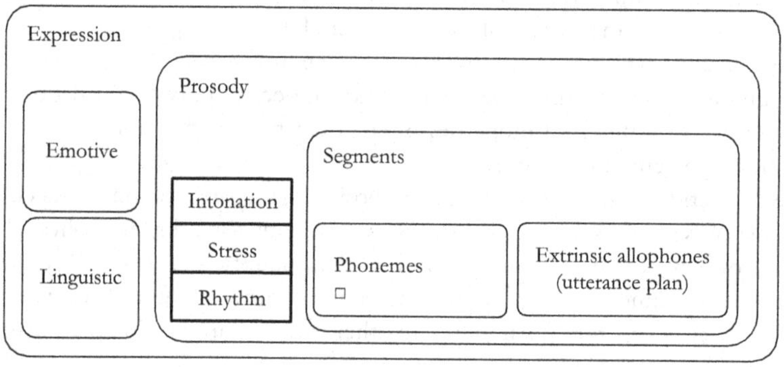

Figure 15.2 The wrapper format: expression wraps prosody, which in turn wraps segmental processing.

However, this representation as it stands cannot be input directly to physical processing, whether considered statically in terms of its potential, or as a dynamic system characterizing particular utterances. The most usual method of bridging the cognitive/physical gap is to assume some kind of rerepresentation of the cognitive plan in physical terms that lead directly into a physical model of speech production. Along these lines, questions asked by researchers include:

1. What is the nature of the input to physical rendering of the cognitively derived utterance plan? The physical input to the premotor control system needs to be initiated by a cognitive representation of the intended plan. This plan is derived by cognitive processes (the language's phonology) and is currently expressed as a string of extrinsic allophonic objects appropriately wrapped; that is, embedded in a prosody and a framework of expression (Tatham & Morton, 2006), see Figure 15.2.
2. Are there physical units or objects matching the cognitive objects of the plan? It would seem so. We have a clear idea of the psychological reality of the basic objects contained in the plan—we call them extrinsic allophones (as opposed to the phonetic intrinsic allophones that are unintended variants resulting from coarticulation) (Tatham, 1971). In addition, it

does seem to be the case that movement results from a system input in terms of a sequence of physical target representations (MacNeilage, 1970). It is possible that at both the cognitive and physical levels the units are organized: in the case of the cognitive plan, in terms of hierarchically structured syllable objects sequenced appropriately; and in terms of the physical plan, as functionally similar physical structures. It is easier to show the structure of the cognitive plan than the physical plan, but the hypothesis has proved productive.

There remain a number of questions about what the physical representation looks like. Is it, for example, in terms of hierarchically organized whole objects or it is parametric? Are the sequenced objects wrapped in the sense that they are contained within a broader domain of prosodic features and, even higher, expressive features?

3. What constraints are there in the equivalence of cognitive and physical plans? The physical plan needs to render all extrinsic allophonic features—these are all linguistically significant (or, by definition, they would not be there). In converting from a cognitive plan to a physical plan the system may find it useful to flag certain known problems further down the line—for example, predicted coarticulatory errors (perhaps hierarchically organized in terms of probability in this context, etc.). Any such flagging could be used to feedback to the cognitive level warning of future stabilization or supervision requirements. So, for example, the /s/ and /ʃ/ (sea vs. she) proximity in both production and perceptual spaces could be flagged to alert a possible need for supervision or increased precision of articulation.

Cognitive phonetics requires a way of dynamically operating within the physical limits of the articulatory system. The CPA conducts a systematic supervisory intervention in physical processes based on tacit knowledge the speaker has of the production process. Thus coarticulatory effects are characterized in cognitive phonetics as varying along a vector from maximal constraint to maximal enhancement. A speaker may constrain a universal coarticulatory effect or may enhance the effect. A pivot point of no intervention lets the inertial constraint find its own level.

scale of CPA control from fully enhanced through neutral to fully constrained [enhanced]
1 ← 0 → 1 [constrained]

The mechanisms available to the CPA

The basic unit involved in motor control is the coordinative structure first put forward in speech by Action Theory (Fowler, 1980). Coordinative structures are hierarchically nested groupings of the musculature, and are characterized by their internal ability to allow low level messaging between muscles in the group without reference to higher control. The coordinative structure is able to learn certain configurations of its member muscles and the messaging that determines their temporal behavior. Equations of constraint determine the interplay between muscles that, via the messaging system, maintains stability of gestures (coordinated movement in time) and improves their robustness in the face of external constraints.

Control of a coordinative structure is initiated centrally, but expanded locally by the knowledge embodied in the structure's equations of constraint. Knowledge beyond some basic biological behavior has to be acquired as the child learns language such that much of the detail of the behavior of the vocal tract for utterances is derived at this low level. As learning continues gradually acquired low level specifications take over from complete central specification. This approach contrasts sharply with simple coarticulation theory, which postulated that target specifications for a string of speech sounds were worked out cognitively and then issued to the musculature as a set of commands every time the segment was required. Not only would such a system be very complex, it would also fail to show how speakers readily adapt to environmental constraints like the changing direction of the gravitational force as the head is tilted during an utterance, or a sudden increase in background noise, or the need to speak faster or slower.

Central to the working of coordinative structures is the low level gamma loop feedback system (Matthews, 1964), and it is the gamma circuits that stabilize movement. Efferent signals originating in the motor cortex are available to the gamma system and are used effectively to set the bias of particular behavior—it is this property of the motor control system that enables CPA supervision in the way postulated by cognitive phonetics. Action theory used gamma efferent signals to tune the system, but cognitive phonetics employs this tuning mechanism on a dynamic on-going basis to continuously adjust for coarticulatory effects, constraining or enhancing them as needed.

The utterance plan and its representation

As the concept of the utterance plan is central to cognitive phonetics, we now ask, aside from the generalizations used on static models of speaking, whether there is a cognitively based plan for an instance of speech. And if so, how is this plan represented?

The plan is the output representation of the set of phonological processes. This set of processes is modeled in a static phonology that simultaneously characterizes all the possibilities for a language, and in a dynamic phonology as a subset detailing the processes underlying the instantiation of a particular utterance. As such, the plan's representation reflects phonology in the sense that it consists of a string of phonological objects appropriately wrapped with prosodic and expressive layers. The final derived objects in phonology are extrinsic allophones: these represent potential sound or articulatory targets and embody all the information required for a successful rendering of the plan into sound and its subsequent decoding in the listener. The information is linguistic and may reflect contrastive requirements (e.g., this vowel vs. that vowel) derived from underlying modeling of morpheme structure (basic phonemes) or idiosyncratic noncontrastive requirements (two different /l/ targets, for example, in English in words like leaf vs. feel).

The CPA intervention can optimize or extend the inventory of cognitive objects available for use in a language.

1. The inventory of a language's extrinsic allophonic objects (objects used to specify the utterance plan) must by definition exclude objects unable to be physically rendered under ideal conditions. That is, the inventory consists of extrinsic allophones able to be rendered with some or minimal supervision.
2. The system that sets up the inventory must have access to a model able to predict extrinsic allophones and the degree of supervision they will need when rendered. So, for example, knowing about the aerodynamics of controlling sudden air outflow following a plosive release enables the system to postulate several possible allophones of a plosive by noting that stable objects can be created from the coarticulatory process by CPA intervention. So, we can have prevoiced [b] (the vocal cords start way before the [b] is released), or somewhat prevoiced [b] (the vocal cords start a little before [b] release), or regular [b] (the vocal cords start just after [b] release), or somewhat aspirated [p] or "normally" (minimally supervised) aspirated [p], or [p] with enhanced aspiration, or [p] with very enhanced aspiration. These are stable at normal rates of delivery and at a useful range of rates from slow to very fast and within a useful range of loudness or overall airflow. Once the perceptual thresholds for these various objects are known (the predictive perceptual model) unusable objects can be filtered out to leave the useful ones. In this way a language builds up additional segments to include phonological objects not possible without CPA intervention.

Supervision

Supervision uses CPA intervention as its mechanism for controlling the precision of utterances. Ongoing adjustment of articulation at the muscular and coordinative structure levels is crucial to cognitive phonetics.

Speech gestures are produced in response to an utterance plan, specifying how an utterance is intended to be. As such, it derives from high level abstract "sound" objects designed to keep words separate to avoid confusion of meaning (called phonemes in classical phonetics) and lower level abstract sound objects that reflect phonological pressures such as assimilation (the cognitively based tendency for one of these abstract objects to succumb to contextual effects from its neighbors), idiosyncratic pressures due to pronunciation niceties specific to the language (such as the use of two different /l/ sounds in English)—all designed to facilitate perception. These variants are the extrinsic allophones to be used in utterance instantiation.

Coarticulatory constraints occurring after the plan has been assembled and environmental constraints, such as noise levels impinging on the acoustic signal, or even physical effects detracting from ideal articulation, such as a sore throat, tend to degrade the acoustic signal—ultimately making it, if severe enough, unintelligible to the listener. Listeners regularly repair some damage to the signal, but the effect is limited. However, observations of the acoustic signal show that it varies continuously with respect to its precision (Charles-Luce, Dressler, & Ragonese, 1999; Tatham & Morton, 1980). Precision is the degree to which the signal, for a specific period of time, matches some idealized physical signal corresponding to the abstract plan. Moreover this variation in precision is systematic: it correlates well with listeners' perceptual difficulties, which themselves vary continuously.

Thus, coarticulation is universal, but its extent or degree on many occasions is not universal. We can vary the degree of coarticulation by limiting or enhancing the effect. Constraint and enhancement has been found to be systematic and stable enough that "new" sounds can be created for use by a language's phonology.

Examples:

1. Unconstrained, an alveolar fricative might take an average tongue position varying broadly around [s] and [ʃ], and this works for a phonology requiring just one fricative in this area (e.g. Greek, Spanish), but not for one requiring two (e.g., French, English) in the same area. Here, precision of articulation must be tightened, or its variability constrained, to ensure that perceptual confusion is minimized.
2. An example of coarticulation enhancement occurs in languages that manipulate the aerodynamic coarticulatory effect of VOT for the purposes of increasing the phonological inventory to include more plosive consonants. Such a language is Hindi (Ladefoged & Maddieson, 1996).
3. An example of constraining the same VOT aerodynamic coarticulatory effect occurs in a number of languages that need to specify the supervision of vocal cord vibration in voiced stops that would otherwise "lose" their target voiced specification; English is an example since VOT occurs only in a constrained way following /b, d, g/. Constraint is necessary to avoid perceptual confusion with /p, t, k/. French extends this supervision to minimise VOT in voiceless stops and preserve vocal cord vibration more fully in voiced stops and fricatives. Loss of target voice specification is enhanced in German and Russian where we find, respectively, bund with final /t/, and хлеб (transliterated as khljeb) with final /p/; examples of a coarticulatory effect so consistently able to be supervised as to attain full phonological status of planned extrinsic allophone (Morton & Tatham, 1980), rather than unplanned intrinsic (coarticulated) allophones in other languages.

Production for perception

Cognitive phonetics introduces the idea that speech production is a managed process; it is supervised toward a particular goal—that of optimal perception (Nooteboom, 1983; Tatham, 1970). Optimal perception does not mean perfect perception; it means perception that works satisfactorily for both speaker and listener. Supervision involves CPA intervention to achieve better precision when the speaker predicts potential failure of the perceptual repair mechanism in dealing with signal error. Actual dynamic speech production is not driven solely by what a speaker wants to say and how they want to say it (speaker plans of utterances and expressive content for those utterances), but also by how well it is predicted the overall communication system will behave at any one moment. Speech production in this theory incorporates a running predictive model of the environment and its constraints and also of the perceptual process and its constraints.

CPA intervention

For CPA supervision of the articulatory rendering of the utterance plan the mechanism of cognitive intervention requires:

1. A predictive model of production robustness and sources of error; and
2. A predictive model of perception robustness and sources of error.

Both of these models need to be static to capture the overall general case of supervision, and dynamic to capture the current rendering within a continuously varying context of constraints external to the utterance plan (Tatham & Morton, 2006). The principle of supervision goes beyond any simple mechanism of intervention because it is organized in the context of speech production, and is itself continuously variable. Supervision depends on the current situation, and the actual degree of intervention necessary cannot be wholly determined in advance since every utterance instantiation is different. A set of continuously varying parameters interact in an ever changing way to determine locally the current instantiation and how it is constrained.

For example, in pulling in information on the current physical performance of the production process, supervision employs all three major possibilities for feedback (slow auditory, medium speed tactile, and fast intramuscular). Locally, coordinative structures are able to be set or tuned to tighten or relax the behavioral precision of an entire group or nested group of muscles in the structure. It is in this way that supervision allows rapid response to changes in mood during conversation, and so on.

Perception

The theory of speech perception addresses the general question: What cognitive processing is involved in interpreting the soundwave the listener is hearing (Pardo & Remez, 2006)?

It is widely felt that once the analyzed physical auditory signals cross to the cognitive domain a number of processes are involved in their interpretation. What must be remembered is that the "meaning" of the utterance is not directly encoded in the acoustic signal: it is pointless to attempt to find linguistic/cognitive objects like phonemes in the signal. They could not exist in an acoustic waveform because, of course, they are abstractions. Phonemes and all linguistic units are symbolic objects existing in the linguist's model and, it is hypothesized, perhaps have some psychological reality in the speaker/listener.

The task of perceptual interpretation of the incoming signal is to assign to it (not find within it) a symbolic representation that will ultimately enable the listener to be aware of the speaker's intended utterance. Various proposals have been made as to how this might be done. These include identification of the incoming signal by consulting a dictionary memory of signals heard in the past, so that the signal can be found and identified.

All such lookup table procedures fail partly because of the theoretically infinite possibilities of the acoustic signal in representing any utterance (so the template knowledge base would have to be vast or categorized in some way, and a means of data reduction would have to be found that did not label each incoming signal as unique), and partly because of the near certainty that the incoming acoustic has been degraded in some way. It is easily observed that the signal can be repaired by the listener to some meaningful and less degraded version, and that the repair of identical signals is often different for different languages or even accents of the same language.

The data that needs to be explained by a theory of perception includes the listener's ability to repair damaged signals, and recover, by assignment, a symbolic representation associated with the speaker's intentions. The recovered symbolic representation matches the speaker's utterance plan, and is an idealized or error free representation of the original intention. In addition, listeners usually realize when they have made an assignment error, then go back and reinterpret a buffered version of the original signal (Hartsuiker, Pickering, & de Jong, 2005).

The listener is in effect not interpreting the original signal but a version of that signal recovered from memory—as such the recovered version has no error, is stable, and has no variability. Prosodic and expressive interpretation proceeds along the same lines. This is why listeners are unaware of variants below the extrinsic allophonic level—they are no longer there: the listener is perceiving their own reconstructed version of the signal.

Theories of perception

Theories of perception within the domain of speech production/perception fall basically into two major types: passive and active.

1. Passive theories involve no, or very little, interpretation. The hypothesis here is that there is sufficient information within the signal to enable perception to proceed without active addition of information by the listener. The general theory is called Direct Perception (Gibson, 1954), and the main theory within speech is called Direct Realism (Fowler, 1986). The main argument against passive theories is their inability to explain the contextually dependent variation in meaning of identical signals even within a single language.
2. Active theories involve varying degrees of interpretation of the signal. To do this the listener must include:
   (a) Knowledge of the special nature of the speech signal required [explains the ability to affirm: I know this is human speech];
   (b) A model of how speech is produced [explains: The speaker said "X"].

Minimally active theories include the Motor Theory of Speech Perception (Cooper, 1966), the Revised Motor Theory (Liberman & Mattingly, 1985), and the Analysis by Synthesis Theory (Stevens & Halle, 1967).

Fully active theories must include:

(a) A means of hypothesizing that a production or transmission error has occurred [explains: His speech is not coming out right or There's too much noise, I can't quite hear].
(b) A means of recovery and reconstruction of the intended signal underlying any degraded version reaching the listeners ears [explains: He must have meant "X"].

(c) A means of accessing a stored idealized signal to replace the actual heard signal, thereby removing errors [explains: I know he said "X,"] when analysis of the acoustic signals shows that X is not exactly what it looks like.
(d) A means of buffering and reiterating the error repair process to cope with realization that a repair error has occurred.

Among the more active theories able to detect and repair errors of production or transmission degradation is the Associative Store Theory (incorporated within cognitive phonetics), which proposes a mechanism for dynamic matching of a defective incoming signal with the inventory of symbolic representations (Tatham & Morton, 2006).

Questions for the model of perception

Contemporary models of speech perception need to address a number of critical questions.

1. Is perception a mirror image of production? Perception seems to depend on the listener's having reference to some model of speech production to be able to anticipate what the speaker is doing. For us, it seems clear that to linguistically interpret the representation assigned to a cognitive version of the incoming acoustic signal, the listener must have reference to a static phonological model capable in principle of characterizing all possible utterances in the language at all the segmental and prosodic/expressive levels.
2. Is the recovered signal represented as a reconstruction of the speaker's plan—a plan the perceiver could have if they were the speaker? This would make an active mirroring of the speaker an essential part of the general perceptual process.
3. What is the role of the perceiver's own production phonology in this reconstruction? Evidence from mis-hearing, say, of a foreign accent: If I myself had made this sound I would be trying to make "X."
4. What is the precise nature of the representation in the listener's mind?
   (a) Is the representation expressed in phonological terms; that is, does it match the production phonology?
   (b) Is the representation segmental rather than continuous? At an abstract cognitive level the representation only makes sense if it is segmental. A continuous representation would have all representations different; technically, an infinity of representations would be possible. The representation must take a "reduced" symbolic form, a form devoid of nonlinguistic variability.
   (c) Cognitive phonetics suggests a continuity between segment and prosody. Standard models add prosody, whereas cognitive phonetics wraps the segment string in a hierarchical arrangement:
      i. The plan's prosodic environment—wraps the segmental plan;
      ii. The plan's expressive environment—wraps the prosody.

For a full explanation of the wrapper format for the model that relates the components formally, seeTatham & Morton, 2006.

(a) The representation is wrapped in much the same way as the production process(es).
   i. Is there a recovery hierarchy mirroring the production wrapper layers?
   ii. The perceptual system actively assigns expression, prosody, and segmental elements. If these form a wrapped package, then we presume that the unwrapping would show a hierarchical perceptual strategy—expression first (because tone of voice can sometimes be perceived before the actual words), segments last because they are perceived within the expression (and production-wise are the most wrapped, least deep, elements).

The wrapper format for the dynamic model is diagrammed in Figure 15.2.

Variability

In any theory of speech it is necessary to account for variability in production and how it is dealt with in perception. Some variability occurs deliberately, as with essential variant phonemes to distinguish words (e.g., cat /kæt/ vs. cap / kæp/), some occurs deliberately, as with nonessential extrinsic variant allophones (e.g., leaf /ljif/ vs. feel /filw/, palatalized and velarized /l/s, respectively), and some occurs mostly involuntarily (e.g., lad /læd°/, devoiced /d/), symbolically, intrinsic allophones.

Types of variability

Early researchers working with classical phonetic recognized variability in speech. They were particularly concerned with allophonic variants of phonemes and their descriptions often noted contextual variations due to assimilation. Variation arises under the influence of linearly juxtaposed phonemes in their model. The picture was confused, however, until two types of allophonic variability were modeled:

1. Extrinsic allophones, which are derived deliberately in cognitively based phonological processing for inclusion in the utterance plan; and
2. Intrinsic allophones, which are derived largely involuntarily during physical phonetic rendering of the plan (Tatham, 1971; Wang & Fillmore, 1961).

The plan's extrinsic allophones can become, according to coarticulation theory, seriously degraded as a result of time constraints on mechanical and aerodynamic processes, and perhaps also on some neurophysiological processes. Even the mood of speakers can distort their physiology to cause changes in the acoustic signal; this occurs, for example, in the tenseness associated with extreme anger.

Expressive features, both emotive and linguistic, dominate the rendering of the intended segmental pattern of the utterance as set out in the utterance plan (see the diagram above). These features are said to wrap the utterance and influence it prosodically for the most part using variations in timing or rhythm, intonation, and stress.

A final type of variability is quite simply randomness, noise, or jitter in the physical system. The degree of variability here can be quite wide, but within certain limits does not interfere with the perceptual system's recovery procedures too badly. By definition the idealized abstract cognitive objects of phonology in either production or perception cannot exhibit random variability: variability of this type belongs strictly to the physical world.

It is important to note that speakers and listeners are only aware in any linguistic sense of the symbolic representations in terms of extrinsic allophones and phonemes. The system pivots on the speaker's extrinsic allophonic utterance plan and on the perceiver's recovered interpretation. Neither speakers nor listeners are aware of intrinsic allophones (unless enhanced or constrained—in which case they have achieved extrinsic allophonic status), nor of any variability due to jitter in the system. The listener's recovery process, within its limitations, is so robust and efficient that it almost completely negates any awareness of error, unless it is gross.

Control of variability

Variability in rendering the utterance plan is principally controlled by manipulating precision (Charles-Luce et al., 1999; Tatham & Morton, 1980). Clearly people can control the precision of their articulations, and do so often without knowing that anything has altered.

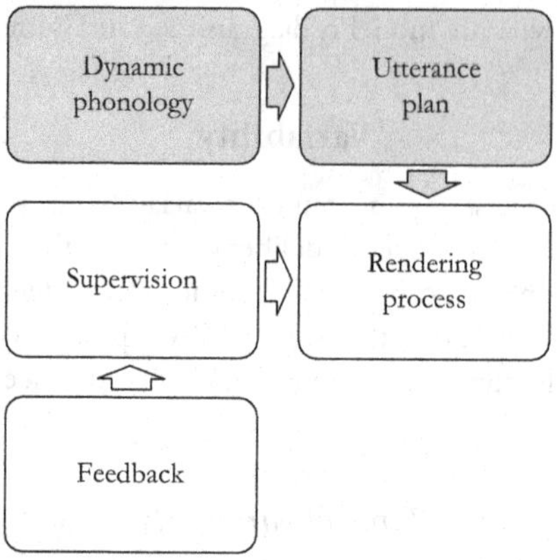

Figure 15.3 Diagram showing how feedback from production is one input to supervision of the rendering process. Supervision also benefits from access to the underlying utterance plan.

Regularly what is involved is a change in delivery tempo: a decrease eases degradation due to time constrained coarticulatory effects. Tightening up on target specifications further attempts to deliver near ideal articulations. Supervision of articulation control is intensified based on local fast intramuscular feedback and reference to the original intended target (see Figure 15.3).

The required degree of precision can clearly vary. Many factors including local phonological contrast (Did you say "sea" or "she"?), environmental constraints such as a noisy channel (a bad phone circuit or high ambient noise), social constraints (the feeling that we need to speak more carefully to nonnative speakers or listeners perceived to be less intelligent than ourselves). Thus variation of precision can have an effect on a whole conversation and can change from syllable to syllable.

Applications modeling

Applications models can be thought of as models that can be put to practical use in addressing particular problems. They are derived from more general underlying theories and models in the relevant disciplines, and arise in response to the need to solve problems in special instances. No underlying comprehensive integrated speech production/perception model has been developed (Fowler & Galantucci, 2005; Tatham & Morton, 2006). Practitioners are therefore faced with the necessity to develop sections of an incomplete but idealized integrated speech production/perception model.

Language production and perception (including the subset of speech production/perception) is described according to principles operating in two different domains: cognitive and physical (Tatham & Morton, 2006). Applications models can draw on research in these two domains, the cognitive including linguistics (semantics, syntax, phonology) and cognitive psychology, and the physical including physiology (neuromuscular movement, the hearing system) and the anatomically oriented parts of classical phonetics. In addition, some models cross domain boundaries: cognitive phonetics, auditory scene analysis (Bregman, 1990), and some phonology/phonetic modeling.

The medium of transmission of ideas and feelings—the speech waveform—is relevant to language/speech disorders since it is the physical event associated with the end product of speaking. The waveform provides the acoustic features that trigger perceptual interpretation.

Production and perception

We speak in order to be listened to and understood. It is therefore reasonable to expect that an awareness of the listener is important to the speaker (see p. 303, Production for Perception).

Applications models might include such a concept to take account of some variability in disordered speech that might be because of modifying what can be produced to take account of the listener. Here some variability may be introduced by the emotive stance of the speaker and their attitude toward the person they are speaking to, or to what that person has to say—part of the general social context. Speaking to a friend may result in different characteristics from speaking to a therapist. The range of variability allowed is limited (see p. 307, Variability), and the model builder should ideally take this into account.

Much applications work is not explicitly theory bound, but based on empirically derived hypotheses. In such cases feedback from observation, together with formal empirical procedures, can provide evidence for claims made by the underlying disciplines (see Tatham & Morton, 2006).

Classical phonetics and applications

Phonetic descriptions based on classical phonetics:

- Provide linear descriptions of someone's speech, usually based on the IPA transcription system in combination with the subjective interpretation of the labeller; idealization in the subjective approach confines this to static modeling—dynamic variability is seldom considered;
- Enable inferences about the listener's phonological perceptions; and
- Allow annotation of departures from expected norms of speech—suggesting possible disorders.

We have suggested a possible format for applications models based on classical phonetics (Tatham & Morton, 2006).

Cognitive phonetics and applications

In addition to the descriptions provided by classical phonetics, cognitive phonetics addresses

- The requirement for linking underlying linguistic events (the phonology, including the prosodic features of rhythm, intonation and stress) to descriptions of the waveform. It puts speech processes into a larger language framework, incorporating the derived utterance plan—the intended linguistic shape for the final utterance prior to phonetic rendering.
- The relationship between cognitive and physical phenomena in an active way within a dynamic model through the pivotal mechanism of the utterance plan.
- Variability as a cognitive influence on the waveform, taking into account expressive and emotive effects.
- A focus for the model based on the listener through the principle of "production for perception."
- The listener's ability to reduce variability to meaningful categories by a process of assignment of idealized representations to analyzed waveforms, and by procedures that can repair damage to the intended waveform.
- The need for an integrated speech production and perception model in which errors can be more precisely specified than they can using the classical phonetics model's surface and linear descriptions.

Conclusion

In this chapter we have contrasted two distinct theories of speech: classical phonetics and cognitive phonetics. Classical phonetics remains useful as a means of describing subjective observations about articulation and listeners' reactions to the resultant soundwave. Classical phonetics also brought us a comprehensive symbolic representation to record these observations in alphabetic form. Classical phonetics is, however, a strictly linear approach to what we now understand to be a highly complex hierarchically organized system. Consequently it fails to explain the surface observations it seeks to characterize.

Cognitive phonetics is typical of a more rigorous contemporary approach to speech production and perception as exemplified by Keating (1990, 2006). It recognizes the hierarchical structure of language and attempts to model the relationship between cognitive and physical processes in speech production and perception. This model also relates earlier attempts to characterize language in a static way to capture generalizations optimally and a more dynamic modeling that can relate individual instantiations to the underlying generality. This last property seems to increase the usefulness of the model in applications, but also in attempting to answer interdisciplinary questions.

The rigorous computational format of cognitive phonetics (Tatham & Morton, 2005) draws out gaps in the theory, leading straight to hypotheses for guiding future thought and experimental work.

Further reading

Kim, D., Clayards, M., & Kong, E. J. (2020). Individual differences in perceptual adaptation to unfamiliar phonetic categories. *Journal of Phonetics*, *81*, 100984.

Tatham, M., & Morton, K. (2006). *Speech production and perception*. New York: Palgrave Macmillan.

Volenec, V., & Reiss, C. (2017). Cognitive phonetics: The transduction of distinctive features at the phonology-phonetics interface. *Biolinguistics*, *11*, 251–294.

References

Abercrombie, D. (1967). *Elements of general phonetics*. Edinburgh: Edinburgh University Press.

Baer, T., Gore, J. C., Gracco, L. C., & Nye, P. W. (1991). Analysis of vocal tract shape and dimensions using magnetic resonance imaging: Vowels. *Journal of the Acoustical Society of America*, *90*(2 Pt 1), 799–828.

Bregman, A. S. (1990). *Auditory scene analysis*. Cambridge, MA: MIT Press.

Charles-Luce, J., Dressler, K., & Ragonese, E. (1999). Effect of semantic predictability on children's preservation of a phonemic contrast. *Journal of Child Language*, *26*(3), 505–530.

Cooper, F. (1966). Describing the speech process in motor command terms: Status reports on speech research. *Haskins Laboratories, SR*, *515*, 2.1–2.7.

Cruttenden, A. (2001). *Gimson's pronunciation of English*. London: Hodder Arnold.

Fant, G. (1960). *Acoustic theory of speech production*. The Hague: Mouton.

Fowler, C. (1980). Coarticulation and theories of extrinsic timing. *Journal of Phonetics*, *8*(1), 113–133.

Fowler, C. (1986). An event approach to the study of speech perception from a direct-realist perspective. *Journal of Phonetics*, *14*(1), 3–28.

Fowler, C., & Galantucci, B. (2005). The relation of speech perception and production. In D. B. Pisoni & R. Remez (Eds.), *The handbook of speech perception* (pp. 633–652). Oxford: Blackwell.

Garland, A., & Alterman, R. (2004). Autonomous agents that learn to better coordinate. *Autonomous Agents and Multi-Agent Systems*, *8*(3), 267–301.

Gibson, J. (1954). A theory of pictorial perception. *Audio Visual Communication Review*, *1*, 3–23.

Hardcastle, W., & Hewlett, N. (Eds.). (1999). *Coarticulation: Theory, data, and techniques*. Cambridge: Cambridge University Press.

Hartsuiker, R., Pickering, M., & deJong, N. (2005). Semantic and phonological context effects in speech error repair. *Journal of Experimental Psychology: Learning, Memory and Cognition*, *31*(5), 921–932.

Higgins, M., Netsell, R., & Schulte, L. (1998). Vowel-related differences in laryngeal articulatory and phonatory function. *Journal of Speech, Language, and Hearing Research*, *41*(4), 712–724.

Keating, P. (1990). The window model of coarticulation: Articulatory evidence. In J. Kingston & M. Beckman (Eds.), *Papers in laboratory phonology I* (pp. 451–470). Cambridge: Cambridge University Press.

Keating, P. (2006). Phonetic encoding of prosodic structure. In J. Harrington & M. Tabain (Eds.), *Speech production: Models, phonetic processes, and techniques* (pp. 167–186). Macquarie Monographs in Cognitive Science. New York and Hove: Psychology Press.

Ladefoged, P., & Maddieson, I. (1996). *Sounds of the world's languages*. Oxford: Blackwell.

Liberman, A., & Mattingly, I. (1985). The motor theory of speech perception revised. *Cognition*, *21*(1), 1–36.

Lisker, L., & Abramson, A. (1964). A cross-language study of voicing in initial stops: Acoustical measurements. *Word, 20*(3), 384–422.
MacNeilage, P. (1970). Motor control of serial ordering of speech. *Psychological Review*, 77(3), 182–196.
MacNeilage, P., & De Clerk, J. (1969). On the motor control of coarticulation in CVC monosyllables. *Journal of the Acoustical Society of America, 45*(5), 1217–1233.
Matthews, P. (1964). Muscle spindles and their motor control. *Physiological Review, 44*, 219–288.
Matthies, M., Perrier, P., Perkell, J., & Zandipour, M. (2001). Variation in coarticulation with changes in clarity and rate. *Journal of Speech, Language, and Hearing Research, 44*, 552–563.
Morton, K., & Tatham, M. (1980). Production instructions. In *Occasional papers* 23 (pp. 14–16). Colchester: University of Essex.
Nooteboom, S. (1983). Is speech production controlled by speech perception? In M. van den Broecke, V. van Heuven, & W. Zonneveld (Eds.), *Studies for Antonie Cohen: Sound structures* (pp. 183–194). Dordrecht: Foris Publications.
Pardo, J. S., & Remez, R. E. (2006). The perception of speech. In M. Traxler & M. A. Gernsbacher (Eds.), *Handbook of psycholinguistics* (2nd ed., pp. 201–248). New York: Academic Press.
Rubin, P., & Vatkiotis-Bateson, E. (1998). Measuring and modelling speech production. In S. L. Hopp, M. J. Owren, & C. S. Evans (Eds.), *Animal acoustic communication* (pp. 251–290). New York: Springer-Verlag.
Stevens, K., & Halle, M. (1967). Remarks on analysis by synthesis and distinctive features. In W. Wathen-Dunn (Ed.), *Models for the perception of speech and visual form* (pp. 88–102). Cambridge, MA: MIT Press.
Tatham, M. (1970). Coarticulation and phonetic competence. In *Occasional papers* 8. Colchester: University of Essex.
Tatham, M. (1971). Classifying allophones. *Language and Speech, 14*(2), 140–145.
Tatham, M. (1984). Towards a cognitive phonetics. *Journal of Phonetics, 12*(11), 37–47.
Tatham, M. (1990). Cognitive phonetics. In W. Ainsworth (Ed.), *Advances in speech, hearing and language processing 1* (pp. 193–218). London: JAI Press.
Tatham, M. (1995). The supervision of speech production. In C. Sorin, J. Mariani, H. Meloni, & J. Schoentgen (Eds.), *Levels in speech communication: Relations and interactions* (pp. 115–125). Amsterdam: Elsevier.
Tatham, M., & Morton, K. (1980). Precision. In *Occasional papers* 23 (pp. 104–113). Colchester: University of Essex.
Tatham, M., & Morton, K. (2002). Computational modelling of speech production: English rhythm. In A. Braun & H. Masthoff (Eds.), *Phonetics and its applications: Festschfrift for Jens-Peter Köster on the occasion of his 60th birthday* (pp. 383–405). Stuttgart: Franz Steiner Verlag.
Tatham, M., & Morton, K. (2005). *Developments in speech synthesis*. Chichester: Wiley & Sons.
Tatham, M., & Morton, K. (2006). *Speech production and perception*. Basingstoke: Palgrave Macmillan.
Wang, W., & Fillmore, C. (1961). Intrinsic cues and consonant perception. *Journal of Speech and Hearing Research, 4*, 130–136.

16

PSYCHOLINGUISTIC VALIDITY AND PHONOLOGICAL REPRESENTATION

Ben Rutter and Martin J. Ball

Introduction

Psycholinguistic theories have had several important insights for speech-language pathologists. Models of speech production and perception have added to the ways in which researchers and clinicians can conceptualize, analyze, and treat a multitude of speech and language disorders. Linguistic models rationalized using psychological or cognitive principles, often based on experimental findings, are appealing because they offer the potential for both explanatory as well as descriptive adequacy (Stackhouse & Wells, 1997). On the other hand, the application of theoretical ideas from strictly descriptive linguistic theories has not always been able to claim such explanatory power. Rather, theories from generative approaches to syntax or phonology, for example, have often provided new and interesting ways to visualize and label clinical data, but any explanation is often heavily couched in theory internal principles.

In this chapter we explore the concept of abstract phonological representations, the kind discussed in most mainstream phonological theories ranging from the seminal work in generative grammar (Chomsky & Halle, 1968), autsoegmental phonology (Goldsmith, 1976, 1990), and more recent generative phonology (Kenstowicz, 1994). We consider the justification for positing highly abstract, single-entry mental representations for lexical items and evaluate the extent to which they have any potential explanatory power for the analysis of disordered speech. We suggest that, like many imports from purely descriptive linguistic theories, abstract phonological representations should not be conflated with genuine attempts to model speech processing and performance. While they are no doubt useful tools for analyzing clinical linguistic data, and perhaps uncovering sound patterns that lie within, their explanatory power for the clinician may in fact be extremely weak. We speculate that the reason lies in the fact that mainstream phonological theories have long concerned themselves purely with linguistic competence, whereas clinical linguists and speech-language pathologists are interested first and foremost in speech performance. What is more, many of the concepts found in phonological theories often take on a slightly different meaning when applied in speech pathology. Our conclusion, however, looks to the possibilities for the future and the development of a more far-reaching application of multiple entry, phonetically rich mental representations of lexical items, as suggested by exemplar theory, and the work of Bybee (2001). We predict, like Ball (2003) and Sosa and Bybee (2007), that clinical applications of such a phonological theory may have much to offer the clinical arena.

The structure of the chapter is as follows. We begin with a brief outline of clinical phonology, focusing on its aims as a discipline. We argue that if clinical phonology is to be anything more than

DOI: 10.4324/9781003204213-18

an exercise in describing clinical data using a set of terms, labels, and diagrams borrowed from mainstream phonology, it must offer the clinician at least some objective explanatory power and some insight into remediation. With this in mind, the next section provides a brief tour of the various definitions of a phonological representation, in both descriptive linguistics and speech pathology. We then trace the gradual evolution of phonological representation, including the conception of the phoneme, distinctive feature, and the autosegment, and then outline a more recent approach to phonological representations, that of usage-based phonology. Following that we suggest that the adoption of usage-based phonology might offer clinical phonology a great deal, and we conclude by summarizing our position, and looking to the future of clinical phonology.

The aim of clinical phonology

Clinical phonology (see, for example, Grunwell, 1987; Ball & Kent, 1998; Ball, Müller, & Rutter, 2009) arose from the revolution of applying linguistic theories, usually reserved for the formulation of grammars based on the analysis of normal speakers alone, to clinical data. As with clinical linguistics in general, clinical phonology is usually cited as having two main aims (see, for example, the preface of Ball, Müller, & Rutter 2009). Firstly, informing the assessment and treatment techniques of the clinician, and, secondly, the testing of the linguistic theories themselves using novel and challenging types of data (so-called "talking back to theory"). Therefore, clinical phonology, as opposed to many branches of purely descriptive phonology, takes as its aim the analysis, primarily, of the speech *performance* of individuals. Descriptive phonology, on the other hand, is the business of analyzing the various systems and patterns of sounds found in specific languages. While these two pursuits clearly have similarities, not least the fact that a speech disorder is defined according to the characteristics of a specific language, their differences should not be overlooked (Ball & Müller, 2002). For example, clinical linguists are typically interested in describing, and then possibly accounting for, the difference between a client's speech output and the expected speech output of a normal speaker. Descriptive linguists are, on the whole, concerned with the description of entire languages. A consequence of this disparity is that many of the concepts found in descriptive theories have taken on a double meaning in clinical phonology. Kent (1998, p. 3) sums this up particularly well:

> The discipline of linguistics is concerned primarily with the structure of language. The disciplines of psychology and speech pathology are concerned primarily with the processing of language – with its formulation and its reception. The linguistic study of language structure has influenced the study of language processing, and, to some degree, the reverse is true as well. Descriptions of language processing often use terms, such as syntax, semantics, phonology, and phonetics, that denote traditional areas of linguistic study. These terms have come to have a dual usage, one referring to structure another to processing.

If the above is true, we should always be careful that the concepts we borrow from descriptive linguistics are truly appropriate for the study of speech performance. It might be the case that, in the domain of phonology, for instance, techniques devised for the description of data are not necessarily appropriate for describing what speakers do. A useful comparison can be drawn with sociolinguistics, which, we would argue, has experienced a similar such tension. Sociolinguists are generally concerned with the variability observed in speech when individuals engage in functional communication. This variability is often related to factors other than lexical meaning; social variables such as age, class, and gender, for example. Because phonology is concerned solely with lexically significant details, many of the theoretical ideas that abound in mainstream phonology are inapplicable to the study of sociolinguistic variation. Unsurprisingly, sociolinguists have not always found the theoretical ideas of descriptive linguistics to be particularly revealing for their interests, and Kerswell and Shockey (2007) describe the phonology/sociolinguistics interface specifically as an "uneasy coexistence" (p. 52).

Unless clinical linguists are to occupy themselves with purely lexically contrastive material in the speech signal, they too must consider whether abstractionist phonological theories are suitable for describing disordered speech data. Our aim in this chapter is to explore this issue by asking whether abstract, single-entry phonological representations can be considered a psycholinguistically valid concept. More specifically, we propose the following questions: what do the abstract phonological representations of traditional (i.e., generative) theories of phonology denote? Put simply, what are phonological representations? And, likewise, do they represent the same thing in the parlance of descriptive linguistics as in clinical phonology?

The extent to which these questions are answered by researchers is often limited, particularly in applied fields such as child language acquisition and speech pathology, where the phonemic principle[1] is often taken as a given. However, we will argue that research teams and speech-language pathologists must take seriously the possibility that the foundations on which many of the assumptions we make about speech disorders are based not on psychological reality but in fact on early attempts to simplify transcription methods.

What are phonological representations? And what do they represent?

The phonetics-phonology interface is perhaps the most widely discussed of the linguistic interfaces and is a division that is far from fixed. Defining the distinction is no easy task, but it seems generally agreed upon that a characterization using the notion of levels is essential. This is routinely adopted in textbook definitions of the distinction. Giegerich (1992, p. 31) provides a particularly good definition of the classical phonetics-phonology interface when he states that "[A] phonological analysis entails two levels of representation – a concrete (phonetic) one and an abstract (underlying) one – as well as statements on how the units on one level are connected with corresponding units on the other level."

While this definition is not a comprehensive one, and such a definition would be impossible to find, it is successful in identifying the two critical characteristics of the phonetics-phonology distinction: levels and abstraction.[2] The notion of levels and, importantly, of abstraction, is likely to feature in most, if not all, definitions of the interface. The need for abstraction is argued by citing the vast phonetic variability observable in speech performance. With the same lexeme exhibiting the potential to be produced in multiple ways, it is often suggested that an abstract level of representation is needed to avoid encoding a potentially infinite degree of variability in storage. Therefore, phonological representations employ a finite number of phonological primes with which the lexical representations of words can be written out. The primes are symbolic, as they "stand for" a set of (potentially) infinite phonetic realizations along a continuum.

Therefore, phonology recognizes abstract categories which comprise phonetically distinct but functionally equivalent places along a phonetic continuum. Cohn (2006) uses this as the basis for a schema of the phonetics-phonology distinction (see Figure 16.1).

The notion of levels, of a hierarchical ordering, of representations very much suggests a relationship between this distinction and some physical correlate, be it cognitive or neurological. The

phonology	=	discrete, categorical
≠		
phonetics	=	continuous, gradient

Figure 16.1 A schema of the phonetics-phonology distinction adapted from Cohn (2006, p. 26).

history of such a distinction, however, does not have its roots in attempts at psycholinguistic validity or even models of articulatory planning. Rather, the phonetics-phonology distinction can, and probably should, be seen as originating from different approaches to the transcription of speech. This is suggested in the *Handbook of the International Phonetic Association* itself:

> the International Phonetic Association has aimed to provide 'a separate sign for each distinctive sound; that is, for each sound which, being used instead of another, in the same language, can change the meaning of a word'. This notion of a 'distinctive sound' is what became widely known in the twentieth century as the phoneme.
>
> *(IPA, p. 27)*

The phoneme, then, arose from early attempts to reduce the amount of detail needed in phonetic transcriptions that were only intended to convey the differences between words. Phonetic variation that did not contribute to word meaning was not a desirable feature of such transcriptions. Consequently, two forms of representation of speech arose, a phonetic, also called allophonic or narrow, representation, and a phonological, also called phonemic or broad, representation. It was this distinction that led to the phonetics-phonology distinction, and to the notion of a phonological representation.

> Historically, the IPA has its roots in a tradition of phonology in which the notions of the phoneme, as a contrastive sound unit, and of allophones, as its variant phonetic realizations, are primary; and in which utterances are seen as the concatenation of the realization of phonemes. The use of an alphabetic notation underlines the conceptualization of speech as a sequence of sounds.
>
> *(IPA, p. 37)*

It has been suggested elsewhere that the concept of a phonological representation not only stems from early transcription practices, but also that it has been unduly influenced by the conventions of written language (see Coleman, 1998, p. 47; Linell, 2005). Regardless, it is very much apparent that phonological representations were initially ways of representing speech on paper and were not intended as mental objects. However, in many circles they seem to have come to mean just that.

The mental status of phonological representations

Investigating the mental status of phonological representation is both a challenging and important endeavor. Are phonological representations intended to be mental objects, perhaps templates or scripts for speech organization and production? Are they perceptual targets, strings of abstract units onto which highly variable incoming speech forms are mapped? Or are they merely graphical images that appear on paper to help us better understand sets of data? Coleman (1998, p. 11) discusses the relationship between linguistic representations and cognitive representations and suggests that generative phonological representations can constitute a number of possible things. These include articulatory scripts, mental scripts, or purely theoretical objects; convenient but fictitious.

Perhaps more important for our endeavor is the intended value of phonological representations in speech pathology, and it seems that for speech pathologists the phonological representation denotes something quite different still. It is not uncommon to come across the suggestion that (underlying) phonological representations are in fact something approaching the target, or adult, form of the word a child is attempting to say. For example, Grunwell (1987, p. 171) notes that in a generative approach to disordered phonology "adult pronunciations … form the 'input' to the phonological rules; the 'output' is the child's pronunciation." This is radically different to what underlying representations are in standard generative phonology (Kenstowicz, 1994). Most importantly, underlying forms in generative phonology are abstract whereas surface forms are concrete.

Presumably, both underlying and surface forms in Grunwell's model are concrete, differing only in the extent to which they map onto one another. Moreover, if the input to phonological rules in clinical generative phonology are akin to adult forms, then they must be sociolinguistically accurate and include fine phonetic detail. That is, they must exhibit the phonetic detail that the child is being exposed to and attempting to learn, with sociolinguistic variables such as geographical region and socioeconomic status considered. As a result, they must be written out in the same way the output is, in allophones. However, because clinical generative phonology adopts the machinery of standard generative phonology the input is written out in phonemes and the output in allophones. Hence, there exists a clear disconnect between the intended usage of rules and representations, and their adoption in the clinical realm.

Phonological representations: theoretical approaches

The evolution of the notion of phonological representation over the last three-quarters of a century is worth tracing for a number of reasons. Firstly, it demonstrates the somewhat uneasy relationship between phonology and phonetics, and the trend for phonological representations to be firmed up, tying them more closely to something pronounceable. Secondly, it reflects the changing approaches to the study of speech disorders in clinical phonology. As new theoretical approaches have emerged in mainstream phonology, so too has their application in clinical settings.

We start first with the splitting of the phoneme into its composite distinctive features and then discuss the autosegmental revolution of the 1970s.

Distinctive features

Chomsky and Halle's seminal work *The Sound Pattern of English* (1968) introduced a number of concepts into the mainstream of phonological theory. Referred to as SPE, the book adopted the two-way phonetics-phonology distinction, outlined above, but divided phonological segments into so-called distinctive features. These were the properties of the segments that were responsible for differentiating them from other segments. Because distinctive features were based on those properties of a sound that distinguish lexical oppositions, which themselves are based on binary opposition, distinctive features were binary in nature. In terms of lexical distinctiveness, a sound is either voiced or voiceless, for example, in the same way that a word is either "pin" or "bin"; there is no middle ground. Therefore, for a given feature [X] a segment would be specified as either [+X] or [-X], often displayed as [±X].

Distinctive feature analysis has been adopted in speech pathology, primarily as a means of quantifying speech errors (see discussion and exemplification in Ball, Müller, & Rutter, 2009). However, there are problems is using this approach (see also Grunwell, 1987). For example, errors that seem phonetically closely linked to the target may show a larger number of feature errors than other less closely related due to the limits of a binary, phonological system. Also, there is no way of showing that a change in features in one direction (e.g., /s/ to [t]) is a frequently occurring error, whereas the opposite (/t/ to [s]) is an unusual error, without resorting to a theory of markedness added on to distinctive feature theory. (Even then markedness conventions may not always reflect patterns found in disordered speech as it is predicated on normal.)

Autosegmental representations

While the distinctive feature approach to phonological representations reduced the size of the unit of analysis to below the level of the segment, the theory of Autosegmental Phonology (Goldsmith, 1976), regarded by many as the next generation of generative phonology, tackled the problem of the "absolute slicing hypothesis". The notion that, at the phonological level at least, speech should be represented as a series of serially ordered segments. Goldsmith's motivations were initially the treatment of tone languages, but autosegmental analysis was soon expanded to incorporate features such as [nasal] and place features.

Importantly, the approach of using autosegmental *graphs* as a means of phonological representation, be it for normal or disordered speech, leads to a radically different idea as to what constitutes a phonological segment. In autosegmental representations, segments are simply the minimal unit of organization on their respective tiers and behave *autonomously* (hence the name *auto*segment). What emerges is a picture of phonology quite different to that found in *SPE*, one with several simultaneous tiers of segments, related to each other through association lines, but ordered independently.

Several researchers have applied the insights from this nonlinear approach to phonology to the analysis of disordered speech (see, for example, Bernhardt, 1992a, b; Bernhardt & Gilbert, 1992; Dinnsen, 1997). However, as with classical SPE phonology, it is not clear whether devices such as autosegments and different layers of representation are simply convenient analytic tools, or are intended to have some kind of psycholinguistic or physical reality (see Goldsmith's 1976 comment referred to above). Further, studies such as Bernhardt (1992b), demonstrate that it is not straightforward to transfer the nonlinear analysis of a disordered speaker into nonlinear means of therapeutic intervention: the therapy recommended still has to deal with individual sounds or sound classes, it cannot target an abstract non-pronounceable autosegment.

Government Phonology

A move towards a more phonetically concrete phonology, yet still within the broad bounds of generative linguistics, can be found in Government Phonology (Kaye, Lowenstamm, & Vergnaud, 1985, 1990; Harris, 1990, 1994; Harris & Lindsey, 1995). Government Phonology eschews the abstractness of underspecification in generative phonology (e.g., Archangeli, 1988), and required that its phonological primes, called "elements" (unary and privative rather than the binary, equipollent, distinctive features we referred to earlier), all be phonetically realizable (i.e., each element has an actual pronunciation; though it is hard to work out how the laryngeal elements are supposed to be pronounced). The theory allows different governing relations between elements, and these combinations can account for the range of segmental units in a language. Changes in governing relations can illustrate diachronic or synchronic sound changes. For example, lenition can be characterized as the gradual removal of different elements and/or changes in governing relations between elements from one sound to the next lenited sound (e.g., /t/ to /s/; /s/ to /h/ etc.).

In the same way, disordered speech can be characterized as changes in the relations between elements, or changes in the actual elements between the target and the realization. Harris, Watson, and Bates (1999) and Ball (2002) both apply Government Phonology to disordered vowel systems (See Ball, Müller, & Rutter, 2009, for full details of these elements).

Government Phonology is, then, a step away from the abstractness often associated with generative phonology. However, in terms of direct input into remediation, we still have to test the status of the claimed basic elements and consider how therapy could deal with combining elements into specific governing relations. We also need to recall that this model retains a derivational process from underlying to surface forms – an assumption that has been challenged in recent "cognitive" models of phonology (see below).

Optimality Theory

Still within the tradition of generative phonology, recent work on theoretical phonology has centered on constraint-based approaches to phonological description (see Prince & Smolensky, 1993, Archangeli & Langendoen, 1997) within a model of language termed "Optimality Theory".

Constraint-based phonology, as the name suggests, has constraints only, and is overtly non-rule-based. By this last point we mean that phonological descriptions do not set out to derive a surface realization from an underlying general phonological description through a set of rules, but rather the relation between the input and the output of the phonology is mediated by the ranking of a set of constraints. The set of phonological constraints is deemed universal, their ranking (and possible violability) is language specific.

Optimality Theory operates as follows. GEN, short for generator, takes some underlying form, called the input, and generates a set of possible candidates for its surface form. The candidate set is then evaluated, by EVAL, according to which constraints of the language each candidate violates. Candidates are then ranked according to *relative harmony*. That is, the higher ranked the constraints they violate, the least harmonic they are. The optimal candidate is hence at the top of the relative harmonic ranking and is said to best fit the constraint ranking of the language in question.

As applied to disordered speech (e.g., Dinnsen & Gierut, 2008), constraints can be re-ordered to account for the client's differences from the target phonology. The candidate set is presumably held to be the same, but the differences in constraint rankings yield a different optimal candidate. It is unclear whether those working with the clinical applications of OT believe that the input is the same as it would be for a normal speaker of English, and that the difference in constraint ranking yields the different output form; or whether the input for a client is the target form, i.e., the output for normal speakers. Dinnsen and Gierut (2008) seem to suggest the latter, but this would be completely altering the way OT is claimed to work.

Again, we are left with the question of whether this approach is attempting to model psycholinguistic activities. A leading researcher in the field has answered this question. In addressing the requirement that the GEN component of OT generates an infinite number of possible inputs to the EVAL component, which would seem to disqualify the theory as an actual attempt to model speech production, McCarthy (2002) states clearly that OT does not aim to model the performance of speech production. OT, therefore, does not appear to get us closer to an explanatory model.

Gestural Phonology

Gestural, or articulatory, phonology addresses the problem of phonological organization from a phonetic perspective and proposes the notion that "phonology is a set of relations among physically real events" (Browman & Goldstein, 1992, p. 156). These real events are called "gestures" in articulatory phonology and constitute the prime of the theory. They are neither feature nor segment but represent "the formation and release of constrictions in the vocal tract" (156). The gesture is distinct from the feature in a number of ways and yields a quite different approach to phonological analysis from traditional feature-based theories.

Broadly speaking, a gesture is the formation of some degree of constriction at some place in the vocal tract. In this sense, the gesture is substantiated through articulatory activity. Distinctive features, on the other hand, are properties of a segment that are responsible for phonological contrast. They are atemporal and are defined in a "present or absent" manner. Gestural Phonology defines gestures according to a series of tract variables. A tract variable defines one element of the formation of a constriction in the vocal tract. The tract variables (lip protrusion, lip aperture, etc.) and the articulators that are involved in conducting them (upper and lower lips, jaw, tongue tip, etc.) are described in Browman and Goldstein (1992, p. 157).

A crucial difference between Gestural Phonology and feature based systems is the fact that gestures have internal duration. This allows gestures to vary in how they co-occur. Crucially, it means gestures can overlap not at all, partly, or indeed completely. Gestures will not always align with each other in an absolute fashion and may well overlap. In application to disordered speech (see, for example, Ball, Rutter, & Code, 2008), we can use this facility to show how gestures may be uncoupled from one another (e.g., to show loss of aspiration in stops), gestures can be removed altogether (denasalization), or how one gesture can be removed and a remaining one realigned (e.g., the loss of a nasal stop with concomitant nasalization of the vowel).

Clearly, this approach to phonology is extremely concrete, and should prove useful to clinicians wishing to describe the nature of speech disorders. It does not attempt to provide insights into cognitive processes underlying the disorder, but if coupled with a cognitive approach to phonology it would seem to be potentially of considerable worth.

Usage-based Phonology

Following the work of Goldinger (1997), Johnson (1997), and Bybee (2001), a model of phonology that can loosely be described as *usage-based* is gradually emerging. Based on the principle that (i) both language use and experience play a significant role in shaping a speaker's knowledge of phonology, and that (ii) all experiences of lexical items are stored whole, the theory is very much influenced by, and compatible with, an exemplar account of lexical storage (see Pierrehumbert, 2001). Bybee's book *Phonology and Language Use* (2001) drew together many of the concepts, and subsequent applications have been forthcoming. Bybee's (2001) model claims that mental representations of linguistic objects have the same properties as mental representations of other objects. That is, every instance of a speaker's experience with a word is stored as a fully concrete object, along with the contextual information that came with it. This is radically different from the abstractionist theories above, which are based on single, abstract entries for each lexical item, with only the distinctive information contained in them. In usage-based phonology, the problem of explaining phonetic variability, the original motivation for positing an abstract level of representation, is dealt with through a system of organized storage. Words are stored in a fully specified form, with both fine and coarse phonetic detail, and are associated with the context in which they were encountered.

The application of exemplar theory and "cognitive phonology" to clinical data is still developing, however both Ball (2003) and Sosa and Bybee (2007) have speculated as to what insights this approach to phonological description might have in the clinical arena. Ball, Müller, and Rutter (2009) introduce the basic apparatus of the theory from a clinical perspective adopting Bybee's suggestion of using the formalism of Gestural Phonology (see above). Hatchard (2015) demonstrates how a usage-based approach to language generally can be useful for the analysis of aphasia. Finally, Patrick et al.'s study (2022) represents the first application of usage-based phonology to inform the treatment of cleft palate speech.

Conclusion

As discussed above, clinical phonology is a sub-discipline of clinical linguistics that takes as its aim the explanation of speech sound difficulties in such a way as to inform both treatment and linguistic theory. As the developments in phonological theory that are discussed above have come about, their application to clinical data has generally followed. Ball, Müller, and Rutter (2009) summarize the application of both generative and non-generative phonological theories to clinical data and demonstrate the far-reaching possibilities for modeling the organization of sound patterns.

By far the most influential phonological model in speech pathology has been generative phonology and a very strict phonetics-phonology separation. This has influenced the study of speech disorders in two important ways. Firstly, it has led to the distinction between a phonetic, or *articulatory*, disorder and a phonological, or underlying, disorder. A decision as to which of these two problems should be diagnosed is based on analysis of the client's productions. In other words, if a client uses the wrong phonological unit, be it an entire phoneme or some distinctive feature of that phoneme, from the target language, this is deemed to be a phonological error, whereas if a wrong variant of the unit is used, or if a sound from outside the language altogether is employed, this is deemed to be an articulatory (or phonetic) error.

The second major sense in which phonological representations have influenced the description of phonological disorders is through the use of theories of phonology to describe various symptoms of, for example, child language production. As suggested above, such accounts run the risk of leading to an explanation of the *cause* of the disorder not being due to any physical, be it motoric or neurological, factor but stemming directly from the principles of the theory. As an example, the use of autosegmental representations to explain, for example, consonant harmony, can lead to an analysis that is driven by the constraints on the graphs of the theory rather than any physiological reason. The cause of the symptom, harmonizing word endings with word beginnings, for example, is explained through positing a violation of the no-crossing constraint rather than a problem with the speech production mechanism.

It is perhaps for this reason that the import of theoretical constructs from descriptive linguistics, often via clinical linguistics, into speech-language pathology has not always brought about any real explanatory success. In phonology, specifically, the state of the art has often been used to cast speech disorders in new and interesting ways, explaining them using constraints as opposed to rules, for example, but the real benefit for the therapist has not always been clear. This is summarized well by Locke, when discussing the role of articulation disorders in clinical phonology:

> In Speech-Language Pathology we have a tradition of borrowing from other fields, and I am afraid we also have borrowed this tendency to label instead of explain, and to take our labels as explanations.
>
> *(Locke, 1983, p. 341)*

We do not intend this chapter to be a criticism of clinical phonology; it has offered much to speech-language pathology. However, we suggest that it is important for the concept of a phonological representation of speech, as it is used in a clinical setting, to be reviewed. For one, the mental status of phonological representations is questionable to begin with. It is not clear whether they constitute scripts for articulation, targets for incoming percepts, or purely theoretical objects. It seems certain, though, that the notion of a phonological representation of speech has its roots in the transcription practices of the early 20th century, and not any attempt to model motor execution or speech perception. Secondly, phonological representations are often used in clinical phonology to mean something quite different from standard generative phonology; something approaching an adult, or target, form. This would presumably have to be specific in terms of sociophonetic detail, however the underlying representations in clinical phonology are still written in phonemes, not in fine phonetic detail.

Considering recent developments in non-generative phonology, it might well be the case that the lexicon comprises multiple phonetic entries for a single lexicon item, with the phonological representation of a word functioning essentially like a lexeme. As exposure to more phonetic variability increases, a speaker's ability to map incoming forms onto the correct item increases. This is very much the model proposed by exemplar theory (Johnson, 1997) and probabilistic approaches to phonology (Pierrehumbert, 2003). The result would be that the phonological representation of a word is merely the sum of the experienced surface forms. In terms of production, speakers are likely to adapt their own production to something approximating the trace with the highest frequency of occurrence. This would succinctly explain how speakers' productions of words can change over time, both during acquisition, and as part of ongoing language change. It would also account for the gradience observed in language change (Bybee, 2001).

Such a model of phonology has quite radical but very exciting implications for the way in which we regard a disorder of speech production. It would be more heavily grounded in phonetic, or articulatory, evidence, and rely less on abstract segments. It would also involve the role of experience, and the extent to which a child is capable of storing instances of language use, and then generalizing across them, coming to the forefront of research, assessment, and remediation (see, for example, Patrick et al., 2022). This may well represent a step forward for research as well as clinical practice.

Notes

1 At its simplest, the notion that two distinct levels of representation can be identified, one being concrete, or phonetic, the other being abstract, or phonological.
2 A third possible element could be added to this list in the form of segmentation, and the idea that at the phonological level, at least, it is possible to represent speech as a series of discrete segments.

Further reading

Bybee, J. (2010). *Language, usage and cognition*. Cambridge: Cambridge University Press.
Kaye, J. (2013). *Phonology: A cognitive view*. London: Routledge.
Sande, H., Jenks, P., & Inkelas, S. (2020). Cophonologies by ph(r)ase. *Natural Language and Linguistic Theory, 38*(4), 1211–1261.

References

Archangeli, D. (1988). Aspects of underspecification theory. *Phonology, 5*(2), 183–208.
Archangeli, D., & Langendoen, T. (1997). *Optimality theory. An overview*. Oxford: Blackwell.
Ball, M. J. (2003). Clinical applications of a cognitive phonology. *Phoniatrics, Logopedics, Vocology, 28*(2), 63–69.
Ball, M. J., & Gibbon, F. (Eds.) (2002). *Vowel disorders*. Woburn: Butterworth-Heinemann.
Ball, M. J., & Kent, R. D. (Eds.) (1998). *The new phonologies*. San Diego: Singular.
Ball, M. J., & Muller, N. (2002). The use of the terms phonetics and phonology in the description of disordered speech. *Advances in Speech-Language Pathology, 4*(2), 95–108.
Ball, M. J., & Muller, N., & Rutter, B. (2009). *Phonology for communicative disorders*. Mahwah: Lawrence Earlbarn.
Ball, M. J., Rutter, B., & Code, C. (2008). Phonological analyses of a case of progressive speech degeneration. *Asia-Pacific Journal of Speech, Language and Hearing, 11*(4), 305–312.
Bernhardt, B. (1992a). Developmental implications of nonlinear phonological theory. *Clinical Linguistics and Phonetics, 6*(4), 259–281.
Bernhardt, B. (1992b). The application of nonlinear phonological theory to intervention with one phonologically disordered child. *Clinical Linguistics and Phonetics, 6*(4), 283–316.
Bernhardt, B., & Gilbert, J. (1992). Applying linguistic theory to speech-language pathology: The case for nonlinear phonology. *Clinical Linguistics and Phonetics, 6*(1–2), 123–145.
Bernhardt, B., & Stemberger, P. (1998). *Handbook of phonological development*. San Diego: Academic Press.
Bernhardt, B. H., & Stemberger, J. P. (2000). *Workbook in nonlinear phonology for clinical application*. Austin: Pro-Ed.
Browman, C., & Goldstein, L. (1992). Articulatory phonology: An overview. *Phonetica, 49*(3–4), 155–180.
Bybee, J. (2001). *Phonology and language use*. Cambridge: Cambridge University Press.
Chomsky, N., & Halle, M. (1968). *The sound pattern of English*. New York: Harper & Row.
Cohn, A. (2006). Is there gradient phonology? In G. Fanselow, C. Fery, R. Vogel, & M. Schlesewsky (Eds.), *Gradience in grammar: Generative perspectives* (pp. 25–44). Oxford: Oxford University Press.
Coleman, J. (1998). *Phonological representations: Their names, forms and powers*. Cambridge: Cambridge University Press.
Dinnsen, D. (1997). Nonsegmental phonologies. In M. J. Ball & R. D. Kent (Eds.), *The new phonologies* (pp. 77–125). San Diego: Singular.
Dinnsen, D., & Gierut, J. (2008). Optimality theory: A clinical perspective. In M. J. Ball, M. Perkins, N. Müller, & S. Howard (Eds.), *Handbook of clinical linguistics* (pp. 439–451). Oxford: Blackwell.
Docherty, G. J., & Foulkes, P. (2000). Speaker [speech], and knowledge of sounds. In N. Burton-Roberts, P. Carr, & G. J. Docherty (Eds.), *Phonological knowledge: Conceptual and empirical issues* (pp. 105–129). Oxford: Oxford University Press.
Giegerich, H. J. (1992). *English phonology*. Cambridge: Cambridge University Press.
Goldinger, S. D. (1997). Echoes of echoes? An episodic theory of lexical access. *Psychologial Review, 105*(2), 251–279.
Goldsmith, J. (1976). *Autosegmental phonology* [Ph.D. Dissertation]. Cambridge, MA: MIT.
Goldsmith, J. (1990). *Autosegmental and metrical phonology*. Oxford: Blackwell.

Goldsmith, J. A. (1990). *Autosegmental and metrical phonology*. Oxford: Basil Blackwell.
Grunwell, P. (1987). *Clinical phonology* (2nd ed.). London: Chapman and Hall.
Harris, J. (1994). *English sound structure*. Oxford, England: Blackwell.
Harris, J., & Harris, J. (1990). Segmental complexity and phonological government. *Phonology*, 7(1), 255–300.
Harris, J., & Lindsey, G. (1995). The elements of phonological representation. In J. Durand & F. Katamba (Eds.), *Frontiers of phonology* (pp. 34–79). London: Longmans.
Harris, J., Watson, J., & Bates, S. (1999). Prosody and melody in vowel disorder. *Journal of Linguistics*, *35*(3), 489–525.
Hatchard, R. (2015). *A construction-based approach to spoken language in aphasia* [Doctoral Thesis]. Sheffield: University of Sheffield.
International Phonetic Association (1999). *Handbook of the International Phonetic Association: A guide to the use of the International Phonetic Alphabet*. Cambridge: Cambridge University Press.
Johnson, K. (1997). Speech perception without speaker normalization: An exemplar model. In K. Johnson & J. W. Mullennix (Eds.), *Talker variability in speech processing* (pp. 145–165). San Diego/London: Academic Press.
Kaye, J., Lowenstamm, J., & Vergnaud, J.-R. (1985). The internal structure of phonological elements: A theory of charm and government. *Phonology Yearbook*, *2*(1), 305–328.
Kaye, J., Lowenstamm, J., & Vergnaud, J.-R. (1990). Constituent structure and government in phonology. *Phonology*, 7(1), 193–232.
Kenstowicz, M. (1994). *Phonology in generative grammar*. Cambridge, MA: Blackwell.
Kent, R. D. (1998). Normal aspects of articulation. In J. E. Bernthal & N. W. Bankson (Eds.), *Articulation and phonological disorders* (pp. 1–59). Boston: Allyn & Bacon.
Kerswell, P., & Shockey, L. (2007). The production and acquisition of variable phonological patterns: Phonology and sociolinguistics. In M. Pennington (Ed.), *Phonology in context* (pp. 51–75). Basingstore: Pelgrave Macmillan.
Linell, P. (2005). *The written language bias in linguistics: Its nature, origins and transformations*. London & New York: Routledge.
Locke, J. (1983). Clinical phonology: The explanation and treatment of speech sound disorders. *Journal of Speech and Hearing Disorders*, *48*(4), 339–341.
McCarthy, J. (2002). *A thematic guide to optimality theory*. Cambridge: Cambridge University Press.
Patrick, K., Fricke, S., Rutter, B., & Cleland, J. (2022, July11). Treatment of cleft palate speech using usage-based electropalatography: A within participant case series [Conference presentation]. 14th International Cleft Congress, Edinburgh, Scotland, July15).
Pierrehumbert, J. (2001). Exemplar dynamics: Word frequency, lenition, and contrast. In J. Bybee & P. Hopper (Eds.), *Frequency effects and the emergence of lexical structure* (pp. 137–157). Amsterdam: John Benjamins.
Pierrehumbert, J. (2003). Probabilistic phonology: Discrimination and robustness. In R. Bod, J. Hay, & S. Jannedy (Eds.), *Probabilistic linguistics* (pp. 177–228). Cambridge, MA: MIT Press.
Prince, A., & Smolensky, P. (1993). *Optimality theory: Constraint interaction in generative grammar*. RuCCs Technical Report #2. Piscataway: Rutgers University Center for Cognitive Science.
Rutter, B. (2008). *Acoustic characteristics of dysarthric conversational speech: An interactional phonetic study* [Ph.D. Dissertation]. LA: University of Louisiana at Lafayette.
Sosa, A.V., & Bybee, J. (2007). A cognitive approach to clinical phonology. In M. J. Ball, M. Perkins, N. Müller, & S. Howard (Eds.), *Handbook of clinical linguistics*. Oxford: Blackwell.
Stackhouse, J., & Wells, B. (1997). *Children's speech and literacy difficulties: A psycholinguistic framework*. London: Whurr.

17

FROM PHONOLOGY TO ARTICULATION

A neurophonetic view

Wolfram Ziegler, Hermann Ackermann, and Juliane Kappes

Introduction

In this chapter, we present a neurophonetic perspective on how phonological representations transform into speech movements during verbal communication. Our "neurophonetic view" approaches speech production from its bottom end, not from the top, and the empirical evidence presented here will predominantly relate to neurologic conditions and brain imaging work. Consequently, we consider phonological and phonetic processes to be constrained by the properties of the vocal tract motor system, on the one hand, and the auditory system, on the other. We start out by describing some crucial elements of a tripartite model of normal and impaired spoken language production, and then sketch the representations operating at each processing stage. In the last section of this chapter, we will delineate the neuroanatomic basis of speech production, from motor execution processes up to the level of cortical auditory-somatosensory-motor integration, with a focus on properties fundamental to the emergence of phonological structure.

A tripartite architecture of speech production

Phonological impairment, apraxia of speech, dysarthria

Neurolinguistic and neurophonetic investigations of phonetic–phonological operations and speech motor processes are centered around the observation that brain lesions may compromise verbal communication at different levels of the speech production chain. A fundamental distinction has been made—at least since the work by Marie—between "language" and "motor" deficits of spoken language. Within the clinical domain, this classical demarcation line separates the two syndromes of phonological paraphasia as a linguistic impairment and dysarthria as a plain motor disorder. The term phonological (better: phonemic) paraphasia refers to a class of symptoms characterized by the substitution, omission, addition, or metathesis of one or several phonemes of a word. As an example, a patient suffering from acquired brain damage might say [da:bel] instead of [ga:bel] (English: fork) with perfectly fluent and clear articulation of each segment of the produced nonword. A popular and straightforward symbolic interpretation of such a paraphasic error is that during the encoding of the target word the patient has mis-selected a [d] for a [g] (e.g., Alexander & Hillis, 2008). The units implicated in this encoding failure could equally well represent syllables ([da:] for [ga:]), distinctive phonetic features ([alveolar] for [velar]), or even articulatory gestures (tongue tip for tongue back). Connectionist theories would ascribe such errors to an inefficient transmission of

DOI: 10.4324/9781003204213-19

activation across the nodes of a neural network or to reduced decay rates (Dell, Schwartz, Martin, Saffran, & Gagnon, 1997). "Dual-origin" models of phonological impairment postulate these errors of spoken language to arise either at the level of lexical representation or during postlexical processing steps (Schwartz, Wilshire, Gagnon, & Polansky, 2004). Irrespective of any details, these models assume subsequent speech motor control processes to be uncompromised. As a consequence, the speaker produced a well-articulated but phonemically inaccurate sound category.

By contrast, the term dysarthria refers to a class of disorders characterized, at the bottom end of the speech production chain, by impaired movement execution due to paresis, ataxia, akinesia, tremor, or any other pathological condition of motor control mechanisms (Duffy, 2005). The word [ga:bel] produced by a dysarthric speaker comes out—depending on the specific variant of this syndrome—with overall imprecise consonant articulation, reduced or increased mouth opening, rough, strained, or breathy voice quality, hypernasality, and so on. Nevertheless, a preserved phonemic structure still can be recognized behind these motor implementation problems.

Since Broca's time, a third kind of speech disorder has emerged between these two syndromes. Broca had assumed damage to the posterior component of the left inferior frontal gyrus, a region now bearing his name, to give rise to a distinct variant of speechlessness ("aphemia"): These patients were not "paralyzed" (in our terms: not dysarthric) but appear to have lost the "memory of the procedures that must be followed in the articulation of words" (Broca, 1861). More specifically, he envisaged an impairment of the faculty of speaking (i.e., a loss of the overlearned motor routines pertaining to a speech motor memory). Liepmann, a German neurologist who worked on apraxic disorders of limb movements, later characterized aphemia, which was then called "motor aphasia" or "Broca's aphasia," as an "apraxia of the language muscles" (Liepmann, 1900), suggesting that aphemic patients have "a correct concept of what they ought to do" (here: to say), "but cannot transform the image of the intended action into appropriate motor commands" (Liepmann, 1907). This characterization of aphemia has almost literally entered modern descriptions of a syndrome that is now—following a proposal by Darley (1968)—called "apraxia of speech" (e.g., Hillis et al., 2004, p. 1479). A patient with mild or moderate apraxia of speech, confronted with the task of producing [ga:bel], would typically display problems initiating this word, grope for the initial [g] and eventually produce some sound in between [g] and [d] or [g] and [k] or often even a plain phonemic substitution, try a new start, and finally articulate the word in a disfluent manner, with varying misarticulations, phonemic errors, and repeated self-corrections. By contrast to dysarthria syndromes, none of the pathomechanisms known from neurological movement disorders (such as paresis, ataxia, tremor, etc.) is recognizable behind the behavioral pattern of apraxia of speech. Furthermore, even moderately impaired apraxic speakers may at times produce stretches of unimpaired speech, a phenomenon that cannot be explained within the framework of dysarthric impairments. Unlike phonological disorders, on the other hand, apraxic speech is not well-articulated and shows a markedly nonfluent character, phenomena that led clinicians and researchers to allocate this constellation to the motor domain.

Phonological encoding, phonetic planning, articulation

The classification of neurogenic speech impairments into phonological impairment, apraxia of speech, and dysarthria largely parallels the architecture of psycholinguistic information processing models of spoken language production, especially of the model proposed by Levelt, Roelofs, and Meyer (1999). In this model, the words stored in a speaker's mental lexicon are considered to be composed of a serially ordered set of phonemes. During production of a lexical item, the respective phonemes are read out in their correct order and, in Levelt's theory, are syllabified according to universal syllabification rules. In interactive activation theories of word production (e.g., Dell et al., 1997), the sequence of phonemes of a lexical item is generated by forward and backward activation flows within a network of nodes representing words, syllables, syllable constituents, and phonemes.

The two approaches referred to have in common that the phonological stage of word production ends up with an ordered set of discrete phonemes (Dell) or phonological syllables (Levelt), providing the input to the phonetic encoding stage or the motor component of speech production.

How do these strings of phonological units translate into movements? In Levelt's theory, the phonological syllables of a word activate motor programs stored in a repository of syllable-sized "phonetic plans." At this point, a motor learning concept enters the scene, since the entries of a speaker's "mental syllabary" are considered to represent crystallized speech motor routines, acquired through extensive exercise during language learning (Levelt et al., 1999). This suggestion is reminiscent of Broca's idea of a "memory" of speech motor procedures (see above). The retrieved phonetic plans encompass the "gestural scores" that specify the articulatory movements required for the production of the syllables of a word.

The theoretical accounts mentioned so far consider phonemes the smallest units of word form encoding. However, this basic assumption of phoneme-based approaches is obviously incompatible with the surface characteristics of speech movements and acoustic speech signals. As a fundamentally different approach, articulatory phonology postulates that the word forms housed in a speaker's mental lexicon consist of abstract gestures rather than segments. Gestures are defined as goal-directed vocal tract actions of the speech organs (i.e., lips, tongue tip, tongue body, velum, and glottis). They have a temporal extension and are characterized by the type and location of vocal tract constrictions underlying the formation of speech sounds. Furthermore, the gestures of a word are organized across parallel tiers, with different "bonding strengths" between them. The coherence between two gestures is expressed by their relative timing, technically, by the phase relationship that governs the coupling of two moving masses. Unlike phoneme-based theories, articulatory phonology makes no distinction between a phonological and a phonetic encoding level (Goldstein, Byrd, & Saltzman, 2006). As a consequence, this theory would not propose a fundamental difference between aphasic phonological impairment and apraxia of speech, but rather explain the well-articulated phonemic errors of aphasic patients and the sound distortions of apraxic speakers by similar mechanisms of impaired selection or coupling of articulatory gestures.

All the theoretical accounts mentioned so far assume the final stage of spoken language production to encompass the mechanisms of speech motor execution. These processes, however, are not further specified beyond the suggestion that the commands conveyed to the articulators to move in a phonetically meaningful are prescribed, for instance, by the syllabic gestural scores created by Levelt's phonetic encoder, by the segmental phonetic features activated at the bottom level of connectionist-type models, or by the abstract phonetic gestures that constitute a word in articulatory phonology. More specifically, it is not known how detailed the motor signals sent to the "vocal apparatus" must be in order to allow for accurate and smooth movement sequences. Among others, theories of the motor execution component of speech production should delineate the interplay between sensory-afferent and motor-efferent functions and also account for the adjustment of speech movement parameters to faster or louder speaking modes. Current computational theories of speech motor control are based on feedforward and feedback mechanisms involving orosensory and auditory afferent information, emerging from an extensive adaptive entrainment during a babbling period of language learning (e.g., Guenther & Perkell, 2004). On these grounds, impaired motor execution in dysarthria would reflect a downscaling of movement parameters (paretic or hypokinetic syndromes), intermittent derailments of scaling parameters (hyperkinetic or dyskinetic variants), or a misadaptation of motor commands to afferent sensory information (ataxic dysarthria).

The nature of phonological, phonetic, and motor representations

Classical aphasiology considers the linguistic and the motor domains of speech production as entirely disjunct or mutually "irrelevant" processing stages (e.g., Alexander & Hillis, 2008). Within this traditional account, phonological impairment pertains to the linguistic realm and, therefore, must be assigned—like agrammatism or semantic disorders—to the aphasic syndrome complex. On the other hand, speech motor deficits, including apraxia of speech, are considered part of the nonlinguistic world, relating to a peripheral instrument rather than language proper. This strict dichotomy of linguistic versus motor disorders of spoken language is grounded in implicit assumptions concerning the computational structure (representations, operations) of the phonological, phonetic, and motor levels of speech production, especially the view of an impermeable demarcation between a symbolic-phonological and a physical-motor domain. The following paragraphs discuss some of the properties that must be ascribed to data structures of each of the three stages of speech production.

The discrete nature of phonological representations

The observation that phonemic paraphasias are discrete phenomena has been invoked as an argument for a symbolic nature of the substitution-, deletion-, or addition-mechanisms underlying aphasic phonological impairments. Discreteness of word forms is an indispensable requirement since words refer to—concrete or abstract—discrete objects in our environment (e.g., to knives or forks), hence our vocal motor apparatus must be capable of generating discrete and separable acoustic signals referring to these concepts. As an example, [ga:bel] (fork) must be sufficiently distinct from [ka:bel] (cable) to serve its referential function, and therefore the onsets of these two similar sounding words must differ by at least one discrete feature. Phonological theories congruently assume that words consist of discrete sub-lexical "atoms," though they may differ in their assumptions on the nature and size of these entities (e.g., Goldstein et al., 2006). This particulation of word forms constitutes the basis of our ability to create a potentially infinite number of verbal messages from a small number of primitives (Levelt, 1998).

An important question arising at this point is how discreteness of phonological form can emerge from continuous physical processes such as muscle contractions, mass movements, or aerodynamic events. The ancient dictum *natura non facit saltus* (i.e., nature does not change in leaps) would suggest that a fundamental dualism must exist between discrete phonology, on the one hand, and gradual movements, on the other, and would force us to postulate a purely symbolic nature of phonological representations.

Yet, nature does behave discontinuously and does make leaps. As a first fundamental source of discreteness, speech motor activity involves distinct articulatory organs (i.e., the lips, tongue, velum, etc.). Hence, vocal tract movements inject discreteness into speech production and, reciprocally, we perceive the contributions of discrete articulators when listening to speech. A parallel can be found in general action theory, especially in accounts of how we perceive and imitate actions of the upper extremities (e.g., the hand). Some authors assume action perception to be in general mediated by a body part coding mechanism, supporting the recognition or imitation of the motor actions of other organisms (Goldenberg, in press).

Notwithstanding the fractionation of motor behavior into contributions of separate body parts, even the trajectories of single moving organs are considered to demonstrate—for purely mechanical reasons—instabilities or attractor states, respectively. These biomechanical properties surface into discrete behavioral patterns. Dynamic field theories or coupled oscillator accounts of biological motion provide the theoretical framework for a description of these phenomena, assuming, for example, movement planning models to be based on nonsymbolic representations that by virtue of their nonlinear physical properties exhibit discontinuous behaviors (Erlhagen & Schöner, 2002).

Further sources of emergent discreteness can be found in the aerodynamic processes associated with spoken language. For instance, a small gradual change in transglottal airflow rate may give rise to a discrete bifurcation between oscillating and nonoscillating vocal folds, hence, between voiced and voiceless consonants. Or an equally small gradual step may turn a turbulent into a laminar airflow (i.e., a fricative into an approximant). Finally, our auditory-perceptual system imposes a great deal of discreteness by fine-tuning its acuity to language-specific, discriminative features of the acoustic signal.

Taken together, there is no sufficient reason to maintain a strict dualism between the discreteness of phonological units and the gradedness of speech movement parameters. The movement-to-sound transformations that underlie human speech embrace a variety of mechanisms that generate discreteness within the domains of motor behavior and sound production, providing a basis for particulation in phonology. As a consequence, discreteness of the units implicated in phonemic paraphasia is by far not incompatible with the view that paraphasic errors arise at some abstract level of speech motor control.

Phonetic representations: from gestures to rhythms

Given that phonological primitives are discrete entities, how are they combined in order to specify the input to the speech motor execution system? Psycholinguistic theories converge on the notion that the phonetic plans for speaking are linear strings of phonetic primitives; that is, syllables (in Levelt's model) or phonemes (in connectionist accounts such as Dell's proposal). As a consequence, the unfolding speech movements operate on information chopped into linearly ordered fragments. In Levelt's model, for instance, articulation of the word [ga:bel] is based on two motor programs, one for each syllable, which are implemented one-by-one in a serial fashion by the motor execution system. As concerns Dell's account, the phonological network would generate five phonemes for [ga:bel], each specified by its distinctive features, which are then fed into the neural motor apparatus of spoken language.

This architecture leaves a large part of the "articulation work" unspecified, delegating it to lower level mechanisms of motor execution. Levelt's syllable-based phonetic plans, for example, do not contain any information concerning the concatenation of two or more syllables to form a word, or any suprasyllabic information concerning its rhythmical structure. These shortcomings loom even larger in case of phoneme-based motor programs, in which all coarticulation processes and any prosodic modulation is left to the motor implementation component.

From the perspective of speech motor planning impairment (i.e., apraxia of speech), linear concatenation models of phonetic planning make very clear predictions: if all motor programming work were encapsulated in the syllables or the phonemes of a word, the number of speech errors of a patient in an utterance would depend solely on the number of phonetic units the utterance contains, but would not be influenced by structural properties from above or below the supposed phonetic unit. If, for instance, Levelt's view is adopted and phonetic representations are conceived of as strings of syllables, the pattern of apraxic errors occurring in a stretch of speech should depend on the number of syllables, but not on their subsyllabic architectures or their metrical parsing (Ziegler, Thelen, Staiger, & Liepold, 2008).

Yet, empirical data are at variance with this prediction. When we count apraxic errors, we find that their frequency in fact depends on syllable number, but also on the complexity of syllable structure (more errors on complex than on simple syllables) and on the grouping of syllables into metrical feet (more errors on two stressed syllables than on a trochee). This implies that phonetic representations (or motor plans) of speech utterances have a complex, hierarchical architecture (Ziegler et al., 2008).

The probability of phonetic encoding to fail in patients with apraxia of speech can be modeled rather efficiently by metrical tree structures of phonological words, with "phonetic gestures" at the bottom level and metrical feet at the top level (Figure 17.1).

The structure in Figure 17.1 is reminiscent of the connectionist network postulated in Dell's phonological encoding model (Dell et al., 1997), with the difference that it extends to the level of phonetic gestures and that it is designed to describe the makeup of motor programs, as inferred

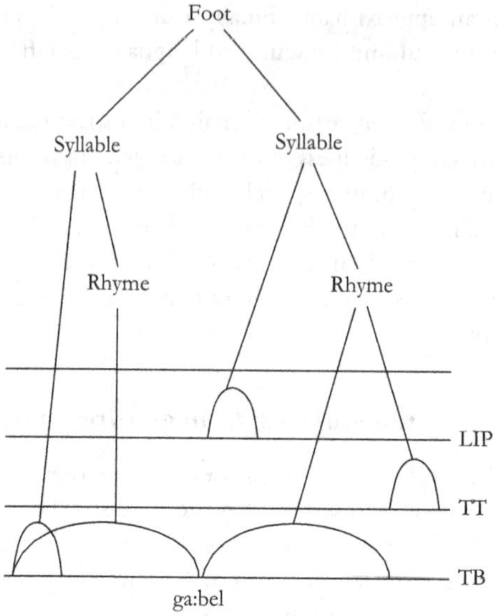

Figure 17.1 Gestural and metrical structure of the word [ga:bel] (engl.: fork), as a model of the non-linear architecture of its phonetic plan.

from the behaviors of patients with speech motor programming disorders. The model depicted in Figure 17.1 also borrows from articulatory phonology in that it uses vocal tract gestures as its primitives and parameterizes the bonding strengths between them (cf. Goldstein et al., 2006). It thereby creates phonetic representations that integrate the signature of the evolving movement sequence from the gestural to the rhythmical level.

By such a model, we were able to predict the errors of a large sample of apraxic speakers on a large variety of word forms (Ziegler, 2009). The prediction was by far better than predictions based on linear string models. The coefficients of the resulting nonlinear model indicated that consonantal gestures in the onset of a syllable or multiple consonants within a syllable constituent impose a high load on phonetic encoding, whereas the consonants in a syllabic rhyme and the syllables in a trochaic foot are less vulnerable than one would predict on purely combinatorial grounds (Ziegler, 2005, 2009). These results suggest that low "bonding strengths" exist between the phonetic gestures at syllable onset and within consonant clusters, and that syllabic rhymes and trochaic feet are highly integrated motor patterns. Hence, if an apraxic patient substitutes [d] for [g] in the onset of [ga:bel], which is not an unlikely event, this may be due to a weak coupling of the velar gesture to the syllabic rhyme of the first syllable.

Overall, the model depicted in Figure 17.1 gives credit to the suggestion that phonetic gestures are basic units of speech motor planning, and it also recognizes that the coupling of these units to form increasingly larger motor patterns, up to the level of metrical feet, must be part of the phonetic information that is finally handed down to the speech motor execution apparatus.

To what extent is speech motor control nonlinguistic?

At the bottom end of the speech production cascade, the vocal tract movements generating the sounds of a word unfold in space and time. According to conventional theories, the neural machinery controlling the speech motor apparatus is prepared to execute all kinds of movement specifications in the same, universal manner. Therefore, lesions to this system are expected to cause motor impairments (e.g., ataxia, paresis, apraxia, etc.), irrespective of the specific motor act to be performed (Ballard, Granier, & Robin, 2000).

Yet, from a clinical perspective this hypothesis must be rejected. It is true that impairments of speech and nonspeech vocal tract movements often co-occur, but numerous clinical reports have also documented instances of brain lesions that compromised speech production, but left other oral motor functions unimpaired. Vice versa, neurologic disorder may interfere with motor activities like swallowing, smiling, tongue protrusion, and so on, sparing spoken language, however. Such clinical dissociations suggest a task-specific perspective on vocal tract motor control, which postulates different neural organizations for autonomous metabolic motor functions (breathing, swallowing), emotional expression (laughter, smiling, sobbing, crying, etc.), nonspeech voluntary motor activities (imitation of mouth movements, visuomotor tracking, etc.), and speech (Bunton, 2008; Ziegler, 2003).

The clinical dissociation between voluntary vocal tract movements, on the one hand, and emotionally expressive facial or laryngeal movements, on the other, has a clear neural basis that will be sketched in a later section. The control of vegetative-autonomous motor functions like breathing or swallowing by distinct neural "pattern generators" in the brainstem is also relatively well understood. Yet, dissociations obviously also exist between different types of voluntary vocal tract actions, on the one hand, and speaking, on the other (Connor & Abbs, 1991; McAuliffe, Ward, Murdoch, & Farrell, 2005; Ziegler, 2002). One of the core arguments for a specific neural organization of speech as compared to nonspeech voluntary vocal tract movements implies that verbal communication is based on a lifelong motor learning process that, through mechanisms of experience-dependent neural plasticity, creates a motor network specifically tuned to the control of speech (see below). As a result, the motor processes at the bottom end of the speech production chain are not at all exclusively nonlinguistic phenomena. They are patterned in a way unique to speech, integrate respiratory, laryngeal, and articulatory muscles in a characteristic manner that is not seen in any other motor activity, are tuned toward the goal of producing sounds, and are entrained over many years, through extensive daily exercise, to subserve this specific goal. Motor control of spoken language must, therefore, be considered an extension of the human language faculty into the periphery of its vocal execution apparatus (Ziegler, 2006).

From articulation to phonology: neural correlates

As outlined above, one of the most salient properties that distinguish human spoken language from vocal communication in subhuman primates is the generative nature of the speech code. Macaques or squirrel monkeys produce calls of a holistic and largely invariant acoustic structure, highly contingent upon specific stimulus constellations and rigidly bound to distinct social functions. As a consequence, monkeys and apes show very limited vocal learning capabilities (Fitch, 2000). In contrast, human verbal communication is based upon patterned signals: the lexical signs of human speech consist of separable and recombinable units, which is fundamental to our capacity to expand our lexicon by learning or creating new words for new concepts (Levelt, 1998). In the following paragraphs, we briefly sketch the neural basis of this capacity, with a particular emphasis on some of the functional properties that distinguish human speech from primate vocal signaling.

Motor execution

A dual-route system of vocal communication in humans

Vocal behavior of monkeys and apes, on the one hand, and human speech, on the other, are mediated by largely different neural networks. The monkey vocal motor system is based on a limbic-mesencephalic-bulbar pathway, which plays only a subordinate role in human communication.

Vice versa, human speech is supported by a neocortical-bulbar motor system, extended by two subcortical pathways, which also exists in subhuman primates, but is "silent" in these species.

The primate vocal motor system has been investigated most extensively in the squirrel monkey model (Jürgens, 2002). Spontaneous calls of these animals arise from neuronal activity in the anterior cingulate gyrus, a cortical structure on the mesial surface of the frontal lobes. The anterior cingulate gyrus is part of the limbic system and is considered to be associated with motivational and affective aspects of behavior. The primate vocal pathways descend from this structure via the midbrain periaqueductal grey to the reticular formation and the vocal tract motor nuclei in the brainstem, eliciting, ultimately, vocalization-related contractions of the laryngeal and supralaryngeal muscles. This system also exists in humans, where it is considered to mediate intrinsic vocalizations like laughter or crying (Ackermann & Ziegler, 2009.

However, the neural pathway conveying volitional vocal tract motor control in humans is almost entirely separate from the limbic vocalization pathway of sub-human primates. It originates from rolandic motor cortex on the anterior bank of the central sulcus and the precentral gyrus, from where it descends to the brainstem motor nuclei. The various vocal tract muscles are represented within the lower third of the lateral precentral motor strip. As a consequence, intraoperative electrical stimulation of this cortical area has been found to elicit vocalizations and facial movements. Bilateral lesions to the face, mouth, and larynx region of primary motor cortex or the descending cortico-bulbar fiber tracts yield a severe dysarthric syndrome, eventually even complete aphonia and anarthria, indicating that this neural pathway plays a crucial role in human speech. In monkeys, on the contrary, complete bilateral destruction of lower sensorimotor cortex does not compromise vocal behavior, although it renders the animals unable to chew, lick, and swallow.

Remarkably, patients who are severely dysarthric or entirely mute after bilateral corticobulbar lesions often display preserved or even exaggerated facial and laryngeal motor patterns in emotionally expressive behavior such as laughter or crying (Ackermann & Ziegler, 2009). Moreover, unilateral lesions of motor cortical pathways projecting on the facial nucleus yield a similar dissociation of emotional and volitional motor behavior. The patients are unable to abduct the contralesional side of their mouth when instructed to volitionally spread their lips, whereas emotional stimuli may elicit an entirely symmetrical spontaneous smile (volitional facial paresis). The reverse pattern of a unilateral emotional facial paresis has also been described. This syndrome is characterized by a preserved volitional abduction of the mouth on the contralesional side, but an asymmetric spontaneous smile (Hopf, Müller-Forell, & Hopf, 1992). As a conclusion, these clinical observations demonstrate that human volitional and emotional vocal motor functions are mediated by distinct neural pathways. As will be outlined below, the specific properties of the neocortical, volitional vocal motor pathway are fundamental to the emergence of a communication system based on particulated vocal signals.

Fractionation and dexterity of the corticobulbar motor system

The vocal motor responses elicited through electrical stimulation of inferior precentral gyrus in humans are not speech-like or well-articulated. This system conveys only fractionated gestural elements of sounds or syllables rather than phonologically structured information. More generally, primary motor cortex activity is considered to be implicated in controlling gestural fractions of complex motor acts rather than holistic actions, which is considered an important basis of the fractionated architecture of skilled motor activity (Brooks, 1986). As we have seen, gestural fractionation is also a salient feature of phonological structure, especially from the perspective of articulatory phonology, in which words are considered to be composed of coordinated vocal tract gestures (Goldstein et al., 2006).

Importantly, the human vocal motor pathway contains direct, monosynaptic fibers projecting onto the vocal tract motor nuclei of the brainstem, including the laryngeal motor nucleus (nucleus ambiguus). The nucleus ambiguus is remarkable, because in monkeys and apes this nucleus lacks a direct, monosynaptic connection with cortical motor cells (Kuypers, 1958). In humans, this direct projection entails that the human laryngeal muscles, like the muscles of the face and mouth, can be addressed directly by cortical signals and may therefore be implicated in versatile vocal motor activity. This allows for a laryngeal contribution to articulated speech, for example, through rapid ad- and abductions of the vocal folds for the distinction between voiced and voiceless consonants, or through a fine-tuning of vocal fold stiffness in the control of pitch for the expression of accent and intonation.

Plasticity of the vocal tract motor system

Unlike the limbic motor system of intrinsic vocalizations, the motor network involved in human speech motor control is characterized by a high functional and structural plasticity. Studies in monkeys and humans have shown that motor exercise of the extremities leads to a structural and functional reorganization at the level of the primary motor cortex. The mechanisms of motor cortical plasticity are mainly characterized by a restructuring of connections between motor cortical neurons and a modulation of synaptic processes. These mechanisms can be triggered by motor learning and motor exercise. The dynamic architecture of primary motor cortex and its resulting functional plasticity are viewed as an important prerequisite of behavioral flexibility and adaptivity (Sanes & Donoghue, 2000). Practice-related plasticity is not confined to the hand area of the motor strip, but in humans has also been shown for cortical vocal tract muscle representations, especially the tongue (Svensson, Romaniello, Wang, Arendt-Nielsen, & Sessle, 2006). Therefore, the cortical maps for the control of speech movements in adults must be viewed as the result of a long-lasting vocal motor learning process, with the consequence that vocal tract movements for speaking have their own specific motor cortical representation.

Learning-induced plasticity extends beyond primary sensorimotor cortex and also encompasses the two subcortical motor loops subserving volitional movement control (i.e., the basal ganglia and the cerebellar loop). The basal ganglia and cerebellum are even considered to play an important active role in the acquisition of motor skills, and their contribution to movement control itself is continuously modulated throughout the motor learning process (Ungerleider, Doyon, & Karni, 2002). Again, this knowledge comes from investigations of manual functions, but there is no reason to assume that the results of these studies do not also apply to vocal tract movements.

As a conclusion, the plasticity of the human vocal tract motor system entails that over the many years of language acquisition motor execution for the production of speech attains a high degree of linguistic specificity. The acquired routines lend themselves to the emergence of phonological representations for the control of speech movements.

Motor planning

As mentioned above, the corticobulbar pathways—in cooperation with cerebellar and striatal motor loops—operate as a speech motor execution system. Bilateral functional organization represents one of the salient features of this neural circuitry. Besides this network, a further cerebral system has been identified that is lateralized to the language-dominant hemisphere and is assumed to subserve speech motor planning processes. Based on observations in patients with severe speech production deficits after damage to the "foot of the third frontal convolution" of the left hemisphere, Broca proposed this area to represent the seat of the "faculty of spoken language" (Broca, 1861, 1865). Since Broca's time, both the status of the disorder we now call apraxia of speech as well as the location of the respective lesions have been disputed passionately. Besides Broca's area, dysfunctions of the white matter underlying left anterior inferior frontal gyrus, of the left anterior insular cortex, and of the oral-facial region of the left primary motor strip have been reported to give rise to apraxia of speech (Ziegler,

2008). Despite the many controversies revolving around this syndrome, one finding has stood the test of time: apraxia of speech is bound to a lesion of the left hemisphere, more specifically, of the anterior peri- and/or subsylvian regions of the language-dominant cortex.

Brain imaging studies have repeatedly identified left anterior insular cortex and ipsilateral inferior frontal gyrus as components of the cerebral network of motor aspects of speech production (for an overview see Riecker, Brendel, Ziegler, Erb, & Ackermann, 2008). Their role within the hierarchical organization of the speech production process was specified in an fMRI-study by Riecker et al. (2005), who identified the left dorsolateral premotor and left anterior insular cortex as part of a "premotor" network whose activation precedes activation of the motor execution pathways mentioned above and is considered to be responsible for higher-order motor planning processes. In Broca's understanding, the left posterior inferior frontal cortex houses the implicit memories for the motor procedures constituting the faculty of spoken language (see above), in Levelt's theory this region would be considered as the neural substrate of a store of syllabic motor plans, still others have used the terms planning, programming, or orchestration of articulation to describe its role. More specifically, Broca's area has been assumed to participate in hierarchical sequential processing (Fiebach & Schubotz, 2006), functions crucially engaged in motor planning processes, as described in Figure 16.1. Furthermore, the ventral premotor cortex and Broca's area play a key role as target areas in the mapping of sensory onto motor representations (see below).

Although the Broca homologue of macaque monkeys seems to take part in the control of orofacial and jaw muscles (Petrides, Cadoret, & Mackey, 2005), electrical stimulation of this region neither evokes nor interrupts vocalizations in subhuman primates, but reliably interferes with speaking in humans. Therefore, the contribution of this region distinguishes human speech from vocal communication behaviors of subhuman species. The existence of this network lends support to the notion of a phonetic planning component in speech production, which is distinct from the bilaterally organized motor execution system.

Auditory-motor integration

While limb movements navigate us through visual space, speaking unfolds in acoustic space. When we learn to speak, we learn to steer our vocal tract organs in a way that they produce intelligible and natural speech sound sequences. This is not a trivial task, since spoken language requires mastery of a complex tool for the generation of air pressure, regulation of airflow, control of resonances, and creation of noises. There is high flexibility and adaptivity of this system, in the sense that a great variety of different patterns of muscle contractions can be used to bring about the same sound under different circumstances (Guenther, Hampson, & Johnson, 1998). Development and maintenance of such a system requires a high degree of integration of motor and auditory processes, since speech movements are exclusively tuned to the generation of sound sequences.

The guidance of movement through perceptual goals has been a major topic in theories of visuomotor action control. Skillful limb motor activity is considered to involve a "dorsal stream" system, by which visual mental images of a movement are transformed into actual movements. This concept goes back to Liepmann, who identified the "idea" of a movement with an internally generated "movement formula" in terms of some abstract visual image of the movement. Liepmann's concept was taken up and refined in modern neuropsychology, with the persistent view that the left inferior parietal lobe plays a crucial role as an interface between occipital visual and frontal motor areas. In these theories, the parietal lobe is assumed to house mental representations of intended motor actions (for a critical discussion see Goldenberg, 2009).

Hickok and Poeppel (2004) transferred the dorsal stream concept into the motor domain of speech production by postulating the existence of a bidirectional "dorsal" pathway involved in the mapping of sound to movement. This concept is reminiscent of a long-standing connectionist tradition, tracing back to Wernicke, based upon the existence of a fiber tract system (i.e., the arcuate fascicle), which projects from posterior superior temporal gyrus toward inferior parietal and dorsolateral inferior frontal cortex. The dorsal stream system of the left hemisphere plays an obvious role in tasks like word repetition, where the acoustic signal must be transformed into a speaker's own movements (Peschke, Ziegler, Kappes, & Baumgärtner, 2009), but appears to be engaged in various other modalities of speech production as well. For example, overlapping hemodynamic activation of left inferior frontal and posterior temporal regions has been found in brain imaging studies both during perceptual and expressive tasks, an observation that highlights the perceptual-motor integrative role of this system. According to a more refined analysis of the dorsal stream, the posterior superior temporal plane of the left temporal lobe is characterized as a device that matches the speech signal with stored auditory templates, in order to disambiguate the incoming acoustic signal and to extract a sequence of speech-specific auditory representations. These data are then mapped onto motor representations, constrained by the auditory input, and further onto the speech motor plans stored within inferior frontal cortex (Warren, Wise, & Warren, 2005).

A dorsal "do-system" based on auditory information appears also to be present in nonhuman primates and, thus, is not restricted to speech production. Yet, the auditory dorsal stream used in producing and perceiving speech has several specific properties that may explain its key role in the development of a phonological communication system in humans. One is that the lateralization of this network to the dominant hemisphere begins early in childhood. This may indicate its specification as a basis for auditory-vocal learning in human infants. Second, its subcomponents, including the auditory and the motor component, are shaped by mechanisms of experience-dependent plasticity, which is fundamental to the generative properties of the phonological architecture of speech. Third, the system also encompasses left inferior parietal regions that may be considered, in analogy to the visual motor system, to make an important contribution to the mapping of auditory "images" of sounds, syllables, or words onto representations of intended movements. Taken together, this neural architecture can be expected to house an embodiment of the sound generating "tool" of the vocal tract with its rather abstract physical relationships between movement and sound. The representations generated by this system acquire a strong potential of being utilized, beyond speaking and listening, in cognitive operations of many other kinds, such as mental imagery of speech, verbal working memory, or alphabetic script.

Summary and conclusion

The path from phonology to articulation during verbal communication was characterized here as a processing chain, unfolding from abstract representations of intended motor acts via hierarchical motor plans to motor executive functions. Despite the tripartite fragmentation of this process in psycholinguistic models, our knowledge about the exact specification of motor information at each stage is still limited, and there is still considerable disagreement about the separation of phonological from phonetic encoding or of phonetic planning from motor execution stages, respectively. The transitions between the three processing levels distinguished here are continuous, and the motor nature of the information is visible on even the highest stage. We emphasized the functional coherence of the phonology-to-articulation interface by highlighting that phonological representations specify motor information at the upper end of the processing chain, and the motor processes are shaped by linguistic form at its bottom end.

The neural substrate of the phonology-to-articulation system has its origin in a left perisylvian cortical auditory-motor integration network, which is at the core of human vocal communicative behavior. This dorsal stream system targets a lateralized premotor system, considered to store acquired "motor knowledge" about the makeup of speech movements for words and phrases. As a subsequent step of speech production, a bilaterally organized system subserving voluntary control of vocal tract movements is activated. All components of this system are characterized by a high potential for experience-related plasticity, fundamental to the generative potential of particulation in phonology.

The connectivity of the components of this system is well established, which makes the whole network identifiable as the basis of human auditory-vocal linguistic behavior. In the light of the coherent architecture of this system, there is no room for a strict demarcation between linguistic and motor speech processing, or between aphasic phonological and non-aphasic speech impairments.

Further reading

Aichert, I., Lehner, K., Falk, S., Franke, M., & Ziegler, W. (2021). In time with the beat: Entrainment in patients with phonological impairment, apraxia of speech, and Parkinson's disease. *Brain Sciences*, *11*(11), 152–154.

Haas, E., Ziegler, W., & Schölderle, T. (2021). Developmental courses in childhood dysarthria: Longitudinal analyses of auditory perceptual parameters. *Journal of Speech, Language, and Hearing Research*, *64*(5), 1421–1435.

Haas, E., Ziegler, W., & Schölderle, T. (2022). Intelligibility, speech rate, and communication efficiency in children with neurologic conditions. A longitudinal study on childhood dysarthria. *American Journal of Speech-Language Pathology*, *31*(4), 1817–1835.

Lehner, K., Ziegler, W., & KommPaS-Study Group (2022). Indicators of communication limitation in dysarthria and their relation to auditory-perceptual speech symptoms: Construct validity of the KommPaS WebApp. *Journal of Speech, Language, and Hearing Research*, *65*(1), 22–42.

Schölderle, T., Haas, E., & Ziegler, W. (2022). Childhood dysarthria: Auditory-perceptual profiles against the background of typical speech motor development. *Journal of Speech, Language, and Hearing Research*, *65*(6), 2114–2127. [bibtex]. https://doi.org/10.1044/2022_JSLHR-21-00608

Ziegler, W., Aichert, I., Staiger, A., Willmes, K., Baumgärtner, A., Grewe, T., Floeel, A., Huber, W., Rocker, R., Korsukewitz, C., & Breitenstein, C. (2022). The prevalence of apraxia of speech in chronic aphasia after stroke: A bayesian hierarchical analysis. *Cortex*, *151*, 15–29.

References

Ackermann, H., & Ziegler, W. (2009). Brain mechanisms underlying speech. In W. J. Hardcastle (Ed.), *The handbook of phonetic sciences* (2nd ed.). Oxford, UK: Blackwell.

Alexander, M. P., & Hillis, A. E. (2008). Aphasia. In G. Goldenberg & B. Miller (Eds.), *Handbook of clinical neurology* (pp. 287–309). London, UK: Elsevier.

Ballard, K. J., Granier, J. P., & Robin, D. A. (2000). Understanding the nature of apraxia of speech: Theory, analysis, and treatment. *Aphasiology*, *14*(10), 969–995.

Broca, P. (1861). Remarks on the seat of the faculty of articulate language; followed by an observation of aphemia. *Bulletins de la Societé d'Anatomie*, *36*, 330–357.

Broca, P. (1865). On the seat of the faculty of articulate language in the left hemisphere of the brain. *Bulletins de la Societé d'Anthropologie*, *6*, 377–393.

Brooks, V. B. (1986). *The neural basis of motor control*. New York: Oxford University Press.

Bunton, K. (2008). Speech versus nonspeech: Different tasks, Different neural organization. *Seminars in Speech and Language*, *29*(4), 267–275.

Connor, N. P., & Abbs, J. H. (1991). Task-dependent variations in Parkinsonian motor impairments. *Brain*, *114*(1A), 321–332.

Darley, F. L. (1968). Apraxia of speech: 107 years of terminological confusion. Paper presented at the Annual Convention of the ASHA.

Dell, G. S., Schwartz, M. F., Martin, N., Saffran, E. M., & Gagnon, D. A. (1997). Lexical access in aphasic and nonaphasic speakers. *Psychological Review*, *104*(4), 801–838.

Duffy, J. R. (2005). *Motor speech disorders: Substrates, differential diagnosis, and management* (2nd ed.). St. Louis: Elsevier Mosby.

Erlhagen, W., & Schöner, G. (2002). Dynamic field theory of movement preparation. *Psychological Review*, *109*(3), 545–572.

Fiebach, C. J., & Schubotz, R. I. (2006). Dynamic anticipatory processing of hierarchical sequential events: A common role for Broca's area and ventral premotor cortex across domains? *Cortex*, *42*(4), 502.

Fitch, W. T. (2000). The evolution of speech: A comparative review. *Trends in Cognitive Sciences*, *4*(7), 258–267.

Goldenberg, G. (2009). Apraxia and the parietal lobes. *Neuropsychologia*, *47*(6), 1449–1459.

Goldstein, L., Byrd, D., & Saltzman, E. (2006). The role of vocal tract gestural action units in understanding the evolution of phonology. In M. A. Arbib (Ed.), *Action to language via the mirror neuron system* (p. 215). Cambridge, UK: Cambridge University Press.

Guenther, F. H., & Perkell, J. S. (2004). A neural model of speech production and its application to studies of the role of auditory feedback in speech. In B. Maassen, R. Kent, H. Peters, P. van Lieshout, & W. Hulstijn (Eds.), *Speech motor control in normal and disordered speech* (pp. 29–49). Oxford and New York: Oxford University Press.

Guenther, F. H., Hampson, M., & Johnson, D. (1998). A theoretical investigation of reference frames for the planning of speech movements. *Psychological Review, 105*(4), 611–633.

Hickok, G., & Poeppel, D. (2004). Dorsal and ventral streams: A framework for understanding aspects of the functional anatomy of language. *Cognition, 92*(1–2), 67–99.

Hillis, A. E., Work, M., Barker, P. B., Jacobs, M. A., Breese, E. L., & Maurer, K. (2004). Re-examining the brain regions crucial for orchestrating speech articulation. *Brain, 127*(7), 1479–1487.

Hopf, H. C., Müller-Forell, W., & Hopf, N. J. (1992). Localization of emotional and volitional facial paresis. *Neurology, 42*(10), 1918–1923.

Jürgens, U. (2002). Neural pathways underlying vocal control. *Neuroscience and Biobehavioral Reviews, 26*(2), 235–258.

Kuypers, H. G. J. M. (1958). Some projections from the peri-central cortex to the pons and lower brainstem in monkey and chimpanzee. *Journal of Comparative Neurology, 110*(2), 221–255.

Levelt, W. J. M. (1998). The genetic perspective in psycholinguistics or where do spoken words come from. *Journal of Psycholinguistic Research, 27*(2), 167–180.

Levelt, W. J. M., Roelofs, A., & Meyer, A. S. (1999). A theory of lexical access in speech production. *Behavioral and Brain Sciences, 22*(1), 1–38.

Liepmann, H. (1900). The clinical pattern of apraxia ("motor asymbolia"), based on a case of unilateral apraxia (I). *Monatsschrift für Psychiatrie und Neurologie, VIII*, 15–41.

Liepmann, H. (1907). Two cases of destruction of the lower left frontal convolution. *Journal für Psychologie und Neurologie, IX*, 279–289.

McAuliffe, M. J., Ward, E. C., Murdoch, B. E., & Farrell, A. M. (2005). A nonspeech investigation of tongue function in Parkinson's disease. *Journals of Gerontology, 60A*(5), 667–674.

Peschke, C., Ziegler, W., Kappes, J., & Baumgärtner, A. (2009). Auditory-motor integration during fast repetition: The neuronal correlates of shadowing. *Neuroimage, 47*(1), 392–402.

Petrides, M., Cadoret, G., & Mackey, S. (2005). Orofacial somatomotor responses in the macaque monkey homologue of Broca's area. *Nature, 435*(7046), 1235–1238.

Riecker, A., Brendel, B., Ziegler, W., Erb, M., & Ackermann, H. (2008). The influence of syllable onset complexity and syllable frequency on speech motor control. *Brain and Language, 107*(2), 102–113.

Riecker, A., Mathiak, K., Wildgruber, D., Erb, M., Hertrich, I., Grodd, W., & Ackermann, H. (2005). fMRI reveals two distinct cerebral networks subserving speech motor control. *Neurology, 64*(4), 700–706.

Sanes, J. N., & Donoghue, J. P. (2000). Plasticity and primary motor cortex. *Annual Review of Neuroscience, 23*, 393–415.

Schwartz, M. F., Wilshire, C. E., Gagnon, D. A., & Polansky, M. (2004). Origins of non-word phonological errors in aphasic picture naming. *Cognitive Neuropsychology, 21*(2), 159–186.

Svensson, P., Romaniello, A., Wang, K., Arendt-Nielsen, L., & Sessle, B. J. (2006). One hour of tongue-task training is associated with plasticity in corticomotor control of the human tongue musculature. *Experimental Brain Research, 173*(1), 165–173.

Ungerleider, L. G., Doyon, J., & Karni, A. (2002). Imaging brain plasticity during motor skill learning. *Neurobiology of Learning and Memory, 78*(3), 553–564.

Warren, J. E., Wise, R. J., & Warren, J. D. (2005). Sounds do-able: Auditory-motor transformations and the posterior temporal plane. *Trends in Neuroscience, 28*(12), 636–643.

Ziegler, W. (2002). Task-related factors in oral motor control: Speech and oral diadochokinesis in dysarthria and apraxia of speech. *Brain and Language, 80*(3), 556–575.

Ziegler, W. (2003). Speech motor control is task-specific. Evidence from dysarthria and apraxia of speech. *Aphasiology, 17*(1), 3–36.

Ziegler, W. (2005). A nonlinear model of word length effects in apraxia of speech. *Cognitive Neuropsychology, 22*(5), 603–623.

Ziegler, W. (2006). Distinctions between speech and nonspeech motor control. A neurophonetic view. In M. Tabain & J. Harrington (Eds.), *Speech production: Models, phonetic processes, and techniques* (pp. 41–54). New York: Psychology Press.

Ziegler, W. (2008). Apraxia of speech. In G. Goldenberg & B. Miller (Eds.), *Handbook of clinical neurology* (pp. 269–285). London: Elsevier.

Ziegler, W. (2009). Modelling the architecture of phonetic plans: Evidence from apraxia of speech. *Language and Cognitive Processes, 24*(5), 631–661.

Ziegler, W., Thelen, A.-K., Staiger, A., & Liepold, M. (2008). The domain of phonetic encoding in apraxia of speech: Which sub-lexical units count? *Aphasiology, 22*(11), 1230–1247.

SECTION II

Developmental disorders

18

TEMPORAL PROCESSING IN CHILDREN WITH LANGUAGE DISORDERS

Martha Burns

Introduction

Scientists have attempted to understand the seemingly effortless process of language acquisition in infants for decades. Despite the acoustic complexity of speech input and apparent limited neurological processing resources of an immature neonatal brain, most infants master their native language in a few years. To accomplish this, the infant must extract from the continuous auditory signals in the environment meaningful segments that constitute phonemes, syllables, and words and determine how they combine into meaningful strings (Dehaene-Lambertz et al., 2006). The process proceeds predictably and effortlessly despite variability in language exposure or culture (Kuhl, 2000). This ease with which children acquire language and the uniformity across languages led Chomsky in 1986 to propose that human infants must possess an innate neurological capacity to acquire language (Chomsky, 1986). The exact nature of this "language acquisition device" has been debated and researched ever since. Yet, as Kuhl states in a thorough review of the research on language acquisition mechanisms, "cracking the speech code is child's play for human infants but [remains] an unsolved problem for adult theorists and our machines" (Kuhl, 2004). Even more perplexing, perhaps, is why a small proportion (6–7%) of children, without sensory, motor, or nonverbal cognitive deficits, fail to develop normal language skills despite exposure to their native language (Tomblin, Records, & Zhang, 1996).

Historical perspective on issues of causation in language disorders

Although the cause(s) of problems learning language might seem an important issue for those scientific disciplines that study normal language acquisition as well as those that treat language disorders, the issue of causation has been mired in controversy and led to divisions within and between those scientific disciplines for over 40 years. In the 1960s, the relatively new fields of speech pathology and audiology began to back away from "etiologic" approaches to classification of communicative disorders in general in an abandonment of the "medical model" that biased research and training toward finding and curing disease (Irwin, 1964). Marge, in a chapter in one of the early books on language disorders written in the early 1970s, further elaborated on the need to deemphasize etiology in understanding language disorders, citing a primary reason that it implies that there might be a single cause that, if identified, could be corrected and the disability eliminated (1972). But perhaps a greater influence on attempts to find and treat causes of language

DOI: 10.4324/9781003204213-21

disorders came from the impact of two scientific disciplines that dramatically influenced language research in the late 1950s and continue to influence research on language pathology to this day. The first was behavioral psychology, Skinner's reaction to Gestalt psychology, which predominated discussions of language learning beginning in the late 1950s. He attributed language learning to stimulus-response contingencies, and advocated for measurement (and by implication treatment) of only observable phenomenon (Skinner, 1957). The second, which stood in opposition to Skinner's behaviorist explanations of language development, was linguistics, where Chomsky's seminal theories of generative grammar (1959) revolutionized the study of language as a solely human capacity and focused on the study of language structure (1957). As he developed his theory, Chomsky's underlying assumption was that although language performance may not be error free, humans possess an innate capacity to learn and use language, a "language competence" that consists of a set of finite computational "rules" that allow children to acquire language quickly, easily, and effortlessly and allow for infinite and creative use of language to express complex ideas (1964).

Chomsky's theories revolutionized not only the field of linguistics, but also cognitive psychology and speech pathology. The study of language acquisition changed from attempts to "measure language skill" milestones (such as Templin's norms for specific speech sound use or vocabulary counts) to specifying the hierarchy for how word order and grammatical form are acquired (Brown, 1973). Instead of relying on vague quantitative measures to gauge language development, one could analyze phrase structure, average length of utterance, and acquisition of specific grammatical and morphological forms (Lee, 1974). Transformational grammar, and the developmental studies that applied it, also provided a framework for systematically analyzing language disorders and treating the presumed underlying hierarchical linguistic deficits using a developmental model. The availability of a developmental model and tests that provided objective measures of syntactical comprehension and use reduced the concern over identification of etiology. Chomsky's theories ultimately led to the emergence of a new scientific discipline, psycholinguistics (Boden, 2006), which focused the fields of cognitive science and psychology on the importance of language to human cognition. This, in turn, provided an enormous boost to the field of speech pathology by emphasizing the need for identification and remediation of language problems in children; ultimately leading in 1978 to the addition of Language in the name of the professional organization ASHA (from the American Speech and Hearing Association to the American Speech-Language-Hearing Association), and resulting in an approximate fivefold increase in certified ASHA members during the same time period (www.asha.com).

However, despite the decreased interest in and emphasis on causation in linguistics and speech–language pathology, others scientific disciplines continued to seek causative explanations for language disorders in children. The field of learning disabilities, for example, was initially rooted in neurological explanations for language disorders (Johnson & Myklebust, 1967). Similarly, some cognitive psychology researchers continued to seek causal explanations for language disorders. Tallal and Piercy were among the most influential researchers in the field of psychology to explore nonverbal auditory processing disturbances that might underlie problems learning language (1973). Yet, because of the profound influence of Chomsky during the period when their original research was published and the prevailing viewpoint that language was an innate human capacity, many psycholinguists originally dismissed their findings, maintaining that nonverbal processing could not play a significant part in a neurological faculty innately derived through a "language acquisition device" (Burns, 2007). Today, although some controversy persists regarding the importance of auditory processing in language acquisition (Bishop, Carlyon, Deeks, & Bishop, 1999), the prevalence of interdisciplinary research involving developmental psycholinguistics, clinicians, and neuroscientists has led to a resurgence of interest in causal mechanisms of language disturbance and recognition of the importance of timing and synchrony in neurological cognitive systems (Boden, 2006).

In this regard, what is now often referred to as the "temporal processing hypothesis," stemming from the research of Tallal and Piercy in the 1970s, has been refined and studied extensively in recent years. Essentially the hypothesis asserts that some language impaired children have difficulty processing rapidly changing acoustic details, which interferes with their ability to adequately parse incoming language signals into phonemes and thereby have an increased risk of developing speech, language, and/or reading problems (Tallal & Piercy, 1974; Tallal & Stark, 1981). This explanation essentially views the capacity to process rapidly changing sensory inputs as a probable core neurological component of phonological processing. How this core capacity is understood by neuroscience and the role it may play in language acquisition is an unfolding scientific inquiry. This chapter will attempt to review and clarify the current state of neuroscience research that led to and supports the temporal processing hypothesis and will review research on assessment and the remediation value to auditory training of temporal processing skills. However, the viewpoint of this chapter is that the consideration of the role of temporal processing in language learning does not necessitate rejecting Chomsky or the vast accumulation of psycholinguistic research on language learning and language disorders. Rather, it is the perspective of this author, that understanding temporal processing adds to what some might consider the top-down influence of language and conceptual knowledge on learning by specifying co-occurring bottom-up processes that influence language learning as well.

Origins of the temporal processing hypothesis

All scientific disciplines begin with a set of underlying principles that define the science. Boden, a preeminent archivist of historical perspectives in cognitive science, has recently likened the child learning language to the scientist,who "formulates theories and hypotheses which suggest what to look for, and where to look for it" (Boden, 2006, p. 647). As speech–language pathologists, audiologists, and psychologists, our science is based in behavior. We tend to study the observable behavioral outcomes to controlled stimuli. In general, we attempt to conduct group research studies where we test hypotheses about factors we theorize may lead to specific behavioral outcomes. Neuroscience is a relatively new scientific discipline that is an outgrowth of medicine (neurology), cognitive science, psychology, and computational studies of neurophysiology that blends all disciplines in an attempt to understand brain function (Bishop, Carlyon, Deeks, & Bishop, 1999). Cognitive neuroscience, for example, uses physical data from brain imaging of various types to attempt to understand the brain processes that underlie specific behaviors. The Temporal Processing Hypothesis is an outgrowth cognitive neuroscience research that seeks to identify neurological processing characteristics that may define and underlie cognitive development. To that end, cognitive neuroscientists distinguish bottom-up from top-down neurological factors in neurological information processing, and seek to define those processes that seem critical to acquisition of any cognitive skill.

Top-down versus bottom-up attentional and perceptual processes

Imagine you are on a bus in a foreign country for the first time and you hear a stream of dialogue in a foreign tongue that you have never experienced before. At the same time, you are aware that the speakers, sitting just across from you, are having a very animated discussion about what appears to be a minor accident in the street. Chances are, as an adult with a well-developed knowledge of how language is organized and years of experience using nonverbal pragmatic cues to guide comprehension, you would begin to use context, gestures, intonation, and facial expression to figure out some of the content of the conversation. You could, for example, probably very easily discern whether the speakers are happy, angry, or sad; in agreement or disagreement; friends or strangers; and so on. If they are pointing or looking at the scene outside the bus, you may also be able to extract meaning from some of their spoken words, especially if spoken with expression and if they resemble words of your own language. That ability to use past knowledge and experience to extract meaning from a sensory event is referred to in neuroscience as "top-down" processing. It has been described and researched thoroughly in the visual processing neuroscience literature (Corbetta & Schulman, 2002) and applied to conceptualization and research on auditory processing disorders in children (Chermak & Musiek, 1998). If on the other hand you wanted to say or repeat words or phrases that were spoken by the foreign speakers, with no prior experience with that language, you would need to attend to different aspects of the conversation. As an adult you would struggle to attend to the internal details of the words. As linguists we could describe that task as determining the phonological composition of the words. As acousticians we might describe the process as identifying and discriminating the relevant temporal or spatial acoustic events that signal differences in meaning. Cognitive neuroscientists and audiologists refer to that "data driven" analysis of incoming sensory events as "bottom-up" processing (Chermak & Musiek, 1998).

In most human sensory processing, both top-down and bottom-up processing is thought to occur simultaneously, through distributed neuronal networks that allow application of past knowledge and experience to the task of attending to and learning from novel sensory information. Fortunately, through advances in neuroimaging technology, scientists can now observe these processing systems at work by carefully controlling sensory events and responses and documenting how the brain changes its strategy to handle top-down versus bottom-up tasks (Cabeza, Ciaramelli, Olson, & Moscovitch, 2008). One component of bottom-up processing of auditory information gleaned from neuroscience research that appears to be essential for learning language is the ability to process rapidly changing sensory inputs (Tallal, 2004). To understand how this relates to language acquisition a discussion of neurological processing of sensory information is helpful.

How the brain processes sensory information

To explain neuroscience exploration of perception, one has to review a few principles of neurological processing. First, although a neuron essentially has only two ways to respond to a stimulus, fire or not fire, the firing rate of serial spikes is likely the mechanisms neurons use to convey information. This is often referred to in systems neuroscience as the "neural code" (Van Vreeswijk, 2006). Therefore, single neurons probably do not convey much information in isolation, but rather form networks by connecting to other neuron groups that work together to fire in patterns (Mesulam, 2000). Just as a single instrument in a symphony orchestra might not play a recognizable melody by itself, the combined contribution of all of the instruments yields a recognizable composition (Kenet, Arieli, Tsodyks, & Grinvald, 2006). Following that analogy, neurons fire in patterns that must combine to convey information. But what are these patterns?

Neuroscientists have discovered through several different methods of studying neuronal firing patterns that neurons, similar to musical instruments in a band or orchestra, seem to convey information by their firing rate and rhythm. Rate and rhythm are temporal (timed) aspects of a signal. If a person claps out the rhythm of "Happy Birthday," without humming the melody or singing the words, most people who know the song can identify it just from the rhythm. But if the rhythm gets distorted by clapping some of the measures too quickly in relation to the others, omitting some of the claps, or inserting pauses or extra claps where they do not belong, then the rhythm becomes unidentifiable. It is no accident that the temporal lobe of the brain is responsible for perception of sound; perception of sound requires analysis of the temporal aspects of the acoustic signal that are referred to as temporal acoustic cues. When one observes the brain at work, processing speech for example, there are regions of the left frontal lobe that appear to be essential when decoding requires handling rapidly changing temporal events (Temple et al., 2000). There is recent evidence that abnormal processing in that area correlates with reading disability (Nagarian et al., 1999), and, of perhaps greater importance, is remediable (Merzenich et al., 1996), and when remediated, improves language (Tallal et al., 1996) and reading skills (Gaab, Gabrieli, Deutsch, Tallal, & Temple, 2007). This research points to the importance of understanding this neurological capacity to process information in a temporal array, and how that contributes to bottom-up processing required for language acquisition and reading skill.

Temporal processing and language acquisition

Speech is, of course, a flow of rapidly changing acoustic events. As stated above, "temporal processing" refers to the ability to process rapidly changing temporal events, both in a stream of speech and also in nonspeech acoustic events. From a neurological perspective, rapid changes are those that occur in tens of milliseconds. In speech, acoustic cues that we use to discriminate phonemes, like voice onset time and place of articulation, for example, are signaled by such rapidly occurring changes in the acoustic signal. Neuroscientists have found that those rapid changes in the physical properties of sound are represented by rapid neurological firing patterns in the primary auditory cortex that can be directly measured through various psychophysical and physiological methods. These cortical representations have been shown to differ in adults with reading problems when compared to those with no history of reading problems (Nagarijan et al., 1999) as well as infants as young as three months old who have immediate family members with language problems (Benasich et al., 2006).

Tallal and Piercy's finding that problems processing rapidly successive auditory changes are correlated with language problems does not by itself support the contention that language acquisition is dependent on the fidelity of this processing system. Some authors over the past two decades have questioned the possibility of a causative relationship between temporal processing and language acquisition because most individuals with reading problems, especially, ultimately develop adequate phonological production and do not appear to have altered aural speech recognition abilities (Bishop et al., 1999), and that studies of children with language problems suggest that the auditory processing issues may be the result of immature patterns that resolve naturally over time (Bishop & McArthur, 2004). These authors and others believe that the failure to master language and/or reading is more likely due to problems with top-down ability to segment words into sounds and syllables (phonological awareness) or other deficits in higher-level aspects of language learning, perhaps affected by working memory or other cognitive constraints (Snowling, 1990; Swan & Goswami, 1997). But interdisciplinary cognitive scientists and developmental psychologists are asserting that, given the abundance of research supporting both scientific contentions, both bottom-up and top-down processing are necessary for normal language acquisition (Thomas & Karmiloff-Smith, 2003).

Assessment of temporal processing disorders

Fortunately, audiologists who specialize in diagnosing auditory processing disorders (APD) have developed a battery of tests that can be used to diagnose temporal processing. The original research of Tallal and Piercy used a two-tone temporal sequencing task to measure temporal processing in children with language disorders (see Figure 18.1). The test, later named the Tallal Repetition Test, involved asking children to sequence two tones in which the interstimulus interval (the period of time between the two tones) decreased from slightly over four seconds between tones (4,062 ms) to less than a 100th of a second (8 ms). This is the task that has been consistently shown to distinguish children with language problems from those developing language normally.

Rawool has recently provided an excellent summary of tasks used by audiologists to assess temporal processing (2007). The tests include gap detection, backward masking, temporally degraded speech, masking level differences, and many others. It is beyond the scope of this chapter to describe the tests that are used by audiologists to diagnose differing temporal processing disorders and it is not known which of those tests are best at identifying the temporal processing difficulties that distinguish children with language problems from those with normal language. However, it is

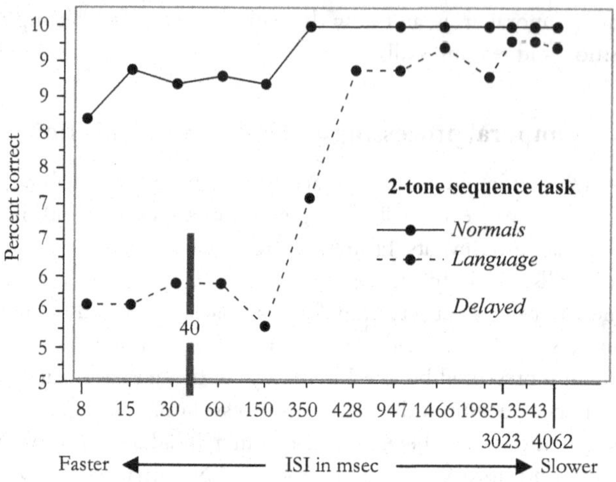

Figure 18.1 Normal vs. language impaired seven-year-old's percentage correct on a two-tone sequencing task as interstimulus interval decreases (right to left) from just over four seconds to eight ms.

recommended that children with speech language or literacy problems for whom speech discrimination, phonic decoding, phonological awareness, or auditory working memory are present receive a thorough auditory processing evaluation by a qualified audiologist to determine the degree to which temporal processing problems may be contributing to the difficulties.

Temporal processing and remediation of language problems

The final issue to be addressed with respect to the Temporal Processing Hypothesis and language disorders is twofold: can temporal processing problems be remediated and if so, what is the effect on language skills? The first controlled research studies that demonstrated the value of temporal processing intervention with language impaired children was published in 1996. The first study reported by Merzenich et al. was conducted with seven children, ages 5.9–9.1 with language learning impairments who participated in two 20-minute temporal processing exercises (one very similar to the two-tone sequencing task of Tallal and Piercy, the other a phonetic element recognition exercise) five days a week for four weeks. At the conclusion of the training the children showed significant gains in temporal processing as measured by the Tallal Repetition Test as well as significant gains in speech discrimination as well as averaging 1.5 years' gain in measures of language development (Merzenich et al., 1996; Tallal, et al., 1996).

A second study was then conducted using a larger sample of 22 language impaired children who were divided into two groups matched for nonverbal intelligence and receptive speech and language skills. Four exercises were used for training the experimental group, the initial two exercises that had been improved for ability to maintain the children's attention and two other exercises that stressed categorical perception of sounds in syllables and the other, a minimal pairs forced choice task. The control group played video games. Both groups received language intervention, but the experimental group had exposure to speech that had been digitally modified to enhance rapid temporal elements and the control group had the same exercises without the acoustic enhancement. Both groups showed benefit from the language intervention, but the experimental group showed significantly greater improvement in language and temporal processing skills (Merzenich et al., 1996; Tallal, et al., 1996). Taken together these two studies provided further evidence that temporal processing deficits were a factor in language disorders and that remediation of temporal processing could be achieved through practice with temporal processing tasks and speech sound discrimination activities. But of great import was the finding of the second study showing that when temporal processing tasks and acoustically modified speech are included in a treatment protocol it enhances the therapeutic outcomes significantly.

Several studies have been conducted since the original 1996 research that have reported positive effects of the intervention protocol developed by Merzenich, Tallal, and colleagues subsequently published as Fast ForWord and later Fast ForWord Language, with children who have cochlear implants (Schopmeyer, Mellon, Dobaj, Grant, & Nipapko, 2000), adults with aphasia (Dronkers et al., 1999), adults with dyslexia (Temple et al., 2003), and children with dyslexia (Gaab, et al., 2007; Temple, et al., 2003). There has been a study reported where Fast ForWord Language was not shown to be more effective than computerized remediation without the temporal processing components of acoustically modified speech (Cohen et al., 2005), and another with a small group of reading impaired children with half from impoverished socioeconomic environments (Pokorni, Worthington, & Jamison, 2004).

Recently, Gillam and associates reported on a three-year randomized controlled trial comparing Fast ForWord Language with other interventions including one-on-one language therapy, other computerized language interventions with language impaired children showing that all the interventions, when administered in an intensive two hour per day, five day a week protocol during eight-week summer sessions resulted in significant language improvements with no significant differences between the groups. In addition, using backward masking as a measure of temporal processing the authors reported that all the groups showed improvements in the backward masking measures as well (Gillam et al., 2008). When combined, the research conducted to this date supports the view that both top-down and bottom-up approaches to language intervention, when conducted using an intensive treatment protocol five days a week for several consecutive weeks have a significant impact on language skills, and perhaps temporal processing skills as well.

Summary and conclusions

Temporal processing is a bottom-up component of neurolinguistic processing that is impaired in many children with language disorders. The degree to which it is a predisposing factor in language disorders is still being debated, but the research to date is persuasive that temporal processing disorders do increase the risk of problems with language development for some children.

The intensive treatment approaches that include remediation of temporal processing deficits have been shown through replicated random controlled studies to result in significant improvements in language skills and temporal processing skills in a short period of time. However, it is clear that other intensive interventions that work directly on language structure and function (top-down approaches) are also effective when used intensively. Future research is needed that will begin to differentiate those patterns of language impairment and temporal processing impairment that benefit preferentially from top-down versus bottom-up approaches or a combination of both. In the meantime, the research overwhelmingly supports the value of intensive language interventions that combine bottom-up (perceptual and temporal processing exercises) and top-down (language structure, function, and use) for children with language disorders.

Further reading

Burns, M. S. (2021). *Cognitive & communication interventions: Neuroscience applications for speech-language pathologists*. San Diego: Plural Publishers.

Jain, C., Priya, M. B., & Joshi, K. (2020). Relationship between temporal processing and phonological awareness in children with speech sound disorders. *Clinical Linguistics and Phonetics, 34*(6), 566–575.

Meilleur, A., Foster, N. E., Coll, S. M., Brambati, S. M., & Hyde, K. L. (2020). Unisensory and multisensory temporal processing in autism and dyslexia: A systematic review and meta-analysis. *Neuroscience and Biobehavioral Reviews, 116*, 44–63.

References

American Speech-Language-Hearing Association. Retrieved from www.asha.org

Benasich, A., Choudbury, N., Friedman, J., Realpe-Bonilla, T., Chojnowska, C., & Gou, Z. (2006). The infant as a prelinguistic model for language learning impairments: Predicting event-related potentials to behavior. *Neuropsychologia, 44*(3), 396–411.

Bishop, D.V. M., & McArthur, M. (2004). Immature cortical responses to auditory stimuli in specific language impairment: Evidence from ERPs to rapid tone sequences. *Developmental Science*, 7(4), 11–18.

Bishop, D.V. M., Carlyon, R. P., Deeks, J. M., & Bishop, S. J. (1999). Auditory temporal processing impairment: Neither necessary nor sufficient for causing language impairment in children. *Journal of Speech and Hearing Research, 42*(6), 1295–1310.

Boden, M. (2006). *Transforming linguistics. The mind as machine: A history of cognitive science.* Oxford, UK: Oxford University Press.

Brown, R. A. (1973). *First language: The early stages.* Cambridge, MA: Harvard University Press.

Burns, M. (2007). Auditory processing disorders and literacy. In D. Geffner & D. Ross-Swain (Eds.), *Auditory processing disorders: Assessment, management and treatment* (p. 973). San Diego: Plural.

Cabeza, R., Ciaramelli, E., Olson, I., & Moscovitch, M. (2008). The parietal cortex and episodic memory: An attentional account. *Nature Reviews. Neuroscience, 9*(8), 613–625.

Chermak, G., & Musiek, F. (1998). *Central auditory processing disorders: New perspectives.* New York: Singular.

Chomsky, A. N. (1957). *Aspects of language.* The Hague, The Netherlands: Mouton.

Chomsky, A. N. (1964). *Aspects of the theory of syntax.* Cambridge, MA: MIT Press.

Chomsky, A. N. (1986). *Knowledge of language: Its nature, origin and use.* New York: Praeger Publishers.

Chomksy, A. N., & Skinner, B. F. (1959). Review of B. F. Skinner, Verbal behavior. *Language, 35*(1), 26–58.

Cohen, W., Hodson, A., OíHare, A., Boyle, J., Durrani, T., McCartney, E., … & Watson, J. (2005). Effects of computer-based intervention through acoustically modified speech (Fast ForWord) in severe mixed receptive–expressive language impairment: Outcomes from a randomized controlled trial. *Journal of Speech, Language, and Hearing Research, 48*(3), 715–729.

Corbetta, M., & Schulman, G. (2002). Control of goal-directed and stimulus-driven attention in the brain. *Nature Reviews. Neuroscience, 3*(3), 201–215.

Dehaene-Lambertz, G., Hertz-Pannier, L., Dubois, J., Mériaux, S., Roche, A., Sigman, M., & Dehaene, S. (2006). Functional organization of perisylvian activation during presentation of sentences in preverbal infants. *Proceedings of the National Academy of Sciences, 103*(38), 14240–14245.

Dronkers, N., Husted, D., Deutsch, G., Taylor, K., Saunders, G., & Merzenich, M. (1999). Lesion site as a predictor of improvement after "Fast ForWord" treatment in adult aphasic patients. *Brain and Language, 69*, 450–452.

Gaab, N., Gabrieli, J., Deutsch, G., Tallal, P., & Temple, E. (2007). Neural correlates of rapid auditory processing are disrupted in children with developmental dyslexia and ameliorated with training: An fMRI study. *Restorative Neurology and Neuroscience, 25*(3–4), 295–310.

Gillam, R. B., Loeb, D. F., Hoffman, L. M., Bohman, T., Champlin, C. A., Thibodeau, L., Widen, J., Brandel, J., & Friel-Patti, S. (2008). The Efficacy of Fast ForWord Language Intervention in School-Age Children With Language Impairment: A Randomized Controlled Trial. *Journal of Speech, Language & Hearing Research, 51*(1), 97–119. https://doi.org/10.1044/1092-4388(2008/007)

Irwin, J. (1964). Comments. In A. House (Ed.), *Proceedings of the conference on communicating by language: The Speech process.* Bethesda, MA: National Institute of Child Health and Human Development, NIH.

Johnson, D. J., & Myklebust, H. R. (1967). *Learning disabilities: Educational principles and practices.* New York: Grune and Stratton.

Kenet, T., Arieli, A., Tsodyks, M., & Grinvald, A. (2006). Are single cortical neurons soloists or are they obedient members of a huge orchestra? In J. L. van Hemmen & T. J. Sejnowski (Eds.), *23 Problems in systems neuroscience* (pp. 160–181). Oxford, UK: Oxford University Press.

Kuhl, P. K. (2000). A new view of language acquisition. *Proceedings of the National Academy of Sciences, 97*(22), 11850–11857.

Kuhl, P. K. (2004). Early language acquisition: Cracking the speech code. *Nature Reviews. Neuroscience, 5*(11), 831.

Lee, L. (1974). *Developmental sentence analysis.* Evanston, IL: Northwestern University Press.

Marge, M. (1972). The general problem of language disabilities in children. In J. Irwin & M. Marge (Eds.), *Principles of childhood language disabilities* (pp. 75–98). New York: Appleton-Century-Crofts.

Merzenich, M., Jenkins, W., Johnston, P., Schreiner, C., Miller, S., & Tallal, P. (1996). Temporal processing deficits of language-learning impaired children ameliorated by training. *Science, 271*(5245), 77–81.

Mesulam, M.-M. (2000). *Principles of behavioral neurology.* Oxford, UK: Oxford University Press.

Nagarian, S., Mahncke, H., Salz, T., Tallal, P., Roberts, T., & Merzenich, M. (1999). Cortical auditory signal processing in poor readers. *Proceedings of the National Academy of Sciences, 96*(11), 6483–6488.

Pokorni, J. L., Worthington, C. K., & Jamison, P. J. (2004). Phonological awareness intervention: Comparison of Fast ForWord, Earobics, and LiPS. *Journal of Educational Research, 97*(3), 147–157.

Rawool, V. (2007). Temporal processing in the auditory system. In D. Geffner & D. Ross-Swain (Eds.), *Auditory processing disorders: Assessment, management and treatment* (pp. 117–138). San Diego, CA: Plural.

Schopmeyer, B., Mellon, N., Dobaj, H., Grant, G., & Nipapko, J. (2000). Use of Fast ForWord to enhance language development in children with cochlear implants. *Annals of Otology, Rhinology, and Laryngology, Supplement, 85*, 96–98.

Skinner, B. F. (1957). *Verbal behavior*. New York: Appleton-Century-Crofts.

Snowling, M. (1990). *Dyslexia: A cognitive developmental perspective*. Oxford, UK: Blackwell.

Swan, D., & Goswami, U. (1997). Phonological awareness deficits in developmental dyslexia and the phonological representations hypothesis. *Journal of Experimental Child Psychology, 66*(1), 18–41.

Tallal, P. (2004). Improving language and literacy is a matter of time. *Nature Reviews. Neuroscience, 5*(9), 721–728.

Tallal, P., & Piercy, M. (1973). Deficits of non-verbal auditory perception in children with developmental aphasia. *Nature, 241*(5390), 468–469.

Tallal, P., & Piercy, M. (1974). Developmental aphasia: Rate of auditory processing and selective impairment of consonant perception. *Neuropsychologia, 12*(1), 83–93.

Tallal, P., & Stark, R. E. (1981). Speech acoustic-cue discrimination abilities of normally developing and language-impaired children. *Journal of the Acoustic Society of America, 69*(2), 568–574.

Tallal, P., Miller, S., Bedi, G., Byma, G., Wang, X., Srikantan, S., … & Merzenich, M. (1996). Language comprehension in language-learning impaired children improved with acoustically modified speech. *Science, 271*(5245), 81–84.

Temple, E., Deutsch, G., Poldrack, R., Miller, S., Tallal, P., Merzenich, M., & Gabrieli, J. D. (2003). Neural deficits in children with dyslexia ameliorated by behavioral remediation: Evidence from functional MRI. *Proceedings of the National Academy of Sciences, 100*(5), 2860–2865.

Temple, E., Poldrack, R., Protopapas, A., Nagarajan, S., Salz, T., & Tallal, P. (2000). Disruption of the neural response to rapid acoustic stimuli in dyslexia: Evidence from functional MRI. *Proceedings of the National Academy of Sciences, 97*(25), 13907–13912.

Thomas, M., & Karmiloff-Smith, A. (2003). Connectionistic models of development, developmental disorders, and individual differences. In R. J. Sternberg, J. Lautrey, & T. I. Lubart (Eds.), *Models of intelligence: International perspectives* (pp. 133–150). Washington, DC: American Psychological Association.

Tomblin, J. B., Records, N. L., & Zhang, X. (1996). A system for the diagnosis of specific language impairment in kindergarten children. *Journal of Speech and Hearing Research, 39*(6), 1284–1294.

Van Vreeswijk, C. (2006). What is the neural code? In J. L. van Hemmen & T. J. Sejnowski (Eds.), *23 problems in systems neuroscience* (pp. 143–159). Oxford, UK: Oxford University Press.

19

LANGUAGE PROCESSING IN CHILDREN WITH LANGUAGE IMPAIRMENT

Bernard Grela, Beverly Collisson, and Dana Arthur

Introduction

It is estimated that approximately 7% of the general population has a syndrome known as specific language impairment (Tomblin et al., 1997). The term specific language impairment (SLI) is used to identify children who have difficulty with the acquisition and use of language. When compared to their typically developing peers, these children's scores on standardized measures of language development fall greater than one standard deviation below the mean, yet their cognitive abilities are within normal limits, they have normal hearing acuity, no frank neurological impairment, and no social-emotional problems (Leonard, 1998; Stark & Tallal, 1981). The acquisition and use of grammatical morphology appears to be the aspect of language most severely affected in children with SLI and they often produce grammatical markers less frequently than younger, typically developing children matched for mean length of utterance (MLU; e.g., Leonard, 1998; Rice & Wexler, 1996). The morphemes that appear to be most problematic for children with SLI include inflectional markers (e.g., third person singular: s, regular past tense: ed, contractible copula and auxiliary forms of to be) and functional words (e.g., uncontractible copula and auxiliary forms of to be). These morphemes may be completely absent or produced inconsistently across utterances (Leonard, Eyer, Bedore, & Grela, 1997; Miller & Leonard, 1998). When errors do occur, children with SLI are more likely to make omission rather than commission errors (Leonard et al., 1997; Rice & Wexler, 1996). Furthermore, they often have problems with other aspects of language such as phonology, vocabulary, and syntax (e.g., Leonard, 1998; Rice, 2004). Recent studies of language intervention have shown that while these children do show progress in their acquisition of language as a result of intervention, they are resistant to mastery of language in a timely manner (Bishop, Adams, & Rosen, 2006; Ebbels, van der Lely, & Dockrell, 2007; Leonard, Camarata, Pawlowska, Brown, & Camarata, 2008; Rice & Wexler, 1996). This difficulty with language may persist into adulthood (van der Lely, 1997, 2005).

Although numerous studies have identified the language characteristics of children with SLI, relatively little is known about the underlying cause of this impairment. This has been complicated by the findings that children with SLI comprise a heterogeneous group (Bishop, Bright, James, Bishop, & van der Lely, 2000; Leonard, 1998; van der Lely, 2005). Furthermore, the symptoms associated with the disorder may have different underlying causes, or a combination of factors (Bishop, 2002; McArthur & Bishop, 2004). This provides a challenge for researchers and clinicians who strive to find the best assessment and intervention practices for children with SLI. Our goals as language interventionists are to identify measures that are highly sensitive in isolating the

DOI: 10.4324/9781003204213-22

cause of the disorder and to develop intervention techniques that are effective in ameliorating the symptoms associated with the disorder. These assessment and intervention procedures will be most effective if we can identify the underlying cause, or causes, of the disorder. The focus of this chapter is to review evidence that children with SLI have a limitation in processing linguistic information. In addition, the implications for assessment and intervention will be discussed.

Theories of SLI

Several theories have been proposed that attempt to explain the cause of SLI. The theories can be divided into two opposing perspectives with each consisting of several related but distinct theories of SLI. The first perspective assumes that children with SLI have a problem with the innate structures of grammar that prevents the application of productive morphosyntactic rules or leads to erroneous parameter settings for a language (e.g., Crago & Gopnik, 1994; Rice & Wexler, 1996; van der Lely, 1994). This faulty linguistic system inhibits the children from determining the linguistic parameters that are appropriate for the language they are learning. When grammatical morphemes are produced correctly, it is assumed that the children have either memorized a specific linguistic form (Crago & Gopnik, 1994) or set a tense optional grammar when tense is obligatory (Rice & Wexler, 1996). The commonality of this set of theories is that children with SLI are exposed to acceptable examples of linguistic input from their care-givers, but they are unable to correctly hypothesize the linguistic rules of their ambient language because of a faulty underlying grammar.

The second perspective proposes that children with SLI have an intact underlying grammatical structure, but processing systems (e.g., working memory, attention, general processing) that are essential for the acquisition of language function less than optimally (Bishop, 1994; Johnston, 1991; Kail, 1994; Leonard et al., 1997). These systems are affected by a processing capacity limitation, which prevents children with SLI from acquiring grammatical rules as efficiently and rapidly as their typically developing peers. During the process of acquisition, children with SLI may develop weak representations of grammatical structures that result in within individual variation in the use of these structures at any one point in development (Leonard et al., 1997; Miller & Leonard, 1998). Therefore, a child may produce a grammatical morpheme in one situation (e.g., The dog's running), but omit it in another (e.g., The dog chasing the cat). Therefore, grammatical structures may be used productively, but not in every situation where they are required. This differs from a deficit in linguistic knowledge perspective, which proposes that children with SLI use grammatical markers because they memorize them in particular contexts.

Assumptions of processing capacity limitations

It is well recognized that the human brain functions as a system that processes and organizes incoming sensory information to make sense of the world. However, it is also known that the brain has a limited capacity for processing incoming information and so it can perform only a limited amount of work within a specific period of time (Johnston, 1991, 1994). When the processing system is taxed, information is lost because of an inability to cope with an overwhelming amount of information. This would be similar to composing an email while conversing on the phone. These tasks are difficult to accomplish simultaneously and often lead to frustration on the part of the person to whom we are talking. We may be able to switch from one task to the other rapidly, but we have difficulty processing several sources of information at the same time. In this scenario, our processing system is receiving and encoding more information than our brain is capable of managing, resulting in a loss of information.

There are several factors that must be considered when taking into account the amount of information that the brain is capable of processing within a given period of time. These include the familiarity of the information, the attentional resources required for processing, and the type of processing that will be necessary (Bishop, 2000). When a new skill is being learned, controlled processing is required. Controlled processing consumes a large percentage of available attentional resources and makes the completion of a task difficult and effortful. As a result, few attentional resources are available to perform other tasks. On the other hand, automatic processing occurs after a skill has been mastered through practice. This mastered skill consumes few attentional resources and can be completed automatically. Automatic processing frees up the processing resources so that other tasks can be performed simultaneously.

In addition, the operational resources available for processing information efficiently are thought to be dependent on at least three other factors: speed of processing, space available for processing, and energy available to drive the processing system (Leonard, 1998; Leonard et al., 2007). These factors have been divided into functional- (speed of processing) and structural-based (space and energy) systems of processing (Montgomery & Windsor, 2007). According to the functional-based perspectives, if information is presented too rapidly, our ability to process the information is compromised (Hayiou-Thomas, Bishop, & Plunkett, 2004). It would follow that if the processing system is abnormally slow, then information will be lost when it is presented at a normal rate (Kail, 1991). In contrast, structural-based systems emphasize the amount of space allocated for processing (Daneman & Carpenter, 1983). It seems logical that a large volume processor should be capable of handling more information within a specific period of time than a small volume processor. Furthermore, a small volume processor may be overwhelmed if too much information is presented within a particular time frame in comparison to a large volume processor. A final way of thinking about information processing is to consider the amount of energy that is required to complete a task (Lapointe, 1985). This perspective assumes that a processing system requires energy in order to complete a task or several tasks simultaneously. If there is insufficient energy to complete the task, only a portion of it will be accomplished. If this involves information processing, a portion of that information will be missing because the energy source required to finish the task will be depleted.

The three factors listed above may contribute to a processing capacity limitation. They may occur in isolation, but are more likely to be codependent factors (Ellis Weismer et al., 2000; Lahey, Edwards, & Munson, 2001). For example, a small volume processor will take longer to process large volumes of information. A combination of reduced space and speed will have an impact on the amount of information that can be processed within a given timeframe. Finally, a large volume of information may take more energy than is available to complete a task. Therefore, any of these factors combined may contribute to a processing capacity limitation.

A major assumption of the processing capacity limitation perspectives for children with SLI is that these children have an intact grammatical structure. An intact grammatical structure has the potential for learning the linguistic rules of a child's ambient language. However, it needs an appropriate flow of linguistic information in order to acquire these rules. If this flow of information is incomplete, degraded, or interrupted due to an improperly functioning processing system, then it will take children with SLI a longer time to acquire language.

There are several reasons to suspect that children with SLI have difficulty processing linguistic information. Physiologically based studies have used functional magnetic resonance imaging (fMRI; e.g., Ellis Weismer, Plante, Jones, & Tomblin, 2005; Hugdahl et al., 2004) and event related potentials (ERPs; e.g., Bishop & McArthur, 2005; McArthur & Bishop, 2004) to examine brain function in children with SLI. The fMRI studies found less activation in the areas of the cortex critical for language processing in children with SLI (Ellis Weismer et al., 2005; Hugdahl et al., 2004). These included the parietal regions, the pre-central gyrus, and inferior frontal gyrus. The ERP studies examined processing at a lower level of processing in the auditory cortex (Bishop & McArthur, 2005; McArthur & Bishop, 2005). These authors argue that children with SLI have immature processing systems. However, the auditory system eventually matures and processes information as efficiently as typically developing children.

The advantage of the physiological studies is that they do not require behavioral responses from the children and may be more sensitive in identifying differences between children with SLI and their typically developing peers. However, the disadvantages are that these procedures are expensive and in many cases can only be used on older disordered populations. Therefore, a large percentage of studies on children with SLI have used behavioral observations including reaction times, comprehension tasks, and production tasks. The next section describes these studies and the different hypotheses suggesting the underlying cause of SLI. Some of the theories assume a general processing capacity limitation for language, while others identify specific systems that result in degraded linguistic input to the grammatical system. The general consensus behind these theories is that the brain has a limited processing capability and when the processing system is taxed, information is lost. These processing limitations have a significant impact on children's abilities to acquire the grammar of their ambient language.

Specific theories of processing capacity limitation in children with SLI

Generalized slowing hypothesis

According to the generalized slowing hypothesis (Kail, 1994), the amount of work that can be accomplished within a given period of time is determined by speed. It then follows that individuals who perform a task slowly complete less work within a specified period of time than individuals who perform a task rapidly. Using a meta-analysis procedure, Kail (1994) found that children with SLI took longer to complete a variety of linguistic (e.g., object naming) and nonlinguistic (e.g., judging picture similarity) tasks when compared to typically developing peers. Furthermore, the response times of the children with SLI increased linearly in comparison to the response times of the typically developing children. Kail concluded that the slower response times of the children with SLI was not specific to any particular task, but more general across both linguistic and nonlinguistic domains. Thus, children with SLI were slower at a variety of tasks including the comprehension and production of language. Kail believes that this reduced speed of processing accounts for the delayed acquisition of language.

Several recent studies have attempted to replicate Kail's results (Hayiou-Thomas et al., 2004; Miller, Kail, Leonard, & Tomblin, 2001; Miller et al., 2006). Miller and colleagues (2001) examined the response times of third grade children with SLI across a variety of linguistic and nonlinguistic tasks. The linguistic tasks included lexical decision making, grammaticality judgment, and phonological awareness. The nonlinguistic tasks included motor response, visual scan, and mental rotation. The results of this study were consistent with Kail's (1994) findings that children with SLI responded more slowly than their typically developing peers across all task domains. They argued that the slower reaction times by the children with SLI provided evidence for a general processing deficit in comparison to their typically developing peers. Several years following the Miller et al. (2001) study, the same tasks were administered to a group of 14-year-old children with SLI (Leonard et al., 2007; Miller et al., 2006). Again, a strong relationship between performance on language tasks and speed of processing was found. They concluded that children with SLI continue to lag behind their typically developing peers in speed of performance as they age. Other studies have reported similar findings for other areas of nonlinguistic processing such as slower visual processing, attentional orientation, and motor responses on the part of children with SLI (Schul, Stiles, Wulfeck, & Townsend, 2004; Windsor & Hwang, 1999). Therefore, there is evidence to suggest that speed of processing is correlated with the language difficulties of children with SLI.

Surface hypothesis

The surface hypothesis as described by Leonard and colleagues (Leonard & Bortolini, 1998; Leonard et al., 1997; Leonard, McGregor, & Allen, 1992) assumes that children with SLI have a general processing capacity limitation. Therefore, they process information at a slower rate than their typically developing peers. In addition, the theory emphasizes the physical properties of language in that morphemes of low phonetic substance are vulnerable to decay when the processing system is taxed. Leonard (1998) defines low phonetic substance as grammatical morphemes that are brief in duration. These include grammatical morphemes consisting of single consonants or weak syllables that occur in sentence positions where they are less likely to be lengthened. When these morphemes are encountered in an utterance, children must perceive them and then hypothesize their grammatical function while subsequent auditory and linguistic information continues to be heard and processed. In children with SLI, some verbal input will be lost because they cannot process the information quickly enough to store it in long-term memory. The information likely to be lost includes forms consisting of low phonetic substance. As a result, it is likely that the information contained within these grammatical morphemes decays from memory before it can be completely processed. Thus, it will take children with SLI longer to determine the function of these grammatical markers and they are less likely to build a productive rule for their use in comparison to their peers.

Studies examining children's ability to perceive grammatical morphemes have lent support to the surface hypothesis (Montgomery & Leonard, 1998, 2006). Montgomery and Leonard (1998) found that children with SLI showed sensitivity to morphemes of high phonetic substance but not to morphemes of low phonetic substance. Their typically developing peers matched either for age or receptive language showed sensitivity to both high and low phonetic substance morphemes. A later study (Montgomery & Leonard, 2006) included a condition where morphemes of low phonetic substance were manipulated by increasing the duration and intensity of these morphemes. The results of this study showed that the children with SLI performed as well on the enhanced morphemes as they did on the morphemes of high phonetic substance. The results of these two studies suggest that the children with SLI have more difficulty processing morphemes of low phonetic substance and provide support for the surface hypothesis.

Deficit in temporal processing

Comprehending language involves the perception of complex and rapidly changing acoustic information. According to Tallal and colleagues (Tallal, 1980; Tallal & Piercy, 1974, 1975), children with developmental language disorders (such as SLI) cannot respond to rapidly changing acoustic events as are found in consonant to vowel transitions in speech. This inability results in difficulty with speech perception that in turn has a significant impact on language acquisition. To test this hypothesis, Tallal and colleagues (Tallal, 2004; Tallal, Miller, & Fitch, 1993; Tallal, Sainburg, & Jernigan, 1991; Tallal, Stark, & Mellits, 1985) described several tasks where children with SLI were asked to detect the difference between two tones presented with either short interstimulus intervals (ISI) or with tones of short duration. The children with SLI had difficulty detecting differences between the tones when the ISIs were short and when the tones were of brief duration. However, they performed as well as their typically developing peers when the ISI between tones and the length of tones were increased. Similar results were found when the children were presented with verbal stimuli that included consonant-vowel (CV) syllables (i.e., /ba/ vs. /da/; Burlingame, Sussman, Gillam, & Hay, 2005; Tallal & Piercy, 1974, 1975). The children with SLI had difficulty identifying the CV pairs when the formant transitions were presented at a normal rate, but improved when the formant transitions were lengthened. Tallal and colleagues argued that this showed evidence of a temporal processing disorder on the part of the children with SLI.

Working memory limitations

Montgomery (2003) provides a comprehensive description of two models of working memory and how they relate to children with SLI. The first model of working memory has been referred to as phonological working memory (PWM; Baddeley, 1986). PWM consists of a central executive and a phonological loop. The central executive functions to regulate the flow of information, the retrieval of information from other memory systems, and the processing and storage of information. The phonological loop consists of a capacity limited system that subvocally rehearses auditory information for a short period of time while information is processed in the central executive. It is thought that the phonological loop is problematic for children with SLI (Adams & Gathercole, 1995; Archibald & Gathercole, 2006b; Gathercole & Baddeley, 1995; Gathercole, Willis, Baddeley, & Emslie, 1994). Therefore, they are not able to rehearse and maintain information in the phonological loop long enough for information to be stored in long-term memory. As a result, it will take children with SLI longer to learn vocabulary, grammatical morphology, and other grammatical forms. Evidence for a problem with the phonological loop has been found in various nonword repetition tasks (Adams & Gathercole, 1995; Archibald & Gathercole, 2006a, b; Archibald & Gathercole, 2007; Dollaghan & Campbell, 1998; Ellis Weismer et al., 2000; Gathercole et al., 1994). In nonword repetition tasks, children are required to repeat nonsense words ranging from one to four syllables in length. These studies have found that children with SLI both tend to make more errors overall and make more errors as the number of syllables per word increases in comparison to their typically developing peers (Dollaghan & Campbell, 1998; Gathercole et al., 1994; Roy & Chiat, 2004). This may be because words with more syllables take longer to rehearse in the phonological loop.

The second model of working memory has been referred to as functional working memory (FWM). This model assumes that information must be held in memory while other processing operations take place (Just & Carpenter, 1992). FWM is similar to PWM, except that the existence of a phonological loop is deemphasized while the relationship between the storage and processing of information is emphasized. In this model, the central executive has a limited capacity and the tasks of storing and processing information must share a limited pool of resources. When the working memory system is taxed, there is a trade-off between attentional resources required for storage and those required for retrieval. To assess the dual function of working memory, Daneman and Carpenter (1983) devised a task where adult participants were asked to answer questions about sentences while remembering the last word of each sentence. This task was modified and used as a measure of working memory in school age children (Gaulin & Campbell, 1994). This procedure was adopted for use in children with SLI to assess their ability to process and store information simultaneously (Ellis Weismer, Evans, & Hesketh, 1999). Ellis Weismer et al. (1999) found that children with SLI responded to questions about the sentences as well as typically developing children matched for age, but were unable to recall as many sentence final words as their peers. This experimental design was later used to assess adolescent children with SLI using both behavioral and fMRI data (Ellis Weismer et al., 2005). The results of this study supported previous findings (Ellis Weismer et al., 1999) that children with SLI recalled fewer words than their typically developing peers. In addition, the fMRI results indicated that the children with SLI had lower levels of activation in areas of the brain responsible for attentional, memory, and language processing. The results of these studies were used to support the argument that children with SLI have structural deficits in verbal working memory that affect their acquisition and use of language.

Phonological deficit hypothesis

It has been suggested that the general processing capacity limitations of children with SLI result in an impairment in the processing of speech that has a significant impact on the development of good phonological representations. These degraded phonological representations are thought to be the central cause of delayed acquisition of morphology and syntax because children with SLI have difficulty translating the auditory forms of words and morphemes into a phonological code necessary for learning these forms (Criddle & Durkin, 2001; Joanisse, 2004; Joanisse & Seidenberg,

2003). This may be the case as children with SLI often have phonological impairments as well as problems with syntax and morphology (e.g., Leonard, 1998; Leonard et al., 1997; Rice, 2004). Adopting a connectionist model, Joanisse (Joanisse, 2004; Joanisse & Seidenberg, 2003) suggested that the phonological form of grammatical morphemes is degraded during exposure and as a result the productive rules for use of inflectional markers take longer to learn. Therefore, the deficit in inflectional morphology is secondary to a phonological impairment. One of the assumptions of connectionist modeling is that knowledge is a distributed and interactive system. So if there is an impairment in one aspect of the system other aspects within the system are also affected. Joanisse (2004) created a network model to simulate degraded phonological representations. The network acquired some of the knowledge for use of inflections so occasionally they were produced. His results were remarkably similar to the language profiles of children with SLI where omission errors are more frequent than commission errors. Therefore, a general processing capacity limitation resulting in poor phonological representations may have a significant impact on the acquisition and use of grammatical morphology.

Linguistic complexity

Linguistic complexity can be thought of as the amount of linguistic information bundled within a particular linguistic structure. More complex structures consist of more linguistic features and require a greater number of mental computations to encode or produce an utterance (e.g., Grela, 2003b; Grela, Snyder, & Hiramatsu, 2005). Therefore, if children with SLI have limited processing capabilities for language, then linguistic structures that have higher levels of complexity should be problematic for these children. This may be due to limited space available for mental computations of these structures or limited energy to complete the computations. Several studies have examined linguistic complexity as a contributing factor to comprehension problems and production errors characteristic of children with SLI (Dick, Wulfeck, Krupa-Kwiatkowski, & Bates, 2004; Grela, 2003a; Grela & Leonard, 2000; Grela et al., 2005; Marton, Schwartz, Farkas, & Katsnelson, 2006). Some of the complex linguistic structures that have been examined include argument structure (Grela, 2003a; Grela & Leonard, 2000), novel root compounds (Grela et al., 2005), verb particles (Juhasz & Grela, 2008; Watkins & Rice, 1991), number of propositions per utterance (Johnston & Kamhi, 1984), and clausal imbedding (Dick et al., 2004). In general, these studies have found that children with SLI tend to make more errors or use fewer linguistic features than their typically developing peers as complexity levels increase.

Johnston and Kamhi (1984) found that children with SLI produced fewer propositions per utterance in comparison to typically developing children matched for MLU. Therefore, even when sentence length was a controlled factor, the children with SLI produced fewer idea units, suggesting that they were limited in the amount of information that could be contained within each utterance. More recently, a study examining use of grammatical morphology associated with phonological mean length of utterance (PMLU), as opposed to MLU in morphemes, found that children with SLI used fewer grammatical structures in comparison to children matched for PMLU (Polite & Leonard, 2006). In other words, when children with SLI attempt to produce utterances of similar length, or of increasing length, they make more grammatical errors than their typically developing peers (Marton et al., 2006). This provides evidence of a grammatical system that reaches its limits at relatively lower levels of linguistic complexity in comparison to typically developing children.

When linguistic complexity has been manipulated, children with SLI have been found to have difficulty comprehending and producing grammatical sentences (Dick et al., 2004; Grela, 2003b; Grela & Leonard, 2000; Grela et al., 2005). These studies have shown that children with SLI make more grammatical errors as argument structure complexity increases (Grela, 2003a, 2003b; Grela & Leonard, 1997, 2000). For example, Grela and Leonard (2000) found that children with SLI omitted more auxiliary verbs when attempting ditransitive sentences (e.g., The boy is giving the ball to the witch) than when producing intransitive (e.g., The boy is jumping) or transitive (e.g., The boy is pushing the car) sentences. Similar results were found for the omission of subject arguments of sentences (Grela, 2003a, 2003b). A study of French-speaking children with SLI found that they were likelier to omit grammatical morphemes in obligatory contexts as more complex argument structures were attempted (Pizzioli & Schelstraete, 2008). In addition, children with SLI were found to have difficulty interpreting the meaning of sentences when clausal imbedding was used to add complexity to sentences (Dick et al., 2004).

Linguistic complexity may have a significant impact on the mechanisms involved in the comprehension (e.g., working memory) and production of linguistic structures. The arguments have been that if children with SLI are presented with too much information while learning, the processing mechanisms are overwhelmed and information is compromised resulting in a slower rate of learning (Ellis Weismer et al., 1999; Gathercole et al., 1994; Johnston, 1994; Montgomery, 2000). It is also possible that during production, children with SLI may reach their processing limitations earlier than typically developing children. This is thought to be true when children with SLI have weak representations of grammatical structures (Grela & Leonard, 2000; Leonard, 1998; Leonard et al., 1997, 2000; Miller & Leonard, 1998). More specifically, the information that needs to be retrieved for sentence production may overwhelm the children's production "buffer" resulting in more grammatical errors as the demands associated with linguistic complexity increases (Grela, 2003a, 2003b; Grela & Leonard, 2000). To support this hypothesis, Leonard and colleagues (2000) devised an experiment where children with SLI were primed for the production of a targeted morpheme. The children with SLI produced more grammatical morphemes when the prime and the target sentence contained the same syntactic frame and prosodic structure (Prime: The birds are building the nest, Target: The horse is kicking the cow) than when they differed (Prime: The doctor smiled, Target: The horse is driving the car). They suggested that the matching prime and target reduced the processing load associated with the retrieval of the syntactic structure and grammatical morphemes required for sentence production. Therefore, linguistic complexity may have a significant impact on the learning and use of grammatical structures.

Implications for assessment

Clearly there is evidence to support processing capacity limitations for at least some children with SLI. Therefore, thoughtful evaluation of processing capacity should become an integral part of any assessment battery for children with SLI. Furthermore, these measures should have sufficient sensitivity to identify an existing language impairment and, ideally, have some evidence of construct validity for assessing processing capacity limitations (Hutchinson, 1996; McCauley & Swisher, 1984; Plante & Vance, 1994; Spaulding, Plante, & Farinella, 2006). It is also important that clinicians and researchers use guidelines to help differentiate children with SLI from other types of language impairments (Leonard, 1998; Stark & Tallal, 1981).

This being said, the assessment of processing ability in children can present particular challenges to clinicians and researchers. Few standardized measures of processing capacity are available (Montgomery, 2003), and not every purported test of processing or memory is created equally. In fact, many tasks labeled as working memory measures tap other memory systems as well (Dehn, 2008). Conversely, tasks designed to evaluate language can tax any, and all, of the facets of processing discussed above. For example, a test requiring children to imitate sentences of increasing length and/or complexity may place a strain on working memory, while a timed test may indirectly measure processing speed. To evaluate the nature and severity of processing capacity limitations in children with SLI—a crucial step toward creating an intervention plan—an effort must first be made to understand the strengths and limitations of the assessment tools available (Hutchinson, 1996; Spaulding et al., 2006). Therefore, it is critical that clinicians and researchers carefully read test manuals to determine if the test items are indeed assessing processing capacity or some other aspect of language.

Tests of processing capacity

Even though few standardized measures of processing capacity exist, some specific tasks have emerged in the literature as assessments of processing capacity and short-term memory. Some can be found as subtests of larger language assessment batteries, such as the nonword repetition subtest of the Comprehensive Test of Phonological Processing (CTOPP; Wagner, Torgeson, & Rashotte, 1999), or Gaulin and Campbell's Competing Language Processing Test (CLEP; Gaulin & Campbell, 1994), which may be adapted as an informal measure of processing ability.

Nonword repetition tests

One of the more promising measures for identifying SLI is the nonword repetition task (also known as CNRep or NRT; Dollaghan & Campbell, 1998; Gathercole et al., 1994). Children with SLI have significant difficulties with nonword repetition compared to their typically developing peers (e.g., Archibald & Gathercole, 2007; Dollaghan & Campbell, 1998; Ellis Weismer et al., 2000). Even compared to younger children matched for language level, children with SLI perform significantly worse on this task (Ellis Weismer et al., 2000). Furthermore, Montgomery and Windsor (2007) found that performance on the NRT predicted significant unique variance on the Clinical Evaluation of Language Fundamentals (CELF-R; Semel, Wiig, & Secord, 1987), suggesting a strong relationship between verbal working memory and direct tests of language ability. When dealing with non-words, children cannot rely on long-term representations or vocabulary knowledge. Therefore, the task of recalling and repeating each item falls primarily on the child's working memory. Children with SLI, working at a reduced processing capacity, are unable to keep up with the demands of the task.

Despite its seeming utility in detecting processing capacity limitations in children with SLI, some researchers caution against its use as a primary determiner of such limitations (Conti-Ramsden, Botting, & Faragher, 2001; Gathercole et al., 1994). One such caution centers around the shared nonword repetition deficit between children with SLI, children at risk for dyslexia, and children with poor working memory abilities, but appropriate oral and written language (Bishop, 2002; Conti-Ramsden et al., 2001). Therefore, the ability of nonword repetition tasks to differentially identify SLI from children who are at risk for language problems comes into question.

A second caution centers on the skills assessed by the nonword repetition task itself. Phonological working memory, while it may loom large as an underlying skill contributing to nonword repetition, is not the only skill brought to bear on this task. Long-term lexical knowledge, according to some researchers (Archibald & Gathercole, 2006a, b; Gathercole et al., 1994), is also at work in nonword repetition despite the seeming unfamiliarity of the nonword items. Specifically, when presented with a nonword item, subjects may draw on their semantic knowledge as well as their working memory in order to repeat it. This may be particularly true when a nonword is similar in phonological structure to a familiar word (Gathercole et al., 1994). If a nonword item is too similar to a real word, children may be able to draw on their long-term representation of the real word to mitigate the strain on working memory. To support this argument, Estes, Evans, and Else-Quest (2007) found significant variability among nonword repetition tasks and cited word likeness as a contributing factor to this variability. With these cautions in mind, nonword repetition cannot be viewed as a strictly nonverbal task, purely assessing children's processing abilities. Clinically, nonword repetition may be a task best utilized as a screening tool and not as the primary assessment of processing limitations.

Sentence repetition tasks

How are we to fill the gaps in assessment left by nonword repetition tasks? Another type of repetition task, sentence repetition, shows promise as an assessment tool for processing capacity limitations and identification of SLI. The Recalling Sentences subtest of the CELF-R (Semel, Wiig, & Secord, 1987) presents children with sentences that increase in length and complexity. The child's task is to repeat the sentences verbatim. Children with processing capacity limitations, such as SLI, should perform poorly as the complexity of the sentences increases. Conti-Ramsden and colleagues (2001) compared several assessment tasks, including nonword repetition and sentence repetition in terms of their potential as phenotypic markers of SLI. Sentence repetition was found to be the most accurate measure studied, showing both high accuracy and predictive value.

Complex span tasks

Gaulin and Campbell's (1994) Competing Language Processing Task (CLPT) was designed specifically to assess processing trade-offs in children as young as six years of age. The CLPT presents the child with groups of short sentences and requires a truth-value response to each. At the same time, the child must recall the final word of each sentence. This requires concurrent processing of meaning and retention of words in working memory, thus forcing the central executive to compete for processing resources involved in storage and processing. Ellis Weismer et al. (1999) revealed that the CLPT was far more taxing for children with SLI than for their typically developing peers.

Processing involvement in other language tasks

Despite the critical role that processing capacity is thought to play as the underlying cause of SLI, assessment of these limitations should in no way be viewed as a complete assessment of SLI. Direct measures of language ability remain necessary, particularly given the heterogeneous nature of the SLI population. Tasks like nonword repetition, or the CLPT, can reveal the presence of limitations on processing, but only broader testing can show how these limitations are manifested in a child's linguistic system.

The need for additional language testing is far from a burden. In fact, it can be considered a remedy for the relative dearth of standardized processing assessment measures. Tasks in formal language testing usually draw on some aspect of processing, and each can tax the capacity of the child's system in different ways. By analyzing the tasks of a standardized assessment battery, the clinician–researcher can observe how a child's processing capacity affects overall language performance. For example, the Token Test for Children (Revised; DiSimoni, Ehrler, & McGhee, 2007), was originally designed to assess comprehension of verbal commands. However, as those commands become increasingly long and complex, it is easy to see the influence that limited processing capacity has on a child's performance. Processing can play more subtle roles as well. Rapid naming tests, popular for assessing expressive vocabulary, can demonstrate weaknesses in the child's processing speed, as can any timed assessment. In the end, nearly any task employed by formal testing has a processing component. By examining each task carefully, standard language batteries can provide useful information about a child's processing capacity limitations.

The dynamic assessment paradigm

The most effective method of evaluating processing capacity in children with SLI may lie not with the specific measure used, but with the overall assessment paradigm employed. Dynamic assessment (DA) moves the focus of the evaluation from the answer that the child provides to the process the child uses to reach that answer. Instead of determining the level at which the child can perform a task without help, this paradigm interactively assesses what the child can do given strategic adult assistance (e.g., Gutierrez-Clellen & Peña, 2001; Hasson & Joffe, 2007; Peña & Gillam, 2000; Peña, Iglesias, & Lidz, 2001; Peña, Quinn, & Iglesias, 1992). By focusing on the process children with SLI use to approach evaluation tasks, the DA paradigm can provide specific information about how their processing ability differs from their typically developing peers. Thus, a DA approach can fill in the gaps that may be left by formal testing. Further, DA provides insight into a child's stimulability and potential for positive change (e.g., Gutierrez-Clellen & Peña, 2001; Hasson & Joffe, 2007). Dynamic assessment provides us with the opportunity to carefully employ various intervention strategies during testing, in order to determine what will provide the most benefit to the child.

Implications for intervention

In this chapter, we have explored SLI from a processing limitation perspective. This perspective provides the framework from which intervention approaches will be discussed. Within the language domain itself, children and adolescents with SLI may experience difficulty with one or more of the various aspects of spoken and written language: phonology, semantics, grammatical morphology, syntax, and pragmatics (Leonard, 1998). Further, evidence suggests that factors in the related areas of speed of processing (Kail, 1994), working memory (Gathercole et al., 1994; Montgomery, 2003), phonological quality (Joanisse, 2004), executive functioning, and attentional capacity (Im-Bolter, Johnson, & Pascual-Leone, 2006) contribute to poor language learning.

A critical component of selecting an intervention program is to consider the theoretical construct underpinning the intervention procedure to ensure that it is consistent with the hypothesized underlying cause of the language impairment. Second, the intervention program chosen should demonstrate evidence of effectiveness and efficacy in ameliorating the characteristics of the language problem in the population with which it is being used (Dollaghan, 2007; Gillam & Gillam, 2006). Finally, the intervention approach should focus on the content, form, and use of language within pragmatically appropriate contexts (Fey, Long, & Finestack, 2003). For children with processing capacity limitations, the interventionist strives to make the acoustic signal more salient and to decrease processing demands placed on children with SLI. These are key elements for children who demonstrate deficits in their ability to store and process information. For example, teaching new forms in old contexts allows the clinician to control the amount of new information to the child's existing level of prior knowledge (Fey, 1986), this in turn allows for increased storage and better coordination of executive processes. Reducing processing demands may free cognitive resources necessary for new skill acquisition.

Based on their results that both verbal processing speed and working memory are differentially implicated in language impairment and the important role that nonlinguistic/nonverbal factors take, Leonard et al. (2007) suggested that clinicians develop intervention goals for children with SLI that not only target the desired linguistic forms, but encompass nonlinguistic targets as well. Activities that promote both linguistic goals and the organization/regulation of material previously attained serve to promote the relationship between information processing and language learning. Ultimately, the goal in intervention for children with SLI is to simultaneously enhance language performance and the efficiency of information processing. Therefore, an intervention program will endeavor to decrease the amount of controlled processing that occurs and increase the automatic processing in children with SLI. This should free up attentional resources and allow the children to learn new information more efficiently. The following intervention practices are meant to serve as illustrations of a broad range of language treatment methods that serve to make the language signal more salient, to decrease processing demands, or to compensate for these processing limitations by training meta cognitive strategies.

Decreasing processing demands and making the signal salient

If children with SLI have difficulty processing the speech signal, the signal must be made more salient. One way to deliver more salient input is to alter the manner in which it is presented. The supersegmental features of a language can be altered by modifying intonation, stress, pause time, or rate of delivery (Montgomery, 2005; Montgomery & Leonard, 2006). Montgomery and Leonard (2006) found that children with SLI were more sensitive to morphemes of low phonetic substance when the intensity and duration of these morphemes was increased. Clinicians may use auditory trainers to increase the intensity of the acoustic signal and reduce background noise for children with SLI. This may function to enhance morphemes of low phonetic substance.

Ellis Weismer and Hesketh (1993, 1996, 1998) conducted a number of investigations to identify the linguistic variables that had an influence on children's language learning. One study examined the influence of varying speaking rate on novel word learning (Ellis Weismer & Hesketh, 1996). Children with SLI and typically developing children were taught two sets of novel words under three speaking rates: a slow rate, a normal rate, and a fast rate. It was found that children with SLI were able to produce fewer of the target words that had been introduced in the fast rate than at the normal rate; however, presentation of the target words at the slow rate did not assist the children with SLI learn the novel words. The authors concluded that fast rates of presentation for children with SLI be avoided. Further they suggested that a slower speaking rate may be beneficial to some children with SLI; however, they were not able to make this claim for the entire group of children with SLI in their investigation. The role of speaking rate, as in other manipulations of input, may demonstrate differential effects on the divergent group of children with SLI. It is important to carefully examine the influence of these modifications on each child individually.

Using the same experimental paradigm as their other investigations of linguistic input modification, Ellis Weismer and Hesketh (1998) examined the role of emphatic stress in word learning. Both typically developing children and children with SLI were exposed to single syllabic words produced with either neutral or emphatic stress. Both groups appeared to benefit from marking the novel lexical term with emphatic stress when tested for production ability. Coupling these findings with other investigations Ellis Weismer (1997) conjectured that emphatic stress does play a role in promoting language learning and this practice can be extended to real words in a clinical setting.

Focused stimulation

Focused stimulation refers to the technique in which a target linguistic form is made highly salient to a child by modeling it at a high frequency rate in a natural context. The child is not required to repeat the form; however, opportunities to produce the target are provided by carefully arranging the environment to promote it in an expected context (Fey, 1986; Fey, Cleave, Long, & Hughes, 1993). A number of treatment studies delivered by both clinicians and parents (e.g., Cleave & Fey, 1997; Girolametto, Pearce, & Weitzman, 1996) that promote both lexical and grammatical targets have demonstrated the effectiveness of this treatment approach with delayed language learners.

Conversational recasts

A recast is a response to a child's inaccurate or immature utterance that both corrects the utterance and includes additional phonological, semantic, and/or grammatical information (Camarata & Nelson, 2006). An example of a recast would be, "The baby is sleeping" in response to a child's observation, "Baby sleep." While making the input more salient, the adult tailors his response directly to the child's production. Experimental investigations comparing the relative effectiveness of the conversational recast technique with the direct imitation technique have demonstrated the effectiveness of conversational recasts to develop both absent and partially mastered grammatical structures in the language of children with SLI (Camarata, Nelson, & Camarata, 1994; Nelson, Camarata, Welsh, & Butkovsky, 1996). The investigators in these treatment studies hypothesized that the conversational recast technique allowed the children with SLI to exploit the meaningfulness of the discourse to aid in the processing of the target structure.

Self-talk and parallel talk

Self-talk and parallel talk are both techniques that fall under the umbrella of child-centered approaches (Fey, 1986). Typically, clinicians and parents facilitate general linguistic development while engaged with a child in play. These techniques may be extended to other contexts in which caregivers find themselves at any time of the day. A linguistic target is not selected for directed reinforcement, rather the conversational partner bases his comments on his or the child's particular activity in that moment in time. Self-talk describes the clinician's or parent's enthusiastic comments on or description of what the parent is engaged in while playing with a child. This serves as a language model for the child. Parallel talk shifts the focus of the adult's comments to what the child is engaged in. Parallel talk was one of several child-centered techniques used in a treatment study successfully targeting the linguistic and social skills of toddlers with delayed language development (Robertson & Weismer, 1999). Toddlers who were not yet using words were provided with a verbal description of their actions (e.g., "Hug the bear"), which in combination with a number of additional child-oriented techniques successfully moved the toddlers forward both linguistically and socially.

Elicited imitation

Elicited imitation is an intervention technique that directs a child's attention to a target form by highlighting it in contrast to another syntactic target form (Cleave & Fey, 1997; Connell, 1987; Connell & Stone, 1992). This serves to make the target more salient by focusing the child's attention to the target, providing opportunity for the child to produce the features of the target and illuminating the grammatical function of the target (Fey, Long, & Finestack, 2003). To promote success with this technique, the target form should be contrasted with a competing grammatical target in a pragmatically appropriate context (Cleave & Fey, 1997). This technique has been used to successfully promote new language forms by children with SLI (Connell, 1987; Connell & Stone, 1992) and as a beneficial component of a treatment study that facilitated the acquisition of grammatical forms in children with language impairments (Fey et al., 1993).

Modifying the speech input

Computer modification of the speech signal provides a way to make the signal perceptually more salient for children with SLI. Tallal, Miller, Bedi, Wang, and Nagarajan (1996) introduced modified speech that temporally prolonged the signal and amplified the phonetic contrasts in the ongoing speech signal in order to assist children with language impairment to enhance speech discrimination and overall language comprehension abilities. Half of the children in this study were exposed to prerecorded acoustically modified speech using computer games, audio tapes, and CD-ROMS designed for this study for approximately five hours each day over a four-week period. The other half of the children received the same training; however, the speech input was not modified. The authors concluded that training children with a temporally prolonged and emphasized speech signal led to significant improvement in measures of speech discrimination, language processing, and grammatical comprehension. Further, testing at six weeks postintervention revealed that the gains the children made during the intervention were maintained. Based on the positive results of this study, a number of the modified speech computer games introduced by Tallal et al. (1996) were packaged as a commercially available software program called Fast ForWord® Language (FFW-L; Scientific Learning Corporation. 1998).

A number of researchers have closely examined the success of intervention in children with SLI when modifications have been made to the speech signal. Cohen et al. (2005) evaluated the efficacy of adding the FFW-L software to the treatment programs of children with severe mixed receptive expressive SLI in a randomized controlled trial. The children who participated in this study received either: (a) FFW-L intervention delivered at home by each child's parents, (b) a number of language learning computer programs that did not contain modified speech delivered at home by each child's parents, and (c) a control group who received no additional home intervention. During the study, all of the children continued to receive their regular speech and language intervention programs at school. The children made significant gains in language outcome measures, but did not demonstrate any significant benefit among any of the three groups. The authors concluded that the inclusion of a modified speech signal into an existing intervention regime did not offer additional benefit.

Bishop, Adams, and Rosen (2006) examined the efficacy of computer training with and without modified speech on the grammatical comprehension abilities of children with receptive language impairments. The children participated in one of three possible intervention groups aimed at enhancing grammatical comprehension of constructs already known to the children: (a) grammatical training using slow speech developed by inserting pauses before critical words, (b) grammatical training using both slow speech and modified speech based on an algorithm used in FFW-L, and (c) an untrained control group. The children in the two intervention groups received anywhere from 6 to 29 sessions consisting of 15-minute training blocks. The results of this intervention study revealed that none of the children in any of the groups demonstrated improved proficiency of the grammatical constructions targeted. The authors were not able to demonstrate any benefit of delivering the stimuli using modified speech.

Gillam and colleagues (2008) conducted a randomized controlled study of the efficacy of FFW-L that included 216 children over a span of three years. In this trial, the authors compared the language and auditory processing outcomes of children with language impairments assigned to one of four treatment groups. The interventions included: (a) the FFW-L computer program using modified speech designed to develop temporal processing abilities (Scientific Learning Corporation. 1998), (b) a language learning computer program designed to promote the same skills targeted by FFW-L without a modified speech signal, (c) a series of academic enrichment computer games not designed to improve language or auditory processing skills, and (d) a clinician-delivered language intervention program. Following a summer program of intervention in one of the four conditions, all the children with language impairments demonstrated a significant improvement in both the language and the auditory processing measures from pre- to post-test and follow up testing at both three and six months later. The children who received FFW-L intervention and a similar computer program without a modified speech signal performed better on a subtest of phonological performance than did the children in the other two treatment conditions. The authors suggest that children should demonstrate improvement in language and auditory processing skills when they receive a time intensive intervention that requires that they focus on and immediately respond to verbal input, coupled with feedback from attentive adults and interactions with peers. In a comprehensive review of intervention practices, Cirrin and Gillam (2008) concluded that use of modified speech to improve language processing abilities is not superior to other forms of intervention including computer software programs without modified speech or clinician-based treatment.

Teaching memory strategies

It is accepted that the role of memory in intervention is compensatory in nature. Thus, rather than trying to increase memory capacity, intervention serves to improve performance through enhancing the efficiency of memory resources (Dehn, 2008). It is difficult to separate memory intervention from language intervention (Gillam, 1997). Children with SLI require strategies that allow them to remember information long enough to use it for learning or for academic demands (Gill, Klecan-Aker, Roberts, & Fredenburg, 2003). Gill et al. (2003) compared three memory strategies in their intervention study that employed 30 school aged children with SLI. Each child was seen twice weekly for a 30-minute period that was divided between 15 minutes of expressive language activities and 15 minutes of following directions. During the following directions components, children received instruction that included: (a) traditional direction following instruction that included teaching prepositional phrases and vocabulary, as well as commercially available worksheet exercises, (b) imposed rehearsal where the children were instructed to repeat the clinician's instructions aloud (i.e., "copy me" or "say what I say" before the child performed the direction), or (c) both rehearse the direction (as above) as well as visualize the instruction (i.e., "see it happen" or "imagine the task finished"). Following five weeks of intervention, the children who received either imposed rehearsal or imposed rehearsal and visualization performed significantly better on a post-treatment measure of following directions than children who received traditional following directions instructions. Eight months following the treatment study, however, only children who received imposed rehearsal and visualization intervention maintained a significant difference from the traditional direction instruction suggesting that this intervention was superior to imposed instruction alone at maintaining the ability to follow directions after the period of direct instruction ended. Importantly, this intervention study demonstrated that children with SLI are able to successfully learn and apply a strategy of rehearsal.

Adolescents with language learning disabilities (LLD) can improve their learning performance after being taught metacognitive strategies (Wynn-Dancy & Gillam, 1997). Dehn (2008) identifies key aspects of metacognitive instruction including teaching skills, such as awareness of processing deficits and strengths, accurate selection of appropriate strategies to match the situation or task, self-monitoring and self-evaluation, and ability to revise or change strategies when necessary. Wynn-Dancy and Gillam (1997) describe two metacognitive strategies (ARROW and BRIDGE). However, they caution that adolescents with LLD not only require direction strategy instruction, but also need to be taught how to act strategically in applying these learning strategies.

Summary and conclusions

The original classification of SLI was developed to help differentiate this population from children with other language related problems such as intellectual disability (Stark & Tallal, 1981). However, as we learn more about children with SLI it has become obvious that they comprise a heterogeneous group with potentially different underlying causes of the language disorder. One possible subgroup of children with SLI displays strong evidence of a processing capacity limitation that contributes to their language learning problem. There are several different processing theories about SLI, but they have at least one factor in common. That is that children with SLI have an intact underlying grammatical structure, but the systems involved in the processing of language prevent these children from acquiring language as efficiently as their typically developing peers. Some theories emphasize a functional problem associated with slow speed of processing while others support a structural disorder that emphasizes reduced space for processing or insufficient energy for processing. The general, or specific, systems responsible for processing acoustic and linguistic information are unable to respond to the rate or volume of information as rapidly as the systems of their typically developing peers. As a result, language development is impaired in children with SLI.

Continued research within this population is essential to help shed light on the causal factors of processing limitations and how they influence language development. Identification of the underlying cause of language impairments is critical for developing sensitive assessment measures and effective intervention procedures for children with SLI. Assessment of processing capacity (such as nonword repetition and CLPT tasks) will assist in identifying children with, or at risk for, SLI. These types of assessment procedures are relatively short in duration and easy to administer. It is unlikely that they identify those components of language that are affected or qualify children for intervention services. However, they will help determine why language learning is affected in this population. This information can be used to help establish what intervention procedures are most likely to be appropriate for children with processing problems, how to use appropriate compensatory strategies, or provide ideas of how to modify the communication environment so that the children receive the maximum benefit from language intervention. There is still much more research that needs to be completed on this population. Recent technological advances (e.g., ERP, fMRI, genetic mapping) are likely to drive research endeavors into areas that were not possible in the past. Indeed, more advanced research designs will continue to enlighten our knowledge of this group of children with language problems. For a comprehensive overview of specific language impairment, *Specific Language Impairment* by Leonard (1998) is recommended reading for anyone interested in this population. In addition, Grela has collaborated with colleagues (Savako et al. 2017) to consider the use of non-verbal IQ when matching children with SLI to typically developing children.

Further reading

Adlof, S. M. (2020). Promoting reading achievement in children with developmental language disorders: What can we learn from research on specific language impairment and dyslexia? *Journal of Speech, Language, and Hearing Research, 63*(10), 3277–3292.

Graham, S., Hebert, M., Fishman, E., Ray, A. B., & Rouse, A. G. (2020). Do children classified with specific language impairment have a learning disability in writing? A meta-analysis. *Journal of Learning Disabilities, 53*(4), 292–310.

Larson, C., Kaplan, D., Kaushanskaya, M., & Weismer, S. E. (2020). Language and inhibition: Predictive relationships in children with language impairment relative to typically developing peers. *Journal of Speech, Language, and Hearing Research, 63*(4), 1115–1127.

References

Adams, A. M., & Gathercole, S. E. (1995). Phonological working memory and speech production in preschool children. *Journal of Speech and Hearing Research, 38*(2), 403–414.

Archibald, L. M. D., & Gathercole, S. E. (2006a). Nonword repetition: A comparison of tests. *Journal of Speech, Language, and Hearing Research, 49*(5), 970–983.

Archibald, L. M. D., & Gathercole, S. E. (2006b). Short-term and working memory in specific language impairment. *International Journal of Language and Communication Disorders, 41*(6), 675–693.

Archibald, L. M. D., & Gathercole, S. E. (2007). Nonword repetition in specific language impairment: More than a phonological short-term memory deficit. *Psychonomic Bulletin and Review, 14*(5), 919–924.

Baddeley, A. (1986). *Working memory*. New York: Clarendon Press/Oxford University Press.

Bishop, D. V. M. (1994). Grammatical errors in specific language impairment: Competence or performance limitations? *Applied Psycholinguistics, 15*(4), 507–550.

Bishop, D. V. M. (2000). How does the brain learn language? Insights from the study of children with and without language impairment. *Developmental Medicine and Child Neurology, 42*(2), 133–142.

Bishop, D. V. M. (2002). The role of genes in the etiology of specific language impairment. *Journal of Communication Disorders, 35*(4), 311–328.

Bishop, D. V. M., & McArthur, G. M. (2005). Individual differences in auditory processing in specific language impairment: A follow-up study using event-related potentials and behavioural thresholds. *Cortex, 41*(3), 327–341.

Bishop, D. V. M., Adams, C. V., & Rosen, S. (2006). Resistance of grammatical impairment to computerized comprehension training in children with specific and non-specific language impairments. *International Journal of Language and Communication Disorders, 41*(1), 19–40.

Bishop, D. V. M., Bright, P., James, C., Bishop, S. J., & van der Lely, H. K. J. (2000). Grammatical SLI: A distinct subtype of developmental language impairment? *Applied Psycholinguistics, 21*(2), 159–181.

Burlingame, E., Sussman, H. M., Gillam, R. B., & Hay, J. F. (2005). An investigation of speech perception in children with specific language impairment on a continuum of formant transition duration. *Journal of Speech, Language, and Hearing Research, 48*(4), 805–816.

Camarata, S. M., & Nelson, K. E. (2006). Conversational recast intervention with preschool and older children. In R. J. McCauley & M. E. Fey (Eds.), *Treatment of language disorders in children* (pp. 237–264). Baltimore, MD: Paul H Brookes Publishing.

Camarata, S. M., Nelson, K. E., & Camarata, M. N. (1994). Comparison of conversational-recasting and imitative procedures for training grammatical structures in children with specific language impairment. *Journal of Speech and Hearing Research, 37*(6), 1414–1423.

Cirrin, F. M., & Gillam, R. B. (2008). Language intervention practices for school-age children with spoken language disorders: A systematic review. *Language, Speech, and Hearing Services in Schools, 39*(1), 110–137.

Cleave, P. L., & Fey, M. E. (1997). Two approaches to the facilitation of grammar in children with language impairments: Rationale and description. *American Journal of Speech-Language Pathology, 6*(1), 22–32.

Cohen, W., Hodson, A., O'Hare, A., Boyle, J., Durrani, T., McCartney, E., & Watson, J. (2005). Effects of computer-based intervention through acoustically modified speech (Fast ForWord) in severe mixed receptive-expressive language impairment: Outcomes from a randomized controlled trial. *Journal of Speech, Language, and Hearing Research, 48*(3), 715–729.

Connell, P. J. (1987). An effect of modeling and imitation teaching procedures on children with and without specific language impairment. *Journal of Speech and Hearing Research, 30*(1), 105–113.

Connell, P. J., & Stone, C. A. (1992). Morpheme learning of children with specific language impairment under controlled instructional conditions. *Journal of Speech and Hearing Research, 35*(4), 844–852.

Conti-Ramsden, G., Botting, N., & Faragher, B. (2001). Psycholinguistic markers for specific language impairment (SLI). *Journal of Child Psychology and Psychiatry, 42*(6), 741–748.

Crago, M. B., & Gopnik, M. (1994). From families to phenotypes: Theoretical and clinical implications of research into the genetic basis of specific language impairment. In R. V. Watkins & M. L. Rice (Eds.), *Specific language impairments in children* (pp. 35–51). Baltimore: Paul H Brookes Publishing.

Criddle, M. J., & Durkin, K. (2001). Phonological representation of novel morphemes in children with SLI and typically developing children. *Applied Psycholinguistics, 22*(3), 363–382.

Daneman, M., & Carpenter, P. A. (1983). Individual differences in integrating information between and within sentences. *Journal of Experimental Psychology: Learning, Memory, and Cognition, 9*(4), 561–584.

Dehn, M. (2008). *Working memory and academic learning: Assessment and intervention* (1st ed.). Hoboken: John Wiley & Sons.

Dick, F., Wulfeck, B., Krupa-Kwiatkowski, M., & Bates, E. (2004). The development of complex sentence interpretation in typically developing children compared with children with specific language impairments or early unilateral focal lesions. *Developmental Science*, 7(3), 360–377.

DiSimoni, F., Ehrler, D. J., & McGhee, R. L. (2007). *Token test for children (Rev.)*. Greenville: Super Duper Publications.

Dollaghan, C. A. (2007). *The handbook for evidence-based practice in communication disorders*. Baltimore: Paul H Brookes Publishing.

Dollaghan, C. A., & Campbell, T. F. (1998). Nonword repetition and child language impairment. *Journal of Speech, Language, and Hearing Research, 41*(5), 1136–1146.

Ebbels, S. H., van der Lely, H. K. J., & Dockrell, J. E. (2007). Intervention for verb argument structure in children with persistent SLI: A randomized control trial. *Journal of Speech, Language, and Hearing Research, 50*(5), 1330–1349.

Ellis Weismer, S. E. (1997). The role of stress in language processing and intervention. *Topics in Language Disorders, 17*(4), 41–52.

Ellis Weismer, S. E., & Hesketh, L. J. (1993). The influence of prosodic and gestural cues on novel word acquisition by children with specific language impairment. *Journal of Speech and Hearing Research, 36*(5), 1013–1025.

Ellis Weismer, S. E., & Hesketh, L. J. (1996). Lexical learning by children with specific language impairment: Effects of linguistic input presented at varying speaking rates. *Journal of Speech and Hearing Research, 39*(1), 177–190.

Ellis Weismer, S., & Hesketh, L. J. (1998). The impact of emphatic stress on novel word learning by children with specific language impairment. *Journal of Speech, Language, and Hearing Research, 41*(6), 1444–1458.

Ellis Weismer, S. E., Evans, J. L., & Hesketh, L. J. (1999). An examination of verbal working memory capacity in children with specific language impairment. *Journal of Speech, Language, and Hearing Research, 42*(5), 1249–1260.

Ellis Weismer, S. E., Plante, E., Jones, M., & Tomblin, J. B. (2005). A functional magnetic resonance imaging investigation of verbal working memory in adolescents with specific language impairment. *Journal of Speech, Language, and Hearing Research, 48*(2), 405–425.

Ellis Weismer, S. E., Tomblin, J. B., Zhang, X., Buckwalter, P., Chynoweth, J. G., & Jones, M. (2000). Nonword repetition performance in school-age children with and without language impairment. *Journal of Speech, Language, and Hearing Research, 43*(4), 865–878.

Estes, K. G., Evans, J. L., & Else-Quest, N. M. (2007). Differences in the nonword repetition performance of children with and without specific language impairment: A meta-analysis. *Journal of Speech, Language, and Hearing Research, 50*(1), 177–195.

Fey, M. E. (1986). *Language intervention with young children.* San Diego: College-Hill Press.

Fey, M. E., Cleave, P. L., Long, S. H., & Hughes, D. L. (1993). Two approaches to the facilitation of grammar in children with language impairment: An experimental evaluation. *Journal of Speech and Hearing Research, 36*(1), 141–157.

Fey, M. E., Long, S. H., & Finestack, L. H. (2003). Ten principles of grammar facilitation for children with specific language impairments. *American Journal of Speech-Language Pathology, 12*(1), 3–15.

Gathercole, S. E., & Baddeley, A. D. (1995). Short-term memory may yet be deficient in children with language impairments: A comment on van der Lely & Howard (1993). *Journal of Speech and Hearing Research, 38*(2), 463–466.

Gathercole, S. E., Willis, C. S., Baddeley, A. D., & Emslie, H. (1994). The children's test of nonword repetition: A test of phonological working memory. *Memory, 2*(2), 103–127.

Gaulin, C. A., & Campbell, T. F. (1994). Procedure for assessing verbal working memory in normal school-age children: Some preliminary data. *Perceptual and Motor Skills, 79*(1 Pt 1), 55–64.

Gill, C. B., Klecan-Aker, J., Roberts, T., & Fredenburg, K. A. (2003). Following directions: Rehearsal and visualization strategies for children with specific language impairment. *Child Language Teaching and Therapy, 19*(1), 85–101.

Gillam, R. B. (1997). Putting memory to work in language intervention: Implications for practitioners. *Topics in Language Disorders, 18*(1), 72–79.

Gillam, R. B., Loeb, D. F., Hoffman, L. M., Bohman, T., Champlin, C. A., Thibodeau, L., ... & Friel-Patti, S. (2008). The efficacy of Fast ForWord language intervention in school-age children with language impairment: A randomized controlled trial. *Journal of Speech, Language, and Hearing Research, 51*(1), 97–119.

Gillam, S. L., & Gillam, R. B. (2006). Making evidence-based decisions about child language intervention in schools. *Language, Speech, and Hearing Services in Schools, 37*(4), 304–315.

Girolametto, L., Pearce, P. S., & Weitzman, E. (1996). Interactive focused stimulation for toddlers with expressive vocabulary delays. *Journal of Speech and Hearing Research, 39*(6), 1274–1283.

Grela, B. G. (2003a). The omission of subject arguments in children with specific language impairment. *Clinical Linguistics and Phonetics, 17*(2), 153–169.

Grela, B. G. (2003b). Production based theories may account for subject omission in normal children and children with SLI. *Journal of Speech-Language Pathology and Audiology, 27*, 221–228.

Grela, B. G., & Leonard, L. B. (1997). The use of subject arguments by children with specific language impairment. *Clinical Linguistics and Phonetics, 11*(6), 443–453.

Grela, B. G., & Leonard, L. B. (2000). The influence of argument-structure complexity on the use of auxiliary verbs by children with SLI. *Journal of Speech, Language, and Hearing Research, 43*(5), 1115–1125.

Grela, B. G., Snyder, W., & Hiramatsu, K. (2005). The production of novel root compounds in children with specific language impairment. *Clinical Linguistics and Phonetics, 19*(8), 701–715.

Gutierrez-Clellen, V. F., & Peña, E. (2001). Dynamic assessment of diverse children: A tutorial. *Language, 32*(4), 212–224.

Hasson, N., & Joffe, V. (2007). The case for dynamic assessment in speech and language therapy. *Child Language Teaching and Therapy, 23*(1), 9–25.

Hayiou-Thomas, M. E., Bishop, D.V. M., & Plunkett, K. (2004). Simulating SLI: General cognitive processing stressors can produce a specific linguistic profile. *Journal of Speech, Language, and Hearing Research, 47*(6), 1347–1362.

Hugdahl, K., Gundersen, H., Brekke, C., Thomsen, T., Rimol, L. M., Ersland, L., & Niemi, J. (2004). fMRI brain activation in a Finnish family with specific language impairment compared with a normal control group. *Journal of Speech, Language, and Hearing Research, 47*(1), 162–172.

Hutchinson, T. A. (1996). What to look for in the technical manual: Twenty questions for users. *Language, Speech, and Hearing Services in Schools, 27*(2), 109–121.

Im-Bolter, N., Johnson, J., & Pascual-Leone, J. (2006). Processing limitations in children with specific language impairment: The role of executive function. *Child Development, 77*(6), 1822–1841.

Joanisse, M. F. (2004). Specific language impairments in children: Phonology, semantics, and the English past tense. *Current Directions in Psychological Science, 13*(4), 156–160.

Joanisse, M. F., & Seidenberg, M. S. (2003). Phonology and syntax in specific language impairment: Evidence from a connectionist model. *Brain and Language, 86*(1), 40–56.

Johnston, J. R. (1991). Questions about cognition in children with specific language impairment. In J. Miller (Ed.), *Research on child language disorders* (pp. 299–307). Austin: Pro-Ed.

Johnston, J. R. (1994). Cognitive abilities of children with language impairment. In R. Watkins & M. Rice (Eds.), *Specific language impairments in children* (pp. 107–121). Baltimore: Paul H. Brookes Publishing Co., Inc.

Johnston, J. R., & Kamhi, A. G. (1984). Syntactic and semantic aspects of the utterances of language impaired children: The same can be less. *Merrill-Palmer Quarterly, 30*(1), 65–85.

Juhasz, C., & Grela, B. G. (2008). Verb particle errors in preschool children with specific language impairment. *Contemporary Issues in Communication Sciences and Disorders, 35*(Spring), 76–83.

Just, M. A., & Carpenter, P. A. (1992). A capacity theory of comprehension: Individual differences in working memory. *Psychological Review, 99*(1), 122–148.

Kail, R. (1991). Developmental change in speed of processing during childhood and adolescence. *Psychological Bulletin, 109*(3), 490–501.

Kail, R. (1994). A method for studying the generalized slowing hypothesis in children with specific language impairment. *Journal of Speech and Hearing Research, 37*(2), 418–421.

Lahey, M., Edwards, J., & Munson, B. (2001). Is processing speed related to severity of language impairment? *Journal of Speech, Language, and Hearing Research, 44*(6), 1354–1361.

Lapointe, S. G. (1985). A theory of verb form use in the speech of agrammatic aphasics. *Brain and Language, 24*(1), 100–155.

Leonard, L. B. (1998). *Children with specific language impairment.* Cambridge, MA: MIT Press.

Leonard, L. B., & Bortolini, U. (1998). Grammatical morphology and the role of weak syllables in the speech of Italian-speaking children with specific language impairment. *Journal of Speech, 41*(6), 1363–1374.

Leonard, L. B., Camarata, S. M., Pawlowska, M., Brown, B., & Camarata, M. N. (2008). The acquisition of tense and agreement morphemes by children with specific language impairment during intervention: Phase 3. *Journal of Speech, Language, and Hearing Research, 51*(1), 120–125.

Leonard, L. B., Eyer, J. A., Bedore, L. M., & Grela, B. G. (1997). Three accounts of the grammatical morpheme difficulties of English-speaking children with specific language impairment. *Journal of Speech, Language, and Hearing Research, 40*(4), 741–753.

Leonard, L. B., McGregor, K. K., & Allen, G. D. (1992). Grammatical morphology and speech perception in children with specific language impairment. *Journal of Speech and Hearing Research, 35*(5), 1076–1085.

Leonard, L. B., Miller, C. A., Grela, B., Holland, A. L., Gerber, E., & Petucci, M. (2000). Production operations contribute to the grammatical morpheme limitations of children with specific language impairment. *Journal of Memory and Language, 43*(2), 362–378.

Leonard, L. B., Weismer, S. E., Miller, C. A., Francis, D. J., Tomblin, J. B., & Kail, R. (2007). Speed of processing, working memory and language impairment in children. *Journal of Speech, Language, and Hearing Research, 50*(2), 408–428.

Marton, K., Schwartz, R. G., Farkas, L., & Katsnelson, V. (2006). Effect of sentence length and complexity on working memory performance in Hungarian children with specific language impairment (SLI): A cross-linguistic comparison. *International Journal of Language and Communication Disorders, 41*(6), 653–673.

McArthur, G. M., & Bishop, D. V. M. (2004). Which people with specific language impairment have auditory processing deficits? *Cognitive Neuropsychology, 21*(1), 79–94.

McArthur, G. M., & Bishop, D. V. M. (2005). Speech and non-speech processing in people with specific language impairment: A behavioural and electrophysiological study. *Brain and Language, 94*(3), 260–273.

McCauley, R. J., & Swisher, L. (1984). Psychometric review of language and articulation tests for preschool children. *Journal of Speech and Hearing Disorders, 49*(1), 34–42.

Miller, C. A., & Leonard, L. B. (1998). Deficits in finite verb morphology: Some assumptions in recent accounts of specific language impairment. *Journal of Speech, Language, and Hearing Research, 41*(3), 701–707.

Miller, C. A., Kail, R., Leonard, L. B., & Tomblin, J. B. (2001). Speed of processing in children with specific language impairment. *Journal of Speech, Language, and Hearing Research, 44*(2), 416–433.

Miller, C. A., Leonard, L. B., Kail, R. V., Zhang, X., Tomblin, J. B., & Francis, D. J. (2006). Response time in 14-year-olds with language impairment. *Journal of Speech, Language, and Hearing Research, 49*(4), 712–728.

Montgomery, J. W. (2000). Verbal working memory and sentence comprehension in children with specific language impairment. *Journal of Speech, Language, and Hearing Research, 43*(2), 293–308.

Montgomery, J. W. (2003). Working memory and comprehension in children with specific language impairment: What we know so far. *Journal of Communication Disorders, 36*(3), 221–231.

Montgomery, J. W. (2005). Effects of input rate and age on the real-time language processing of children with specific language impairment. *International Journal of Language and Communication Disorders, 40*(2), 171–188.

Montgomery, J. W., & Leonard, L. B. (1998). Real-time inflectional processing by children with specific language impairment: Effects of phonetic substance. *Journal of Speech, Language, and Hearing Research, 41*(6), 1432–1443.

Montgomery, J. W., & Leonard, L. B. (2006). Effects of acoustic manipulation on the real-time inflectional processing of children with specific language impairment. *Journal of Speech, Language, and Hearing Research, 49*(6), 1238–1256.

Montgomery, J. W., & Windsor, J. (2007). Examining the language performances of children with and without specific language impairment: Contributions of phonological short-term memory and speed of processing. *Journal of Speech, Language, and Hearing Research, 50*(3), 778–797.

Nelson, K. E., Camarata, S. M., Welsh, J., Butkovsky, L., & Camarata, M. (1996). Effects of imitative and conversational recasting treatment on the acquisition of grammar in children with specific language impairment and younger language-normal children. *Journal of Speech and Hearing Research, 39*(4), 850–859.

Peña, E. D., & Gillam, R. B. (2000). Dynamic assessment of children referred for speech and language evaluations. *Advances in Cognition and Educational Practice, 6*, 543–575.

Peña, E. D., Iglesias, A., & Lidz, C. S. (2001). Reducing test bias through dynamic assessment of children's word learning ability. *American Journal of Speech-Language Pathology, 10*(2), 138–154.

Peña, E. D., Quinn, R., & Iglesias, A. (1992). The application of dynamic methods to language assessment: A nonbiased procedure. *Journal of Special Education, 26*(3), 269–280.

Pizzioli, F., & Schelstraete, M.-A. (2008). The argument-structure complexity effect in children with specific language impairment: Evidence from the use of grammatical morphemes in French. *Journal of Speech, Language, and Hearing Research, 51*(3), 706–721.

Plante, E., & Vance, R. (1994). Selection of preschool language tests: A data-based approach. *Language, 25*(1), 15–24.

Polite, E. J., & Leonard, L. B. (2006). Finite verb morphology and phonological length in the speech of children with specific language impairment. *Clinical Linguistics and Phonetics, 10*, 751–760.

Rice, M. L. (2004). Growth models of developmental language disorders. In M. L. Rice & S. F. Warren (Eds.), *Developmental language disorders: From pheno-types to etiologies* (pp. 207–240). Mahwah, NJ: Lawrence Erlbaum Associates Publishers.

Rice, M. L., & Wexler, K. (1996). Toward tense as a clinical marker of specific language impairment in English-speaking children. *Journal of Speech and Hearing Research, 39*(6), 1239–1257.

Robertson, S. B., & Weismer, S. E. (1999). Effects of treatment on linguistic and social skills in toddlers with delayed language development. *Journal of Speech, Language, and Hearing Research, 42*(5), 1234–1248.

Roy, P., & Chiat, S. (2004). A prosodically controlled word and nonword repetition task for 2-to 4-year-olds: Evidence from typically developing children. *Journal of Speech, Language, and Hearing Research, 47*(1), 223–234.

Sayako, F., Earle, M., Gallinat, E., Grela, B., Lehto, A., & Spaulding, T. (2017). Empirical implications of matching children with specific language impairment to children with typical development on nonverbal IQ. *Journal of Learning Disabilities, 50*(3), 252–260.

Schul, R., Stiles, J., Wulfeck, B., & Townsend, J. (2004). How "generalized" is the "slowed processing". In SLI? The case of visuospatial attentional orienting. *Neuropsychologia, 42*(5), 661–671.

Scientific Learning Corporation (1998). *Fast forward language [computer software]*. Berkeley: Author.

Semel, E., Wiig, E., & Secord, W. (1987). *Clinical evaluation of language fundamentals-revised*. San Antonio: The Psychological Corporation.

Spaulding, T. J., Plante, E., & Farinella, K. A. (2006). Eligibility criteria for language impairment: Is the low end of normal always appropriate? *Language, 37*(1), 61–72.

Stark, R., & Tallal, P. (1981). Selection of children with specific language deficits. *Journal of Speech and Hearing Disorders, 46*(2), 114–122.

Tallal, P. (1980). Language disabilities in children: A perceptual or linguistic deficit? *Journal of Pediatric Psychology, 5*(2), 127–140.

Tallal, P. (2004). Improving language and literacy is a matter of time. *Nature Reviews. Neuroscience, 5*(9), 721–728.

Tallal, P., Miller, S. L., Bedi, G., Wang, X., Nagarajan, S. S., Nagarajan, S. S., ... & Merzenich, M. M. (1996). Language comprehension in language-learning impaired children improved with acoustically modified speech. *Science, 271*(5245), 81–84.

Tallal, P., Miller, S. L., & Fitch, R. H. (1993). Neurobiological basis of speech: A case for the preeminence of temporal processing. In P. Tallal, A. M. Galaburda, R. R. Llinás & C. von Euler (Eds.), *Temporal information processing in the nervous system: Special reference to dyslexia and dysphasia* (pp. 27–47). New York: New York Academy of Sciences.

Tallal, P., & Piercy, M. (1974). Developmental aphasia: Rate of auditory processing and selective impairment of consonant perception. *Neuropsychologia, 12*(1), 83–93.

Tallal, P., & Piercy, M. (1975). Developmental aphasia: The perception of brief vowels and extended stop consonants. *Neuropsychologia, 13*(1), 69–74.

Tallal, P., Sainburg, R. L., & Jernigan, T. (1991). The neuropathology of developmental dysphasia: Behavioral, morphological, and physiological evidence for a pervasive temporal processing disorder. *Reading and Writing, 3*(3), 363–377.

Tallal, P., Stark, R. E., & Mellits, E. D. (1985). Identification of language-impaired children on the basis of rapid perception and production skills. *Brain and Language, 25*(2), 314–322.

Tomblin, J. B., Records, N. L., Buckwalter, P., Zhang, X., Smith, E., & O'Brien, M. (1997). Prevalence of specific language impairment in kindergarten children. *Journal of Speech and Hearing Research, 40*(6), 1245–1260.
van der Lely, H. K. J. (1994). Canonical linking rules: Forward versus reverse linking in normally developing and specifically language-impaired children. *Cognition, 51*(1), 29–72.
van der Lely, H. K. J. (1997). Language and cognitive development in a grammatical SLI boy: Modularity and innateness. *Journal of Neurolinguistics, 10*(2), 75–107.
van der Lely, H. K. J. (2005). Domain-specific cognitive systems: Insight from grammatical-SLI. *Trends in Cognitive Sciences, 9*(2), 53–59.
Wagner, R., Torgeson, J., & Rashotte, C. (1999). *Comprehensive test of phonological processing (CTOPP)* (1st ed.). Bloomington: Pearson Assessment Group.
Watkins, R. V., & Rice, M. L. (1991). Verb particle and preposition acquisition in language-impaired preschoolers. *Journal of Speech and Hearing Research, 34*(5), 1130–1141.
Windsor, J., & Hwang, M. (1999). Testing the generalized slowing hypothesis specific language impairment. *Journal of Speech, Language, and Hearing Research, 42*(5), 1205–1210.
Wynn-Dancy, M. L., & Gillam, R. B. (1997). Accessing long-term memory: Metacognitive strategies and strategic action in adolescents. *Topics in Language Disorders, 18*(1), 32–44.

20

GRAMMATICAL-SPECIFIC LANGUAGE IMPAIRMENT

A window onto domain specificity

Heather van der Lely and Chloë Marshall

Introduction

There has been much debate as to which aspects of language are specific to language rather than shared with other aspects of cognition, and which aspects of language are specific to humans rather than shared with other groups of animals (Hauser, 2001; Hauser, Chomsky, & Fitch, 2002; Pinker & Jackendoff, 2005). In addition, there continues to be much discussion about how this specialized language system is represented and develops in the brain. New insight into this debate comes from studying people with a developmental language disorder, Specific Language Impairment (SLI), and particularly a subtype of this disorder known as Grammatical (G)-SLI. Such insight is bidirectional: our growing understanding of language and brain-systems enhances and directs our line of enquiry into SLI, furthering our knowledge of the underlying nature of both typical and atypical language development. In turn, this informs our enquiries about language and brain systems.

In this context, our chapter reviews the findings from G-SLI, and aims to contribute to our understanding both of specialized cognitive systems, specifically language, and of the nature of typical and atypical language acquisition. We argue that our data provide evidence that certain aspects of grammar are domain-specific and can be selectively impaired.

Theoretical foundations

SLI: what do we agree on?

SLI is a disorder of language acquisition in children, in the absence of any obvious language-independent cause, such as hearing loss, low nonverbal IQ, motor difficulties, or neurological damage (Bishop, 1997; Leonard, 1998). Children, teenagers, or even adults with SLI may produce sentences such as "Who Marge saw someone?" (van der Lely & Battell, 2003) or "Yesterday I fall over" (Leonard, Dromi, Adam, & Zadunaisky-Ehrlich, 2000; Rice, 2003; van der Lely & Ullman, 2001), or may fail to correctly interpret sentences such as "The man was eaten by the fish" (Bishop, 1982; van der Lely, 1996). SLI is one of the most common developmental disorders, affecting around 7% of children in its "pure form" (Tomblin et al., 1997), and the prevalence is even greater when children with co-occurring impairments (e.g., Autism, ADHD) are included.

The disorder heterogeneously affects components of language such as syntax, morphology, phonology, and, often to a lesser extent, the lexicon. It has a strong genetic component as shown by familial aggregation studies (for a review see Stromswold, 1998), twin studies (Bishop & Bishop,

DOI: 10.4324/9781003204213-23

1998), and genetic analyses (Fisher, Lai, & Monaco, 2003). The current view is that SLI is likely to have a complex geno-phenotypic profile, with different genetic forms of the disorder causing different phenotypes and possibly even the same genotype resulting in varied phenotypes (Fisher et al., 2003).

SLI: what don't we agree on?

It is perhaps not surprising that, given the heterogeneous nature of SLI, there is disagreement over two areas: a taxonomy of SLI, and its cause at the cognitive level.

The discussion surrounding the taxonomy of SLI concerns the variation and number of component deficits in children who fall under the broad umbrella of "SLI." Broadly speaking, the following disorders and language component deficits are found in the literature. Note that we are focusing on the 7% of children who fall within the "typical definition" of SLI; that is, those who do not have co-occurring problems. It is the particular combination or specification of component deficits that characterizes the various definitions of SLI, some of which are considered SLI subgroups. On the one hand, Bishop and Snowling (2004) reviewed children with SLI who have a double deficit of phonological deficits plus "language impairments." We understand this to mean some or perhaps any other component impairments within the language system. Therefore, we might expect a range of different profiles in the children they study. In contrast to this group of SLI, a highly restrictive subgroup are those called "Syntactic-SLI," characterized by only syntactic and morphosyntactic impairments (Friedmann & Novogrodsky, 2004). The "Grammatical(G)-SLI" subgroup, however, is defined by similar core impairment in syntax and morphology, but in addition the majority suffer from phonological impairment too (Gallon, Harris, & van der Lely, 2007). Even within these component deficits in syntax, morphology, and phonology, the deficit is restricted to structures that are hierarchically complex, as we will discuss in due course. Interestingly, the distinction between phonology on the one hand and syntax and morphology on the other appears to be relevant to geno-phenotypic associations. Whereas a locus on Chromosome 16, now identified as CNTNAP2, is associated with children with phonological deficits and/or phonological memory deficits, a locus on Chromosome 19 is associated with expressive grammatical impairments, with no significant overlap between the groups (Bishop, Adams, & Norbury, 2006; Vernes et al., 2008).

In contrast, a subgroup who appear to have relative strengths in the grammatical aspects of language are those with "Pragmatic(P)-SLI," who, as their name implies, have impaired pragmatic abilities (Bishop & Norbury, 2002). There is one subgroup—which we shall refer to as Familial-SLI (of which the most famous is the KE family), which has an identified simple genotype—a mutation of the gene FOXP2 with a simple autosomal, dominant inheritance—but which results in a rather complex phenotype (Fisher et al., 2003). Familial-SLI is characterized by not only impairments in language components, most notably morpho-syntax, morphology, phonology, as well as the lexicon, but also outside the language system. Specifically, the impaired family members have an oral dyspraxia concerning problems in motor programming of fine articulatory movements for speech sounds (Fisher & DeFries, 2002; Watkins, Dronkers, & Vargha-Khadem, 2002). It is also of note that some members of the KE family have a low IQ; however low IQ doesn't segregate with the language impairment (Fisher & DeFries, 2002). In other children, low IQ is frequently (but not always) associated with a delayed pattern of language development, which we shall call the "delayed language" subgroup (Rice, 2004). Children in this group often exhibit delayed vocabulary acquisition and immature pragmatic development, alongside other language impairments (Rice, 2004).

In addition, many children with a diagnosis of SLI also have dyslexia, and vice versa. However, these two disorders are not synonymous, and can occur in isolation. For the majority of children with dyslexia, impairments center around the phonological component, either with the phonological representations themselves, or with accessing and/or manipulating those representations

(Ramus & Szenkovits, 2008; Snowling, 2000). Whether such phonological deficits are identical or different to those found in SLI children is the focus of much current research (de Bree, 2007; Marshall, Harcourt-Brown, Ramus, & van der Lely, 2009; Marshall & van der Lely, 2009; and papers in Messaoud-Galusi & Marshall, 2010).

The second area of discussion concerns the cognitive cause of SLI. Given the considerable heterogeneity in the phenotype, it could well be that different cognitive causes and pathways underlie different forms of SLI. But equally, there could be different routes to a particular surface impairment, for example, omission of tense marking. In this context, we now consider the two predominant approaches to the cognitive origins of SLI that can be broadly characterized as the domain-general and domain-specific perspectives.

Domain-General (D-G) deficit proponents identify the primary deficit in general cognitive mechanisms such as temporal discrimination, lower-level sensory processing speed, processing capacity, and short-term memory (Bishop, 1997; Leonard, 1998; Montgomery, 2000; Tallal, 2002). These deficits are considered to impair auditory processing of nonspeech and speech sounds, or alternatively memory and/or general learning. The resulting phonological deficit in turn causes problems in language learning (Joanisse & Seidenberg, 1998). Although the primary source of the domain-general deficit varies across different accounts, they share the common view that the underlying deficit is not in mechanisms specific to grammar, but in lower-level processing or later nongrammatical cognitive processing. Note that whereas temporal deficits alone are proposed by some to be sufficient to cause SLI (Tallal et al., 1996), short-term memory deficits are thought to cause SLI only when found in combination with other impairments (Gathercole, 2006). Within this framework, Joanisse provides perhaps the most clearly specified model starting from an auditory or speech processing deficit, and he describes the resulting developmental trajectory of SLI (Joanisse, 2004; Joanisse, 2007).

Domain-Specific (D-S) deficit proponents, in contrast, claim that in some children the deficit affects the development of neural circuitry underlying the components of grammar (Bishop et al., 2006; Friedmann & Gvion, 2002; Rice, 2003; van der Lely, Rosen, & Adlard, 2004; van der Lely, Rosen, & McClelland, 1998). Thus, although both D-G and D-S mechanisms are likely to contribute to language (Gathercole, 2006; Jakubowicz & Strik, 2008; Marcus, 2004), SLI is thought to be caused by deficits to specialized computational mechanisms underlying grammar processing itself. Although a number of hypotheses have been proposed from this perspective, the Computational Grammatical Complexity (CGC) hypothesis (van der Lely, 2005), provides a framework for our research and investigations of the G-SLI subgroup. Specifically, the CGC claims that the deficit is in hierarchical structural knowledge that is core to the computational grammatical system. Our work reveals that many school-aged children and teenagers with G-SLI lack the computations to consistently form hierarchical, structurally complex forms in one or more components of grammar that normally develop between three and six years of age. This working hypothesis emphasizes the notion that impairments in syntax, morphology, and phonology are functionally autonomous, but cumulative in their effects (Marshall & van der Lely, 2007a, b; van der Lely, 2005).

Figure 20.1 illustrates this model, and in the following sections we will elaborate on the characterization for these three components of grammar, and how they affect language. For the purposes of this paper, Figure 20.1 only shows the arrows that are key to the discussion below. Based on this component model of language impairment the CGC predicts that there is no causal relation between lower-level auditory abilities or short-term memory abilities and grammatical development, although these abilities, as with typically developing (TD) children, contribute to general language performance. Lines rather than arrows show these relations.

We will now consider the CGC in more detail with respect to each of the three impaired grammatical components, syntax, morphology, and phonology, and present evidence that the impairment in the G-SLI subgroup is domain-specific.

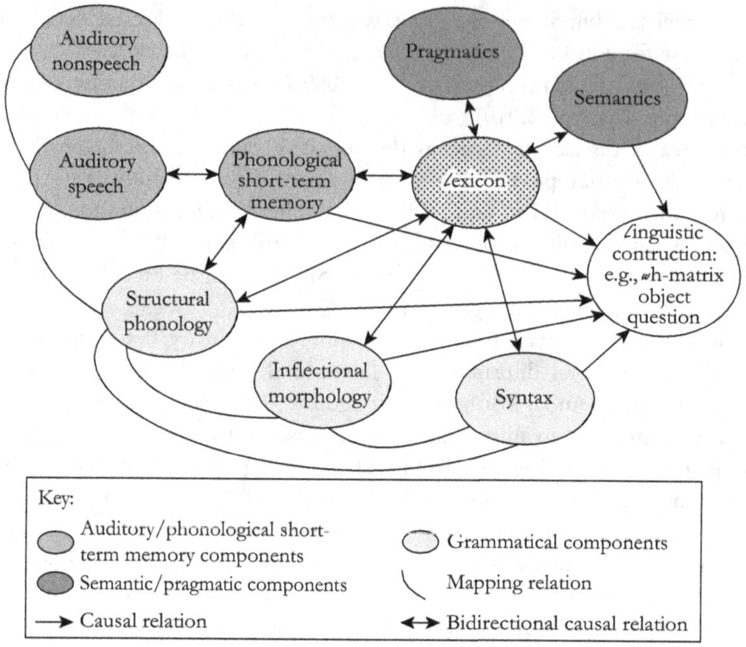

Figure 20.1 A component model of language acquisition and impairment. Note for clarity, only lines pertinent to the discussion have been included. There are clearly many more relations between components than depicted.

Syntax

The CGC claims that the deficit in hierarchical structure is characterized by impairment in syntactic dependencies. Specifically, whereas dependences within the phrase are preserved (e.g., agreement), those outside the phrase but within the clause are impaired. Broadly speaking, this can be characterized by what Chomsky terms "movement" or "feature checking" (Chomsky, 1998) or in current terminology "internal merge" (Chomsky, 2004). The impairment affects a large number of structures. For example, tense marking is impaired, resulting in errors such as "Yesterday I walk to school" (van der Lely & Ullman, 2001). Such errors have been eloquently described and explored by Wexler and Rice and colleagues and have led them to claim that this "extended optional infinitive" phase is the primary impairment within syntax (Rice, Wexler, & Redmond, 1999). However, the CGC claims that, at least for the G-SLI subgroup, their impairment with syntactic dependencies also affects assignment of theta roles, particularly when more general pragmatic and world knowledge is not available to facilitate interpretation, such as in reversible passive sentences (The man was eaten by the fish), or when assigning reference to pronouns or anaphors within sentences (Mowgli said Baloo was tickling him/himself; van der Lely, 1994, 1996; van der Lely & Stollwerck, 1997), as well as embedded sentences and relative clauses. The nature of the G-SLI children's syntactic deficits is clearly illustrated in a series of studies of wh-questions. Object matrix and embedded questions are particularly problematic in English because the wh-word has to move from the end of the sentence to the beginning, and "do support" requires checking of tense and question features.

Thus, G-SLI children produce questions such as "Who Joe see someone?" (van der Lely Battell, 2003) and judge such sentences to be grammatical (van der Lely Jones & Marshall, in press). They also make "copying" errors of the wh-word in embedded questions as in (1) (Archonti, 2003). This pattern is sometimes found in young children (Thornton, 1995), suggesting that such structures are syntactically simpler and easier.

(1) "Who did Joe think who Mary saw?" Furthermore, using a cross-modal priming paradigm, we found that G-SLI children showed no reactivation at the "gap" [marked by "t" in (2)] in preposition object questions in scenarios such as (2), in contrast to age and language matched control groups (Marinis & van der Lely, 2007).

(2) Balloo gives a long carrot to the rabbit. "Who did Balloo give the long carrot to tI at the farm?"

However, we found reactivation for the G-SLI children at the offset of the verb, where subcategorized arguments might be activated, suggesting that, in contrast to their peers, they were using semantic-lexical processing rather than syntactic processing (Marinis & van der Lely, 2007).

Following these findings, our next question was "Is there evidence at the brain level of impaired processing of just these syntactic dependencies, but normal functioning in other language processes?" If this was so, it would provide good evidence for the domain-specificity of this particular syntactic operation. However, the alternative domain-general hypothesis would be supported if brain correlates showed generally slow or abnormal characteristics to all (or most) language and/or auditory processing. To investigate these alternative hypotheses, we recorded electrophysiological time-locked, event-related brain potentials (ERPs) in 18 G-SLI participants aged 10–21 years, plus age-matched, language-matched, and adult controls, when they were listening to questions containing a syntactic violation. The particular syntactic violation we were interested in concerns structural syntactic dependencies at the clause level such as those that occur between a question word (who, what) and the word, which in declarative sentences follows the verb, but typically is absent in questions. In our particular design, the first possible "wh-word-gap" following the verb was filled. Pretesting of the sentences (see (3)(a)) indicated that, at the critical noun following the verb to which our EEG recordings were time-locked, the listener would perceive the word as a violation. This is because, if the gap is filled, the animacy property of the noun should mismatch that of the wh-word (see (3)(b)). Therefore, an animacy match ((3)(a)) was highly unexpected (a syntactic violation), whereas the animacy mismatch ((3)(b)) provided the control condition.

(3) (a) Who did the man push the clown into? (violation)
(b) What did the man push the clown into? (control)

Crucially, the syntactic violation relied on a structural syntactic dependency between two non-adjacent words in the sentence. What is at issue here is not merely to know whether the children noticed the violation/unexpectancy of the noun, but to identify the different functional neural circuitries that are used to detect such a violation/unexpectancy. We found an "Early Left Anterior Negativity" (ELAN), a language-specific neural correlate associated with structural syntactic violations (Friederici, 2002), in all the control groups but not in the G-SLI children. The electrophysiological brain responses revealed a selective impairment to only this neural circuitry that is specific to grammatical processing in G-SLI. The participants with G-SLI appeared to be partially compensating for their syntactic deficit by using neural circuitry associated with semantic processing (N400), and all nongrammar-specific (N400, P600) and low-level auditory neural responses (N1, P2, P3) were normal (Fonteneau & van der Lely, 2008). Thus, we found that the G-SLI children did indeed notice the violation, but they were using a different brain system to do this compared to the control subjects. The findings indicate that grammatical neural circuitry underlying this aspect of language is a developmentally unique system in the functional architecture of the brain, and this complex higher cognitive system can be selectively impaired.

In summary, our syntactic findings from G-SLI show a consistent impairment in syntactic dependencies outside the phrase but within the clause, which are manifest across a broad range of structures. The findings from the cross-modal priming and ERP studies indicated that G-SLI children use semantic mechanisms to compensate for their syntactic deficits. The use of such a semantic system leads to the speculation that the optional pattern of performance for syntax that is commonly reported in the literature results from this imprecise form of sentence processing, rather than an optional functioning of the syntactic mechanism(s). Such imprecise processing may not sufficiently restrict interpretation or production. Further research is warranted to explore this possibility. Note that children who do not necessarily fit the G-SLI criterion exhibit syntactic impairments with similar characteristics in both English speaking children (Bishop, Bright, James, Bishop, & van der Lely, 2000; Norbury, Bishop, & Briscoe, 2002; O'Hara & Johnston, 1997) and languages that are typologically different from English, such as French, Greek, and Hebrew (Friedmann & Novogrodsky, 2004, 2007; Jakubowicz, Nash, & van der Velde, 1999; Stavrakaki, 2001; Stavrakaki & van der Lely, 2010). The largely similar characteristics of the component deficit across different SLI subgroups is also illustrated in morphology and indeed phonology, which we turn to in the next sections.

Morphology

Within the morphology component, the CGC hypothesizes a hierarchical deficit that impacts on morphologically complex forms. Thus, over and above the syntactic deficits that affect both irregular and regular tense marking, regular forms are particularly problematic for children with G-SLI. Investigations using both elicited production (e.g., Every day I walk to school, Yesterday I …) and grammaticality judgments of correct and incorrect forms reveal a lack of the regularity advantage found in typically developing children (van der Lely & Ullman, 1996, 2001). Furthermore, individuals with G-SLI show an atypical pattern of frequency effects for both irregular and regular past tense forms. The Words and Rules model of past tense forms (Marcus et al., 1992; Pinker, 1999) provides a parsimonious explanation for these data: for typically developing children, irregular, morphologically simple forms are stored, which leads to frequency effects, whereas regular, morphologically complex forms are computed online and show no frequency effects. Van der Lely and Ullman (2001) therefore hypothesized that G-SLI children preferentially store regular inflected forms whole, as they do irregular forms. Thus, phonological-to-semantic mapping is key to the learning and processing of both regular and irregular forms.

We report two direct tests of van der Lely and Ullman's hypothesis. The first test explored plural compounds, building on Gordon's study of young children (Gordon, 1985). Gordon showed that three- to five-year-olds use irregular plurals inside compounds, such as mice-eater, but avoid using regular plurals to create forms such as rats-eater. This is because only stored forms can enter the compounding process (Gordon, 1985). Therefore, we hypothesized that if G-SLI children were storing regular plural forms whole, then these would be available to the compounding process, just like irregular plurals. Consistent with our hypothesis, G-SLI children, in contrast to language-matched controls, produced compound forms such as rats-eater (van der Lely & Christian, 2000).

The second test of the hypothesis considered the phonotactics of regular past tense marking, and specifically the clusters formed at the verb end when the suffix is added. Some of these clusters also occur in monomorphemic words, for example, the cluster at the end of missed (mist) and scowled (cold), and we refer to these as "monomorphemically legal clusters." In contrast, some clusters, such as those at the end of slammed, robbed, and loved, only occur in morphologically complex words (past tense or past participles), and we call these "monomorphemically illegal clusters." Because these illegal clusters only occur in inflected words, their frequency is much lower than that of legal clusters. Thus if, as we hypothesized, G-SLI children are storing past tense forms, they should find it harder to inflect verbs when an illegal cluster would be created. On the other hand, if typically developing children are able to compute regular past tense verb forms online, then cluster frequency should have no effect, and they should be equally able to infect the stem whatever the legality of the final cluster.

Re-analysis of the past tense elicitation data collected by van der Lely and Ullman (2001), a new elicitation experiment conducted with a new group of G-SLI children, plus re-analysis of data previously collected by Thomas et al. (2001) confirmed our predictions. Whereas typically developing children from all three studies showed no differences between regular past tense forms containing legal or illegal clusters, the G-SLI children performed consistently worse on verbs containing illegal clusters (Marshall & van der Lely, 2006).

A further investigation of this phenomenon studied past participle forms in online processing of passive sentences, which contained a past participle with either a monomorphemically legal cluster (kissed; see (4)(a)) or a monomorphemically illegal cluster (bathed; see (4)(b)).

(4) (a) I think that the squirrel with the gloves was kissed by the tortoise at his house last weekend.
(b) I think that the squirrel with the gloves was bathed by the tortoise at his house last weekend.

We predicted that typically developing children would be able to use the phonotactic cues provided by an illegal cluster to identify the past participle, and therefore interpret the passive sentence more accurately than when this cue was not available; that is, in the forms with legal clusters. G-SLI children, however, were predicted not to be able to use this parsing cue, and therefore show no advantage for sentences where the past participle contained an illegal cluster. Using a self-passed listening task involving a sentence-picture judgment task, this is exactly what we found: typically developing children were significantly more accurate on their judgments for sentences containing the monomorphemically illegal past participle forms. In contrast, G-SLI children did not show a difference between legal and illegal forms, suggesting that the phonotactic cue to the words' morphological complexity did not facilitate their parsing of the sentence.

Our investigations into the phonotactics of clusters with respect to morphology is at the interface of morphology and phonology. We now turn to the phonology component itself and our findings from G-SLI children.

Phonology

Just as the deficit in G-SLI affects hierarchical structures in syntax and morphology, so it affects hierarchical structures in phonology. Phonological constituents such as syllables and prosodic words are grouped into successively higher levels of the prosodic hierarchy (Selkirk, 1978). Certain aspects of phonological structure cause difficulty for children with G-SLI. Children with G-SLI have clear and fluent speech, and are intelligible for known words. Their phonological deficit manifests as a difficulty with forms that are complex at the syllable and foot levels of the prosodic hierarchy (Gallon et al., 2007). In a nonword repetition task, G-SLI children simplify consonant clusters in all word positions, while unfooted syllables are deleted or cause syllabic simplifications and segmental changes elsewhere in the word (Marshall, 2004; Marshall, Ebbels, Harris, & van der Lely, 2002).

For example, in Gallon et al.'s study, fə. klɛs. tə. lə (where dots indicate syllable boundaries) was repeated by some children as, fə. kɛs. tə. lə with cluster simplification, and by others as fə. kɛs. tə. lə with erroneous voicing of the velar stop and deletion of the final unfooted syllable (Gallon et al., 2007). Furthermore, systematically increasing the complexity of phonological structure resulted in a systematic increase in errors, regardless of the number of syllables, indicating that it is not just the length of phonological material to be retained in phonological short-term memory that is relevant to repetition accuracy, but the arrangement of that material in the prosodic hierarchy. Even monosyllabic nonwords with two clusters (e.g. klɛst) were more difficult for G-SLI children than those with one cluster (e.g., klɛt) or no clusters (e.g., kɛt), and for disyllabic nonwords, a marked initial weak syllable caused weak-strong forms (e.g., bə.dremp) to be more difficult than strong-weak forms (e.g., drɛm.pə). This contrasts with previous studies of nonword repetition in children with SLI, which have not shown group differences between SLI and typically developing children when nonwords are only one or two syllables long.

However, it is how these deficits in phonology and other components of language impact on language processing and production that is of ultimate concern to both researcher and clinician.

The cumulative effect of component deficits

The CGC model hypothesizes that for children with G-SLI, the deficit is in representing linguistic structural complexity in three components of the computational grammatical system—syntax, morphology, and phonology. Deficits in these components impact on a variety of linguistic constructions as a function of their syntactic, morphological, and phonological complexity. The regular past tense deficit that is found not only in children with G-SLI, but also in the vast majority of children with SLI, has been explored most thoroughly. We have already discussed the impact of syntactic and morphological deficits on G-SLI children's realization of tense. Here we complete the picture by considering the effects of phonological complexity. Using an elicitation task we manipulated the phonological complexity of the inflected verb end, and found that, as predicted, phonological complexity impacted on suffixation. G-SLI children were less likely to inflect stems when the suffixed form would end in a consonant cluster, for example, jumped and hugged, compared to when no cluster would result, for example, weighed. Furthermore, stems ending in a cluster (jump) were less likely to be suffixed than stems ending in a single consonant (hug). In contrast, typically developing controls showed no effect of phonological complexity on inflection (Marshall & van der Lely, 2007b).

In another study, we found that morphological and phonological deficits impact even on an aspect of language that is not traditionally noted as being problematic for English-speaking children with SLI—derivational morphology (Marshall & van der Lely, 2007a). We elicited two types of derived forms—adjectives derived from nouns by the addition of -y (sand → sandy, rocks → rocky), and comparative and superlative adjectives (happy → happier, happiest). In the former case, the stimulus was either a singular or a regular plural noun, while in the latter the adjectival stem was either one or two syllables long. G-SLI children almost invariably supplied the -y, -er, and -est suffixes, in stark contrast to their high omission of the past tense suffix. Moreover, increasing the morphological or phonological complexity of the stimulus did not trigger suffix omission, but did result in nontarget forms that were uncharacteristic of typically developing children. Some G-SLI children included -s inside -y when presented with a plural stimulus, producing forms such as holesy, rocksy, and frillsy, whereas typically developing children very rarely did so (holey, rocky, frilly). In forming comparative and superlative adjectives, both G-SLI and typically developing children reduced three-syllable outputs (e.g., happier, narrowest) to two-syllable outputs, providing evidence of a maximal word effect on derivation; that is, pressure to limit the output to the size and shape of a trochaic (strong-weak) foot, a constraint that is characteristic of young English-speaking children. However, the groups responded differently—G-SLI children's favored strategy was to truncate the stem and retain the suffix (happer, narrest), whereas for typically developing children the favored strategy was to omit the suffix and retain the stem-final weak syllable (happy, narrow).

The cumulative impact of independent component deficits in the grammatical computational system is illustrated in Figure 20.2.

Do auditory deficits maintain G-SLI?

One possibility is that an auditory deficit causes and maintains the grammatical impairments found in G-SLI. Evidence of subtle auditory deficits would conflict with domain-specific hypotheses and,

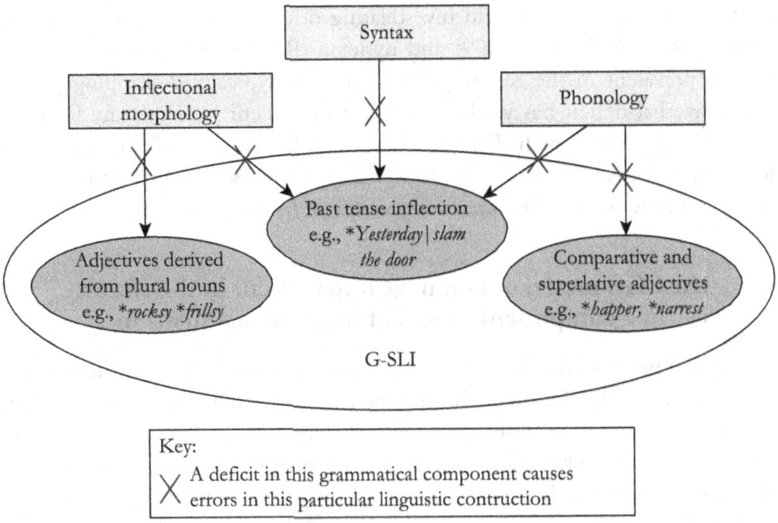

Figure 20.2 The computational grammatical complexity model of G-SLI: the impact of component deficits on different linguistic constructions.

instead, support domain-general perspectives. However, neither behavioral nor electrophysiological data have revealed any consistent auditory deficit in individuals with G-SLI that is independent of their language deficit. First, we explored G-SLI children's auditory perception for speech and nonspeech sounds, at varying presentation rates, and controlling for the effects of age and language on performance (van der Lely et al., 2004). For nonspeech formant transitions, 69% of the G-SLI children showed normal auditory processing, whereas for the same acoustic information in speech, only 31% did so. For rapidly presented tones, 46% of the G-SLI children performed normally. Auditory performance with speech and nonspeech sounds differentiated the G-SLI children from their age-matched controls, whereas speed of processing did not. A further set of experiments looked at "backward masking"; that is, their ability to detect a brief tone in quiet, and in the presence of a following noise (Rosen, Adlard, & van der Lely, 2009). Here group analyses showed that mean thresholds for the G-SLI group were never worse than those obtained for the two younger language control groups, but were higher in both backward and simultaneous masking compared to age-matched controls. However, more than half of the G-SLI group (8/14) were within normal limits for all thresholds. Furthermore, the G-SLI children consistently evinced no relationship between their auditory and phonological/grammatical abilities.

A further possibility is that a more sensitive measure might identify an impairment. To test this, we explored the neural correlates to auditory processing using event related potential techniques. ERPs can measure brain responses with a millisecond precision, and therefore have the time resolution to detect delayed or deviant brain responses. We recorded Auditory Evoked Potentials (AEPs) of G-SLI and age-matched control participants to pure tones in a classical auditory oddball paradigm. Auditory processing elicits early electrophysiological responses known as the N100/P200 (or N1/P2) complex. This complex is associated with perceptual detection of a discrete change in the auditory environment. In addition, they elicit a later P300 component that reflects attentional control processes to detect and categorize a specific event. We discovered that children with G-SLI have age-appropriate waveforms for the N100, P200, and the P300 components (latency, amplitude, distribution on the scalp; Fonteneau & van der Lely, 2008). Our results reveal that G-SLI children have normal auditory processing during the discrimination of pure tones.

These findings, along with those investigating nonverbal cognitive abilities thought to possibly co-occur with, but not cause SLI (or G-SLI; see van der Lely et al., 1998), are consistent with a number of other researchers in the field investigating other SLI subgroups (Bishop et al., 2000; Bishop, Carlyon, Deeks, & Bishop, 1999) and dyslexia (Ramus, 2003). Auditory and nonverbal deficits are more prevalent in the SLI population than in typically developing populations, but no consistent nonverbal deficit has yet been found to co-occur or cause any form of SLI. This, of course, does not mean that such deficits, when they do co-occur, do not have an impact on language development: it is likely that they do to some extent. We set out in the discussion of our model just why and how we see different components of language affecting performance.

The CGC model of language impairment in the context of a component model of language acquisition

Our discussion above provides details of the nature of component deficits within the CGC model, and specifically the nature of the hierarchical deficits within each grammatical component. This model has led to clear predictions with respect to precisely those structures in syntax, morphology, and phonology that will be impaired. In addition, the model has enabled us to predict how component deficits would individually impact on processing of linguistic forms, such as wh-questions, and tense marking. The model provides a parsimonious explanation for the pattern of impairments in G-SLI: cumulative effects of component deficits, alongside compensation by components that potentially function normally. Although the CGC model was originally developed to account for G-SLI, the component nature of this model and the detail within the grammatical components enables it to be applied to other forms of SLI, in both English and other languages, and indeed to typical language acquisition. For example, the model predicts that an auditory speech deficit will impact on phonology (specifically at the segmental level) due to mapping relations between the two, and thereby impact on language. It will not, however, directly cause the basic mechanisms and representations of phonology to be impaired. The CGC differs from domain-general perspectives in this respect, and this is, of course, an empirical issue. However, the specification of the CGC goes some way to helping understand how different components can affect language processing and performance. There is still much to understand about the role of mapping relations between components in normal and impaired acquisition, but we hope that this model will contribute to clarifying these relations.

Conclusion

This chapter has focused on the G-SLI subgroup. It has shown the existence of a relatively pure grammatical impairment that affects syntax, morphology, and phonology, but spares other cognitive abilities. More specifically, the deficit affects particular aspects of the grammatical system: complex hierarchical structure. This deficit in the CGC system manifests itself as an impairment in the computation of syntactic dependencies at the level of clause structure, complex morphological words, involving abstract rules, and complex phonological forms involving, for example, clusters and unfooted syllables. All these aspects of language are those learned through development and vary in interesting ways from language to language. Our data challenge views denying that some forms of language impairment are caused by underlying deficits to highly specialized domain-specific mechanisms that normally develop in the young child to facilitate language learning. The fact that other subgroups of SLI show deficits that have similar characteristics in syntax, morphology, and phonology, regardless of any co-occurring problems (Norbury et al., 2002), points to multiple genetic causes impacting on these components, with some genetic causes being more discrete than others.

Finally, the CGC model explains how processing in many different components of language—some within and some outside the grammatical system—in addition to factors pertinent to language such as phonological memory, contributes to language performance. In other words, processing is a reflection of "multiple processing systems." Our model clarifies how each component impacts on language performance in highly predictable ways. Thus, language performance will depend on both the linguistic characteristics of the material with respect to its complexity in each component, and the basic functioning of each component itself. We have shown how G-SLI children appear to use their strengths in certain components to compensate, at least partially, for deficits in others. Thus, for G-SLI children and perhaps other SLI subgroups too, a relative strength in semantic processing could be targeted to help compensate for their syntactic impairment.

In conclusion, our data from the G-SLI subgroup show how some components in grammar can be selectively impaired, supporting a domain-specific view of at least some cognitive systems. These findings provide a valuable window onto the functional architecture of the brain and the development of uniquely human and specialized higher cognitive systems.

Acknowledgments

We thank the children, parents, schools, and speech and language therapists who have contributed so much to the work reported here. The work was supported by the Wellcome Trust Grant number 063713, the ESRC Grant number RES-000–23–0575, and a Leverhulme Trust Visiting Fellowship to H. van der Lely. Particular thanks are due to the insightful comments and discussion from participants of the Biocomp Workshop on "Specific language impairment and the language faculty" at Harvard University, February 20, 2008, where many of the above issues were discussed.

Further reading

Delage, H., & Frauenfelder, U. H. (2020). Relationship between working memory and complex syntax in children with Developmental Language Disorder. *Journal of Child Language, 47*(3), 600–632.

Jaber-Awida, A. (2018). Experiment in non word repetition by monolingual Arabic preschoolers. *Athens Journal of Philology, 5*(4), 317–334.

Montgomery, J. W., Gillam, R. B., & Evans, J. L. (2016). Syntactic versus memory accounts of the sentence comprehension deficits of specific language impairment: Looking back, looking ahead. *Journal of Speech, Language, and Hearing Research, 59*(6), 1491–1504.

Rombough, K., & Thornton, R. (2019). Subject–aux inversion in children with SLI. *Journal of Psycholinguistic Research, 48*(4), 921–946.

Schaeffer, J. (2018). Linguistic and cognitive abilities in children with specific language impairment as compared to children with high-functioning autism. *Language Acquisition, 25*(1), 5–23.

References

Archonti, A. (2003). *Wh-Question formation in typically developing children and children with Grammatical SLI. Human communication science*. London, UK: UCL.

Bishop, D.V. M. (1982). Comprehension of spoken, written and signed sentences in childhood language disorders. *Journal of Child Psychology and Psychiatry, 23*(1), 1–20.

Bishop, D. V. M. (1997). *Uncommon understanding: Comprehension in specific language impairment*. Hove, UK: Psychology Press.

Bishop, D. V. M., & Bishop, S. J. (1998). "Twin language": A risk factor for language impairment? *Journal of Speech, Language, and Hearing Research, 41*(1), 150–160.

Bishop, D.V. M., & Norbury, C. F. (2002). Exploring the borderlands of autistic disorder and specific language impairment: A study using standardised diagnostic instruments. *Journal of Child Psychology and Psychiatry, 43*(7), 917–929.

Bishop, D.V. M., & Snowling, M. J. (2004). Developmental dyslexia and specific language impairment: Same or different? *Psychological Bulletin, 130*(6), 858–886.

Bishop, D.V. M., Adams, C.V., & Norbury, C. F. (2006). Distinct genetic influences on grammar and phonological short-term memory deficits: Evidence from 6-year-old twins. *Genes, Brain and Behavior, 5*(2), 158–169.

Bishop, D.V. M., Bright, P., James, C., Bishop, S. J., & van der Lely, H. K. J. (2000). Grammatical SLI: A distinct subtype of developmental language disorder? *Applied Psycholinguistics, 21*(2), 159–181.

Bishop, D.V. M., Carlyon, R. P., Deeks, J. M., & Bishop, S. J. (1999). Auditory temporal processing impairment: Neither necessary nor sufficient for causing language impairment in children. *Journal of Speech, Language, and Hearing Research, 42*(6), 1295–1310.

Chomsky, N. (1998). *Minimalist inquiries: The framework Ms.* Cambridge, MA: MIT Press.

Chomsky, N. (2004). Beyond explanatory adequacy. In A. Belletti (Ed.), *Structures and beyond: The cartography of syntactic structures* (Vol. 3, pp. 104–131). Oxford, UK: Oxford University Press.

de Bree, E. (2007). *Dyslexia and phonology: A study of the phonological abilities of Dutch children at-risk of dyslexia.* The Netherlands: University of Utrecht. LOT.

Dromi, A., & Zadunaisky-Ehrlich. (2000). Tense and finiteness in the speech of children with specific language impairment acquiring Hebrew. *International Journal of Language & Communication Disorders, 35*(3), 319–35.

Fisher, S. E., & DeFries, J. C. (2002). Developmental dyslexia: Genetic dissection of a complex cognitive trait. *Nature Reviews. Neuroscience, 3*(10), 767–780.

Fisher, S. E., Lai, C. S., & Monaco, A. P. (2003). Deciphering the genetic basis of speech and language disorders. *Annual Review of Neuroscience, 8*, 8.

Fonteneau, E., & van der Lely, H. K. J. (2008). Electrical brain responses in language-impaired children reveal grammar-specific deficits. *PLOS ONE, 3*(3), e1832.

Friederici, A. D. (2002). Toward a neural basis of auditory sentence processing. *Trends in Cognitive Sciences, 6*(2), 78–84.

Friedmann, N., & Gvion, A. (2002). Modularity in developmental disorders: Evidence from SLI and peripheral dyslexias. *Behavioral and Brain Sciences, 25*(6), 756–757.

Friedmann, N., & Novogrodsky, R. (2004). The acquisition of relative clause comprehension in Hebrew: A study of SLI and normal development. *Journal of Child Language, 31*(3), 661–681.

Friedmann, N., & Novogrodsky, R. (2007). Is the movement deficit in syntactic SLI related to traces or to thematic role transfer? *Brain and Language, 101*(1), 50–63.

Gallon, N., Harris, J., & van der Lely, H. K. J. (2007). Non-word repetition: An investigation of phonological complexity in children with Grammatical SLI. *Clinical Linguistics and Phonetics, 21*(6), 435–455.

Gathercole, S. (2006). Nonword repetition and word learning: The nature of the relationship. *Applied Psycholinguistics, 27*(4), 513–543.

Gordon, P. (1985). Level-ordering in lexical development. *Cognition, 21*(2), 73–93.

Hauser, M. D. (2001). What''s so special about speech? In E. Dupoux (Ed.), *Language, brain and cognitive development: Essays in honor of Jacques Mehler* (pp. 417–433). Cambridge, MA: MIT Press.

Hauser, M. D., Chomsky, N., & Fitch, W. T. (2002). The faculty of language: What is it, who has it, and how did it evolve? *Science, 298*(5598), 1569–1579.

Jakubowicz, C., & Strik, N. (2008). Scope-marking strategies in the acquisition of long-distance wh-questions in French and Dutch. Language and speech: On phonological, lexical and syntactic components of language. *Development, 51*(1–2), 101–132.

Jakubowicz, C., Nash, L., & van der Velde, M. (1999). *Inflection and past tense morphology in French SLI.* Somerville: BUCLD. Cascadilla Press.

Joanisse, M. (2004). Specific language impairments in children: Phonology, semantics and the English past tense. *Current Directions in Psychological Science, 13*(4), 156–160.

Joanisse, M. (2007). Phonological deficits and developmental language impairments. In D. Mareschal, S. Sirois, & G. Westermann (Eds.), *Neuroconstructivism, Vol. 2: Perspectives and Prospects.* Oxford, UK: Oxford University Press.

Joanisse, M., & Seidenberg, M. (1998). Specific language impairment: A deficit in grammar or processing? *Trends in Cognitive Sciences, 2*(7), 240–247.

Leonard, L. (1998). *Children with specific language impairment.* Cambridge, MA: MIT Press.

Leonard, L. B., Dromi, E., Adam, G., & Zadunaisky-Ehrlich, S. (2000). Tense and finiteness in the speech of children with specific language impairment acquiring Hebrew. *International Journal of Language and Communication Disorders, 35*(3), 319–335.

Marcus, G. F. (2004). *The birth of the mind: How a tiny number of genes creates the complexities of human thought.* New York: Basic Books.

Marcus, G. F., Pinker, S., Ullman, M., Hollander, M., Rosen, T. J., & Xu, F. (1992). Overregularization in language acquisition. In *Monographs of the Society for Research in Child Development Series 228.* Chicago, IL: University of Chicago Press.

Marinis, T., & van der Lely, H. K. J. (2007). On-line processing of questions in children with G-SLI and typically developing children. *International Journal of Language and Communication Disorders, 42*(5), 557–582.

Marshall, C. R. (2004). *The morpho-phonological interface in specific language impairment* [PhD Thesis]. London: DLDCN Centre. University College.

Marshall, C. R., & van der Lely, H. K. J. (2006). A challenge to current models of past tense inflection: The impact of phonotactics. *Cognition, 100*(2), 302–320.
Marshall, C. R., & van der Lely, H. K. J. (2007a). Derivational morphology in children with grammatical-specific language impairment. *Clinical Linguistics and Phonetics, 21*(2), 71–91.
Marshall, C. R., & van der Lely, H. K. J. (2007b). The impact of phonological complexity on past tense inflection in children with Grammatical-SLI. *Advances in Speech-Language Pathology, 9*(3), 191–203.
Marshall, C. R., & van der Lely, H. K. (2009). Effects of word position and stress on onset cluster production: Evidence from typical development, SLI and dyslexia. *Language, 85*, 39–57.
Marshall, C. R., Ebbels, S., Harris, J., & van der Lely, H. (2002). Investigating the impact of prosodic complexity on the speech of children with Specific Language Impairment. In R. Vermeulen & A. Neeleman (Eds.), *UCL Working Papers in Linguistics* (Vol. 14, pp. 43–68).
Marshall, C. R., Harcourt-Brown, S., Ramus, F., & van der Lely, H. K. J. (2009). The link between prosody and language skills in children with SLI and/or dyslexia. *International Journal of Language and Communication Disorders, 44*(4), 466–488.
Messaoud-Galusi, S., & Marshall, C. R. (2010). Introduction to this special issue. Exploring the overlap between dyslexia and SLI: The role of phonology. *Scientific Studies of Reading, 14*(1), 1–7.
Montgomery, J. W. (2000). Verbal working memory and sentence comprehension in children with specific language impairment. *Journal of Speech, Language, and Hearing Research, 43*(2), 293–308.
Norbury, C. F., Bishop, D. V. M., & Briscoe, J. (2002). Does impaired grammatical comprehension provide evidence for an innate grammar module? *Applied Psycholinguistics, 23*(2), 247–268.
O'Hara, M., & Johnston, J. (1997). Syntactic bootstrapping in children with specific language impairment. *European Journal of Disorders of Communication, 2*(2), 189–205.
Pinker, S. (1999). *Words and rules: The ingredients of language*. London, UK: Weidenfeld & Nicolson.
Pinker, S., & Jackendoff, R. (2005). The faculty of language: What's special about it? *Cognition, 95*(2), 201–236.
Ramus, F. (2003). Developmental dyslexia: Specific phonological deficit or general sensorimotor dysfunction? *Current Opinion in Neurobiology, 13*(2), 212–218.
Ramus, F., & Szenkovits, G. (2008). What phonological deficit? *Quarterly Journal of Experimental Psychology, 61*(1), 129–141.
Rice, M. (2003). A Unified Model of specific and general language delay: Grammatical tense as a clinical marker of unexpected variation. In Y. Levy & J. Schaeffer (Eds.), *Language competence across populations: Toward a definition of Specific Language Impairment* (pp. 63–95). Mahwah, NJ: Lawrence Erlbaum.
Rice, M. (2004). Language growth of children with SLI and unaffected children: Timing mechanisms and linguistic distinctions. In A. Brugos, L. Micciulla, & C. Smith (Eds.), *Proceeding of the 28th Annual Boston University Conference on Language Development* (Vol. 1, pp. 28–49). Somerville, MA: Cascadilla Press.
Rice, M., Wexler, K., & Redmond, S. M. (1999). Grammaticality judgments of an extended optional infinitive grammar: Evidence from English-speaking children with specific language impairment. *Journal of Speech, Language, and Hearing Research, 42*(4), 943–961.
Rosen, S., Adlard, A., & van der Lely, H. K. J. (2009). Backward and simultaneous masking in children with grammatical specific language impairment: No simple link between auditory and language abilities. *Journal of Speech, Language, and Hearing Research, 52*(2), 396–411.
Selkirk, E. O. (1978). On prosodic structure and its relation to syntactic structure. In T. Fretheim (Ed.), *Nordic prosody* (Vol. 2, pp. 111–140). Trondheim, The Netherlands: TAPIR.
Snowling, M. (2000). *Dyslexia* (2nd ed.). Oxford, UK: Blackwell.
Stavrakaki, S. (2001). Comprehension of reversible relative clauses in specifically language impaired and normally developing Greek children. *Brain and Language*, 77(3), 419–431.
Stavrakaki, S., & van der Lely, H. (2010). Production and comprehension of pronouns by Greek children with specific language impairment. *British Journal of Developmental Psychology, 28*(1), 189–216.
Stromswold, K. (1998). Genetics of spoken language disorders. *Human Biology, 70*(2), 297–324.
Tallal, P. (2002). Experimental studies of language learning impairments: From research to remediation. In D. Bishop & L. Leonard (Eds.), *Speech and language impairments in children* (pp. 131–156). East Sussex, UK: Psychological Press.
Tallal, P., Miller, S. L., Bedi, G., Byma, G., Wang, X., Nagarajan, S. S., … & Merzenich, M. M. (1996). Language comprehension in language-learning impaired children improved with acoustically modified speech. *Science, 271*(5245), 81–83.
Thomas, M. S. C., Grant, J., Barham, Z., Gsödl, M., Laing, E., Lakusta, L., … & Karmiloff-Smith, A. (2001). Past tense formation in Williams syndrome. *Language and Cognitive Processes, 16*(2–3), 143–176.
Thornton, R. (1995). Referentiality and wh-movement in child English: Juvenile D-Linkuency. *Language Acquisition, 1–2*(4), 139–175.

Tomblin, J. B., Records, N. L., Buckwalter, P., Zhang, X., Smith, E., & O'Brien, M. (1997). Prevalence of specific language impairment in kindergarten children. *Journal of Speech, Language, and Hearing Research, 40*(6), 1245–1260.

van der Lely, H. K. J. (1994). Canonical linking rules: Forward versus reverse linking in normally developing and specifically language-impaired children. *Cognition, 51*(1), 29–72.

van der Lely, H. K. J. (1996). Specifically language impaired and normally developing children: Verbal passive vs. adjectival passive sentence interpretation. *Lingua, 98*(4), 243–272.

van der Lely, H. K. J. (2005). Domain-specific cognitive systems: Insight from grammatical-specific language impairment. *Trends in Cognitive Sciences, 9*(2), 53–59.

van der Lely, H. K. J., & Battell, J. (2003). Wh-movement in children with grammatical SLI: A test of RDDR Hypothesis. *Language, 79*, 153–181.

van der Lely, H. K. J., & Christian, V. (2000). Lexical word formation in children with grammatical SLI: A grammar-specific versus an input-processing deficit? *Cognition, 75*(1), 33–63.

van der Lely, H. K. J., Jones, M., & Marshall, C. R. [in press]. Who did buzz see someone? Grammaticality judgement of wh-questions in typically developing and children and children with Grammatical-SLI. *Lingua.*

van der Lely, H. K. J., Rosen, S., & Adlard, A. (2004). Grammatical language impairment and the specificity of cognitive domains: Relations between auditory and language abilities. *Cognition, 94*(2), 167–183.

van der Lely, H. K. J., Rosen, S., & McClelland, A. (1998). Evidence for a grammar-specific deficit in children. *Current Biology, 8*(23), 1253–1258.

van der Lely, H. K. J., & Stollwerk, L. (1997). Binding theory and grammatical specific language impairment in children. *Cognition, 62*(3), 245–290.

van der Lely, H. K. J., & Ullman, M. (1996). The computation and representation of past-tense morphology in normally developing and specifically language impaired children. In The 20th Annual Boston University Conference on Language Development, Vol. 2. Somerville, MA: Cascadilla Press.

van der Lely, H. K. J., & Ullman, M. (2001). Past tense morphology in specifically language impaired children and normally developing children. *Language and Cognitive Processes, 16*, 113–336.

Vernes, S. C., Newbury, D. F., Abrahams, B. S., Winchester, L., Nicod, J., & Groszer, M. (2008). A functional genetic link between distinct developmental language disorders. *New England Journal of Medcine, 359*(22), 2337–2345.

Watkins, K. E., Dronkers, N. F., & Vargha-Khadem, F. (2002). Behavioural analysis of an inherited speech and language disorder: Comparison with acquired aphasia. *Brain, 125*(Pt 3), 452–464.

21

THE DEVELOPING MENTAL LEXICON OF CHILDREN WITH SPECIFIC LANGUAGE IMPAIRMENT

Holly Storkel

Introduction

The mental lexicon refers to "the collection of words stored in the human mind" (Trask, 1997, p. 140) with each entry "detailing the properties of a single lexical item: its pronunciation, its meaning, its word class, its subcategorization behavior, any grammatical irregularities, and possibly other information" (Trask, 1997, p. 130). This chapter will focus on a subset of the properties of lexical items that are frequently incorporated in adult and child models of spoken language processing, namely phonological, lexical, and semantic representations (Dell, 1988; Gupta & MacWhinney, 1997; Levelt, 1989; Luce, Goldinger, Auer, & Vitevitch, 2000; Magnuson, Tanenhaus, Aslin, & Dahan, 2003; McClelland & Elman, 1986; Norris, 1994). The phonological representation includes information about individual sounds, with models varying in the specific information incorporated (e.g., phonetic features, context-specific allophones, phonemes). For simplicity of illustration, phoneme units will be used to illustrate the phonological representation in this chapter. Thus, the phonological representation of the word "cat" would consist of the individual phonemes /k/, /æ/, and /t/ (i.e., three separate units). The lexical representation includes information about the sound structure of the word as an integrated unit. Continuing the illustration, the lexical representation for "cat" would be /kæt/ (i.e., one unit). Lastly, the semantic representation consists of information about the meaning or referent of the word. Here, the semantic representation for "cat" would include, but not be limited to, information such as "four-legged furry pet that purrs."

For the developing mental lexicon, there are two processes of critical importance. The first process involves the actual creation of the mental lexicon. That is, children are not born knowing the words of their language. Instead, words must be learned through exposure to the language during everyday interactions. The second process involves accessing the words in the mental lexicon for language production or comprehension. This is the process that allows children to use the words that they know to communicate. It is critical to understand the potential relationship between these two processes to differentiate different underlying causes of the same behavior. For example, one commonly used paradigm to assess the status of the mental lexicon is to have children name pictures (e.g., Brownell, 2000; Williams, 1997). If a child fails to produce a name for the target picture (i.e., no response is provided), there are at least two possible explanations. The first possible explanation is that the child may not have learned the name for the picture, either because the

DOI: 10.4324/9781003204213-24

child has never encountered that item before (i.e., lack of exposure) or because the child has failed to create an appropriate phonological, lexical, and/or semantic representation for the word despite being exposed to the word (i.e., word learning deficit). The second potential explanation is that the child has created an appropriate phonological, lexical, and semantic representation for the word but is having difficulty accessing those representations to produce a correct response within the time constraints of the test format (i.e., retrieval deficit). It should be clear that these two potential underlying causes of the same observed behavior would lead to different diagnostic conclusions and different treatment approaches.

Models of the lexicon

One of the difficulties in disentangling learning and access in the developing lexicon is that there are few models that incorporate both processes (but see Magnuson et al., 2003). The tendency is for models of word learning to account for patterns observed in learning new words without accounting for patterns observed in production or recognition of known words (e.g., Gupta & MacWhinney, 1997). Likewise, many models of production or recognition of known words do not account for how those words were acquired (e.g., Dell, 1988; Levelt, 1989; Luce et al., 2000; McClelland & Elman, 1986; Norris, 1994). It is not the case that researchers are disinterested in creating models of the lexicon that learn new words and access known words, but rather that the complexities of both processes make an omnibus model somewhat intractable. Although a complete model or theory does not exist, important components can be garnered from existing models of each process.

One critical component in a model that integrates lexical learning and access is to provide some mechanism to trigger learning. That is, when listening to spoken language, the child must have some way of determining whether a word is novel, and thus new lexical and semantic representations need to be created (i.e., learning), or whether a word is known, and thus existing lexical and semantic representations should be accessed so that the word can be produced or recognized. Some types of models include just such a mechanism. Specifically, adaptive resonance theory, which has been used to model a variety of cognitive processes, involves activation of existing representations whenever novel or known information is encountered (e.g., Carpenter & Grossberg, 1987). However, when the information in the environment sufficiently mismatches the representations in memory, learning is triggered. This allows for the creation of new representations in memory as well as modification to existing representations. Thus, when listening to a word, existing representations will be activated. In the case of a novel word, existing lexical and semantic representations will not sufficiently match the novel word, thereby triggering learning. In the case of a known word, an existing lexical and semantic representation will sufficiently match the known word, thereby triggering production or recognition of the word.

Assuming that word learning is triggered, how does it proceed? Here, models of word learning are useful in outlining the process (e.g., Gupta & MacWhinney, 1997). Figure 21.1 offers a schematic of the learning process when the novel word /goʊm/ is encountered. Phonological representations of the individual phonemes comprising the novel word will be activated and may aid in maintaining the sound sequence in working memory while a new lexical representation is created. Likewise, a new semantic representation will be created. Various forms of working memory will likely play a role in temporary storage of information while the semantic representation is being created but this will depend on the details of how the referent is presented (e.g., whether there is a visual referent or not). In addition to creating new lexical and semantic representations, a link must be created between the two new representations to support future production and recognition of the word. Finally, links must be created between the new representations and existing representations in the lexicon so that the new representations are integrated with the old. These new representations and links are accessed upon subsequent exposure to the novel word, allowing

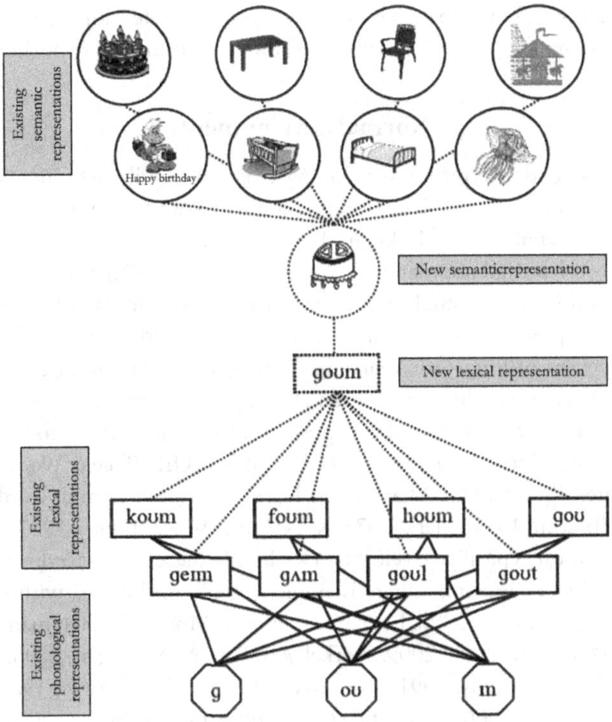

Figure 21.1 Illustration of the word learning process when the novel word /goʊm/ is encountered. Existing representations are depicted by solid lines and new representations are depicted with dashed lines. Pictures of known objects are taken from www.freeclipartnow.com (i.e., jellyfish) and www.clker.com (i.e., all pictures except jellyfish). The picture of the novel object is from Kroll and Potter (1984). Semantic neighbors of the novel object are based on the child data from Storkel and Adlof (2009a). Lexical neighbors of the novel words are based on the child calculator described by Storkel and Hoover (2010).

modification of the representations and links (in the case of incorrectly learned or missing information) as well as strengthening of the representations and links. Thus, word learning is a protracted process with the potential for incorrect or gradient representations prior to mastery (e.g., Capone & McGregor, 2005; Gershkoff-Stowe, 2002; Metsala & Walley, 1998).

Figure 21.1 Illustration of the word learning process when the novel word /goʊm/ is encountered. Existing representations are depicted by solid lines and new representations are depicted with dashed lines. Pictures of known objects are taken from www.freeclipartnow.com (i.e., jellyfish) and www.clker.com (i.e., all pictures except jellyfish). The picture of the novel object is from Kroll and Potter (1984). Semantic neighbors of the novel object are based on the child data from Storkel and Adlof (2009a). Lexical neighbors of the novel words are based on the child calculator described by Storkel and Hoover (2010).

For production or recognition, multiple existing representations are activated until one representation is selected. In the case of spoken word production, activation of semantic representations will be initiated first (e.g., Dell, 1988; Levelt, 1989). In the case of spoken word recognition, activation of form based units, namely phonological and lexical representations, will be initiated first (e.g., Luce et al., 2000; McClelland & Elman, 1986; Norris, 1994). Models differ in the amount of interaction between lexical and semantic activation. Some models hypothesize that activation of one type of representation must be completed before activation of the other is initiated (e.g., Levelt, 1989), whereas others assume that activation of one type of representation influences activation of the other (e.g., Dell, 1988). This debate has not fully reached the developmental literature. Thus, the developmental literature does not necessarily favor one type of model over the other.

Normal development

Past research documents that typically developing children rapidly acquire a lexicon. Following just a single exposure, children are able to associate a novel word form with its referent (Dickinson, 1984; Dollaghan, 1985; Heibeck & Markman, 1987).

This ability has been termed fast mapping (Carey & Bartlett, 1978). It is not assumed that a child has mastered a word following a single exposure but rather has initiated the creation of an initial lexical and semantic representation, which is then refined over time and with repeated exposure to the word. This period of long-term learning is often referred to as extended mapping (Carey & Bartlett, 1978). Typically developing children also are able to create initial lexical and semantic representations of words with relatively few exposures in naturalistic discourse (e.g., television programs), sometimes referred to as quick incidental learning (QUIL; Rice & Woodsmall, 1988). These abilities allow children to rapidly build a lexicon, learning as many as nine words per day by some naturalistic counts (Bloom, 1973; Clark, 1973; K. Nelson, 1973; Templin, 1957).

Additional research on typically developing children has attempted to determine what factors account for this rapid word learning. There is ample research in this area with studies focusing on phonological (Bird & Chapman, 1998; Leonard, Schwartz, Morris, & Chapman, 1981; Schwartz & Leonard, 1982; Storkel, 2001, 2003, 2009; Storkel, Armbruster, & Hogan, 2006; Storkel & Rogers, 2000), prosodic (Cassidy & Kelly, 1991; Cutler & Carter, 1987; Morgan, 1986), lexical (Storkel, 2004a, 2009; Storkel et al., 2006), semantic (Gershkoff-Stowe & Smith, 2004; Grimshaw, 1981; Pinker, 1984; Samuelson & Smith, 1999; Smith, Jones, Landau, Gershkoff Stowe, & Samuelson, 2002; Storkel, 2009; Storkel & Adlof, 2009b), syntactic (Gleitman, 1990; Gleitman & Gleitman, 1992; Landau & Gleitman, 1985), and pragmatic cues (Baldwin, 1993; Baldwin et al., 1996; Sabbagh & Baldwin, 2001; Tomasello, Strosberg, & Akhtar, 1996). Below, some of the research on phonological, lexical, and semantic cues relevant to word learning is highlighted.

One phonological cue that has received recent attention is phonotactic probability. Phonotactic probability is the frequency of occurrence of individual sounds or pairs of sounds such that some legal sound sequences in a language can be identified as common (e.g., /kæt/—"cat") whereas others are classified as rare (e.g., /dag/—"dog"). Phonotactic probability appears to be learned early in development with sensitivity emerging around nine months of age (Jusczyk, Luce, & Charles-Luce, 1994). Phonotactic probability is positively correlated with a lexical cue, namely neighborhood density (Storkel, 2004c; Vitevitch, Luce, Pisoni, & Auer, 1999). Neighborhood density refers to the number of words in a language that are phonologically similar to a given word, such that some words reside in dense neighborhoods (e.g., /kæt/—"cat") with many phonologically similar neighbors (i.e., 27 neighbors for "cat"), whereas others reside in sparse neighborhoods (e.g., /dag/—"dog") with few phonologically similar neighbors (i.e., six neighbors for "dog"). The correlation between phonotactic probability and neighborhood density arises because words with common sound sequences tend to reside in dense neighborhoods (e.g., /kæt/—"cat") and words with rare sound sequences tend to reside in sparse neighborhoods (e.g., /dal/—"dog"). Note that this correlation is not perfect and that is it possible to identify words with common sound sequences residing in sparse neighborhoods (e.g., /dal/—"doll" with nine neighbors) and those with rare sound sequences residing in dense neighborhoods (e.g., /geim/—"game" with 18 neighbors).

Word learning studies of correlated phonotactic probability and neighborhood density show that typically developing preschool children learn common/dense novel words more accurately than rare/sparse novel words, when given limited exposure to the novel words (Storkel, 2001, 2003, 2004b; Storkel & Maekawa, 2005). Recently, the individual effects of phonotactic probability and neighborhood density have been disentangled. In experimental studies of adult and child word learning, both phonotactic probability and neighborhood density appear to influence word learning with each variable affecting a different step of the word learning process (Hoover, Storkel, & Hogan, 2010; Storkel et al., 2006). Specifically, phonotactic probability appears to play a role in triggering word learning, such that novel words with rare sound sequences are learned more accurately than novel words with common sound sequences. It was hypothesized that because rare sound sequences are more unique from other known sound sequences, they create larger mismatches, triggering creation of a new representation immediately. In contrast, common sound sequences are deceptively similar to many other known sound sequences, creating smaller mismatches. This potentially impedes the recognition of the word as novel and delays the triggering of word learning. Neighborhood density appeared to play a role in the integration of a new lexical representation with existing lexical representations. Here, novel words from dense neighborhoods were learned more accurately than novel words from sparse neighborhoods. It was hypothesized that forming links with many existing lexical representations served to strengthen the newly created lexical representation, improving retention of the new representation. Similar results were obtained in a corpus analysis of the words known by typically developing infants (Storkel, 2009).

Recent work has examined a semantic variable similar to neighborhood density, namely semantic set size (Storkel & Adlof, 2009a, 2009b). Semantic set size refers to the number of words that are meaningfully related to or frequently associated with a given word, as determined by discrete association norms (Nelson, McEvoy, & Schreiber, 1998). We collected discrete association data from preschool children and adults for novel objects so that the novel objects could be classified as similar to many other known objects, namely a large semantic set size, or similar to few other known objects, namely a small semantic set size (Storkel & Adlof, 2009a). An experimental word learning study showed that preschool children learned novel words with small and large semantic set sizes equivalently. However, children retained novel words with a small semantic set size better than novel words with a large semantic set size (Storkel & Adlof, 2009b). Note that this finding is counter to the findings for neighborhood density where similarity to many known items facilitated learning. In the case of semantic set size, it was hypothesized that forming links with many existing semantic representations leads to confusion between the newly created semantic representation and existing semantic representations. This likely degraded the newly created representation, impeding retention. Further research is needed to better understand this discrepancy between the influence of lexical versus semantic similarity on word learning; however, one initial hypothesis is that lexical and semantic neighborhoods differ in neighbor diversity and this may impact how these representations influence word learning. Specifically, lexical neighbors always share the majority of phonemes with the new word (i.e., by definition, a neighbor differs by only one sound), whereas semantic neighbors could share few features with the new word and differ by many features, leading to a less focused and cohesive neighborhood.

The studies reviewed to this point have focused primarily on the early stages of learning a word when learning is triggered or when a new representation was recently created or retained over a relatively short delay. There is evidence that these newly created representations may be graded (e.g., Capone & McGregor, 2005; Gershkoff-Stowe, 2002; Metsala & Walley, 1998), such that the representation is incomplete or lacks detail. This hypothesis is supported by empirical study. For example, Storkel (2002) showed that lexical representations of known words from dense neighborhoods were phonologically detailed, whereas lexical representations of known words from sparse neighborhoods were less detailed, particularly for sounds in word final position. Likewise, McGregor and colleagues (McGregor, Friedman, Reilly, & Newman, 2002) showed that semantic representations of known words could be rich and complete or meager and incomplete. Thus, even when a typically developing child knows a word, the underlying lexical and semantic representation may not be as complete and detailed as in the adult lexicon. This, in turn, has consequences for production and recognition. For example, Newman and German (2005) demonstrated that the impact of neighborhood density on spoken word production diminished with development, presumably because the difference in completeness of lexical representations diminishes with development. That is, completeness of lexical representations is hypothesized to vary by neighborhood density in children. In contrast, adults arguably have complete and detailed representations of words in dense as well as sparse neighborhoods. Turning to spoken word recognition, Garlock and colleagues (Garlock, Walley, & Metsala, 2001) showed minimal developmental changes in the recognition of dense words in a gating task but greater developmental changes in the recognition of sparse words. They attribute this developmental pattern to changes in the completeness of lexical representations of words in sparse neighborhoods.

Children with SLI

Children with Specific Language Impairment (SLI) are children who show significant deficits in language acquisition in the absence of any obvious cause (Leonard, 1998). In general, language deficits in children with SLI are noted across all domains of language, although some argue that the most severe deficits occur in morphosyntax (Rice & Wexler, 1996; Rice, Wexler, & Cleave, 1995; Rice, Wexler, & Hershberger, 1998). Prevalence rates for SLI are approximately 7% for kindergarten children (Tomblin et al., 1997). There are a variety of theories about the nature of SLI, with some focusing on limitations in linguistic knowledge and others focusing on general or domain-specific processing deficits (see Leonard, 1998 for review). In terms of the lexicon, children with SLI usually score lower than their age-matched typically developing peers on standardized tests of vocabulary, although their scores may still fall within the normal range (Gray, Plante, Vance, & Henrichsen, 1999). Experimental word learning studies generally show that children with SLI learn fewer words than their same aged typically developing peers, although there is variability across studies and there is evidence of individual differences within the SLI group (specific studies reviewed below). Research by Gray (2004; Kiernan & Gray, 1998) examining individual differences in word learning indicated that approximately 30–73% of children with SLI learned as many words as their typically developing peers. Thus, word learning by 27–70% of children with SLI fell outside the normal range. These estimates of the percentage of children with SLI who exhibit word learning difficulties should be viewed with caution because they are based on small samples of children with SLI. However, these individual differences should be kept in mind when reviewing the results of group studies (see below).

In terms of fast mapping, deficits in fast mapping have been documented in some studies (Dollaghan, 1987; Gray, 2004) but not others (Gray, 2003, 2004). Across studies, there is no evidence that children with SLI have difficulty associating the novel word with a novel object. When difficulties occur, they appear in later comprehending (Gray, 2004) or producing the novel word (Dollaghan, 1987). Deficits are observed more consistently during extended mapping (Gray, 2003, 2004; Kiernan & Gray, 1998; Oetting, Rice, & Swank, 1995; Rice, Buhr, & Nemeth, 1990), with some studies suggesting that children with SLI may need twice as many exposures to achieve the same comprehension and production accuracy as same aged typically developing children (Gray, 2003).

Where in the word learning process do these deficits occur in children with SLI? Triggering of word learning has received less attention in the literature on word learning by children with SLI. The results of at least some fast mapping studies would hint that triggering word learning may not be problematic for children with SLI (Gray, 2003, 2004). However, this conclusion can only be viewed as tentative, given the paucity of research in this area. In contrast, there is clear and consistent evidence that children with SLI have difficulty creating and retaining mental representations of novel words. Moreover, this difficulty appears to impact both lexical and semantic representations. For example, Alt and colleagues (Alt & Plante, 2006; Alt, Plante, & Creusere, 2004) exposed children to novel words paired with novel objects. After exposure, they examined lexical representations by having the children judge whether a sound sequence was the correct name of the novel object (i.e., the name paired with the object during exposure). Children with SLI recognized fewer names than their typically developing peers, suggesting deficits in the creation and/or retention of lexical representations. In addition, Alt and colleagues examined semantic representations by presenting the novel word and asking children whether its referent had certain semantic features. Children with SLI correctly identified fewer semantic features than their typically developing peers, indicating deficits in the creation and/or retention of semantic representations.

Work by Gray provides a similar conclusion, although suggests that these deficits may be true of only certain children with SLI. Gray (2004) identified children with SLI who performed significantly more poorly on the word learning task than the rest of the group. Approximately 35% of the children with SLI were classified as poor word learners. Gray then examined the word learning profiles of these children to identify potential areas of deficit. For each novel word that the child did not learn, lexical representations were viewed as the area of deficit if the child never learned to produce the novel word during training, whereas semantic representations were viewed as the area of deficit if the child drew a poor picture of referent of the novel word after training. For 79% of the unlearned words, lexical representations were implicated whereas semantic representations were implicated for the remaining 21%. Interestingly, both areas of deficit generally were observed for each child. Moreover, Gray (2005) has shown that providing phonological (e.g., initial sound, initial syllable, rhyming word) or semantic cues (e.g., superordinate category, physical characteristics, action or use) during training improves word learning by children with SLI. Presumably, provision of cues improves the child's ability to create a new lexical or new semantic representation, depending on the cue provided.

Even when children are successful in creating a new lexical or semantic representation, there is evidence that they have difficulty retaining these representations over time. Rice and colleagues (Rice, Oetting, Marquis, Bode, & Pae, 1994) examined the influence of amount of exposure on word learning by children with SLI. With three exposures to the novel words, the children with SLI performed more poorly than the typically developing children on an immediate posttest of comprehension. In contrast, with ten exposures to the novel words, children with SLI performed similarly to typically developing children in an immediate posttest of comprehension. Thus, immediate learning by the children with SLI was similar to the typically developing children when greater exposure was provided. However, when the posttest was re-administered one to three days after the ten exposures, group differences emerged with the children with SLI performing more poorly than the typically developing children, especially for verbs. This suggests that children with SLI had greater difficulty retaining new representations over time and implicates the integration of newly created representations with existing representations as a potential area of deficit in children with SLI.

These potential word learning deficits have consequences for spoken word production and recognition by children with SLI. Considering first production and semantic representations, McGregor and colleagues (McGregor, Newman, Reilly, & Capone, 2002) provide evidence that naming by children with SLI is affected by the quality of semantic representations. Children were asked to name pictures and their responses were categorized as correct, semantic error, indeterminate error (e.g., "I don't know"), or other error. Children then were asked to draw pictures and define the same items that they had been asked to name. Analyses compared the quality of drawings and definitions for correct versus semantic errors versus indeterminate errors as a means of examining the quality of the semantic representations of the words in each response category. Results showed that children with SLI named fewer pictures correctly than their typically developing peers. For both groups of children, drawings and definitions for correctly named items were richer and more accurate than those for incorrectly named items, with no differences noted between semantic versus indeterminate errors. McGregor and colleagues (2002) also examined the pattern of responses across tasks for each word and determined that approximately one-third of erred responses were attributable to retrieval failure during naming despite adequate semantic representations (i.e., rich drawing, rich definition, and correct comprehension). Approximately another one-third of erred responses were attributable to sparse semantic representations (i.e., poor drawing, or poor definition, or incorrect comprehension). The final one-third of erred responses was attributable to missing lexical or semantic representations (i.e., poor drawing, poor definition, and incorrect comprehension). Taken together, approximately one-third of naming errors were due to retrieval failures, whereas two-thirds of naming errors were attributable to word learning deficits.

Turning to word recognition and lexical representations, Maillart and colleagues (Maillart, Schelstraete, & Hupet, 2004) provide evidence that recognition by children with SLI is affected by the quality of lexical representations. Children completed a lexical decision task where they were asked to identify auditorially presented stimuli as real words or nonwords. Children with SLI were less accurate than typically developing children in this task. Moreover, children with SLI had much greater difficulty rejecting nonwords that differed only slightly (i.e., a phoneme change rather than a syllable change) from a real word. This pattern suggests that children with SLI may have had more holistic lexical representations of real words leading to confusion between slightly modified nonwords and real words.

Finally, research suggests that the quality of lexical and semantic representations has implications for learning to read and write, placing children with SLI at risk for future academic deficits (e.g., Catts, Adolf, Hogan, & Weismer, 2005; Catts, Fey, Tomblin, & Zhang, 2002; Walley, Metsala, & Garlock, 2003).

Summary and conclusions

The theoretical framework outlined at the onset of this chapter provides a means for investigating and understanding differences in the lexicons of children with SLI and their typically developing counterparts. In terms of the different types of representations in the lexicon, children with SLI exhibit deficits in both lexical and semantic representations. The status of phonological representations has received less attention. Most of the research in this area has focused on accessing phonological representations (e.g., Tallal, Stark, & Mellits, 1985), rather than examining the quality of phonological representations. Turning to the process of word learning, children with SLI appear to have deficits in creating, retaining, and/or integrating new representations in their lexicons. Additional research is needed in this area to more fully differentiate the deficits in each process (i.e., creating vs. retaining vs. integrating). Investigation of variables from studies of normal development (e.g., neighborhood density, semantic set size) may be useful in this endeavor. The process of triggering word learning has not been fully investigated, warranting future study. Considering production and recognition of known words, children with SLI show complex deficits in spoken word production and recognition. At least some of their difficulties in this area can be attributed to problems in accessing detailed representations, whereas others can be attributed to holistic or incomplete representations. This pattern highlights the interplay between word learning and production/recognition in the developing mental lexicon.

While much has been learned about the nature of the developing mental lexicon of children with SLI, clinical methods have not yet been fully informed by this knowledge. Specifically, most diagnostic tools take a global approach to assessment by examining the words that a child has already learned. The words a child has already learned, as revealed by this type of test, is a function of the child's exposure to words, the child's ability to learn words, and the child's ability to produce or recognize the words within the format and time constraints of the test. Thus, most diagnostic tools fail to differentiate environment, learning, and access in their examination of the lexicon. Consequently, if a child performs poorly on such a task, the underlying cause of that poor performance cannot be immediately identified. Moreover, a deficit could be missed because strengths in one (or more) of these areas (environment, learning, access) could mask weaknesses in the other areas. Given this situation, it is important to supplement standardized test scores with clinician developed probes that are informed by theory. Probes that examine the quality of representations (lexical vs. semantic), different stages of learning (triggering learning vs. creation of new representations vs. retention/integration of new representations), and differentiate these from access to representations would be the most informative for treatment planning (see Gray, 2004, 2005, for a potentially clinically adaptable example).

Acknowledgments

Preparation of this chapter was supported by NIH grant DC08095. S. M. Adlof, M. S. Bridges, T. P. Hogan, and J. R. Hoover provided valuable comments on an earlier version of this chapter.

Further reading

Han, M., Storkel, L. H., & Bontempo, D. (2019). The effect of neighborhood density on children's word learning in noise. *Journal of Child Language, 46*(1), 153–169.

Krueger, B. I., & Storkel, H. L. (2022). The impact of age on the treatment of late-acquired sounds in children with speech sound disorders. *Clinical Linguistics and Phonetics*, 1–19.

References

Alt, M., & Plante, E. (2006). Factors that influence lexical and semantic fast mapping of young children with specific language impairment. *Journal of Speech, Language, and Hearing Research, 49*(5), 941–954.

Alt, M., Plante, E., & Creusere, M. (2004). Semantic features in fast-mapping: Performance of preschoolers with specific language impairment versus preschoolers with normal language. *Journal of Speech, Language, and Hearing Research, 47*(2), 407–420.

Baldwin, D. A. (1993). Infants' ability to consult the speaker for clues to word reference. *Journal of Child Language, 20*(2), 395–418.

Baldwin, D. A., Markman, E. M., Bill, B., Desjardins, R. N., Irwin, J. M., & Tidball, G. (1996). Infants' reliance on a social criterion for establishing word-object relations. *Child Development, 67*(6), 3135–3153.

Bird, E. K. R., & Chapman, R. S. (1998). Partial representations and phonological selectivity in the comprehension of 13-to 16-month-olds. *First Language, 18*(52), 105–127.

Bloom, L. (1973). *One word at a time: The use of single word utterances before syntax*. The Hague, The Netherlands: Mouton.

Brownell, R. (2000). *Expressive one-word picture vocabulary test* (third edn.). Novato, CA: Academic Therapy Publications.

Capone, N. C., & McGregor, K. K. (2005). The effect of semantic representation on toddlers' word retrieval. *Journal of Speech, Language, and Hearing Research, 48*(6), 1468–1480.

Carey, S., & Bartlett, E. (1978). Acquiring a single new word. Papers and Reports on Child Language. *Development, 15*, 17–29.

Carpenter, G. A., & Grossberg, S. (1987). A massively parallel architecture for a self-organizing neural pattern recognition machine. *Computer, Vision, Graphics, and Image Processing, 37*(1), 54–115.

Cassidy, K. W., & Kelly, M. H. (1991). Phonological information in grammatical category assignments. *Journal of Memory and Language, 30*(3), 348–369.

Catts, H. W., Fey, M. E., Tomblin, J. B., & Zhang, X. (2002). A longitudinal investigation of reading outcomes in children with language impairments. *Journal of Speech, Language, and Hearing Research, 45*(6), 1142–1157.

Catts, H. W., Adolf, S. M., Hogan, T. P., & Weismer, S. (2005). Are specific language impairment and dyslexia distinct disorders? *Journal of Speech, Language, and Hearing Research, 48*(6), 1378–1396.

Clark, E. (1973). What's in a word? On the child's acquisition of semantics in his first language. In T. Moore (Ed.), *Cognitive development and the acquisition of language* (pp. 65–110). New York: Academic.

Cutler, A., & Carter, D. (1987). The predominance of strong initial syllables in the English vocabulary. *Computer Speech and Language, 2*(3–4), 133–142.

Dell, G. S. (1988). The retrieval of phonological forms [in press]: Tests of predictions from a connectionist model. *Journal of Memory and Language, 27*(2), 124–142.

Dickinson, D. K. (1984). First impressions: Children's knowledge of words gained from a single exposure. *Applied Psycholinguistics, 5*(4), 359–373.

Dollaghan, C. A. (1985). Child meets word: "Fast mapping" in preschool children. *Journal of Speech and Hearing Research, 28*(3), 449–454.
Dollaghan, C. A. (1987). Fast mapping in normal and language-impaired children. *Journal of Speech and Hearing Disorders, 52*(3), 218–222.
Garlock, V. M., Walley, A. C., & Metsala, J. L. (2001). Age-of-acquisition, word frequency, and neighborhood density effects on spoken word recognition by children and adults. *Journal of Memory and Language, 45*(3), 468–492.
Gershkoff-Stowe, L. (2002). Object naming, vocabulary growth, and development of word retrieval abilities. *Journal of Memory and Language, 46*(4), 665–687.
Gershkoff-Stowe, L., & Smith, L. B. (2004). Shape and the first hundred nouns. *Child Development, 75*(4), 1098–1114.
Gleitman, L. (1990). The structural sources of verb meanings. *Language Acquisition, 1*(1), 3–55.
Gleitman, L., & Gleitman, J. (1992). A picture is worth a thousand words, but that's the problem: The role of syntax in vocabulary acquisition. *Current Directions in Psychological Science, 1*, 1–5.
Gray, S. (2003). Word-learning by preschoolers with impairment: What predicts success? *Journal of Speech, Language, and Hearing Research, 46*(1), 56–67.
Gray, S. (2004). Word learning by preschoolers with specific language impairment: Predictors and poor learners. *Journal of Speech, Language, and Hearing Research, 47*(5), 1117–1132.
Gray, S. (2005). Word learning by preschoolers with specific language impairment effect of phonological or semantic cues. *Journal of Speech, Language, and Hearing Research, 48*(6), 1452–1467.
Gray, S., Plante, E., Vance, R., & Henrichsen, M. (1999). The diagnostic accuracy of four vocabulary tests administered to preschool-age children. *Language, Speech, and Hearing Services in Schools, 30*(2), 196–206.
Grimshaw, J. (1981). Form, function, and the language acquisition device. In C. Baker & J. McCarthy (Eds.), *The logical problem of language acquisition* (pp. 183–210). Cambridge, MA: MIT Press.
Gupta, P., & MacWhinney, B. (1997). Vocabulary acquisition and verbal short-term memory: Computational and neural bases. *Brain and Language, 59*(2), 267–333.
Heibeck, T. H., & Markman, E. M. (1987). Word learning in children: An examination of fast mapping. *Child Development, 58*(4), 1021–1034.
Hoover, J. R., Storkel, H. L., & Hogan, T. P. (2010). A cross-sectional comparison of the effects of phonotactic probability and neighborhood density on word learning by preschool children. *Journal of Memory and Language, 63*(1), 100–116.
Jusczyk, P. W., Luce, P. A., & Charles-Luce, J. (1994). Infants' sensitivity to phonotactic patterns in the native language. *Journal of Memory and Language, 33*(5), 630–645.
Kiernan, B., & Gray, S. (1998). Word learning in a supported-learning context by preschool children with specific language impairment. *Journal of Speech, Language, and Hearing Research, 41*(1), 161–171.
Kroll, J. F., & Potter, M. C. (1984). Recognizing words, pictures, and concepts: A comparison of lexical, object, and reality decisions. *Journal of Verbal Learning and Verbal Behavior, 23*(1), 39–66.
Landau, B., & Gleitman, L. (1985). *Language and experience: Evidence from the blind child.* Cambridge, MA: Harvard University Press.
Leonard, L. B. (1998). *Children with specific language impairment.* Cambridge, MA: The MIT Press.
Leonard, L. B., Schwartz, R. G., Morris, B., & Chapman, K. L. (1981). Factors influencing early lexical acquisition: Lexical orientation and phonological composition. *Child Development, 52*(3), 882–887.
Levelt, W. J. M. (1989). *Speaking: From intention to articulation.* Cambridge, MA: MIT Press.
Luce, P. A., Goldinger, S. D., Auer, E. T., & Vitevitch, M. S. (2000). Phonetic priming, neighborhood activation, and PARSYN. *Perception and Psychophysics, 62*(3), 615–625.
Magnuson, J. S., Tanenhaus, M. K., Aslin, R. N., & Dahan, D. (2003). The time course of spoken word learning and recognition: Studies with artificial lexicons. *Journal of Experimental Psychology: General, 132*(2), 202–227.
Maillart, C., Schelstraete, M., & Hupet, M. (2004). Phonological representations in children with SLI: A study of French. *Journal of Speech, Language, and Hearing Research, 47*(1), 187–198.
McClelland, J., & Elman, J. (1986). The TRACE model of speech perception. *Cognitive Psychology, 18*(1), 1–86.
McGregor, K. K., Friedman, R., Reilly, R., & Newman, R. (2002). Semantic representation and naming in young children. *Journal of Speech, Language, and Hearing Research, 45*(2), 332–346.
McGregor, K. K., Newman, R. M., Reilly, R. M., & Capone, N. C. (2002). Semantic representation and naming in children with specific language impairment. *Journal of Speech, Language, and Hearing Research, 45*(5), 998–1014.
Metsala, J. L., & Walley, A. C. (1998). Spoken vocabulary growth and the segmental restructuring of lexical representations: Precursors to phonemic awareness and early reading ability. In J. L. Metsala & L. C. Ehri (Eds.), *Word recognition in beginning literacy* (pp. 89–120). Mahwah, NJ: Lawrence Erlbaum Associates, Inc.
Morgan, J. (1986). *From simple input to complex grammar.* Cambridge, MA: MIT Press.

Nelson, D. L., McEvoy, C., & Schreiber, T. (1998). The University of South Florida word association, rhyme, and word fragment norms. Retrieved from http://www.usf.edu/FreeAssociation/

Nelson, K. (1973). Concept, word and sentence: Interrelations in acquisition and development. *Psychological Review, 81*(4), 267–295.

Newman, R. S., & German, D. J. (2005). Life span effects on lexical factors in oral naming. *Language and Speech, 48*(2), 123–156.

Norris, D. (1994). Shortlist: A connectionist model of continuous speech recognition. *Cognition, 52*(3), 189–234.

Oetting, J. B., Rice, M. L., & Swank, L. K. (1995). Quick incidental learning (QUIL) of words by school-age children with and without SLI. *Journal of Speech and Hearing Research, 38*(2), 434–445.

Pinker, S. (1984). *Language learnability and language development*. Cambridge, MA: Harvard University Press.

Rice, M. L., Buhr, J. C., & Nemeth, M. (1990). Fast mapping word-learning abilities of language-delayed preschoolers. *Journal of Speech and Hearing Disorders, 55*(1), 33–42.

Rice, M. L., Oetting, J. B., Marquis, J., Bode, J., & Pae, S. (1994). Frequency of input effects on word comprehension of children with specific language impairment. *Journal of Speech and Hearing Research, 37*(1), 106–122.

Rice, M. L., & Wexler, K. (1996). Toward tense as a clinical marker of specific language impairment in English-speaking children. *Journal of Speech and Hearing Research, 39*(6), 1239–1257.

Rice, M. L., Wexler, K., & Cleave, P. L. (1995). Specific language impairment as a period of extended optional infinitive. *Journal of Speech and Hearing Research, 38*(4), 850–863.

Rice, M. L., Wexler, K., & Hershberger, S. (1998). Tense over time: The longitudinal course of tense acquisition in children with specific language impairment. *Journal of Speech, Language, and Hearing Research, 41*(6), 1412–1431.

Rice, M. L., & Woodsmall, L. (1988). Lessons from television: Children's word learning when viewing. *Child Development, 59*(2), 420–429.

Sabbagh, M. A., & Baldwin, D. A. (2001). Learning words from knowlegeable versus ignorant speakers: Links between preschoolers' theory of mind and semantic development. *Child Development, 72*(4), 1054–1070.

Samuelson, L. K., & Smith, L. B. (1999). Early noun vocabularies: Do ontology, category structure and syntax correspond? *Cognition, 73*(1), 1–33.

Schwartz, R. G., & Leonard, L. B. (1982). Do children pick and choose? An examination of phonological selection and avoidance in early lexical acquisition. *Journal of Child Language, 9*(2), 319–336.

Smith, L. B., Jones, S. S., Landau, B., Gershkoff Stowe, L., & Samuelson, L. (2002). Object name learning provides on-the-job training for attention. *Psychological Science, 13*(1), 13–19.

Storkel, H. L. (2001). Learning new words: Phonotactic probability in language development. *Journal of Speech, Language, and Hearing Research, 44*(6), 1321–1337.

Storkel, H. L. (2002). Restructuring of similarity neighbourhoods in the developing mental lexicon. *Journal of Child Language, 29*(2), 251–274.

Storkel, H. L. (2003). Learning new words II: Phonotactic probability in verb learning. *Journal of Speech, Language, and Hearing Research, 46*(6), 1312–1323.

Storkel, H. L. (2004a). Do children acquire dense neighbourhoods? An investigation of similarity neighbourhoods in lexical acquisition. *Journal of Applied Psycholinguistics, 25*(2), 201–221.

Storkel, H. L. (2004b). The emerging lexicon of children with phonological delays: Phonotactic constraints and probability in acquisition. *Journal of Speech, Language, and Hearing Research, 47*(5), 1194–1212.

Storkel, H. L. (2004c). Methods for minimizing the confounding effects of word length in the analysis of phonotactic probability and neighborhood density. *Journal of Speech, Language, and Hearing Research, 47*(6), 1454–1468.

Storkel, H. L. (2009). Developmental differences in the effects of phonological, lexical, and semantic variables on word learning by infants. *Journal of Child Language, 36*(2), 291–321.

Storkel, H. L., & Adlof, S. M. (2009a). Adult and child semantic neighbors of the Kroll and Potter (1984) nonobjects. *Journal of Speech, Language, and Hearing Research, 52*(2), 289–305.

Storkel, H. L., & Adlof, S. M. (2009b). The effect of semantic set size on word learning by preschool children. *Journal of Speech, Language, and Hearing Research, 52*(2), 306–320.

Storkel, H. L., & Hoover, J. R. (2010). An on-line calculator to compute phonotactic probability and neighborhood density based on child corpora of spoken American English. *Behavior Research Methods, 42*(2), 497–506.

Storkel, H. L., & Maekawa, J. (2005). A comparison of homonym and novel word learning: The role of phonotactic probability and word frequency. *Journal of Child Language, 32*(4), 827–853.

Storkel, H. L., & Rogers, M. A. (2000). The effect of probabilistic phonotactics on lexical acquisition. *Clinical Linguistics and Phonetics, 14*(6), 407–425.

Storkel, H. L., Armbruster, J., & Hogan, T. P. (2006). Differentiating phonotactic probability and neighborhood density in adult word learning. *Journal of Speech, Language, and Hearing Research, 49*(6), 1175–1192.

Tallal, P., Stark, R. E., & Mellits, E. D. (1985). Identification of language-impaired children on the basis of rapid perception and production skills. *Brain and Language, 25*(2), 314–322.
Templin, M. C. (1957). *Certain language skills in children, their development and interrelationships (Institute of Child Welfare, Monograph Series 26).* Minneapolis, MN: University of Minnesota Press.
Tomasello, M., Strosberg, R., & Akhtar, N. (1996). Eighteen-month-old children learn words in non-ostensive contexts. *Journal of Child Language, 23*(1), 157–176.
Tomblin, J. B., Records, N. L., Buckwalter, P., Zhang, X., Smith, E., & O'Brien, M. (1997). Prevalence of specific language impairment in kindergarten children. *Journal of Speech, Language, and Hearing Research, 40*(6), 1245–1260.
Trask, R. L. (1997). *A student's dictionary of language and linguistics.* London, UK: Arnold.
Vitevitch, M. S., Luce, P. A., Pisoni, D. B., & Auer, E. T. (1999). Phonotactics, neighborhood activation, and lexical access for spoken words. *Brain and Language, 68*(1–2), 306–311.
Walley, A. C., Metsala, J. L., & Garlock, V. M. (2003). Spoken vocabulary growth: Its role in the development of phoneme awareness and early reading ability. *Reading and Writing, 16*(1/2), 5–20.
Williams, K. T. (1997). *Expressive vocabulary test.* Circle Pines, MN: American Guidance Services.

22

SCREENING AND INTERVENTIONS FOR DEVELOPMENTAL FLUENCY DISORDERS

Peter Howell, Clarissa Sorger, Roa'a Alsulaiman, and Zhixing Yang

Introduction

Howell's (2010) chapter on fluency disorders in the previous edition of this handbook looked at the pros and cons of different accounts of stuttering including the Covert Repair Hypothesis (CRH) and the Vicious Cycle account. Both these theories propose that errors in generating language forms are detected by the perception system and speakers correct the utterance. Such accounts link speech production and perception (often called feedback theories), the speech symptoms of stuttering and of fluency failures more generally, reflect breakdown in production planning and repair processes when errors occur. For instance, the CRH maintains that in an utterance such as "I, I spilt," the sentence starts (the first "I") an incorrect word was selected, this was detected internally leading to a pause in speech, the error was repaired covertly (the incorrect verb was not produced) and the sentence restarted and the utterance was then produced fluently. Fluency failures like "I, I" (a whole-word repetition) occur frequently in the speech of people who stutter (PWS) and CRH maintains that this is because PWS make many word selection errors that require repair. A number of problems that feedback theories face were discussed in Howell (2010) and it was argued that a non-feedback perspective was required to account for known features of stuttering and other childhood fluency issues.

To this end, Howell (2010) outlined the EXPLAN theory, which shares some features with feedback theories but which differs, importantly, concerning whether symptoms of fluency breakdown signify underlying (internal) word selection errors that are detected and repaired covertly. According to EXPLAN, "I, I spilt" and "I sspilt" (prolongation of the initial /s/) reflect two distinct types of fluency breakdown in response to the same problem (insufficient time to plan the word "spilt"). One version of EXPLAN applies across languages and first distinguishes words that are short, have limited complexity at onsets, and are comprised of phones that are simple (indicated by early acquisition in the speaker's language) from those words with the converse properties (Howell & Rusbridge, 2011). The two-word classes correspond approximately to content and function words for languages such as English (for simplicity, we use content and function words when reviewing evidence from English and languages that distinguish content and function words). Stutters and fluency failures on content words (such as "sspilt") are reflections of insufficient time being available for generating the complete plan of "spilt" (not a word selection error) and prolonging the /s/ gains time for completing the plan for this word. Another way of gaining time to complete the plan is to hesitate or repeat simple words prior to the content word (as in the func-

DOI: 10.4324/9781003204213-25

tion word repetition "I, I") called here stalling. Stalling avoids up-coming planning-time problems by speech prior to the problem by repeating motor forms of function words that have already been produced.

Evidence for differences between stalls and stutters like prolongations that result from advancing through speech rapidly and the different roles they may play in fluency development has accrued since Howell (2010) and this is presented after EXPLAN is outlined. EXPLAN maintains that fluency problems in early childhood mostly correspond to stalling type patterns and stuttering that persists to later ages involves advancing symptoms that affect onsets of words. Moreover, the early-developmental pattern is a form of fluency problem also commonly seen in children who do not stutter. In this chapter, we discuss alternative forms of fluency failure (e.g., word-finding) that show this specific pattern and raise the practical issues of how to separate this from stuttering in early life (screening in schools). Our work in schools in the UK (screening for word-finding and stuttering) is reviewed. Issues faced in UK schools arise because of the large number of children who start school not speaking English who often experience word-finding problems when required to use this language which is a further reason why procedures are needed for separating these two forms of fluency failure. Our work on equitable assessment of fluency for heterogeneous language groups is reviewed. Also, application of our assessment approach that focuses on children who speak Arabic and English is described. Finally, some experimental interventions for word-finding difficulty (WFD) that have been applied to English and Arabic cohorts are reviewed.

EXPLAN

The speech of PWS contains relatively fluent episodes of speech interspersed with dysfluencies. According to Johnson and associates (1959), the main dysfluencies in stuttered speech are: (1) Interjections (silent or filled pauses); (2) Word repetitions; (3) Phrase repetitions; (4) Part-word repetitions; (5) Prolongations; (6) Broken words; (7) Incomplete phrases (abandonments); and (8) Revisions. Only the first six events are consistent with the ICD-10 definition of stuttering (World Health Organization, 1992) which maintains that speakers know what they wish to say but are unable to do so. None of these six categories includes an overt speech error. This is one reason why EXPLAN does not assume fluency problems are a result of speech errors. Event types (7) and (8) are usually disregarded in fluency assessments.

The first six event-types tend to be associated with particular linguistic structures for English and related languages. Pauses occur, according to different theorists, around the onsets of either grammatical or prosodic units. Word and phrase repetitions occur (again depending on theoretical position) around onsets of prosodic words or at points prior to a presumed word error. Part-word repetitions, prolongations, and broken words occur on content words rather than being linked to the start of syntactic or prosodic units (Howell, 2007).

All these events occur in fluent speakers' speech, although their incidence is low and their distribution differs relative to speakers who stutter (in particular, fluent speakers have a low proportion of event-types (4)–(6), Howell, 2007). The overlap in event-types seen in fluent and stuttered speech makes diagnosis of the disorder difficult. Both fluent children (Clark & Clark, 1977) and children who stutter show a high proportion of word and phrase repetitions, which adds to the problem of differential diagnosis. The incidence of stuttering when Johnson's symptoms (1)–(6) are included is at its peak at ages at which language development is maximal. Thus, modal onset ages of three and five years were reported by Andrews and Harris (1964) and onset around these ages has been confirmed in a number of other studies. Andrews and Harris also reported that the incidence of the disorder up to 15 years was about 5% and recovery rate was about 80%. Recovery rate declines with age (Andrews and Harris's study reported no new cases occurred in their study after age 12). The incidence of different dysfluency events changes over ages as the proportion of event-types (4)–(6) is higher in older, compared to younger, speakers who stutter (Howell, Davis, & Williams, 2008). A satisfactory theory of stuttering should address all these points.

Feedback monitoring of speech for fluency control would only be needed if errors occur frequently whilst speech is generated. However, types (1)–(6) do not contain errors. This is not to deny that occasional errors occur during speech generation (Dell, 1986), some of which could be detected by a feedback monitor like that proposed in CRH. However, the ideas that language is continuously monitored for errors in real time and that speech progresses fluently until one is detected (Levelt, 1989) present many problems (Howell, 2010). If language-monitoring is dismissed as a means of online speech control, the perceptual mechanism need not necessarily be linked to production to achieve speech control. The fundamental distinguishing characteristic of EXPLAN is that it does not require feedback-monitoring for ongoing speech control.

We assume that language planning (PLAN) and speech-motor programming and execution (EX) are independent processes (Levelt, 1989). The term EXPLAN signifies that both processes are implicated in fluent speech control. PLAN generates a symbolic language representation that takes different amounts of time to generate, depending on the complexity of the segments (e.g., whether dealing with difficult content words or easy function words) it contains, and EX implements each representation motorically and realizes it as vocal output.

The independence assumption allows planning for future words to continue whilst a speaker utters the current word. Fluency problems arise when the plan for material is not ready in time. This arises in two ways: (1) If the speaker utters the prior material fast this advances when the problem material is needed; (2) If the problem material is particularly difficult to generate, its plan may not be ready irrespective of the rate on the lead-in sequence. Fluency problems happen more often when both influences apply in a stretch of speech.

Phonological word (PW) units, as originally defined by Selkirk (1984) for English, are a unit within which the interacting processes can be examined. PW consist of an obligatory content word (C) and an arbitrary number of function words preceding and following the content word (F_nCF_m where n and m are positive integers). From the current perspective, the important features of PW for English are: (1) that each PW has a single locus of difficulty (a content word); (2) the difficult word can be preceded by function words which are executed quickly, hence the content word is approached rapidly.

The speaker can deal with the situation where the linguistic plan is not ready in time either by stalling or advancing, each of which leads to characteristic forms of dysfluency associated with them. Stalling delays the move to output the difficult word by pausing prior to the content word or repeating the motor plans for the simple function word or words (the F_n) that have been output previously (leading to whole-word, or phrase, repetitions). In stallings, the speaker deals with the situation where the content word plan is not ready by increasing the time taken up before its execution starts. Advancing arises when speakers start the difficult word with the part of its plan already available. This can result in part-word repetitions, prolongations, and word breaks if the plan runs out. According to EXPLAN, PW incorporate adjustments to motor rate (initial function words) and planning difficulty (on the content word). From this perspective, a PW is a unit that has elements that span between PLAN and EX processes.

Evidence for EXPLAN

Difficulty

In this and the following sub-section, work on the relationship between difficulty (language factor) and speech rate (motor factor) in stuttering in spontaneous utterances is reviewed to determine whether they operate as predicted by EXPLAN. Howell's research group has used phonological and phonetic measures to quantify different levels of difficulty within function and content word classes.

Content words usually contain material that is difficult (phonetically and phonologically). One way of showing the difficulty of content words is by comparison of their phonetic properties with function words. Figure 22.1 shows the incidence of manner, word length, and contiguous consonants, and that these vary across the age range from six years to adulthood as language develops (shown separately for content and function words). Figure 22.1a shows significant increases over ages in use of each factor for content words whilst Figure 22.1b shows no such increase for function words. Figure 22.1a shows that content words that are acquired later are more complex than those acquired earlier.

When words are phonetically difficult, stuttering rate increases for content words. This is shown in Figure 22.2 where phonetic difficulty is represented as the sum total over eight features marked as easy/difficult by Jakielski (1998) in her Index of Phonetic Difficulty (IPC) scheme. An example for one feature is that words containing a contiguous string of consonants score a point, but words with just singletons score zero. There is a significant correlation for content, but not function words.

Figure 22.2 also shows that function words have a more limited range of phonetic difficulty. The lack of correlation with the difficulty measure for the function words underlines the importance of examining word types separately. Similar findings have been reported for the Arabic language; content words are phonologically more complex than function words (Al-Tamimi et al., 2013). To summarize, planning difficulty, as indicated by this phonetic measure, correlates with stuttering rate.

Rate

Variation in speech rate has been examined to see whether it affects stuttering in the way EXPLAN predicts (more problems when speech rate is high). Generally speaking, if speech is slow, there is less

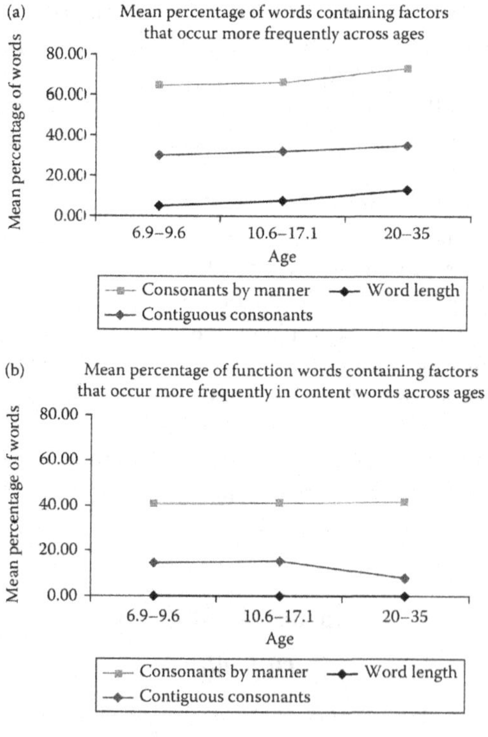

Figure 22.1 Mean percentage of content (section a) and function (section b) words containing difficult manners, long words, or contiguous consonants that occur more frequently in the speech of speakers who stutter aged 18+.

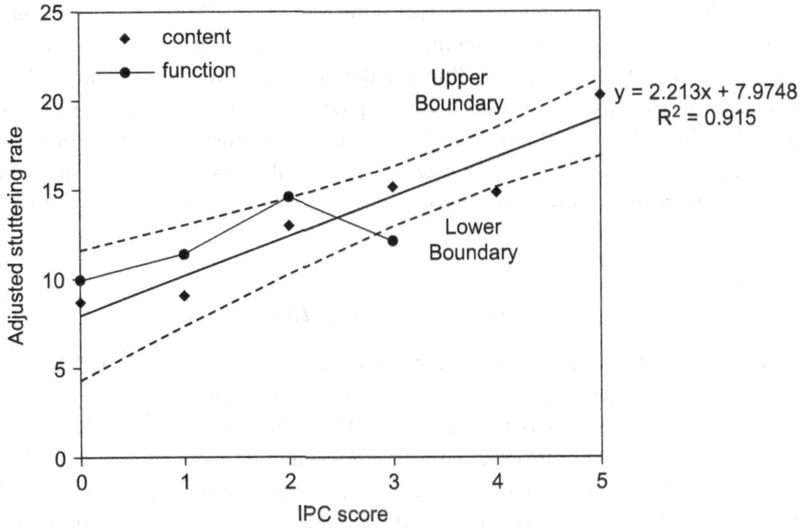

Figure 22.2 Adjusted stuttering rate (ordinate) versus number of times the four factors marked as difficult occurred (abscissa) for speakers aged over 18 years. The straight line is fitted to the content words and the upper and lower bounds around this line are indicated by the dashed line. The function word points are connected by a solid line.

likelihood of planning getting out of alignment with execution. When dysfluencies start to occur, rate adjustments are needed, but only around the points where difficulty is high (local). Global changes are necessary when speakers have to make a long-term adjustment to rate (as, for instance, when a speaker is continuously producing advancings).

Howell, Au-Yeung, and Pilgrim (1999) showed that rate control operates locally in utterances. Spontaneous speech of adults who stutter was segmented into tone units (TU) and these were separated into those that were stuttered and those that were fluent. Syllable rate was measured in the section prior to the stuttering (the whole segment in the case of fluent TU). The TU were classified into fast, medium, and slow rate categories based on the rate in the fluent section. The TU that were spoken slowly had a lower rate of stuttering than those spoken more rapidly. These findings support the idea that fluency problems arise when speech rate is high locally to the content word (possibly because approach rate taxes planning of difficult words).

Howell and Sackin (2000) examined whether local rate change can occur independently of global rate change for conditions known to affect the fluency of speakers who stutter. Fluent speakers repeated the sentence "Cathy took some cocoa to the teletubbies" several times under frequency shifted feedback (FSF), in normal listening conditions, and when speaking and singing. The plosives in the utterance were marked and the duration of the intervals between the first and each of the subsequent plosives was measured. The interval-distributions were plotted for every interval and for all speaking conditions. Global slowing between speaking conditions occurs when the mean of the distribution shifts to longer durations. Local slowing between conditions occurs when there are fewer intervals at the short duration end of the distribution, but no shift in the overall mean. One statistic that reflects shifts at the lower end of the distribution is the duration at which the 25th percentile occurs (towards the lower end of the distribution).

The differences between the means of the distributions were significant for all pairs of speaking conditions (showing global slowing) except speaking versus singing in normal listening conditions. Howell and Sackin then calculated the time where the 25th percentile fell, and repeated the earlier analyses, this time to see whether the fast intervals shifted between the different conditions. Of particular note was the finding that there was a significant shift of the 25th percentile when speaking was compared with singing in normal listening conditions (singing produced local slowing). Thus, local slowing occurred between these conditions, although there had been no global slowing. This suggests that these are two distinct modes of changing rate. EXPLAN specifically requires speakers to have the option of making local rate changes to deal with fluency problems. Singing is known to enhance the fluency of speakers who stutter and this would have to derive from the local rate changes that speakers make in this mode of vocal control. To summarize, difficulty and speech rate operate in the way EXPLAN predicts.

Dysfluency-distribution

The proposal that whole word repetition serves the role of delaying the time at which the following word is produced has been made by several authors working on fluent speech (Blackmer & Mitton, 1991; Clark & Clark, 1977; Maclay & Osgood, 1959; MacWhinney & Osser, 1977; Rispoli, 2003). However, these accounts have not linked such delaying to function words nor examined how word repetition depends on the position they occupy in PW contexts. For word repetition to stall speech, only the function words before the content word should be involved, as reported in a number of studies on stuttering (Au-Yeung, Vallejo, Gomez, & Howell, 2003, for Spanish; Dworzynski, Howell, Au-Yeung, & Rommel, 2004 and Dworzysnki & Howell, 2004, for German; and Howell, Au-Yeung, & Sackin, 1999, for English). Repetition specific to function words prior to content words has been reported for selected constructs for fluent English speakers (Stenström & Svartvik, 1994). The latter authors reported that subject pronouns (which appear before verbs in English, i.e., PW-initial) have a greater tendency to be produced dysfluently than object pronouns (which appear after verbs in English). Overall, word repetitions tend to appear in the position in PW that EXPLAN requires.

Stalling/advancing reciprocity

EXPLAN predicts a reciprocal relationship between stalling on function words and advancing on content words. If a speaker stalls, there should be no need to advance and vice versa. Early findings confirmed this relationship as stalling and advancing occurred rarely in the same PW (Howell, Au-Yeung, & Sackin, 1999).

It has been reported for a number of languages (Au-Yeung et al., 2003; Dworzynski et al., 2004; Howell et al., 1999), that speakers who stutter show more dysfluency on function words (stalling) than on content words (advancing) in early development, but the opposite in later development (termed an exchange relation). This suggests that older speakers stop stalling and start advancing. Howell, Au-Yeung, and Sackin (1999) noted that the exchange to advancing at older ages corresponded with a reduced chance of recovering from stuttering and suggested that the advancing pattern may be a factor implicated in this change.

There are several other ways of characterizing the points where simple and complex material alternate as well as shifts from function to content words which would apply to other languages. For example, Howell (2004) looked at stressed and unstressed words. He reported that stressed function words and unstressed content words produced an exchange relation. From this, it also appears that stressing a word (irrespective of lexical type) can result in the exchange first reported on content and function words. Some authors have argued that word frequency effects could account for the exchange pattern (exchanges would then be expected between low and high frequency items). This account seems problematic in connection with stuttering, since word frequency is particularly difficult to measure in childhood and varies markedly between speakers at these early stages of language development.

The EXPLAN account maintains that exchanges reflect a change from stalling to advancing with age. Consequently, Howell (2007) examined these dysfluency categories directly in a longitudinal study on children who stuttered aged from about eight years up to teenage. They were independently assessed at teenage to see whether they were still stuttering (persistent) or not (recovered). For recovered speakers, the absolute level of dysfluencies decreased as they get older, but the ratio of stallings to advancings remained constant. Speakers whose stuttering persisted, on the other hand, showed a reduced rate of stalling and an increased rate of advancing. This is consistent with the EXPLAN predictions, but not CRH. CRH would predict that the pattern of dysfluencies produced by children whose stuttering persists would always differ from children who recover or who have always been fluent because of speech planning time differences across the groups.

Priming

Priming is a way of manipulating planning time. An auditory sentence or syllable is presented (the prime). Participants then describe a picture (the probe), and speech initiation time (SIT) is measured. When the auditory prime matches some aspect of the probe, the planning time needed for the production of different elements in the phrase is reduced. Past work has shown that SIT is shorter for children who stutter than children who do not stutter for material which is primed phonologically and syntactically (Anderson & Conture, 2004; Melnick, Conture, & Ohde, 2003) but not lexically (Pellowski & Conture, 2005).

All previous priming investigations looked for effects at the language level whereas EXPLAN stresses the importance of PW units that reflect operation at the language-motor interface. Savage and Howell (2008) used PW like "He is swimming" and "She is running" (both consist of two function words followed by a content word) in a priming study that tested EXPLAN. On a trial, a child was primed either with a function word (e.g., they heard and repeated "he is") or a content word (e.g., they heard and repeated "swimming"). A cartoon (the probe) was then displayed depicting an action that had to be described, and SIT and dysfluency rate were measured. When the auditory prime matched an aspect of the probe (e.g., "he is" was primed and the picture was of a boy, or "swimming" was primed and this was the action), the planning time needed for the production of different elements in the phrase would be reduced.

EXPLAN predicts that priming either the function or the content word (the elements in PW) will have opposite effects (Savage & Howell, 2008). Priming a function word should reduce its planning time, allowing it to be produced more rapidly. When rate of production of a function word is increased, pressure is placed on having the content word plan ready earlier. If it is not ready, this increases the chance of stalling or advancing dysfluencies. Priming the content word reduces its planning time. But this time priming should reduce the dysfluency rate on function and content words (priming the content word accelerates planning and decreases the chances of plan-unavailability, which should be reflected in a reduction of stalling and/or advancing). In addition to the asymmetric effects of function and content word priming, EXPLAN predicts that there will be bigger effects in participants who stutter than in fluent controls though both speaker groups should show priming effects.

Savage and Howell (2008) confirmed these predictions in children who stuttered and controls (mean age six years). Priming function words increased dysfluencies on function and content words whereas priming content words reduced dysfluencies on function and content words. The additional prediction that these effects should be true of both groups of speakers was also confirmed and the effects for the children who stutter were greater.

The priming findings suggest that the same process underpins the production of dysfluencies for both children who stutter and controls, and that it takes the form of a timing misalignment between planning and execution. The primed production of a content word immediately before it is used in a picture description reduced the time needed to plan the content word online by activating its plan (so that it was available in advance). This reduced the discrepancy between the time needed to plan the content word (relatively long) and the time needed to execute the function words (relatively short), and in turn decreased the likelihood of speaking dysfluently.

Neuroimaging

Jiang et al.'s (2012) neuroimaging study reported that the activation pattern of one type of stalling (whole-word repetition) differs from that seen for other symptoms of stuttering. They classified types of disfluency into "clear" instances of stuttering (part-word repetitions, prolongations, and pauses), and instances of other dysfluency (phrase repetitions and revisions), and excluded whole-word repetitions. They established a model of brain areas that were active in "clear" instances of stuttering, compared to areas active in other types of dysfluent speech (excluding whole-word repetition). Distinctive brain areas were activated for the "clear" vs. other types of dysfluencies. Subsequently, whole-word repetitions were added into the model as "unknown examples," to see whether they would be associated with clear stuttering or other dysfluencies. Whole-word repetitions showed activation of similar brain regions to those seen in other dysfluent speech (not stuttering), and as mentioned, these patterns differed from brain regions activated when people produced more typical symptoms of stuttering. This provides evidence that whole-word repetition has a different role (EXPLAN would maintain stalling rather than advancing) to clear instances of stuttering.

Symptom-based screening for stuttering

We return now to some of the issues that, as mentioned at the start, should be addressed by an adequate theory of stuttering (screening and intervention in particular). Next, we look at clinical ways of screening for stuttering before we progress to examining how we can apply EXPLAN ideas for the related purpose of screening for fluency issues more generally in school samples which include more children and considerable diversity in language background (Howell et al., 2017).

Clinical assessment

A widely used standardized tool for the identification of stuttering is Riley's Stuttering Severity Instrument "SSI" (Riley, 1994; Riley & Bakker, 2009). Inter- and intra-judge reliability have been reported (Riley, 1994), and good validity is claimed (Davidow, 2021). The SSI is an objective assessment method that focusses on observable behaviour rather than self-reported information. The assessment is usually audio- or video-recorded. Picture materials are used to elicit spontaneous speech comprising a minimum of two hundred syllables (Todd et al., 2014). Three parameters are assessed: the percentage of stuttered syllables (i.e., the frequency of occasions of stuttering), the duration of instances of stuttered speech (by identifying and averaging the time duration of the three longest stuttering events), and physical concomitants, which include distracting sounds, facial grimaces, head movements, and movements of the extremities. An overall score is calculated based on the three parameters; scores correspond to severity of stuttering ranging from "very mild" to "very severe."

The SSI has also been extensively used in large, unselected samples of children, and generally is reported to be sensitive to identifying children who stutter (e.g., Davis et al., 2007; Mirawdeli, 2015) or to differentiate between persistent and recovered stuttering in children when used in combination with caregiver and child (self-)assessment reports (Howell et al., 2008). SSI is also an appropriate measure for use with children who have English as an additional language (Howell, 2013). Such children may be more prone to having word-finding difficulties (WFD) and hence produce a higher occurrence of whole-word repetitions in their speech. SSI does not include whole-word repetitions as events of stuttered speech; hence these children would not be classed as "stuttering."

Reliability

The usefulness and reliability of SSI notwithstanding, there are some criticisms and practical issues with the SSI and practical concerns when considering its use as an assessment tool for stuttering or fluency issues in children starting school. The way in which the SSI classifies stuttered speech has been criticized by some researchers. For example, it has been argued that stuttering events are highly variable and may differ from one day to the next (Constantino et al., 2016). In addition, the percentage of stuttered syllables may not always reflect the severity of an adult's stutter; reports of psychological processes regarding the experience of stuttering can also indicate stuttering severity, but may not always correlate with the percentage of stuttered syllables as measured in SSI (Manning & Beck, 2013). In contrast to these reservations about SSI, one study found that the percentage of stuttered syllables on its own is sufficient (i.e., without the additional SSI measures of duration of dysfluencies and physical concomitants) and more reliable when assessing risk of speech difficulties in children than is SSI (Mirawdeli & Howell, 2016). These exclusions would make SSI a shortened, more clinically viable tool for assessing children.

Most current measures of speech disorders classify a person as having a speech difficulty or not based on specific cut-off criteria. There is no dimensional questionnaire concerning fluency for children and/or adults which provides a general rather than a condition-specific indication of fluency. Furthermore, thresholding is not desirable for those who consider speech disorders as lying on a continuum (Johnson, 1955; Widiger & Samuel, 2005).

There are several additional established and validated questionnaires which focus on specific speech disorders. Examples for assessments of stuttering include the "Overall Assessment of the Speaker's Experience of Stuttering" (OASES) (Yaruss & Quesal, 2006), the "Wright & Ayre Stuttering Self-Rating Profile" (WASSP) (Wright & Ayre, 2000), and the "Communication Attitude Scale" with 24 items (CAS-24) (Andrews & Cutler, 1974).

Most of these reflect the World Health Organization's Classification of Functioning, Disability and Health framework (2007). A notable fact regarding existing instruments is that they were developed and established for English. Whilst translations into some other languages have been done (e.g., Persian SSI; Bakthiar et al., 2010), these may not be fully reliable or valid measures (Karimi et al., 2011). This highlights the lack of resources for use with speakers with diverse language backgrounds.

When screening children in a school environment, there is a need for short and efficient procedures which ideally do not require special training to carry out the assessment (data collection and analysis). Existing types of assessment are labor-intensive and, along with training, can make assessments time-consuming and prohibitive for use in schools. Finally, with the rising numbers of children who speak English as an additional language, there is a need for universally standardized measures of fluency that are easily administered in schools.

SSI does not count whole-word repetitions as stutters and EXPLAN maintains that this is appropriate for identifying stuttering that will persist. The pauses and whole-word repetition that EXPLAN considers as ways of stalling are also indicators of word-finding issues in children (Clark & Clark, 1977). Advancing symptoms can be used as an indication of stuttering that persists, and stalling as an indication of word-finding difficulty, provided no advancing symptoms are present at the same time. Before empirical work on screening is discussed, the link between positioning pauses and whole-word repetitions in PW is considered, as this is crucial for separating symptom types associated with word-finding and stuttering during screening.

Pauses

EXPLAN predicts that pauses should occur prior to the content word in a PW (the positions where they can delay onset of the following content word). To fill this role, pauses should appear around the start of PW more often than they occur at the start of syntactic units (as some other authors have maintained). Pinker (1995) used the examples "[The baby]$_{np}$ [ate [the slug]$_{np}$]$_{vp}$" and "[He]$_{np}$ [ate [the slug]$_{np}$]$_{vp}$" to show that pauses do not occur at syntactic boundaries. He stated that pausing is allowed after the subject NP "*the baby*," but not after the subject NP, in the pronominal "*he*." Note that both these positions involve the same major syntactic boundary, a subject NP, so syntactic factors alone cannot account for this difference in pause occurrence.

It is possible that pauses occur at PW boundaries as they do not always coincide with syntactic boundaries. The PW boundaries in the examples are "[The baby]$_{PW}$ [ate]$_{PW}$ [the slug]$_{PW}$" and "[He ate]$_{PW}$ [the slug]$_{PW}$" respectively. If the PW boundaries in the two sentences are examined, pausing between "*baby*" and "*ate*" is allowed in the first sentence (as Pinker observed), as they are in two separate PW. Pausing should not occur in the second sentence (again as Pinker observed) because there is no PW boundary at the corresponding point. Thus, it seems that PW are preferred units for specifying boundaries where pauses occur. Gee and Grosjean (1983) offer a related analysis to the current one using units related to PW. It has also been proposed that pause-location is determined by both syntactic and prosodic factors (Ferreira, 1993; Watson & Gibson, 2004).

To summarize, based on the link between onset of PWs and pausing, pauses are things that speakers do in anticipation, or as a result of material that is time-consuming to prepare such as the content word in a PW (consistent with EXPLAN).

Whole-word repetitions (WWR)

Researchers such as Johnson (1955) consider WWR to be a symptom of stuttering; however, they might actually be a sign of WFD due to a language barrier when, for example, speaking English as an additional language, rather than a sign of a speech disorder. This highlights the need for tasks for assessing fluency that are applicable to speakers of many languages.

Several studies have suggested that assessments for stuttering might be more accurate when WWR are not considered symptoms of stuttering. A risk factor model for predicting whether stuttering in eight-year-old children would persist or recover by teenage was developed (Howell & Davis, 2011) and adapted to screen school-aged children for risk of stuttering (Howell, 2013). The model showed higher sensitivity and specificity once WWR were excluded in analyses; this is likely due to the fact that WWR are common in all children's speech before vocabulary is fully developed suggesting that WWR are not sensitive indicators of stuttering (Howell, 2013). Recently, a longitudinal study described a measure (stuttering-like disfluency index; SLD) using spontaneous speech samples for assessing the likelihood of persistence in stuttering in children (Walsh et al., 2020). Whilst specific occurrences of stuttered speech such as part-word repetitions or blocks, prolongations, and broken words were significantly more frequent in children whose stutter persisted compared to those who recovered, whole-word repetitions were not specifically associated with persistence (Walsh et al., 2020) as predicted by EXPLAN. This again highlights that assessments arguably should not focus on WWR as indicators of stuttering. The appropriate type of intervention should then be given before the problem exacerbates. Research has shown that interventions are most effective when given early in life (i.e., usually at school age in the case of stuttering; Bercow, 2008; Howell, 2010). Hence, any speech dysfluency should be identified at an early age (Yairi & Ambrose, 1992, 2004)

Practical consideration when screening unselected samples for WFD and stuttering

Failure to identify a disorder may lead to several challenges in terms of educational attainment as well as on a mental health level due to bullying or isolation from others (Antoniazzi et al., 2010). Existing measures of assessment of stuttering have several constraints: they are often labor-intensive, time-consuming, and require training for the person carrying out the assessment, therefore they are not practically appropriate for use in schools.

When analyzing dysfluency, researchers need to consider that incidence of types of dysfluencies differ between children who do and do not stutter. Also, statistical procedures need to be sensitive to non-normally distributed data (e.g., negative binominal distributions of the data) and have to tackle covariates such as gender imbalances (Tumanova et al., 2014).

Recently, the number of children speaking a language other than English as their native language, as well as the number of children who use English as an additional language (EAL; i.e., using English predominantly at school but not at home) in UK schools has increased significantly. Similar situations apply internationally. Many of the affected children will not speak the language spoken in their home country before starting school. For the UK, the percentage of use of additional languages other than English in schools has doubled since 1997, rose to 18.1% in 2013 (Strand et al., 2015), and by 2018, rose again to 21.2% (DfE, 2018).

Children with EAL often have word-finding difficulties (WFD), which are characterized as the difficulties when pronouncing a word whilst being able to identify the referent of that word (e.g., Julie et al., 1998). WFD is frequently associated with whole-word repetitions (WWR) (Clark & Clark, 1977; Westbury & Bub, 1997). This is a different pattern to that in stuttering. A child whose first language is not English might experience word retrieval in their non-native language and produce a high number of whole-word repetitions (WWR). It is important to distinguish WFD from stuttering as the former do not have speech fluency problems (Yan & Nicoladis, 2009) and the two forms require different interventions. Appropriate intervention can be very efficient even after a short period; for example, phonological skills and fluency of EAL children at high risk of dysfluency improve following a two-week working memory intervention (Howell et al., 2020). Effective screening measures that can accurately assess stuttering and WFD in children with various linguistic backgrounds is essential, so that appropriate intervention can be facilitated.

When there is heterogeneity in first languages spoken, a universal test for fluency would be beneficial for use in schools. Most importantly, the needs of teachers and schools need to be taken into consideration, with testing needing to be quick, efficient, and easy to administer for someone not trained as a speech and language pathologist (SLP), so that effective testing and intervention for children can take place (Dockrell, 2001; Dockrell & Lindsay, 2001; Dockrell & Marshall, 2015). To this end, several authors advocate using an alternative assessment (in contrast to symptom-based assessment) such as a non-word repetition task like UNWR (Howell et al., 2017). UNWR is discussed in detail in the following section of this chapter. Such tests may distinguish between stuttering and WFD in children including in samples with diverse language backgrounds.

Non-word repetition (NWR) based methods in English

NWR provides information about potential issues with phonological processing. If a person has difficulties accurately repeating non-words, this can indicate a speech fluency impairment such as stuttering (Howell et al., 2017). However, the performance of a person who has WFD is not expected to be affected in UNWT or other NWR tasks. UNWR is recommended as a screening procedure for children with fluency problems since typical children who use any of the native languages covered would not have NWR problems whereas children who stutter would have problems.

Non-word repetition test (NWR) performance in children who stutter (CWS)

Non-word repetition tests other than UNWR could partially overcome shortcomings of traditional screening methods such as the SSI since NWR procedures are more concise than SSI; children are instructed to repeat non-words immediately after hearing them (e.g., Piazzalunga et al., 2019). Hence, there is no requirement for assessing several components as with SSI, since NWR performance is only based on the accuracy or reaction time (Hakim & Ratner, 2004) of pronunciation of non-words.

The time-efficiency is beneficial for use in schools. On a theoretical basis, it has been suggested that NWR enables schools to assess children's phonological abilities as it imitates the mechanism by which children learn languages, which is the instant repetition of novel sound forms (Archibald, 2008). Studies have also found that repeating the novel non-words involves several underlying processes, including speech perception (Coady & Evans, 2008), motor articulation, phonological processing (Bowey, 1996), and short-term phonological memory (Masoura & Gathercole, 1999). Therefore, children with fluency difficulties are predicted to have NWR deficits due to impaired phonological processing (Gathercole et al., 1994). Several studies have reported deficits in NWR in children who stutter (CWS) compared to control groups of the same age (Anderson & Wagovich, 2010; Bakhtiar et al., 2007; Hakim & Ratner, 2004; Howell et al., 2017). This supports the idea that the NWR test is a sensitive measure for distinguishing CWS and fluent speakers.

NWR languages other than English

NWR tests have been developed and applied with children who stutter (CWS) for several single languages other than English. For example, Bakhtiar et al. (2007) examined NWR performance amongst Persian children. However, their results contradicted previous findings: they found that although CWS performed slightly poorer than children who did not stutter in the NWR test, no significant differences in NWR performance between groups were found. It is not clear whether this was due to the NWR test for Persian having faults or a genuine difference between Persian CWS and those who speak English. The conflicting findings might be due to the stimulus materials and, hence, present low complexity to both groups of children and hence yield no differences. NWR tests have been developed for adoption with other targeted languages, such as Spanish (Summers et al., 2010), Greek (Windsor et al., 2010), and Italian (Schindler, 1962). One study reported the reliability and validity of the Italian version of the NWR test developed by Schindler (1962) for Italian-native children (Piazzalunga et al., 2019). However, since a language-specific NWR test was used it would only be appropriate for children with a monolingual language background. Hence, it might be less sensitive when used for screening children with diverse language backgrounds such as those in the UK with EAL. In support of this, Greek-native children performed more accurately on the Greek version of the NWR test than an English NWR test (Masoura & Gathercole, 1999). Related findings have been reported by Windsor et al. (2010); they noted that Spanish children showed better performance on the Spanish NWR test than peers who spoke English only. However, when the English NWR test was applied, the results reversed. Therefore, the NWR test is not sufficient to satisfy schools' needs where a more sensitive language test that applies to children with diverse language backgrounds is needed.

In sum, previous findings suggest that the NWR test resolves some of the issues encountered by the SSI. However, the practical application of the NWR test among children with diverse language backgrounds is an ongoing challenge. Whilst NWR tests could effectively identify CWS in the forms discussed so far, they are not sensitive when classifying CWS with diverse language backgrounds.

"Universal" non-word repetition test (UNWR)

To address the shortcomings of SSI and traditional monolingual NWR tests, a new form of NWR test ("Universal" *Non-word* repetition (UNWR) test) was developed (Howell et al., 2017). The design of the UNWR test matched schools' demands for a screening test to detect fluency difficulties. It takes into account the phonotactics (i.e., which segments and sounds can be combined in a language) of 20+ languages, hence making it quasi-"universal," and offering a fair screening for many children with EAL.

The UNWR's development included assessing word-likeness between non-word stimuli and words for 20 languages; high word-likeness occurs when non-words have phonotactic constraints that are similar to words in a targeted language, and this could affect NWR performance (Munson et al., 2005). For this reason, word-likeness of non-word stimuli were checked by native speakers of the 20 targeted languages. In addition, the lexicons were also checked computationally for five targeted languages examined in the study. Also, extraneous factors that can bias the UNWR test's performance, such as IQ and lexical knowledge, were controlled for. Archibald (2008) reported that compared to traditional language assessments, which rely heavily on the existing knowledge of languages, assessing children's phonological abilities using non-words can moderate such influences. Conti-Ramsden et al. (2001) also noted no significant correlation between NWR deficit and Intelligent Quotient performance.

UNWR has served as a basis for creating an Arabic-English NWR test to help identify speech dysfluency in speakers of Arabic and English (Alsulaiman et al., 2022), which is described in more detail in the following section of this chapter. All the above highlight the scientific rigor that informed the design of the UNWR, and its reliability.

Practically, the UNWR test also matches schools' needs for a language test that relates to fluency. Schools desire for a brief language test to ensure students' learning time will be little affected. Thus, the stimuli used in the UNWR test were small in number, which only consisted of seven non-words per syllable length (with syllable length ranging from two to five). In addition, to ensure teachers can deliver the test efficiently without the help of professionals, the procedures should be easy to understand, and the equipment used to conduct the test should be minimal. Together these design factors enable the UNWR test to effectively discriminate children with word-finding difficulty, CWS, and those who do not stutter, irrespective of children's language backgrounds, thus facilitating future assessments of people with a range of language backgrounds in clinics or schools (Howell et al., 2017).

As administered at present, the UNWR requires an experimenter who is phonetically trained to score a person's responses on the task as correct or incorrect in real time. Live assessments may not always be accurate, and may be less time-efficient and accurate compared to an automated analysis. Automated scoring processes would provide useful information more quickly and efficiently. Since speech production and speech perception are tightly linked (Casserly & Pisoni, 2010) an automated speech recognition system would need to be highly sensitive to variations in speech production. Despite various previous studies using live-scoring as part of their methodology, none has mentioned the difficulties this might pose, and there is a lack of studies on the assessment of live scoring procedures and what factors might influence live judgments of the person scoring the task. While previous phonetic training will most probably play a role in being able to correctly identify the response of a participant on the UNWR, it is unclear what other underlying factors might contribute to deciding whether a non-word is scored as pronounced correctly or incorrectly. A deeper understanding of manual live scoring techniques is required so that a clearer profile of children's speech, language, and cognitive profiles can be attained, allowing speech and language therapists to target detailed issues, which might have been missed during live scoring, with suited interventions.

Application of screening approach to Arabic

Few instruments are appropriate for assessing speech fluency of speakers of Arabic. As noted, direct translations of English instruments into Arabic without re-standardization is not appropriate (Karimi et al., 2011). Moreover, for existing instruments to be adapted for use in clinics and in research in other languages, they first need to be translated into the target language and the translation needs to be checked. The newly formed instrument then needs to be validated and standard scores re-estimated (Karimi et al., 2011). Generally speaking, re-standardization for target languages is not undertaken when instruments are employed in other languages. For this reason and because Arabic is very different to, for example, the languages UNWR addresses, the above steps need taking for Arabic (i.e., develop tests from scratch).

To this end, an attempt to systematically develop a speech-based fluency measure to account for many unique phonological, morphological, and syntactic features of Arabic has been initiated by

Alsulaiman (2022). It was noted that there were no indications about what to count as disfluency in Arabic, which, if such disfluencies differ from those in English, would require re-standardization of instruments as with Arabic forms of SSI. In other words, there was no scheme for analysis of stuttered speech in Arabic that shows which types of disfluencies should be counted. Therefore, Alsulaiman used the Arabic index of phonetic complexity as a basis (AIPC), which was adapted from the IPC which applies to English (Al-Tamimi et al., 2013). The AIPC was developed to account for the unique phonological, phonotactic, and morphological features of Arabic. It took into consideration the complexity in articulating certain consonant phonemes that are identified as difficult sounds due to either late age mastery or complex articulatory movements that they involve. The idea was to use AIPC to inform parts of speech analysis for the purpose of developing a new disfluency scheme. AIPC was devised as a framework that provides detailed assessment of which Arabic words are phonologically complex. This was achieved by attributing difficulty of words to the phonetic factors that a word may possess, which might make it more susceptible to stuttering. The AIPC then gives an aggregated complexity score based on summing up the number of phonological factors within each word. Additionally, an important feature of AIPC is that it accounts for geminated consonants through a new category "consonants by length." It is worth noting here that gemination has been defined as "the prolongation of the continuants and a longer closure of Stops" (Al-Ani, 1970).

The rationale behind adopting the AIPC was to minimize arbitrary decision making when assessing spontaneous speech samples. An empirical investigation was then carried out to determine (1) what should be counted when measuring stuttering; and (2) what and how disfluency symptoms should be quantified. As a first step, two preliminary algorithms were proposed based on our investigation of syllabic, phonological, and morphological features of the Arabic language. This gave the basis for the development of a formal scheme, which is intended to provide a framework for the characterization of syllabic and phonological structure of words in spontaneous samples. The empirical work involved analysis of conversational speech samples of at least 200 syllables; these were obtained from Arabic adult and child speakers who stutter. Speech samples were transcribed using Arabic orthography and moments of disfluency were marked on the transcripts. The stuttering symptoms used were part-word repetition, prolongation, or a break as in Riley's (1994) stuttering symptoms. The main goal of the analysis was to highlight areas where potential changes in counting the number of syllables and the number of disfluencies is needed to accommodate the requirements of the Arabic language.

With respect to phonological factors, the analysis also took some aspects of AIPC and incorporated those when designing the scheme. A commendable feature of AIPC is that it has a way of deriving a numerical value across all AIPC factors to characterize a word's difficulty. Consequently, two algorithms have been proposed: one for counting the number of syllables and one for counting disfluencies. These were presented with clear guidelines on how they should be applied. Overall, it was deemed advisable to analyze words of different lexical categories separately as these word types tend to have different phonological characteristics and involve different types of stuttering. However, more research on Arabic is needed on the role of different lexical categories to see how it affects stuttering on different parts of speech (e.g., adjectives and adverbs which have specific inflectional structures). To explain, Arabic has unique inflectional structures on different parts of speech that potentially makes the link between word type and stuttering more complex (Vahab et al., 2013). Adjectives and adverbs in Arabic use a system of agreement on number and gender with the noun or pronoun that they modify. That is, this creates lexical flexibility in combining words of different forms, which in turn could have an impact on stuttering rate (Vahab et al., 2013). Furthermore, whilst English has a classic subject-verb object structure, the word order in Arabic is mostly verb-subject- object, but other forms are also acceptable such as the subject-verb-object (Watson, 2007). In fact, in many dialects of Arabic word order usually depends on factors such as the dynamism of the verb. Arabic also accommodates almost all patterns and word-forming processes that are used in inflectional languages, as well as ones that are specific to isolated languages (Vahab et al., 2013). There is obviously a much greater flexibility with respect to the position of the subject in Arabic, which necessitates further investigations on the effect of specific morphological variables on stuttering. It would be of interest also to examine the role of inflections in the forms of suffixes and prefixes on stuttering rate in Arabic.

A non-word repetition task for Arabic and English speakers

UNWR does not apply to the Arabic language; because of its unique phonological structure that varies markedly from English. Alsulaiman et al. (2022) designed and developed a language specific Arabic and English non-word repetition task (AEN_NWR) that can equally assess children who speak either of the languages, or a mixture of both languages. The AEN_NWR is based on the same phonologically informed approach used with UNWR. The list of the stimuli in the AEN_NWR conform to accepted standards for NWR tasks including the following: language-specific phonotactic constraints of Arabic and English, avoiding later-developing consonants, and minimizing potential resemblance between real words and nonwords. The test also does not require knowledge of lexical semantics for either of the two languages.

To assess the AEN_NWR is a reliable measure of phonological skills and speech fluency, the relation between AEN_NWR scores, and the percentage of stuttered syllables (%SS) was examined. AEN_NWR scores were associated with a higher %SS indicating higher levels of stuttering. The strong correlation between AEN_NWE and the %SS was interpreted as an indication that the test has a high potential for identifying preschool children with speech disfluency. At present, no conclusion can be made until the current results are compared with results of a control group. This then would ensure that the AEN_NWR is a sensitive marker of fluency difficulty.

WFD interventions for English and Arabic

The question that may arise is when stuttering is identified and distinguished from WFD, is what can be done to improve word-finding and speech fluency. Children who show stuttering symptoms need to be referred to SLPs for full evaluation and intervention. Procedures for training working memory to enhance fluency could be delivered in schools and should not preclude intervention administered by SLPs whether or not a child has WFD or stutters. For example, Howell et al. (2020) addressed disfluency using WM training. Two-hundred-and-thirty-two reception class children from five primary schools were assessed by obtaining measures of their %SS and %WWR. Twelve were at high-risk of fluency difficulty and received WM training over two weeks. The results showed marked improvements; children's %SS dropped from pre-test to post-test and these improvements lasted for at least a week after the intervention.

WFD can also be addressed by giving them phonological or semantic training. It is unfortunate that despite the negative consequences of WFD, there is a scarcity of well-controlled intervention studies for preschool children. Moreover, the available studies are inconsistent in their methodologies, including participant numbers, intervention intensity and its duration. All of this make it challenging to compare these studies or draw general conclusions. Furthermore, the current WFD interventions are not sensitive to children's specific demands raised by our work (heterogeneous language background) due to the materials being language specific. The majority of research focuses on monolingual English speakers; and there is a need for interventions for children with different languages profiles (Ebbels, 2014). Current and novel treatment procedures for WFD must be rigorously designed to direct treatment practices for this population. For instance, Best et al. (2018) carried out a phase one randomized control trial (n=20) study to demonstrate the effect of a WFD intervention with children with WFD in schools. The study compared phonological and semantic interventions and children were assessed three times before and once after the intervention. The intervention was carried out over six weeks and employed a word-web protocol where children were encouraged to generate semantic or phonological features of words. The intervention was effective in improving retrieval of treated items. Children in the experimental group gained on average four times as many items as the control group. This was a small-scale rigorously designed study that employed a clinically realistic intervention in terms of intensity and duration. Another important aspect of the study was that it took place at a mainstream primary school where WFD is a common problem. It should also be noted that this study has not targeted children with EAL. Children were English speakers who either have been exposed to English at home from birth, or have been in an English speaking nursery at the age of three and continued to be exposed to English after that at home. Moreover, Best et al. (2018) pointed out a critical point concerning factors that may have affected the effectiveness. That is, the child background could have an influence on WFD which might affect their lexical retrieval, which in turn is likely to change over time. This reinforces the idea that WFD is a vocabulary problem (Howell et al., 2017) and that it should be treated separately from stuttering. It is important to emphasize that there are only a few studies on treating WFD, and the results of these studies differ with respect to the appropriateness of phonological vs. semantic training (Wright et al., 1993). This indicates that caution must be exercised before selecting the most suitable treatment. Further support on the equivocal results come from work by Bragard et al. (2012) who stated that the issue about the effectiveness for semantic vs. phonological intervention is open to debate. It is possible that both types of intervention are needed; or it could be that one type of treatment outperforms the other. In Wright et al.'s (1993) study, eight children received semantic training and seven children received phonological training as a WFD intervention. The phonological treatment group made significant improvement post intervention in naming untrained pictures, whilst the semantic group did not. This study focused only on phonological training to treat WFD. This allowed testing of whether phonological training is effective; and whether or not semantic training may also be needed.

The effectiveness of a language-specific phonological training intervention for improving WFD in Arabic children with EAL has been examined in work by Alsulaiman (2022). The training materials were NWR stimuli that are considered difficult because they include English-specific features that are absent from the Arabic language. Thus, the aim was to use the difficult non-words in a phonological training task using the priming effect, and then to determine whether this training transfers to real English words with similar sound structure as the non-word primes. Sixty-three reception class children were tested (31 males, 32 females, M_{age} 5;1). Of the total 63 children, 33 children were in the experimental groups; they were all Arabic speakers with EAL. The control group comprised 30 children who spoke English predominantly, although some had exposure to French through one of their parents. Children's language, literacy, and phonological performance (using the AEN_NWR) were assessed individually at pre-, post-, and follow-up assessments about two weeks post-intervention. The results showed that children in the experimental and control groups generally performed better post intervention: they showed higher accuracy in phonological performance, faster reaction times, and a decline in WFD (as indicated by WWR); and this was partly sustained at the follow-up session. The results also showed that there were no significant changes in %SS over the assessment phases for both groups. This suggests that %SS was not affected by the WFD training, and that the intervention did not improve articulation, but rather it works at the phonological and lexical levels. Thus, as indicated earlier, WFD and speech disfluency are two communication difficulties, and each requires a different type of intervention. The WFD procedure suggested here could be offered in schools. Overall, the intervention showed effects for Arabic children with EAL and for English children. Thus, the study provided a good approach to improving word-finding in preschool EAL children with other first languages, given that the right intervention materials are used, and the procedures could be easily and efficiently administered by teachers.

Conclusions and future work

We started with work that investigated how to characterize stuttering and its development over age by looking at the EXPLAN model and reviewing the evidence that supported it. An important detail that emerged in this evaluation was the different role played by WWR and agree/agreed stutters as supported by various empirical studies. Our original proposal for screening children for stuttering used a symptom set that excluded WWR as suggested by EXPLAN. This showed some success. WWR were not dismissed in our assessments since, it was argued, they could play an important role in identifying WFD. Moreover, WFD is commonly seen in school cohorts where children are required to use non-native languages. We successfully used WWR as a way of identifying children with WFD, including those using English as an additional language. Whilst these symptom-based methods were successful, we went on to seek more concise methods for use in schools. NWR was chosen, but current tests had to be modified to tackle language diversity in schools, which led to the UNWR test. UNWR proved successful at screening children with WFD, CWS, and children with typical fluency. However, issues remain about the robustness of NWR scoring procedures in general which we are addressing. This approach was developed for UK school contexts where English has to be spoken. A parallel procedure has successfully been conducted for children who speak mixed variations of Arabic and English. In-school interventions for children with fluency problems are starting to be examined; however, care should be taken that these procedures do not conflict with anything SLPs might subsequently need to do with a child who is treated.

Further reading

Barrett, L., Hu, J., & Howell, P. (2022). Systematic review of machine learning approaches for detecting developmental stuttering. *IEEE/ACM Transactions on Audio, Speech, and Language Processing.*

Howell, P., Chua, L.Y., Yoshikawa, K., Tang, H. H. S., Welmillage, T., Harris, J., & Tang, K. (2020). Does working-memory training given TO Reception-class children improve the speech of children at risk of fluency difficulty? *Frontiers in Psychology, 11*, 568867.

References

Alsulaiman, R., Harris, J., Bamaas, S., & Howell, P. (2022). Identifying stuttering in Arabic speakers who stutter: Development of a non-word repetition task and preliminary results. *Frontiers in Pediatrics, 10*, 750126–750126. https://doi.org/10.3389/fped.2022.750126

Alsulaiman, R. M. (2022). *Arabic fluency assessment: Procedures for assessing stuttering in Arabic preschool children* ([Doctoral Dissertation]. UCL (University College London)).

Al-Ani (1970). *Arabic phonology: An Acoustical and Physiological Investigation* (Vol. 61). Berlin: De Gruyter, Inc.

Al-Tamimi, F., Khamaiseh, Z., & Howell, P. (2013). Phonetic complexity and stuttering in Arabic. *Clinical Linguistics and Phonetics, 27*(12), 874–887.

Anderson, J. D., & Conture, E. G. (2004). Sentence-structure priming in young children who do and do not stutter. *Journal of Speech, Language, and Hearing Research, 47*(3), 552–571. https://doi.org/10.1044/1092-4388(2004/043)

Anderson, J. D., & Wagovich, S. A. (2010). Relationships among linguistic processing speed, phonological working memory, and attention in children who stutter. *Journal of Fluency Disorders, 35*(3), 216–234.

Andrews, G., & Cutler, J. (1974). Stuttering therapy: The relation between changes in symptom level and attitudes. *Journal of Speech and Hearing Disorders, 39*(3), 312–319.

Andrews, G., & Harris, M. (1964). *The syndrome of stuttering: Clinics in developmental medicine 17*. London: Heinemann

Antoniazzi, D., Snow, P., & Dickson-Swift, V. (2010). Teacher identification of children at risk for language impairment in the first year of school. *International Journal of Speech-Language Pathology, 12*(3), 244–252.

Archibald, L. M. D. (2008). The promise of nonword repetition as a clinical tool. *Revue Canadienne d'Orthophonie et d'Audiologie, 32*(1), 21–27.

Au-Yeung, J., Gomez, I.V., & Howell, P. (2003). Exchange of disfluency with age from function words to content words in Spanish speakers who stutter. *Journal of Speech, Language, and Hearing Research, 46*(3), 754–765.

Au-Yeung, J., Howell, P., & Pilgrim, L. (1998). Phonological words and stuttering on function words. *Journal of Speech, Language, and Hearing Research, 41*(5), 1019–1030.

Bakhtiar, M., Dehqan, A., & Sadegh, S. (2007). Nonword repetition ability of children who do and do not stutter and covert repair hypothesis. *Indian Journal of Medical Sciences, 61*(8), 462–470.

Bakhtiar, M., Seifpanahi, S., Ansari, H., Ghanadzade, M., & Packman, A. (2010). Investigation of the reliability of the SSI-3 for preschool Persian-speaking children who stutter. *Journal of Fluency Disorders*, 35(2), 87–91.

Bercow, J. (2008). The Bercow report: A review of services for children and young people (0–19) with speech. *Language and Communication Needs*. Nottingham: DCSF Publications.

Best, W., Hughes, L. M., Masterson, J., Thomas, M., Fedor, A., Roncoli, S., & Kapikian, A. (2018). Intervention for children with word-finding difficulties: A parallel group randomised control trial. *International Journal of Speech-Language Pathology, 20*(7), 708–719.

Blackmer, E. R., & Mitton, J. L. (1991). Theories of monitoring and the timing of repairs in spontaneous speech. *Cognition, 39*(3), 173–194.

Bowey, J. A. (1996). On the association between phonological memory and receptive vocabulary in five-year-olds. *Journal of Experimental Child Psychology, 63*(1), 44–78.

Bragard, Schelstraete, M.-A., Snyers, P., & James, D. G. H. (2012). Word-finding intervention for children with specific language impairment: a multiple single-case study. *Language, Speech, and Hearing Services in Schools, 43*(2), 222–234. https://doi.org/10.1044/0161-1461(2011/10-0090)

Casserly, E. D., & Pisoni, D. B. (2010). Speech perception and production. *Wiley Interdisciplinary Reviews: Cognitive Science, 1*(5), 629–647.

Clark, H. H., & Clark, E. V. (1977). *Psychology and language: An introduction into psycholinguistics*. New York: Harcourt Brace.

Coady, J. A., & Evans, J. L. (2008). Uses and interpretations of non-word repetition tasks in children with and without specific language impairments (SLI). *International Journal of Language and Communication Disorders, 43*(1), 1–40.

Constantino, C. D., Leslie, P., Quesal, R. W., & Yaruss, J. S. (2016). A preliminary investigation of daily variability of stuttering in adults. *Journal of Communication Disorders, 60*, 39–50.

Conti-Ramsden, G., Botting, N., & Faragher, B. (2001). Psycholinguistic markers for specific language impairment (SLI). *Journal of Child Psychology and Psychiatry, 42*(6), 741–748.

Davidow, J. H. (2021). Reliability and similarity of the stuttering severity instrument-and a global severity rating scale [Speech]. *Language and Hearing, 24*(1), 20–27.

Davis, S., Shisca, D., & Howell, P. (2007). Anxiety in speakers who persist and recover from stuttering. *Journal of Communication Disorders, 40*(5), 398–417.

Dell, G. S. (1986). A spreading-activation theory of retrieval in sentence production. *Psychological Review, 93*(3), 283.

DfE (2018). Schools, pupils and their characteristics: January 2018. Statistics N, editor.

Dockrell, J. E. (2001). Assessing language skills in preschool children. *Child Psychology and Psychiatry Review, 6*(2), 74–85.

Dockrell, J. E., & Lindsay, G. (2001). Children with specific speech and language difficulties—The teachers' perspective. *Oxford Review of Education, 27*(3), 369–394.

Dockrell, J. E., & Marshall, C. R. (2015). Measurement issues: Assessing language skills in young children. *Child and Adolescent Mental Health, 20*(2), 116–125.

Dworzynski, K., & Howell, P. (2004). Predicting stuttering from phonetic complexity in German. *Journal of Fluency Disorders, 29*(2), 149–173.

Dworzynski, K., Howell, P., Au-Yeung, J., & Rommel, D. (2004). Stuttering on function and content words across age groups of German speakers who stutter. *Journal of Multilingual Communication Disorders, 2*(2), 81–101.

Ebbels, S. (2014). Effectiveness of intervention for grammar in school-aged children with primary language impairments: A review of the evidence. *Child Language Teaching and Therapy, 30*(1), 7–40.

Ferreira, F. (1993). Creation of prosody during sentence production. *Psychological Review, 100*(2), 233.

Gathercole, S. E., Willis, C. S., Baddeley, A. D., & Emslie, H. (1994). The Children's Test of Nonword Repetition: A test of phonological working memory. *Memory (Hove, England)*, 2(2), 103–127.

Gee, J. P., & Grosjean, F. (1983). Performance structures: A psycholinguistic and linguistic appraisal. *Cognitive Psychology, 15*(4), 411–458.

Hakim, H. B., & Ratner, N. B. (2004). Nonword repetition abilities of children who stutter: An exploratory study. *Journal of Fluency Disorders, 29*(3), 179–199.

Howell, P. (2004). Assessment of Some Contemporary Theories of Stuttering That Apply to Spontaneous Speech. *Contemporary Issues in Communication Science and Disorders*: CICSD, 31, 122–139.

Howell, P. (2007). Signs of developmental stuttering up to age eight and at 12 plus. *Clinical Psychology Review, 27*(3), 287–306.

Howell, P. (2010). Language processing in fluency disorders. In J. Guendouzi, F. Loncke & M. Williams (Eds.), *The handbook on psycholinguistics and cognitive processes: Perspectives on communication disorders* (pp.437–464). London: Taylor & Francis.

Howell, P. (2011). *Recovery from stuttering*. New York: Psychology Press.

Howell, P. (2013). Screening school-aged children for risk of stuttering. *Journal of Fluency Disorders, 38*(2), 102–123.

Howell, P., & Davis, S. (2011). Predicting persistence of and recovery from stuttering by the teenage years based on information gathered at age 8 years. *Journal of Developmental and Behavioral Pediatrics, 32*(3), 196–205.

Howell, P., & Rusbridge, S. (2011). The speech and language characteristics of developmental stuttering in English speakers. *Multilingual Aspects of Fluency Disorders, 5*, 93.

Howell, P., & Sackin, S. (2000). Speech rate modification and its effects on fluency reversal in fluent speakers and people who stutter. *Journal of Developmental and Physical Disabilities, 12*(4), 291–315.

Howell, P., Au-Yeung, J., & Sackin, S. (1999). Exchange of stuttering from function words to content words with age. *Journal of Speech, Language, and Hearing Research, 42*(2), 345–354.

Howell, P., Chua, L.Y., Yoshikawa, K., Tang, H. H. S., Welmillage, T., Harris, J., & Tang, K. (2020). Does working-memory training given TO Reception-class children improve the speech of children at risk of fluency difficulty? *Frontiers in Psychology, 11*, 568867.

Howell, P., Davis, S, & Williams, R. (2008). Late childhood stuttering. *Journal of Speech, Language, and Hearing Research, 51*(3), 669–687.

Howell, P., Tang, K., Tuomainen, O., Chan, S. K., Beltran, K., Mirawdeli, A., & Harris, J. (2017). Identification of fluency and word-finding difficulty in samples of children with diverse language backgrounds. *International Journal of Language and Communication Disorders, 52*(5), 595–611.

Jakielski, K. J. (1998). *Motor organization in the acquisition of consonant clusters* [PhD Thesis] [UMI Dissertation] services. Ann Arbor: University of Texas at Austin.

Jiang, J., Lu, C., Peng, D., Zhu, C., & Howell, P. (2012). Classification of types of stuttering symptoms based on brain activity. *PLOS ONE*, 7(6), e39747.

Johnson, W. (1955). *Stuttering*. Hagerstown, Maryland: WF Prior Company.

Johnson, W. (1959). *The onset of stuttering: Research findings and implications/Wendell Johnson and associates*. University of Minnesota Press.

Julie, D., David, M., Rachel, G., & Gillie, W. (1998). Notes and discussion children with word-finding difficulties-prevalence, presentation and naming problems. *International Journal of Language and Communication Disorders, 33*(4), 445–454.

Karimi, H., Nilipour, R., Shafiei, B., & Howell, P. (2011). Translation, assessment and deployment of stuttering instruments into different languages: Comments arising from Bakhtiar et al., investigation of the reliability of the SSI-3 for preschool Persian-speaking children who stutter. *Journal of Fuency Disorders, 36*(3), 246–248 [*Journal of Fluency Disorders* 2010, 35(2), 87–91].

Levelt, W. J. (1989). *Speaking: From intention to articulation*. Cambridge, MA: MIT Press.

Maclay, H., & Osgood, C. E. (1959). Hesitation phenomena in spontaneous English speech. *Word, 15*(1), 19–44.

MacWhinney, B., & Osser, H. (1977). Verbal planning functions in children's speech. *Child Development*, 978–985.

Manning, W., & Gayle Beck, J. (2013). The role of psychological processes in estimates of stuttering severity. *Journal of Fluency Disorders, 38*(4), 356–367.

Masoura, E.V., & Gathercole, S. E. (1999). Phonological short-term memory and foreign language learning. *International Journal of Psychology, 34*(5–6), 383–388.

Melnick, K. S., Conture, E. G., & Ohde, R. N. (2003). Phonological priming in picture naming of young children who stutter. *Journal of Speech, Language, and Hearing Research, 46*(6), 1428–1443.

Mirawdeli, A. (2015). Identifying children who stutter or have other difficulties in speech production in school reception classes. *Procedia-Social and Behavioral Sciences, 193*, 192–201.

Mirawdeli, A., & Howell, P. (2016). Is it necessary to assess fluent symptoms, duration of dysfluent events, and physical concomitants when identifying children who have speech difficulties? *Clinical Linguistics and Phonetics, 30*(9), 696–719.

Munson, B., Edwards, J., & Beckman, M. E. (2005). Relationships Between Nonword Repetition Accuracy and Other Measures of Linguistic Development in Children With Phonological Disorders. *Journal of Speech, Language, and Hearing Research*, 48(1), 61–78.

Pellowski, M. W., & Conture, E. G. (2005). Lexical priming in picture naming of young children who do and do not stutter. *Journal of Speech, Language, and Hearing Research, 48*(2), 278–294.

Piazzalunga, S., Previtali, L., Pozzoli, R., Scarponi, L., & Schindler, A. (2019). An articulatory-based disyllabic and trisyllabic Non-Word Repetition test: Reliability and validity in Italian 3-to 7-year-old children. *Clinical Linguistics and Phonetics, 33*(5), 437–456.

Pinker, S. (1995). Why the Child Holded the Baby Rabbits: A Case Study in Language Acquisition. In D. N. Osherson, L. R. Gleitman, M. Liberman, & E. E. Smith. (Eds.). *An Invitation to Cognitive Science: Language* (pp. 107–133).

Riley, G. (1994). *Stuttering severity instrument-3 (SSI-3).* Austin, TX: Pro Ed. In: Inc.

Riley, G., & Bakker, K. (2009). Stuttering severity instrument / Glyndon D. Riley. In (4th ed., p. SSI-4). Austin, TX: Pro-Ed.

Rispoli, M. (2003). Changes in the nature of sentence production during the period of grammatical development. *Journal of Speech, Language, and Hearing Research, 46*(4), 818–830

Savage, C., & Howell, P. (2008). Lexical priming of function words and content words with children who do, and do not, stutter. *Journal of Communication Disorders, 41*(6), 459–484.

Schindler, O. (1962). *Manuale di Audiofonologopedia. Propedeutica.* Torino, Italy: Omega Edizioni.

Selkirk, E. (1984). *Phonology and syntax: The relation between sound and structure.* Cambridge, MA: MIT Press.

Stenström, A. B., & Svartvik, J. (1994). Repeats and other nonfluencies in spoken English. *Corpus-Based Research into Language: In Honour of Jan Aarts, 12*, 241.

Strand, S., Malmberg, L., & Hall, J. (2015). *English as an Additional Language (EAL) and educational achievement in England: An analysis of the National Pupil Database.* London, UK: Education Endowment Foundation & Unbound Philanthropy; Cambridge, UK: The Bell Foundation.

Summers, C., Bohman, T. M., Gillam, R. B., Peña, E. D., & Bedore, L. M. (2010). Bilingual performance on nonword repetition in Spanish and English. *International Journal of Language & Communication Disorders*, 45(4), 480–493.

Todd, H., Mirawdeli, A., Costelloe, S., Cavenagh, P., Davis, S., & Howell, P. (2014). Scores on Riley's Stuttering Severity Instrument versions three and four for samples of different length and for different types of speech material. *Clinical Linguistics and Phonetics, 28*(12), 912–926.

Tumanova, V., Conture, E. G., Lambert, E. W., & Walden, T. A. (2014). Speech disfluencies of preschool-age children who do and do not stutter. *Journal of Communication Disorders, 49*, 25–41.

Vahab, M., Zandiyan, A., Falahi, M. H., & Howell, P. (2013). Lexical category influences in Persian children who stutter. *Clinical Linguistics and Phonetics, 27*(12), 862–873.

Van Borsel, J., Maes, E., & Foulon, S. (2001). Stuttering and bilingualism: A review. *Journal of Fluency Disorders, 26*(3), 179–205.

Walsh, B., Bostian, A., Tichenor, S. E., Brown, B., & Weber, C. (2020). Disfluency characteristics of 4-and 5-year-old children who stutter and their relationship to stuttering persistence and recovery. *Journal of Speech, Language, and Hearing Research, 63*(8), 2555–2566.

Watson, D., & Gibson, E. (2004). The relationship between intonational phrasing and syntactic structure in language production. *Language and Cognitive Processes, 19*(6), 713–755.

Watson, J. C. (2007). *The phonology and morphology of Arabic.* Oxford: Oxford University Press.

Westbury, C., & Bub, D. (1997). Primary progressive aphasia: A review of 112 cases. *Brain and Language, 60*(3), 381–406.

Widiger, T. A., & Samuel, D. B. (2005). Diagnostic categories or dimensions? A question for the Diagnostic and statistical manual of mental disorders--. *Journal of Abnormal Psychology, 114*(4), 494.

Windsor, J., Kohnert, K., Lobitz, K., & Pham, G. (2010). Cross-language nonword repetition by bilingual and monolingual children. *American Journal of Speech-Language Pathology.* American Speech-Language-Hearing Association, *19*(4), 298–310.

World Health Organization (1992). *The ICD-10 classification of mental and behavioral disorders: Clinical descriptions and diagnostic guidelines.* Geneva: World Health Organization.

World Health Organization (2007). *International classification of functioning, disability, and health: Children & youth version: ICF-CY.* Geneva: World Health Organization.

Wright, S. H., & Ayre, A. (2000). *WASSP: The Wright and Ayre stuttering self-rating profile/Louise Wright, Anne Ayre.* Bicester: Winslow Press.

Wright, S. H., Gorrie, B., Haynes, C., & Shipman, A. (1993). What's in a name? Comparative therapy for word-finding difficulties using semantic and phonological approaches. *Child Language Teaching and Therapy, 9*(3), 214–229.

Yairi, E., & Ambrose, N. (1992). A longitudinal study of stuttering in children: A preliminary report. *Journal of Speech, Language, and Hearing Research, 35*(4), 755–760.

Yairi, E., & Ambrose, N. G. (2004). Early childhood stuttering. In *PRO-ED, Inc. 8700.* Austin, TX: Shoal Creek Blvd.

Yan, S., & Nicoladis, E. (2009). Finding le mot juste: Differences between bilingual and monolingual children's lexical access in comprehension and production. *Bilingualism: Language and Cognition, 12*(3), 323–335.

Yaruss, J. S., & Quesal, R. W. (2006). Overall assessment of the speaker's experience of stuttering (OASES): Documenting multiple outcomes in stuttering treatment. *Journal of Fluency Disorders, 31*(2), 90–115.

23

AN APPROACH TO DIFFERENTIATING BILINGUALISM AND LANGUAGE IMPAIRMENT

Sharon Armon-Lotem and Joel Walters

Introduction

Bilingualism presents a weighty challenge to clinical assessment in general and to the analysis of language impairment and neurological disorders in particular. A wide range of linguistic and social phenomena converge in the bilingual person in ways which are often difficult to differentiate. Simply analyzing and comparing the two languages of a bilingual may be insufficient for identifying disorder (although this alone would be a major improvement of much current practice which generally addresses only a single language, often, the second language). From a research perspective, clinical disorders offer numerous challenges to the study of bilingualism, in particular what it means theoretically to know a language, the notion of completeness in linguistic knowledge, and the relationship between a language user's two languages. From a practitioner's point of view, theory and method in bilingualism can help inform clinical decisions which may make a large difference in people's lives.

This chapter on bilingualism and neurolinguistic disorders centers on whether diagnosis is necessary in both languages or whether it is sufficient to look at a single language. The two populations we choose to look at here, children with Developmental Language Disorder (DLD) and adults with schizophrenia (SZ), share the fact that impairment is manifested in both languages. A further question arises as to whether bilingualism exacerbates the linguistic manifestation of the impairment, i.e., whether it makes linguistic performance worse or makes it harder to diagnose, etc. The two populations potentially differ in several ways: (1) age (children vs. adults); (2) the nature of the impairment (for children with DLD – more grammatically indicated/diffuse across linguistic domains, for schizophrenia – more focused on lexical/pragmatic phenomena); (3) different manifestation due to typological differences (DLD) vs. similar manifestation (schizophrenia). It will be argued that it may be sufficient to diagnose and treat a single language in adult schizophrenics, but it is crucial to look at both languages in the case of DLD.

Two sets of questions for the study of bilingualism and language impairment

At the outset we contrast two perspectives: bilinguals with a disorder or individuals with a disorder who happen to be bilingual. The researcher in bilingualism is drawn to the former; the clinician/educator naturally gravitates to the latter. We are motivated here to integrate these two perspectives in an attempt toward dialogue between researchers and clinicians.

One set of questions relates to social aspects of bilingualism, in particular to social identity and attitudes. Again we ask: are we talking about bilinguals with language disorders or individuals with

DOI: 10.4324/9781003204213-26

language disorder who happen to be bilingual? These alternative formulations of the question bring us to the heart of the difference/deviance debate. In the study of bilingualism, especially subtractive bilingualism in children (Lambert, 1990) but also the relative prestige of a bilingual's two languages, the relevant constructs include ethnolinguistic vitality, language status, and attitudes towards the second language and its speakers (e.g., Allard & Landry, 1994). In the area of language-related learning disabilities, intentions and goals are critical notions for proper assessment, along with affective factors, such as self-esteem and self-confidence.

In bilingual acquisition, Pearson (2007) reviews a variety of studies (e.g., Pearson et al., 1997; de Houwer, 2003) in search of social factors to explain why approximately 25% of bilingual children from bilingual environments do *not* acquire the home/minority/heritage language. The factors examined include input, language status, access to literacy, immigrant status, and community support. She concludes that "quantity of input has the greatest effect on whether a minority language will be learned," but that both status and attitudes also make a difference. In showing the importance of language status, i.e., the difference between minority and majority languages, Pearson presents the intuitive observation: "if one does not speak a language well, one will not use it. If one reports using a language often, we can infer the person has some skill in that language." But then she goes on to show that this adage may not be true for the majority language, citing Hakuta and d'Andrea (1992) who showed language attitudes to be a better predictor of language use than proficiency in Mexican-American teenagers. Finally, in the context of community support for the minority language and the economic benefits of ethnolinguistic enclaves, Pearson states that "It is crucial to have contact with monolingual speakers of the minority language," but goes on to report that "the effect of language of instruction at school could more than counterbalance the effect of less Spanish in the home." She argues strongly for either simultaneous bilingualism or early second language acquisition both as a means to maintaining the minority language and for its presumed cognitive, social, and affective benefits (Bialystok, 2001; Bialystok & Senman, 2004; Cummins, 1976; Pearson, 2008).

Questions on social aspects of bilingualism and language impairment include:

(a) How are both bilingualism and language impairment expressed in a speaker's social identity?
(b) How do positive attitudes to a bilingual's native and/or second language and its speakers contribute to achievement in L2 (additive bilingualism)? How do negative attitudes to L1 and its speakers and positive attitudes to L2 and its speakers contribute to or impede achievement in L2 (subtractive bilingualism)?
(c) What are some of the goals and beliefs of bilinguals with language disorders about their bilingualism and language disabilities, and how are those goals and beliefs expressed in their perceptions of self, in the way they conceive of language and communication, and in their language behavior. In particular, how do the intentions and speech acts of bilingual language disordered individuals reflect their social identities, attitudes, goals, and beliefs?

A second set of questions attempts to disentangle bilingualism and language impairment (LI) by identifying the relative contribution of each to language performance. For bilingual DLD, these questions have been addressed by COST Action IS0840 "Language Impairment in a Multilingual Society: Linguistic Patterns and the Road to Assessment" (Armon-Lotem et al., 2015). In doing so, we hope to shed light on theoretical issues in bilingualism and neurolinguistics as well as on clinical practice, asking:

a. How can linguistic indicators of LI be identified in both languages in DLD/schizophrenia? More specifically, to what extent are the manifestations of LI similar/different across the two languages?

b. How can the manifestations of LI and typically developed (TD) bilingualism be differentiated given the fact that some of the same linguistic markers are characteristic of both bilingualism and LI?

The motivation for these questions is both practical and methodological. Practically, we are interested in knowing what to recommend to teachers and clinicians regarding educational planning and programming for children or family members. A second motivation comes from our research bias favoring individual analysis, personal design, and case studies and rejecting approaches which rely on large samples, group means, and comparisons of monolinguals and bilinguals. We do not expect that answers to these questions will be easy to attain, certainly not as easy as the "monolingual" solution, recommending that the child be spoken to in one language only at home or at school.

To address these questions, we ideally need demographic and ethnographic information about language use, language choice, language preferences, and language attitudes in the home, neighborhood, and school environments in *both* languages, sampling a range of topics, with a variety of listeners/interlocutors. We need to combine this information with a variety of language tasks, conducted in *both* languages, including spontaneous speech and focused probes of a range of morphosyntactic, lexical, syntactic, and pragmatic stimuli, tasks, and response measures. Within this mass of data, we pay special attention to bilingual phenomena such as codeswitching, interference, and fluency and how they interact with pragmatic phenomena such as certainty and confidence, insecurity and defensiveness.

Representation and processing in bilingualism

Two theoretical constructs inform this work: representation and processing. Representation of syntactic and lexical structure may be incomplete or different for both bilingual children and children with DLD, but are assumed to be unimpaired in schizophrenia. Processing of linguistic information, however, may differ for both groups. DLD in children has been considered a result of impaired representations and/or impaired processing in terms of duration, rate, and salience, but there is no consensus as to whether impaired representation is the source of processing difficulty or whether impaired processing leads to compromised representations. The phenomena show up in DLD as difficulties in temporal integration, word-finding, morphosyntactic substitution, syntactic permutation errors, and in tasks with heavy memory demands. Schizophrenic language processing difficulties have been reported primarily in the lexical and pragmatic domains as word salad, an overabundance of lexical rather than anaphoric cohesion, and prevalence of exophoric reference. Developing bilinguals may show evidence of linguistic representations which differ from those of monolinguals, and may also experience difficulties in processing related to their lexical knowledge or reduced exposure to each language. Adult second language learners, however, are assumed to transfer linguistic representations from L1, especially with regard to morphology and syntax; lexical knowledge and declarative memory are said to be more involved in adult language learning than grammatical knowledge and procedural memory (Ullman & Pierpont, 2005). Representation has not been addressed in the literature on SZ.

Linguistic representations and processing of linguistic structures are central constructs in cognitive theories of bilingualism and second language acquisition (e.g. Universal Grammar, Usage Based models, Dynamic Systems Theory). They are non-existent in most sociocultural approaches. Highlighting the work of Kroll and Green, this section selectively reviews research on representation and processing as background for an approach which is exceptional for taking into account both psycholinguistic/cognitive and sociolinguistic/sociopragmatic dimensions of bilingualism. The section concludes with a review of three issues deemed most relevant to the study of bilingualism and language disorder: typological differences, codeswitching, and code interference.

Focus on bilingual lexical representation

Lexical representation has been widely investigated in bilingualism, in particular to address the question of shared vs. separate representational systems. Kroll's model of bilingual lexical production (Kroll & de Groot, 1997; Kroll & Tokowicz, 2005; Kroll et al., 2010) contains multiple levels of representation for concepts, lemmas, and phonology. Language specific information is claimed to be available at the conceptual level in the form of language cues (cf. language tags) and at the lemma level, where language information is "distinct for words in each of the bilingual's languages" (p. 539). The phonological level consists of features shared between the two languages, activating representations from both languages. This model argues for an integrated set of lemmas to account for comprehension processes in word recognition.

Kroll and Tokowicz (2005) criticize some models of bilingualism for not distinguishing "among different levels of representation," maintaining that bilingualism does not need to be represented in the same way at each level. Their review analyzes studies from a wide range of linguistic domains (e.g., orthography, phonology, lexical semantics). Bilingual stimuli in these studies included cognates, translation equivalents, interlingual homographs, orthographic neighbors, semantically related words, and concrete and abstract nouns. Tasks included word recognition, priming, lexical decision, Stroop-type picture-word production, translation, word association, and semantic ratings. In contrast to morphology and syntax, where typological differences (see below) may argue for more separate systems (Emmorey et al., 2008; Meisel, 2004, Paradis & Genesee, 1997), Kroll and Tokowicz (2005) amass a broad range of support on behalf of the notion that the "lexicon is integrated across languages, and that lexical access is parallel and non-selective" (p. 534).

Processing models in bilingualism

In terms of processing, the most prevalent constructs in bilingual research are storage and retrieval/access, activation/inhibition, language selection, and control. There is widespread consensus (e.g., Costa et al., 2016; Kroll et al., 2015; Kroll, Bobb, & Hoshino, 2016) that the two languages of bilinguals are both activated even when only a single language is needed for a particular task. This argument holds for recognition as well as production in lexical as well as sentence contexts and across bilinguals of varying proficiencies. Co-activation is said to lead to phenomena variously described as interference, competition, cross-language intrusion errors, and has been explained by more general cognitive mechanisms, in particular inhibition and control (Kroll et al., 2015; Green, 1998).

Green (1998, 2000) poses the parallel activation question in bilingual processing as a problem of control under conditions of multi-tasking, comparing bilingual production to a Stroop task. Phrased differently: how do bilinguals avoid speaking in L1 when they want to speak in L2? Green's (1993) model proposes to account for a broad range of bilingual data, including involuntary speech errors, interference, and fluent codeswitching and for findings in a variety of different tasks.

The core structural constructs in the model are lemmas and language tags. The model involves two processes, *activation* of the lemma and *retrieval* of the lexeme, with *control* specified as one of three states of activation. The processing notions in control include competition, selection, and inhibition as well as schemas and goals. The multi-level nature of control is explained as follows: "first, one level of control involves language task schemas that compete to control output; second, the locus of word selection is the lemma level...and selection involves the use of language tags; third, control at the lemma level is inhibitory and reactive." Two conditions are involved in control: explicit intentions and language tags on both word meanings (lemmas) and word forms (lexemes). Green discusses how this works for steady state production in a second language and for codeswitching, arguing: in L2 production, activation of both lemmas and lexemes in L2 is increased, while L1 lexemes are suppressed when phonological information is retrieved. In codeswitching, there is competition at the stage of phonological assembly, and the lexeme that "reach[es] threshold first" is the one produced.

In Green's model, an executive processor, the Supervisory Attentional System (SAS), activates language task schemas (e.g., for translation and word naming), which compete to control output. These schemas exercise control by activating and inhibiting language tags at the lemma level via functional control circuits. The "functional control circuits" regulate activation and inhibition to handle competition between language task schemas. Green illustrates this process with an example of a bilingual aphasic who was able to translate into a language he could not speak spontaneously. The functional control circuit for this phenomenon is called a translation schema (L1=>L2) which increases activation of a word production schema (for L2) and suppresses L1. Codeswitching "costs" in studies of numeral naming (Meuter & Allport, 1999) are also explained in terms of inhibitory control. He cites experimental research on translation, codeswitching, Stroop effects, and cross-language competitive priming as further evidence for his model.

Green takes this work a quantum step forward in his Control Process Model (Green & Wei, 2014) and its extended version (Green, 2018) to account for various types of codeswitching – alternations, insertions and dense CS/congruent lexicalisations (Muysken, 2000) in a theory of bilingual processing which goes from intention to utterance planning to production. The model distinguishes between competitive language control where only one language is produced and two types of cooperative language control, coupled control to account for insertional CS and open control to account for dense CS. The CPM is based on a neurocomputational account of sentence production at the level of subcortical processes and goes beyond the sentence level to include conversational/discourse processes.

Our work differs in several ways. We focus on morphosyntactic rules and typological differences across languages in language disorder in children and in lexical as well as pragmatic issues in schizophrenia. The model presented below offers a broader view of bilingual representation, including sociopragmatic as well as psycholinguistic information in a single framework as well as a different perspective on processing.

Representation and processing in a sociopragmatic-psycholinguistic model

Representation

The Sociopragmatic Psycholinguistic (SPPL) model of bilingualism (Walters, 2005) contains seven structural components/information sources and a set of processing mechanisms to describe how information flows between these components during bilingual speech. Two modules, which extend from input to output, aim to show that L1 and L2 *language choice* and *affective* information are available at every stage of language production. Interaction of the *language choice* module with the other information components provides an account for codeswitching, code interference, and fluency. Sociopragmatic information is represented at the beginning of the process with psycholinguistic information closer to the output stage. The sociopragmatic-psycholinguistic partition distinguishes impairment which is more communicative, e.g., in schizophrenia, from language disorders which are focused on linguistic indicators, as with Developmental Language Disorder (DLD).

The *language choice module* is responsible for making L1 and L2 information available to the bilingual speaker (1) for expressing one's social identity, (2) in the choice of where to speak and in preferences for interlocutors and genres, (3) in conceiving intentions, (4) in retrieving and formulating concepts and words, and finally, (5) in articulating an utterance. The language choice module selects, regulates, and retrieves information from these components and integrates them with the speaker's linguistic choices. This module has been used to account for a distinction between sociopragmatically and psycholinguistically motivated codeswitching in healthy bilingual adults (Altman, Schrauf, & Walters, 2012), in sequential bilingual children (Altman, Walters, & Raichlin, 2018), and in bilingual children with language impairment (Iluz-Cohen & Walters, 2012).

The *affective module* has an analogous framework for distinguishing sociopragmatically motivated discourse markers and those which are used to convey fluency and other discourse formulation functions. At the level of formulation and articulation, this module characterizes differences between affectively motivated slips of the tongue (of the Freudian type) and phonetically and phonologically based tip-of-the-tongue phenomena.

Five structural components represent information sources and stages in language production, moving from expression of social identity to articulatory output.

(1) *Social identity* information, the initial component, shows that bilingualism is grounded in the social world of the speaker. Social identity is constructed when the bilingual makes new friends, switches jobs, and integrates language choices regarding accent, names, and greetings with these elements of social life. Social identity information is relevant to both language impairment in adult schizophrenia due to social ostracizing and to DLD in accounting for aspects of identity grounded in communication difficulties.

(2) The *contextual/genre component* specifies setting, participants, topic, and genre information in conversational interaction. It addresses the classical sociolinguistic question of "who speaks which language to whom, where, and about which topic" (Fishman, 1965). It accounts for bilingual code alternation between immigrant parents and their native-born children. The genre subcomponent distinguishes scripted language, e.g., in doctor-patient exchanges, from spontaneous conversation. For both DLD and schizophrenia, this component accounts for language choices, with preferences for "safe" listeners, topics, and perhaps more scripted language than spontaneous conversation.

(3) The central component of the model is responsible for identifying *speaker intentions* and their bilingual features. It is informed by Speech Act theory (e.g., Austin, 1962) and research on discourse markers (e.g., *well, like, ya' know*), greetings, and lexical choice. Intentions are bridges between sociopragmatic and psycholinguistic sources of information. A speaker's intention (to request, promise, apologize, deceive, or blame) is peppered with bilingual information, from subtle indicators of the speaker's identity latent in discourse markers or the prosodic shape of the utterance to lexical preferences influenced by psycholinguistic factors such as interference, lexical gaps, and word frequency.

(4) The *formulator*, locus of most psycholinguistic research on bilingual processing, gets at the heart of lexical representation, or how words are stored and retrieved. In contrast to monolingual models of lexical processing, lexical formulation in the SPPL Model contains pragmatic information as well as structural features from ***both*** languages. Representations are highly variable, both within and across speakers. In addition to lexical information, the formulator specifies discourse patterns to handle relevance, cohesion, and sequencing of information. It is discourse which has been shown to be a marker of impairment in SZ (Fine, 2006).
   a. The SPPL approach to formulation accounts for variability and incompleteness in a bilingual's knowledge of language. All bilinguals (and even monolinguals) experience lexical near-misses, which the listener perceives as malapropisms. The model attempts to characterize this variability by incorporating pragmatic and discourse information in the formulator and by making bilingual information available from the language choice module.

(5) Finally, the bilingual *articulator* accounts for the fact that bilinguals, even those without a trace of an accent, show evidence (sometimes only via precise acoustical measurements) of a merged system of sounds (e.g., Caramazza et al., 1973; Obler, 1982). The SPPL Model and its bilingual articulator attempt to characterize this uniqueness as well as variability within and across speakers.

Processing in SPPL

Four general cognitive processing mechanisms are found in the SPPL framework: imitation, variation, integration, and control. Their generality enables an account of both sociopragmatic and psycholinguistic information. These mechanisms are supported by a set of basic processes, including attention, discrimination, recognition, identification/recall, classification/sorting, and categorization. Imitation and variation, grounded conceptually in linguistics, are elaborated on here. Integration and control draw from Anderson's (1996) Functional Theory of Cognition and Powers' (1973, 1978) Perceptual Control Theory, respectively, and are beyond the scope of this chapter (but see Walters, 2005).

Imitation drives both sociopragmatic and psycholinguistic information. Language production begins with an innate representation which is defined by a set of structural features, i.e., phonemes, morphemes, syntactic and semantic structures. These features are selected, copied, and adapted, in order to express social, psychological, and linguistic preferences. Among the basic level processes which support this mechanism, *recognition* and *recall* are prominent.

By way of example, the selection of names and use of greetings are among the most salient ways to project *social identity*. If schizophrenics are impaired in the social domain, their impairment could be manifested in the imitation mechanism. In contrast, language impaired children may show use of lexical imitation, e.g., use of social routines or a fixed verb stem, as a strategy to compensate for limitations in morphosyntactic processing.

Imitation is also vital in generating *intentions*. A speech act selected to encode an intention is assumed to involve social identity, contextual, and genre information. It is conceived here as having been copied from a mental inventory of available intentions and integrated with appropriate propositional content. In bilingual processing, copies of L1 speech act forms are sometimes combined with L2 propositional content (or vice versa) to yield utterances with code interference. When the Israeli speaker of English responds "Not right" in order to express mild disagreement, imitation is at work in replicating the speech act and propositional content from each of the bilingual speaker's languages. Intentions are not expected to be impaired in either schizophrenia or DLD, but the expression of intentions in terms of speech act form and its link to propositional content should present different kinds of problems for each population.

In the *formulator*, imitation is the processing mechanism which takes the abstract information in a concept and lemma and copies or maps it onto morphophonological information to yield the lexeme. In bilingual lexical processing, information can be said to be copied from different linguistic levels and integrated to yield transfer errors, i.e., forms with code interference as well as codeswitching. For example, Hebrew does not lexicalize the difference between process and result like English does in the distinction between "*study*" and "*learn*." Thus, native Hebrew speakers of English typically use the word "learn" in a context which requires use of the word "study" (e.g., "I am learning English at school."). In terms of the imitation mechanism, the speaker has selected the syntactic and semantic information from the Hebrew lemma "*lmd*" (to learn) and copied it onto the English lexeme, resulting in the word "learn." Studies of codeswitching might ignore this phenomenon, since on the surface only a single language appears in the example above. In the present context, codeswitching and code interference show evidence of the same underlying imitation process.

Variation. The approach to variation taken here builds on notions of diversity or richness of linguistic forms, strategies, and patterns from sociolinguistics, adding a psycholinguistic perspective on variation as a mechanism in language use. The claim is: richer variation will allow a speaker to generate more language, more varied language and in more contexts. When the bilingual speaker produces codeswitching or code interference, a variant is produced. The mechanism by which choices are made is variation – variation in presentation of self, in deciding who to interact with, in choosing a topic, in selecting a speech act, in accessing a lexical representation. The variation mechanism allows the speaker to select from a range of linguistic options and manipulate them to fit his/her social identity and specific intentions. The variation mechanism is grounded in the basic processes of *discrimination* and *classification*.

In both schizophrenia and DLD, processing demands in other domains (e.g., lexical selection in schizophrenics, temporal integration in DLD) may lead to impairment in the variation mechanism, which in turn may have similar or different manifestations in the two phenomena.

Representation and typological differences

Insight into abstract linguistic representations can be attained by taking advantage of contrasting typological differences between a bilingual's two languages, particularly in the areas of morphology and syntax. For example, English is morphologically "sparse" and requires an overt sentence subject, whereas Russian, Hebrew, and Spanish are relatively rich in their inflectional morphologies. Russian has a rich morphological case system; English, Hebrew, and Spanish do not. All four languages have prepositions, some which are governed by verbs (and obligatory) and others used to introduce adverbial prepositional phrases, such as locatives, temporals, and instrumentals. Syntactically, English, Russian, Hebrew, and Spanish are all SVO languages, but show different degrees of freedom in word order, with English and Spanish less flexible than Russian and Hebrew. Russian, Hebrew, and Spanish all allow null subjects, but English does not. The use of null subjects in Hebrew is more limited than its use in Spanish. On the borders of syntax, semantics, and pragmatics, English and Spanish have both definite and indefinite articles, Hebrew has only a definite article, and Russian has neither, but marks definiteness by demonstratives and changes in word order.

These typological differences lead to code interference in bilinguals. Zdorenko and Paradis (2008) and Schönenberger et al. (2011) report that bilingual children who speak a home language with articles/determiners (like Hebrew) outperform children whose home language does not have articles (like Russian) when acquiring the article system in English. Russian speakers' omission of definite articles in English and Hebrew suggests that a slot for this morpheme is missing in their underlying representation. Inappropriate insertion of definite articles in these languages may be attributed to interference of semantic and pragmatic constraints from the home language (see Zdorenko & Paradis, 2008) or show that a speaker has acquired a representation for grammatical definiteness, but may not yet have acquired all of the semantic and pragmatic constraints on their use, as found in monolingual acquisition (Armon-Lotem & Avram, 2005).

Typological differences have also been found in the clinical markers for DLD. In English, root infinitives are clinical markers for DLD (Rice & Wexler, 1996), whereas in Hebrew, children with DLD show weakness in some aspects of the inflectional system, but this is not a diagnostic for DLD. A combination of inflectional and derivational factors seems to offer a better diagnostic (Dromi et al., 1999; Ravid et al., 2003). For Hebrew-English bilingual children, use of root infinitives in English and difficulties with Hebrew verb morphology could be the result of code interference between very different systems rather than indicators of language impairment, as is reported for learners of English with different first languages (Paradis, 2007).

The interface of bilingualism and language impairment requires that we distinguish processing from representation, and more specifically, differentiate cross-linguistic influence in competing bilingual processing from clinical markers of DLD (Armon-Lotem, 2017). Typological variation can lead to different manifestations of (impaired) linguistic representation and can be differentiated from bilingual competing processing by the quantity and quality of errors. Impaired representation results in omission errors (of phonemes in cluster reduction, morphemes in root infinitives, or sentence fragments), while bilingual competing processing was found to yield substitutions due to shared storage. In contrast, bilingual schizophrenics should present a relatively intact morpho-syntactic system in their native language and the same kind of code interference as non-impaired bilinguals in their second language.

Code switching and code interference

Codeswitching, a unique feature of bilingualism, is the use of two languages in a single utterance, across utterances and across speakers. Sociolinguistically, codeswitching reflects a speaker's social awareness of the setting, topic and language background of the people addressed. Pragmatically, it marks emphasis, focus or topic shifts, and is used to maintain fluency or to compensate for difficulties in lexical retrieval. Motivations for codeswitching can be distinguished in terms of intentionality and directionality. For example, a Russian immigrant to the US might codeswitch into English to show how much she understood about her new job but would codeswitch back to Russian to describe a particular kind of existential frustration because English doesn't have a term with Russian flavor. Similarly, an Argentinian-born ivy-league professor who feigns a non-native accent in English in order to project her minority identity in faculty meetings, might converse in accentless, idiomatic English with her native English-speaking graduate students. Sociopragmatic codeswitching is goal-driven and motivated by identity as well as external, contextual factors. Structural-psycholinguistic codeswitching stems from individual linguistic and mental factors, in particular difficulties in finding words and lack of structural equivalence across languages, when the bilingual is confronted with word finding and fluency issues. In processing terms, codeswitching is characterized as involving the mechanisms of imitation and variation.

In early bilingual acquisition, codeswitching occurs across speakers and intrasententially. Despite 50 years of scientific research on codeswitching, folk wisdom says that it causes confusion and leads to problems in school. But, as Zentella (1997) states so strongly, the pediatrician, school official, or other "professional" makes this kind of assessment based on very limited data. The child is usually assessed in the majority language. The diversity of patterns of bilingualism and socialization in the home, in the neighborhood, and in the schoolyard are often ignored (but see Bedore & Peña, 2008). This situation has changed somewhat in the past few years (due to new ASHA guidelines, Bilingualism Matters, and research networks like COST Action IS0840), but there is still a long way to go.

Structural properties of codeswitching (e.g., where it occurs syntactically) alone cannot say unequivocally whether a bilingual's two languages are represented in like fashion or whether they are differentiated. Neither can structural and distributional features of codeswitching in the environment, e.g., how much and where family members codeswitch, directionality from L1→L2 or L2→L1, tell the whole story about questions of representation. However, coupled with information about identity, context, genre, and intention, this structural information can offer a wider picture of the role of codeswitching in bilingualism, and as claimed here, as a diagnostic of language impairment. We have found directionality and psycholinguistic motivations for codeswitching to be excellent indicators of language dominance in both schizophrenics and children with DLD (Iluz-Cohen & Walters, 2012; Smirnova et al., 2015; Soesman & Walters, 2021; Soesman & Walters, in press).

Code interference is closely related to codeswitching. Three constructs are relevant here: completeness, fluency, and automaticity. Completeness is grounded in the structural or representational aspects of language. The products of one or both languages in bilinguals are incomplete because their linguistic representations are incomplete. In the lexical domain, bilingual lemmas, perhaps more so than their monolingual counterparts, are not full-scale OED (*Oxford English Dictionary*) entries. Rather, they are potentially "incomplete" – phonologically, syntactically, semantically, and pragmatically.

Fluency and automaticity are processes, reflections of incompleteness. Fluency is linguistically defined; automaticity cuts across perceptual and cognitive domains. Along these lines, dysfluency results when:

- Information from the two languages has not been accurately or appropriately copied from memory (due to deficiencies in storage, search, or retrieval).

- There is underuse, overuse, inappropriate use of the imitation and/or variation mechanisms.
- Imitation and variation are out of balance, i.e., when the control mechanism indicates disturbances (e.g., unstable relations between intentions and perceptions).

Dysfluency manifests itself as hesitations, pauses, false starts, repetitions, use of discourse markers as space fillers and lexical inventions. Two additional bilingual phenomena related to code interference and fluency are *size of lexicon* and *rate of speech*. Bilinguals' vocabulary size, both children and adults, is marked by lexical gaps and size limitations, which lead to word-finding difficulties. Vocabulary size is a structural issue, and rate of speech is a processing phenomenon. Both contribute to fluency.

Research on bilingual DLD and schizophrenia

Our research on bilingualism and language impairment in DLD and schizophrenia is marked by its wide range of linguistic indicators, including morphosyntactic features of verbs and prepositions, lexis, syntax, pragmatics, and social factors. Due to space limitations, we focus on verbal morphosyntax, prepositions, syntactic structures, and narrative abilities in DLD and clinical as well as linguistic indicators in schizophrenia.

Bilingual DLD

Verbal Morphosyntax. For DLD, the bilingual children were all English-Hebrew successive bilinguals, immigrant children with at least two years of exposure to the L2 in Hebrew-speaking preschool programs. In one paper (Armon-Lotem, Adam, & Walters, 2008), we examined use of verbal inflections by 15 English-Hebrew preschool bilinguals, ages four to seven: six typically developing (TD) bilinguals from regular preschools and nine language impaired bilinguals placed in "language preschools" following standardized SLP assessments. All children were screened again, at time of study, identifying four types of bilingual profiles: typical development in both languages (TD), atypical development in both languages (A-TD), and typical development in one language (English: E-TD; Hebrew: H-TD).

Using a case studies approach and multiple tasks (sentence completion, sentence imitation and productions/enactment), we found similar errors for all bilinguals, with a significance difference in quantity across the different groups. In English, both TD bilinguals and E-TD bilinguals tended to use root infinitives in up to 20% of the relevant contexts. By contrast, A-TD bilinguals showed the same kind of errors in 50–60% of the relevant contexts, like monolingual children with DLD. In Hebrew, the TD bilinguals used the wrong person inflection in 16% of the contexts, which targeted verbs inflected for first and second person. A-TD bilinguals substituted first and second person forms like TD bilinguals, but did so in 50–60% of the relevant contexts. By contrast, E-TD children opted for the bare form, omitting person morphology altogether in 50–60% of the relevant contexts.

These findings raised the question as to whether quantitative differences are enough to diagnose language impairment in bilinguals. Is the high ratio of root infinitives indicative of DLD in the A-TD bilinguals? Does this mean that the E-TD group is not DLD? Is the high ratio of person substitution indicative of DLD in the A-TD group? Are the omissions of person morphology in Hebrew indicative of DLD in the E-TD group?

We propose that since the E-TD bilinguals perform like TD children in their L1, they are not DLD by definition, but rather slow second language learners, who have not mastered the inflectional system of their L2. More specifically, their errors reflect a strategy which is unlike Hebrew typical and impaired acquisition. The E-TD bilinguals had difficulties with the uninterpretable person features which are not available in their L1. These features are sensitive to critical period

(White, 2003), and so the E-TD bilinguals show an error pattern that reflects the acquisition of L2 after the critical period. For the A-TD children, though tense-marking may not be a qualitative clinical indicator of DLD in bilingual populations, the quantity of errors, when manifested in both languages, is a potential indicator. That is, quantitative and qualitative differences when found in both languages can be indicative of DLD, while a qualitative difference only in the second language is not.

Prepositions. Twelve children with language impairment (LI) who attended special "language preschools" after being diagnosed as language impaired by a speech clinician and seven with TD who attended regular preschools were tested. Children's ages ranged from four years to seven years and four months, and they all came from the same bilingual neighborhood and same (middle-high) SES. Our case study approach made it possible to start profiling the different groups.

Data were analyzed for quantity of errors, according to the following categories:

- Substitution with code interference: The baby laughed **on** the clown.
- Substitution with no code interference: The baby laughed **to** the clown.
- Omission with code interference: The elephant pulled ***(down)** the zebra's pants.
- Omission with no code interference: The baby laughed ***(at)** the clown.

Both TD and LI children had errors in prepositions due to code interference, but LI children also showed substitutions of prepositions which could not be explained by code interference. This was true for both languages, with verb governed prepositions being more problematic than locatives and temporals in English. There were very few omission errors, which were mostly restricted to the ATD group.

A study of preposition use with 15 children with Language Impairment (LI) who were ATD (six male, nine female) and 11 Typically Developing (TD) children (three male, eight female), showed evidence of code interference for both typically developing and language impaired bilingual children, as manifested by substitution errors. Different performance on obligatory (verb-governed) and free prepositions (locatives and temporals) distinguished LI and TD bilinguals, with LI children performing better on free than obligatory prepositions and TD children showing no difference on these two forms. Moreover, LI children's omissions were not traceable to code interference. In addition, language specific effects emerged in English, with obligatory prepositions posing greater difficulty than the Hebrew prepositions in this category. Finally, sentence length influenced the proportion of bilingual errors but not LI errors. The findings contribute to the discussion of ways to generate bilingual language samples which are comparable across languages despite structural differences and further suggest a possible new indicator for DLD among bilingual children.

- Only LI children omitted prepositions where there was no code interference.
- Both TD and LI children show unsystematic substitutions which are not due to code interference, with a quantitative difference between the two groups.
- Utterance length had a different influence on the two types of prepositions and errors.

Syntactic abilities are addressed with a sentence repetition task. Sentence repetition has been found to provide reliable access to multiple syntactic structures and high accuracy in the assessment of DLD among monolinguals. The LITMUS–SRep task used for the present study (Marinis & Armon-Lotem, 2015) includes a wide range of structures, some which can be assessed in both languages of the studied population (word order, questions, biclausal sentences, relative clauses, and conditionals) and some that are language-specific (case, inflectional morphology). An investigation of the performance on morpho-syntax among 45 Russian-Hebrew sequential bilingual preschool children with and without DLD (30 biTLD and 15 biDLD) in both languages (Meir et al., 2016) revealed "that both the quantity and the quality of errors differentiate the two bilingual groups." In both languages (L1 and L2), bilingual children with TLD outperformed their peers with DLD on eight structures (SOV, OVS, biclausal sentences with subordination, oblique questions, subject relatives, object relatives, real and unreal conditionals). The difficulty with questions and relative clauses was of special interest, since findings for these structures replicate difficulties reported for monolingual children with DLD (e.g., Friedmann & Novogdrodsky, 2004, 2011). Results showed four main error patterns which distinguish children with biSLI from those with biTLD: sentence fragments, omission of coordinators and subordinators, omission of prepositions, and simplification of wh-questions and relative clauses, all of them involving simplification. These specific error patterns on structures shared across the two languages replicate those previously reported for monolingual children with DLD and could not be attributed to L1–L2 influence, while the errors of children in the biTLD group could be traced to cross-linguistic influence (mostly L2 influence on L1).

Narrative and discourse abilities are elicited with multiple stimulus materials, including response to picture books, and retelling of stories presented orally or via interactive role playing. A series of papers (Altman et al., 2016; Fichman et al., 2017; Fichman et al., 2020) analyzed narrative abilities of Russian-Hebrew bilingual preschool children with and without DLD using the LITMUS-MAIN (Multilingual Assessment Instrument for Narratives, Gagarina et al., 2012) protocols which involved storytelling and retelling tasks in both languages. Analyses focused on story grammar elements and causal relations in order to identify macrostructure features which distinguish bilingual children with DLD from those with typical development.

Differences between groups of children with DLD and TLD emerged for the proportion of Goal-Attempt-Outcome sequences across the three episodes of the narratives. For story grammar elements, BiDLD children included fewer elements than BiTD children in the first episode of their stories, but performed similarly to BiTD children in the second and third episodes. Differences between these groups also resulted for the proportion of Enabling, Physical, and Motivational relations. Narratives of children with BiDLD contained fewer Enabling and Physical relations, and differed qualitatively from those of BiTD children. Analyses of causal relations showed the importance of linguistic expressions (mental state terms) in narrative coherence. Mental state terms were used differently by children with BiTD and BiDLD. Children with BiDLD also showed weakness in using adequate referential expressions by omitting antecedents and/or producing ambiguous pronouns to maintain character reference. Such studies show the importance of examining a wider array of macrostructure features in narratives than in previous research.

Schizophrenia in two languages

Our approach to the relation between schizophrenia and bilingualism parallels the work in bilingual DLD. We want to identify linguistic indicators which may be unique to schizophrenia which are not influenced by second language use. We examine clinical indicators (blocking, topic shift) and a range of linguistic markers (exophoric reference, lexical repetition, incomplete syntax, unclear reference) of schizophrenia and two bilingual/discourse phenomena (codeswitching, discourse markers) in order to begin disentangling bilingualism and schizophrenia.

Cognitive dysfunction has been found to correlate better with schizophrenic phenomena than traditional diagnostic criteria such as delusions, hallucinations, and flat affect (Perry et al. 2001; Park et al. 2003). Cognitively, schizophrenia includes executive functions and working memory. Linguistically, the illness is defined and diagnosed by disorganized speech and thought, e.g., topic switching, alogia, derailment, incoherence, blocking, poverty of content of speech, poverty of speech, derailment, thought-disorder, loose associations, incoherence, and word salad. Avolition and affective disturbance are also expressed to some extent in language, leading to social dysfunction. While current thinking in research and clinical practice labels schizophrenia a cognitive disorder, all aspects of the illness involve language behavior (Fine, 2006). Current research offers a number of explanatory proposals which shed light on the role of language in schizophrenia, among them diminished lateralization (Liddle et al., 2007), attention and sequencing difficulties (Docherty, 2005), and impaired ability to build up context verbally and non-verbally.

Since the previous edition of this Handbook (Guendouzi et al., 2010), the literature on SZ and bilingualism has added four systematic review articles (Dugan, 2014; Erkoreka, 2020; Seeman, 2016; Smirnova et al., 2019), but unfortunately only a few empirical studies (Lutz et al., 2021; Samuel & Boeckl, 2022; Smirnova et al., 2015). We describe here the work from our lab as background for the research strategy outlined below.

In one study (Bersudsky et al., 2005) eight diagnosed bilinguals with SZ were matched with healthy bilinguals for age, gender, and educational level, and speech data were collected via sociolinguistic interviews and transcribed for analysis. One clinical measure and four linguistic measures which have shown differences between schizophrenics and different control groups (Caplan et al., 2000; Goren et al., 1995; Rochester & Martin, 1979) were examined.

The clinical measure, blocking (sudden inability to participate in the interview due to word or thought retrieval difficulties), successfully distinguished the two populations, only the schizophrenics showing evidence of blocking. The linguistic measures – incomplete syntax, lexical repetition, and unclear reference – revealed virtually no differences between schizophrenics and healthy bilinguals. One other measure, exophoric reference (to the physical context of the interaction), did appear more in the transcripts of the patient group, but this may have been an artifact of the interview procedure. Thus, based on clinical diagnosis (PANNS) and linguistic measures showing differences between clinical and typical populations, we concluded that our eight schizophrenics were very similar to other immigrant language learners. Next, approaching the data from a second language/bilingual perspective, we looked at three additional indicators from the areas of morphosyntax, lexis and pragmatics/discourse.

Morphosyntax

Structures based on typological similarities and differences between Russian and Hebrew were examined. Gender agreement for nouns and adjectives, preposition use, and verb tense morphology showed appropriate use in both schizophrenics and healthy immigrants. At the other end of the difficulty scale, the definite article does not exist in Russian and thus poses major difficulties due to its presence as a prefix on Hebrew nouns. It is also a highly frequent form in Hebrew. Appropriate use of definite articles in Hebrew, then, is a good indicator of the extent to which Russian native speakers have acquired Hebrew. In the present study, contexts in which the definite article was obligatory were counted and the proportion of appropriate obligatory use was calculated. On the whole, schizophrenics afforded themselves fewer opportunities to use definite articles, and their error patterns (both omissions and substitutions) were very similar to those of the controls. For schizophrenics, appropriate use of definite articles ranged from 13% to 82% of obligatory uses of the article (M=58.9%); for healthy immigrants, appropriate use ranged from 47% to 90% (M=72.6). Individual analyses revealed that four healthy immigrants performed better than the schizophrenics, but four other schizophrenics performed equal to or better than the controls.

Lexis

Type-token ratios, measures of lexical diversity, were calculated for both an overall estimate of diversity and for diversity of content words. In Hebrew, a morphologically rich language, prepositions, pronouns, and determiners appear both as prefixes and suffixes attached to nouns and verbs as well as independent function words. The findings for schizophrenics and healthy L2 learners differed very little, the data showing very similar mean lexical diversity (0.36 vs. 0.39, respectively) and range (0.12 vs. 0.19).

Pragmatics/discourse

Four markers were selected to cover a range of discourse and pragmatic functions (*az* "so," *ze* "this," *em* "um," *eh* "uh"). Only one group difference emerged, schizophrenics producing almost twice as many fluency markers (*eh*) as healthy immigrants. Moreover, a very large proportion of these forms came during blocking, the clinical indicator of schizophrenia. The picture that emerges, then, from these discourse and pragmatic data continues to show that immigrant schizophrenics use language very much like their healthy counterparts.

For the bilingual measure examined (codeswitching), there were again no differences between schizophrenics and healthy language learners, and only six participants (three in each group) codeswitched at all. The very limited use of codeswitching during the interviews attests to the fact that even schizophrenics were well aware of the social norms of the interview situation (despite the fact that they knew the interviewer to be bilingual in Russian and Hebrew). Finally, both groups presented the same range of language learner phenomena, including interference/translation strategies, use of routine phrases, and self-monitoring.

A second study (Smirnova et al., 2015) was aimed to avoid the inherent variability in comparing small numbers of patients with healthy subjects and take advantage of bilingualism as an opportunity to implement a within-subject design.

From a pool of 60 patients diagnosed clinically (PANNS evaluation), ten (eight males and two females) ranging in age from 25 to 59 (M=33.8), who met the following criteria were identified: (1) clear signs of thought disorder in their schizophrenic diagnosis; (2) homogeneity in terms of age, age at the time of immigration, length of residence in Israel; (3) age at the onset/diagnosis of illness. These patients participated in two sessions, one in their preferred language (Russian) and the other in Hebrew/L2, with a bilingual interviewer.

A range of clinical and linguistic indicators of schizophrenia and two bilingual discourse phenomena were examined. Clinical markers of SZ (blocking, topic shifting) were similar in L1 and L2, but four linguistic markers of SZ (incomplete syntax, lexical repetition, exophoric reference, and unclear reference) showed more frequent presentation in L2/Hebrew than in L1/Russian. Thus, despite the patients' relative success in acquiring L2, linguistic markers of SZ were evident in that second language.

The bilingual discourse measures (CS and DMs) showed a high level of individual variation and different manifestations in the two languages. For CS, eight of ten patients codeswitched more from L1/Russian to L2/Hebrew in order to compensate for difficulties in lexical retrieval and to maintain fluency. The other two patients showed disproportionate CS (they had more CS than any of the other patients and did so primarily from L2 to L1). None of their demographic or clinical background could explain this pattern.

Discourse markers also showed more prevalence in L1/Russian than in L2/Hebrew (six times as many occurrences). The finding for DMs belies the fact that patients declared a preference for Russian and the bilingual experimenter who conducted both Russian and Hebrew interview sessions reported proficiency to be better in Russian than in Hebrew. It may, however, hint at impairment in social skills grounded in language. More detailed analyses are needed to clarify this speculation.

The dissociation among clinical, linguistic, and discourse indicators of SZ and different manifestations across the two languages has both research and clinical implications. On the one hand, despite diagnosis, patients with schizophrenia are capable of using and varying two features of language use, CS and DMs, both of which show social awareness of interlocutors as well as awareness of the need to maintain fluency.

Research and assessment strategy

The methodological approach we use is based on large amounts of data, collected with a variety of tasks and procedures from relatively small numbers of subjects from bilingual backgrounds, matched with typically developing bilinguals for age and language for children and for education and occupation for adults. In order to deal with the heterogeneity of bilingualism and neurolinguistic disorders, we conduct within-subject, cross-language case studies of a range of linguistic phenomena. Data analyses proceed in stages, focusing first on the individual subject, with comparisons across languages, linguistic markers, and tasks; next on comparisons of bilingual impaired subjects matched linguistically and chronologically with unimpaired bilingual subjects, and finally on group comparisons, across languages, linguistic features, and tasks. Such studies are then followed by more robust research to check for specificity and sensitivity once the clinical markers have been identified.

Three general principles guide this approach. They have been implemented in the development of the tools for the LITMUS battery within the framework of COST Action IS0840 (Armon-Lotem et al., 2015). One essential requirement is to assess and collect data in *both languages*. This practice follows the principle that language impairment in children and psychiatric disorders in adults should be manifested in both languages of a bilingual. Second, since a bilingual is more than a sum of her two languages, assessing one language can be highly misleading, especially if the assessment is done in the less dominant language. Thus, the individual is the primary unit of analysis, and group data are examined only after labor-intensive analyses of individual cases (see Guendouzi, 2003 on the importance of individual analysis). A third principle is that assessment measures should not be literal translations of words and structures; rather they need to be developed and constructed by taking into account the typological differences and similarities manifested in the two languages.

Beyond these general guidelines, methodological choices in studies of bilingual language acquisition and use involve several sampling decisions. These choices include:

1. The specific linguistic structures to investigate.
2. The tasks and response measures needed to elicit those structures.
3. Which bilingual speakers to choose to examine.

The question of which linguistic structures to examine poses a problem of whether to aim for depth or breadth. Linguistic studies tend to aim for depth in their quest for answers to focused research questions (e.g., Genesee, 2001 for bilingualism; Rice & Wexler, 1996 for DLD), while clinical and psycho-educational studies seek breadth (e.g., Stuart-Smith & Martin, 1999) and tend to use standardized measures. The selection of structures for each language should rely on previous knowledge about the domains that are affected by DLD across languages alongside language specific properties. It is recommended to always begin from a broad set of structures and test them in order to identify a reduced set with greater ecological validity. Once relevant structures and functions in the two languages have been selected, tasks and response measures can be derived from the theoretical constructs. Nevertheless, the comparison of impaired bilinguals and "typically developing bilinguals," still remains, introducing a lot of variance to the study.

The unpredictability in these sources of variance and the inherent confounding in designing studies which can keep track of all of them favor a "bilingual" approach based on large amounts of data, gathered in both languages, from relatively small numbers of bilinguals, each individual offering a relatively self-contained basis for analysis and interpretation. In the terminology of design and statistics, each subject in effect serves as his or her own control. Thus, bilingualism offers a unique opportunity to avoid the pitfalls of group comparisons and between-subject designs which are inevitably victims of the kind of heterogeneity discussed above with regard to defining bilingualism. The remainder of this section outlines the choices we make in terms of identification of participants, selection of stimuli, tasks and procedures, and data analyses.

Participant selection

For the study of bilingual DLD, we focus on children ages four to seven with bilingual backgrounds in English-Hebrew and Russian-Hebrew, conducting cross-linguistic, intra-subject comparisons on a case-by-case basis. Within-subject comparisons reduce the impact of the socio-cultural differences. We choose children from similar SES and from L2 (Hebrew-speaking) preschools with a majority of native speakers of the target language. We use parent questionnaires (Abutbul-Oz & Armon-Lotem, 2022) to gather as much information as possible about the children's linguistic and non-linguistic background and their language experience in both languages, using the parents as agents to learn about the child's language use in natural contexts. We select participants from among LI children since LI children represent a clinically referred population, but at the same time aim at identifying children who show low performance in both languages and have parental concerns about their language development. This approach is motivated by the reported over-representation of bilingual children in language units, and under-diagnosis of DLD among bilingual children in regular schools. Given the heterogeneity in the bilingual population, we have limited our work to simultaneous bilinguals who use both languages at home and early successive bilinguals, where the child is exposed to one language at home and another in pre-school prior to the age of three, i.e., early L2 acquirers. We include only early bilinguals who are able to carry on a conversation in both languages and whose two languages are balanced for a range of linguistic measures (e.g., MLU), excluding late bilinguals who began acquiring L2 after the age of three. Finally, all participants are cognitively, emotionally, and neurologically unimpaired but show primary language disorder, using bilingual standards for normed tests developed in our lab. These standards take into consideration the interaction between chronological age and the age of onset of bilingual exposure in calculating the means and standard deviations for bilingual development (Altman et al., 2021; Armon-Lotem et al., 2021). With these bilingual standards, children are identified with DLD if they are between -1.25SD and -1.5SD (depending on the specifics of the standardized measure and conventional practice in using it) behind typically developing bilinguals for both languages. Where standardized measures do not exist, it is recommended to use a combination of a sentence repetition task and non-word repetition task in both languages to reflect the contrastive structures of the two languages, together with a parent questionnaire (Armon-Lotem et al., 2015).

For schizophrenia, we identify patients from a hospital environment, choosing participants from a larger outpatient pool who have been evaluated with standardized instruments (PANNS) and clinical interviews, focusing on language-based indicators: disorganized speech, derailment, alogia. Language proficiency in both languages is evaluated by bilingual research assistants in three domains: lexis, grammar, and fluency.

Stimulus selection based on contrast across languages

Typological differences and similarities serve as the theoretical basis for development of stimuli. Target structures include those which are similar in both languages and those which are contrastive, allowing investigation of transfer as well as code interference. For example, in the area of verbal morphosyntax we targeted present and past tense morphemes in English, tense, number, gender, and conjugation (pattern) morphology in Hebrew, tense and aspect in Russian. For prepositions, we distinguish "obligatory" prepositions lexically or grammatically selected by the verb from "free" prepositions which introduce adverbial (locative/temporal) preposition phrases with parallel and contrastive stimuli across language pairs. For syntactic structure we have been using the LITMUS-SRep task (Marinis & Armon-Lotem, 2015) in multiple languages, since it is designed precisely along the lines described above with object questions and relative clauses as typologically similar structures and passive vs. topicalization, or auxiliaries vs. negation as language specific properties.

Due to the exploratory nature of research on schizophrenic language and findings of largely intact grammatical systems in the second language, our research has relied primarily on sociolinguistic interviews and narrative recall. Future studies will investigate lexical and pragmatic deficits along the same lines described here for bilingual children with DLD.

Tasks and procedures

Each participant is assessed with a wide range of tasks. In addition to the tasks presented above (e.g. sentence repetition and narrative retelling), we have used the following.

1. The Bilingual Parent Questionnaire (BIPAQ) (Abutbul-Oz & Armon-Lotem, 2022), developed alongside the PaBiQ (Tuller, 2015) from an SLP's perspective, is designed to serve as a protocol for soliciting background information in five sections: (A) demographic information, (B) developmental background, (C) home language abilities, (D) societal language abilities, and (E) quantity and quality of exposure to both home and societal. A scoring system is available for sections (B), (C), and (D) with a cut-off point that indicates risk for DLD. Section (E) quantifies various forms of current and past exposure, where exposure is measured by length of exposure to the societal language-Hebrew (LoE), age of first exposure to the societal language-Hebrew (AoB), exposure to both the home and societal languages during the past year and in the educational setting, and present exposure (hourly week-day child interactions with different interlocutors). Quality of exposure is measured by evaluation of the proficiency of primary caregivers and frequency of specific language-related activities (e.g., reading, singing) in each language as measures of input richness.
2. Guided play with a uniform set of toys in two settings: kitchen and playground, where "kitchen" represents the home environment and is expected to elicit more spontaneous speech in the home language and "playground" represents the school environment and is expected to elicit more spontaneous speech in the societal/school language.
3. A pragmatic-discourse task involving role playing, e.g., a doctor/patient situation. For this task the context is constrained by the role relationship, allowing examination of pragmatic choices and sociolinguistic appropriateness.
4. Social identity as elicited via person perception and ethnolinguistic identity procedures (Armon-Lotem et al., 2013; Walters et al., 2014).

This range of tasks serves as the basis for bilingual profiles, allowing comparison across languages and examination of task effects both within and across languages.

Data analyses: from individual profiles to group patterns

Data analyses include some measures which cut across tasks (e.g., omission and substitution errors) and others which are unique to certain tasks (e.g., story grammar categories for narratives, discourse markers for spontaneous speech). With the individual participant as the primary unit of analysis, comparisons across languages, linguistic markers, and tasks are conducted with a careful eye on individual variation and conservative use of statistics complemented by qualitative linguistic analyses of language use and errors.

(a) Cross-language measures

In order to prepare linguistic data for analyses, we first identify all the obligatory contexts for a particular structure. For verbal morphology and prepositions, these are the contexts in which a particular verb form is expected to appear. For prepositions, the procedure is the same. For narrative structure, obligatory contexts are not as clear-cut, notwithstanding findings from story grammar research. Thus, we transcribe the narratives, pair the subject's utterances with the picture or oral stimuli and then identify the narrative categories. Beyond each separate linguistic domain, we also examine performance across domains, e.g., lexical abilities in spontaneous speech, role playing and narrative; verbal inflections and prepositions in these tasks as well as in story completion, sentence imitation and other tasks which specifically target these structures. Social identity indicators such as names, pronouns, and discourse markers in actual language use are also examined.

Error analyses are particularly useful. We have looked at (1) the quantity of errors, (2) comparisons of omissions and substitutions, (3) qualitative assessment of errors which can be traced to code interference, and (4) errors which are unique and cannot be traced to either of the child's languages.

Additional cross-language measures comparing individual performance for each individual include: (1) proficiency as indicated by standardized language tests; MLU/MPU; verb-based utterances (percentage of verbs per utterance); subjective ratings of lexis, grammar, and fluency; non-word repetition designed to capture typological contrasts in morphophonology; and pragmatic variation (2) structure of the lexicon (e.g., content/function word distributions) and lexical diversity; (3) fluency measures (e.g., pauses, repetitions, discourse markers);

(b) Measures of bilingualism

(i) Codeswitching (analyses based on frequency, grammatical category, locus of the switch, directionality, and motivations) in narrative, retelling, and role playing tasks; (ii) background information including age, gender, birth order, length and amount of exposure to L1 and L2.

Coda

From this modest attempt to disentangle bilingualism from language impairment in DLD and SZ, the constructs of representation and processing, along with our current findings, point us in a number of important directions. First, it is clear we should not compromise on the necessity to examine our participants in both languages. This procedure alone may help distinguish neurogenetic impairment like DLD from more socio-psychiatric conditions. A methodological requirement is to focus on individual case studies, with their accompanying benefits of within-subject, cross-language analyses, avoiding the inherent heterogeneity of group comparisons. In addition, as we saw in our studies of bilingual DLD, a broad range of linguistic features was necessary to assess typological differences and to allow for the possibility that not all features would be clinically relevant. Finally, the societal imperative of research and assessment on bilingual language impairment makes data on identity, attitudes, preferences, language use, and exposure patterns crucial to studies of this type.

References

Abutbul-Oz, H., & Armon-Lotem, S. (2022). Parent Questionnaires in screening for Developmental Language Disorder among bilingual children in speech and language clinics. *Frontiers in Education*, 7, 846111.

Allard, R., & Landry, R. (1994). Subjective ethnolinguistic vitality: A comparison of two measures. *International Journal of the Sociology of Language*, *108*(1), 117–144.

Altman, C., Schrauf, R., & Walters, J. (2012). Crossovers and codeswitching in the investigation of immigrant autobiographical memory. In L. Isurin & J. Altarriba (Eds.), *Memory, language, and bilingualism: Theoretical and applied approaches* (pp. 211–235). Cambridge University Press.

Altman, C., Armon-Lotem, S., Fichman, S., & Walters, J. (2016). Macrostructure, microstructure, and mental state terms in the narratives of English–Hebrew bilingual preschool children with and without specific language impairment. *Applied Psycholinguistics*, *37*(1), 165–193.

Altman, C., Harel, E., Meir, N., Iluz-Cohen, P., Walters, J., & Armon-Lotem, S. (2021). Using a monolingual screening test for assessing bilingual children. *Clinical Linguistics and Phonetics*. https://doi.org/10.1080/02699206.2021.2000644

Anderson, N. H. (1996). *A functional theory of cognition*. Lawrence Erlbaum Associates.

Armon-Lotem, S. (2017). Variations in Phonological Working memory: The contribution of impaired representation and bilingual processing. *Applied Psycholinguistics*, *38*(6), 1305–1313.

Armon-Lotem, S., & Avram, I. (2005). The autonomous contribution of syntax and pragmatic: The acquisition of the Hebrew definite article. In A.-M. Di Sciullo & R. Delmonte (Eds.), *Universal Grammar and the external systems* (pp. 169–182). John Benjamins.

Armon-Lotem, S., Adam, G., & Walters, J. (2008). Verb inflections as indicators of bilingual SLI. In *Proceedings of the reading child language seminar* (pp. 25–36). University of Reading.

Armon-Lotem, S., Joffe, S., Oz-Abutbul, H., Altman, C., & Walters, J. (2013). Ethno-linguistic identity, language exposure and language acquisition in bilingual preschool children from English and Russian- speaking backgrounds. In Th. Gruter & J. Paradie (Eds.), *Input and experience in bilingual development. TILAR Series* (pp. 77–98). John Benjamins.

Armon-Lotem, S., de Jong, J., & Meir, N. (Eds.) (2015). *Assessing multilingual children: Disentangling bilingualism from Specific Language Impairment.* Multilingual Matters

Armon-Lotem, S., Rose, K., & Altman, C. (2021). The development of English as a Heritage Language: The role of chronological age and age of onset of bilingualism. *First Language, 41*(1), 67–89.

Austin, J. (1962). How to Do Things with Words: The William James Lectures delivered at Harvard University in 1955 J. O. Urmson & M. Sbisà (Eds.). Oxford: Clarendon Press.

Bedore, L. M., & Peña, E. D. (2008). Assessment of bilingual children for identification of language impairment: Current findings and implications for practice. *International Journal of Bilingual Education and Bilingualism, 11*(1), 1–29.

Bersudsky, Y., Fine, J., Gorjaltsan, I., Chen, O., & Walters, J. (2005). Schizophrenia and second language acquisition. *Progress in Neuro-Psychopharmacology and Biological Psychiatry, 29*(4), 535–542.

Bialystok, E. (2001). *Bilingualism in development: Language, literacy, and cognition.* Cambridge University Press.

Bialystok, E., & Senman, L. (2004). Executive processes in appearance-reality tasks: The role of inhibition of attention and symbolic representation. *Child Development, 75*(2), 562–579.

Caplan, R., Guthrie, D., Tang, B., Komo, S., & Asarnow, R. F. (2000). Thought disorder in childhood schizophrenia: Replication and update of concept. *Journal of the American Academy of Child and Adolescent Psychiatry, 39*(6), 771–778.

Caramazza, A., Yeni-Komshian, G., Zurif, E., & Carbone, E. (1973). The acquisition of a new phonological contrast: The case of stop consonants in French-English bilinguals. *Journal of the Acoustical Society of America, 54*(2), 421–428.

Costa, A., Pannunzi, M., Deco, G., & Pickering, M. J. (2016). Do bilinguals automatically activate their native language when they are not using it? *Cognitive Science, 41*(6), 1629–1644.

Cummins, J. (1976). The influence of bilingualism on cognitive growth: A synthesis of research findings and explanatory hypotheses. *Working Papers on Bilingualism, 9*, 1–43.

De Houwer, A. (2003). Home languages spoken in officially monolingual Flanders: A survey. In K. Bochmann, P. Nelde & W. Wolck (Eds.), *Methodology of conflict linguistics* (pp. 71–87). Asgard.

Docherty, N. M. (2005). Cognitive impairments and disorded speech in schizophrenia: Thought disorder, disorganization, and communication failure perspectives. *Journal of Abnormal Psychology, 114*(2), 269–278.

Dromi, E., Leonard, L., Adam, G., & Zadunaisky-Ehrlich, S. (1999). Verb agreement morphology in Hebrew-speaking children with specific language impairment. *Journal of Speech, Language, and Hearing Research, 42*(6), 1414–1431.

Dugan, J. E. (2014). Second language acquisition and schizophrenia. *Second Language Research, 30*(3), 307–321.

Emmorey, K., Borinstein, H. B., Thompson, R., & Gollan, T. H. (2008). Bimodal bilingualism. *Bilingualism: Language and Cognition, 11*(1), 43–61.

Erkoreka, L., Ozamiz-Etxebarria, N., Ruiz, O., & Ballesteros, J. (2020). Assessment of psychiatric symptomatology in bilingual psychotic patients: A systematic review and meta-analysis. *International Journal of Environmental Research and Public Health, 17*(11), 4137.

Fichman, S., Altman, C., Voloskovich, A., Armon-Lotem, Sh., & Walters, J. (2017). Story grammar elements and causal relations in the narratives of Russian-Hebrew bilingual children with SLI and typical language development. *Journal of Communication Disorders, 69*, 72–93.

Fichman, S., Walters, J., Melamed, R., & Altman, C. (2020). Reference to characters in narratives of Russian-Hebrew bilingual and Russian and Hebrew monolingual children with Developmental Language Disorder and typical language development. *First Language, 40*, 263–291.

Fine, J. (2006). *Language in psychiatry: A handbook of clinical practice.* Equinox.

Fishman, J. A. (1965). Who speaks what language to whom and when? *Linguistique, 2*, 67–88.

Friedmann, N., & Novogrodsky, R. (2004). The acquisition of relative clause comprehension in Hebrew: A study of SLI and normal development. *Journal of Child Language, 31*(3), 661–681.

Friedmann, N., & Novogrodsky, R. (2011). Which questions are most difficult to understand?: The comprehension of Wh questions in three subtypes of SLI. *Lingua, 121*(3), 367–382.

Gagarina, N., Klop, D., Kunnari, S., Tantele, K., Välimaa, T., Balčiūnienė, I., … & Walters, J. (2012). MAIN: multilingual assessment instrument for narratives. *ZAS Papers in Linguistics*, 1–135.

Genesee, F. (2001). Bilingual first language acquisition: Exploring the limits of the language faculty. *Annual Review of Applied Linguistics, 21*, 153–168.

Goren, A. R., Fine, J., Manaim, H., & Apter, A. (1995). Verbal and nonverbal expressions of central deficits in schizophrenia. *Journal of Nervous and Mental Disease, 183*(11), 715–719.

Grainger, J., & Dijkstra, A. (1992). On the representation and use of language information in bilinguals. In R. J. Harris (Ed.), *Cognitive processing in bilinguals* (pp. 207–220). Elsevier Science Publishers B.V.

Green, D. W. (1993). Towards a model of L2 comprehension and production. In R. Schreuder & B. Weltens (Eds.), *The bilingual lexicon* (pp. 249–277). John Benjamins.

Green, D. W. (1998). Mental control of the bilingual Lexico-semantic system. *Bilingualism: Language and Cognition, 1*(2), 67–81.

Green, D. W. (2000). Concepts, experiments and mechanisms. *Bilingualism: Language and Cognition, 3*(1), 16–18.

Green, D.W. (2018) Language Control and Code-switching. *Languages, 3*, 8.

Green, D. W., and Wei, L. (2014). A control process model of code-switching. Language. *Cognition and Neuroscience 29*, 499–511.

Guendouzi, J. (2003). 'SLI', a generic category of language impairment that emerges from specific differences: A case study of two individual linguistic profiles. *Clinical Linguistics and Phonetics, 17*(2), 135–152.

Guendouzi, J., Loncke, F., & Williams, M. (Eds.). (2010). *The handbook of psycholinguistic & cognitive processes: Perspectives in communication disorders.* Taylor & Francis.

Hakuta, K., & D'Andrea, D. (1992). Some properties of bilingual maintenance and loss in Mexican background high-school students. *Applied Linguistics, 13*(1), 72–99.

Iluz-Cohen, P., & Walters, J. (2012). Telling stories in two Languages: Narratives of bilingual preschool children with typical and impaired language. *Bilingualism: Language and Cognition, 15*(1), 58–74.

Kroll, J. F., & De Groot, A. M. B. (1997). Lexical and conceptual memory in the bilingual: Mapping form to meaning in two languages. In A. M. B. de Groot & J. F. Kroll (Eds.), *Tutorials in bilingualism: Psycholinguistic perspectives* (pp. 169–199). Lawrence Erlbaum Publishers.

Kroll, J. F., & Tokowicz, N. (2005). Models of bilingual processing and representation: Looking back and to the future. In J. F. Kroll & A. M. B. de Groot (Eds.), *Handbook of bilingualism: Psycholinguistic approaches* (pp. 531–554). Oxford University Press.

Kroll, J. F., van Hell, J. G., Tokowicz, N., & Green, D. W. (2010). The revised Hierarchical Model: A critical review and assessment. *Bilingualism: Language and Cognition, 13*(3), 373–381.

Kroll, J. F., Dussias, P. E., Bice, K., & Perrotti, L. (2015). Bilingualism, mind, and brain. *Annual Review of Linguistics, 1*, 377–394.

Lambert, W. E. (1990). Issues in foreign language and second language education. In *Proceedings of the first research symposium on limited English proficient student issues.* Office of Bilingual and Multicultural Education.

Liddle, P., White, T., & Francis, S. (2007). Diminished lateralization and focalization of cerebral function in schizophrenia. *Schizophrenia Research, 98*, 19–20.

Lutz, M., Streb, J., Titze, L., Büsselmann, M., Riemat, N., Prüter-Schwarte, C., & Dudeck, M. (2021). Migrants with schizophrenia in forensic psychiatric hospitals benefit from high-intensity second language programs. *Frontiers in Psychiatry, 12*, 711836.

Marinis, T., & Armon-Lotem, S. (2015). Sentence repetition. In S. Armon-Lotem, N. Meir & J. de Jong (Eds.), *Assessing multilingual children: Disentangling bilingualism from language impairment* (pp. 116–143). Multilingual Matters.

Meir, N., Walters, J., & Armon-Lotem, S. (2016). Bi-directional cross-linguistic influence in bilingual Russian-Hebrew children. *Linguistic Approaches to Bilingualism*, 7(5), 514–553.

Meisel, J. M. (2004). The bilingual child. In T. K. Bhatia & W. C. Ritchie (Eds.), *The handbook of bilingualism* (pp. 90–113). Wiley.

Meuter, R. F., & Allport, A. (1999). Bilingual language switching in naming: Asymmetrical costs of language selection. *Journal of Memory and Language, 40*(1), 25–40.

Muysken, P. (2000). *Bilingual speech: a typology of code-mixing.* Cambridge University Press.

Obler, L. K. (1982). The parsimonious bilingual. In L. K. Obler & L. Menn (Eds.), *Exceptional language and linguistics* (pp. 339–346). Academic Press.

Paradis, J. (2007). Bilingual children with specific language impairment: Theoretical and applied issues. *Applied Psycholinguistics, 28*(3), 512–564.

Paradis, J., & Genesee, F. (1997). On continuity and the emergence of functional categories in bilingual first-language acquisition. *Language Acquisition, 6*(2), 91–124.

Park, S., Puschel, J., Sauter, B. H., Rentsch, M., & Hell, D. (2003). Visual object working memory function and clinical symptoms in schizophrenia. *Schizophrenia Research, 59*(2–3), 261–268.

Pearson, B. Z. (2007). Social factors in childhood bilingualism in the United States. *Applied Psycholinguistics, 28*(3), 399–410.

Pearson, B. Z. (2008). *Raising bilingual children: A parents' guide.* Random House.

Pearson, B. Z., Fernandez, S., Lewedag, V., & Oller, D. K. (1997). Input factors in lexical learning of bilingual infants (ages 10 to 30 months). *Applied Psycholinguistics, 18*(1), 41–58.

Perry, W., Heaton, R. K., Potterat, E., Roebuck, T., Minassian, A., & Braff, D. L. (2001). Working memory in schizophrenia: Transient "online" storage versus executive functioning. *Schizophrenia Bulletin, 27*(1), 157–176.

Powers, W. T. (1973). *Behavior: The control of perception.* Aldine.

Powers, W. T. (1978). Quantitative analysis of purposive systems: Some spadework at the foundations of scientific psychology. *Psychology Review, 85*(5), 417–435.

Raichlin, R., Walters, J., & Altman, C. (2018). Some wheres and whys in bilingual codeswitching: Directionality, motivation and locus of codeswitching in Russian-Hebrew bilingual children. *International Journal of Bilingualism, 23*(2), 629–650.

Ravid, D., Levie, R., & Ben-Zvi, G. A. (2003). The role of language typology in linguistic development: Implications for the study of language disorders. In Y. Levy & J. Schaeffer (Eds.), *Language competence across populations: Toward a definition of specific language impairment* (pp. 171–196). Lawrence Erlbaum Associates Publishers.

Rice, M., & Wexler, K. (1996). Toward tense as a clinical marker of specific language impairment in English-speaking children. *Journal of Speech and Hearing Research, 39*, 1239–1257.

Rochester, S., & Martin, J. (1979). *Crazy talk: A study of discourse of schizophrenic speakers.* Plenum.

Samuel, S., & Boeckle, M. (2022). *Schizotypy and theory of mind in a second language: Evidence from German-English bilinguals.* https://doi.org/10.31234/osf.io/uxmz7

Schönenberger, M., Sterner, F., & Ruberg, T. (2011). The realization of indirect objects and case marking in experimental data from child L1 and child L2 German. In J. Herschensohn & D. Tanner (Eds.). Proceedings of the 11th Generative Approaches to Second Language Acquisition Conference (GASLA 2011). Cascadilla (pp. 143–151).

Seeman, M.V. (2016). Bilingualism and schizophrenia. *World Journal of Psychiatry, 6*(2), 192–198.

Smirnova, D., Walters, J., & Fichman, S. (2019). In J. W. Schwieter (Ed.). *The handbook of the neuroscience of multilingualism* (pp. 625–654). John Wiley & Sons, Ltd.

Smirnova, D., Walters, J., Fine, J., Muchnik-Rozanov, Y., Paz, M., Lerner, V., … Bersudsky, Y. (2015). Second language as a compensatory resource for maintaining verbal fluency in bilingual immigrants with schizophrenia. *Neuropsychologia, 97*, 597–606.

Soesman, A., & Walters, J. (2021). Codeswitching within prepositional phrases: Effects of switch site and directionality. *International Journal of Bilingualism, 25*(3), 747–771.

Soesman, A., Walters, J., & Fichman, S. [in press]. Language control and intra-sentential codeswitching among bilingual children with and without Developmental Language Disorder. *Languages.*

Stuart Smith, J., & Martin, D. (1999). Developing assessment procedures for phonological awareness for use with Panjabi-English bilingual children. *International Journal of Bilingualism, 3*(1), 55–80.

Tuller, L. (2015). Clinical use of parental questionnaires in multilingual contexts. In S. Armon-Lotem, J. de Jong & N. Meir (Eds.), *Assessing Multilingual Children: Disentangling bilingualism from language impairment* (pp. 229–328). Multilingual Matters.

Ullman, M. T. (2001). The neural basis of lexicon and grammar in first and second language: The declarative/procedural model. *Bilingualism: Language and Cognition, 4*(2), 105–122.

Ullman, M. T., & Pierpont, E. I. (2005). Specific language impairment is not specific to language: The procedural deficit hypothesis. *Cortex, 41*(3), 399–433.

Walters, J. (2005). *Bilingualism: The sociopragmatic-psycholinguistic interface.* Routledge.

Walters, J., Armon-Lotem, S., Altman, C., Topaj, N., & Gagarina, N. (2014). Language proficiency and social identity in Russian-Hebrew and Russian-German preschool children. In R. K. Silbereisen, Y. Shavit & P. F. Titzmann (Eds.), *The challenges of diaspora migration in today's societies – Interdisciplinary perspectives from research in Israel and Germany* (pp. 45–62). Ashgate.

White, L. (2003). *Second language acquisition and universal grammar.* Cambridge University Press.

Wiig, E. H., Secord, W. A., & Semel, E. M. (2004). *Clinical evaluation of language fundamentals - Preschool, 2.* Psych Corp.

Zdorenko, T., & Paradis, J. (2008). The acquisition of articles in child second language English: Fluctuation, transfer or both? *Second Language Research, 24*(2), 227–250.

Zentella, A. C. (1997). *Growing up bilingual: Puerto Rican children in New York.* Blackwell.

24

CONSTRAINTS-BASED NONLINEAR PHONOLOGY:

Clinical applications for English, Kuwaiti Arabic, and Mandarin

Barbara May Bernhardt, Joseph Stemberger, Hadeel Ayyad, and Jing Zhao

Introduction

Phonological assessment and intervention has benefited from the application of phonological and psycholinguistic theories. In recent decades, constraints-based nonlinear phonological theories (e.g., Clements & Keyser, 1983; Goldsmith, 1976; McCarthy & Prince, 1993) have influenced phonological descriptions. Nonlinear phonological theories describe the hierarchical representation of phonological form from the phrase to the individual feature. Constraints-based theories contrast possibilities and limitations for output (e.g., codas are possible or impossible) when a speaker attempts to produce a word. The following chapter outlines major characteristics of constraints-based nonlinear phonological theories and their application to phonological assessment and intervention for English, Kuwaiti Arabic, and Mandarin. Following Bernhardt and Stemberger (1998), constraints are grounded in the processing of words and the access of phonological elements during the learning process, where only a subset of a language's possible phonological output forms have yet been learned, and differential accuracy on different elements in the target word lead to the access of some target elements but not others.

Nonlinear phonological theories

Nonlinear phonological theories evolved from "linear" theories in generative phonology. Phonological alternations reflect context: thus, A → B/_C (A is pronounced as B when preceding and contiguous [*adjacent*] to C). Linear theories can explain alternations in *surface*-adjacent sequences. For example, in some languages (e.g., English), nasals in coda clusters share the place of articulation of the following surface-adjacent stop, for example, *limp* [ˈlɪmp] ([Labial]), *lint* [ˈlɪnt] ([Coronal]), *link* [ˈlɪŋk] ([Dorsal]). However, linear theories cannot easily account for patterns which affect interactions of multiple segments (one-to-many), or non-surface-adjacent elements. In accounting for alternations concerning tones, Goldsmith (1976) demonstrated that one-to-many associations between phonological elements can be explained if phonological elements are viewed as hierarchically organized *autosegments*. Clements and Keyser (1983) accounted for distant assimilations (e.g. *baby* |beɪbi| → [bibi]; *take* |tʰeɪk|[1] → [kʰeɪk]) by positing autosegmental tiers (levels) for consonants and vowels; on their own tier, consonants are adjacent to other consonants

DOI: 10.4324/9781003204213-27

(and vowels to vowels) and thus can participate in "not-so-distant" consonant and vowel assimilation. (That is not to say that consonants and vowels cannot interact with each other, because they are surface-adjacent at output.)

The concept of hierarchical representation of independent phonological elements was extended to all aspects of phonological form (see Figure 24.1).

At the highest level, words are grouped into rhythmic phrasal units with various levels of prominence (stress). A phrase is made up of "prosodic words," each of which has one primary stress (level of prominence).

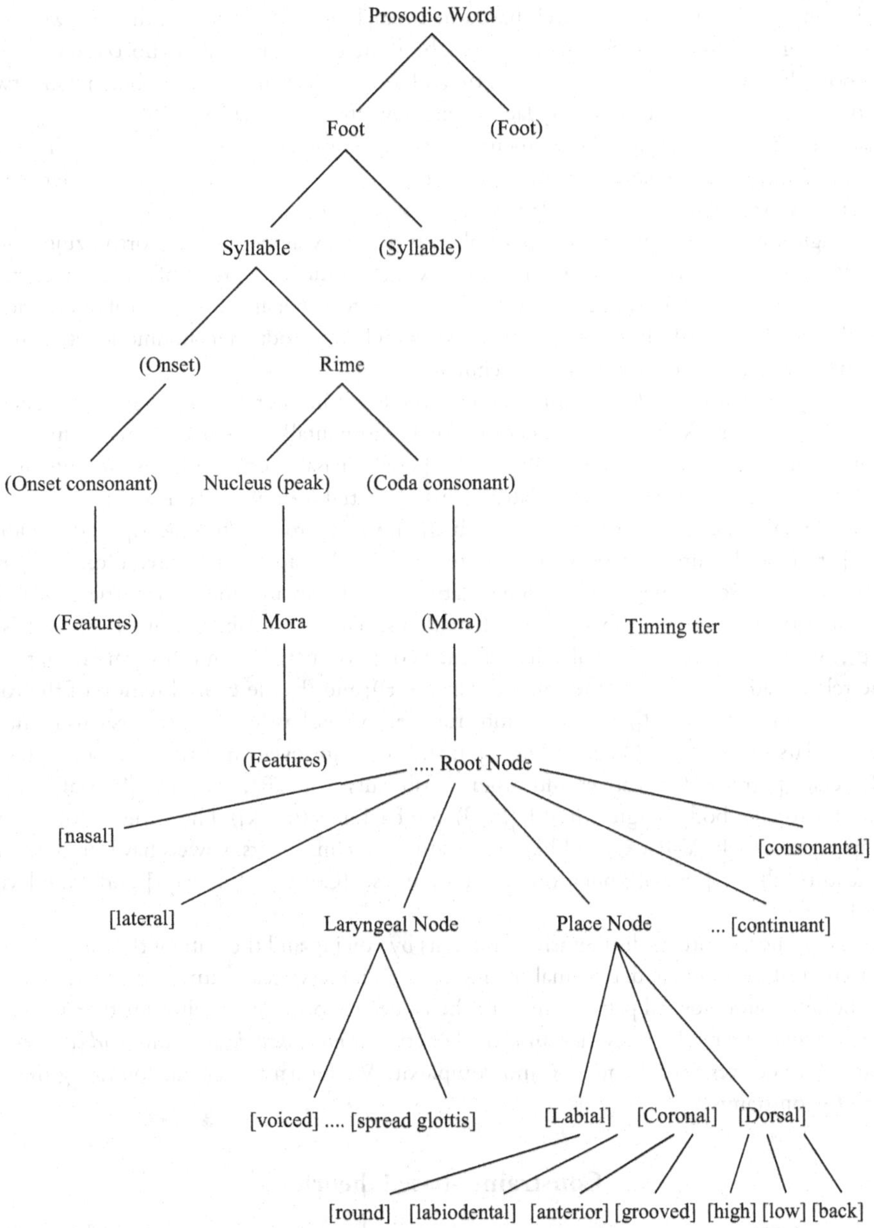

Figure 24.1 Phonological hierarchy from the phrase to the features.

The prosodic word has "feet" (metrical groupings of syllables). In English, a foot can be composed of one syllable (a *degenerate* foot) or up to five (e.g., in *unfortunately*) and is described in terms of the location of prominence, i.e., by which part of the foot is stressed. The left-prominent trochee (Strong-weak/Stressed-unstressed), as in *bucket*, is the most frequent foot cross-linguistically and contrasts with the right-prominent iambic foot (weak-Strong/unstressed-Stressed), as in *bouquet*.

Syllables subdivide into onsets and rimes (Kenstowicz, 1994). The *rime* includes the most sonorous element of the syllable (*nucleus/peak*) and any post-nuclear consonants (*coda*); the *onset* includes all pre-nuclear consonants.

Each segment takes up a unit of time (Hayes, 1995). Rime timing units are designated as "weight units" or "moras"; short vowels have one mora, long vowels and diphthongs, two. In some languages (e.g., English, Arabic), codas can also be moraic, especially after short/lax vowels; e.g., *book* /ˈbʊk/ has two moras, one each for /ʊ/ and /k/. The pronunciation [ˈbʊː] retains two. In *quantity-sensitive* languages, bimoraic syllables generally attract stress (Hayes, 1995).

Below the prosodic tier are the segmental tiers (for consonants and vowels), which are composed of hierarchically organized features (Figure 24.1 and Table 24.1, based on Bernhardt & Stemberger, 1998, 2000; McCarthy, 1988; Sagey, 1986).

Although feature descriptions vary, phonologists generally agree on three organizing features/nodes (Place, Laryngeal, Root [Manner features]), which dominate a group of specific features. The feature groupings reflect how features typically pattern together in phonological alternations. At the level of the Root node, features are linked to the higher prosodic tiers in unique sets of manner, place, and laryngeal combinations (i.e., as segments).

The following feature description is based on English; later we highlight differences for Arabic and Mandarin. Manner features comprise: [consonantal] (consonants versus glides); [continuant] (stops versus fricatives and affricates); [nasal] (nasals versus other sonorants and oral stops); and [lateral] (consonants with lateral versus central airflow). The Place node comprises three single-valued articulatory features: [Labial] (lips), [Coronal] (tongue tip and blade), and [Dorsal] (tongue dorsum). These organizing features are considered privative ("on-off") rather than binary, because the negatively valued feature (i.e., [-Labial]) does not participate in phonological patterns. Under [Labial], [labiodental] distinguishes bilabials from labiodentals, and [round], /w/ from other labials. Subsidiary features of [Coronal] distinguish segments in terms of (a) the relative advancement of the tongue ([anterior]); and (b) the central region of the tongue along the midline ([grooved]), i.e., (a) [+anterior] dentoalveolars (e.g. /t/, /θ/) versus [−anterior] palatoalveolars (e.g. /ʃ/) and palatals (e.g. /j/); and (b) [+grooved] fricatives and affricates (e.g., /s/, ʧ) versus [−grooved] fricatives and other consonants (e.g., /θ/, /n/, /t/). [Dorsal] subsumes features for tongue body height ([high], [low]) and backness ([back]). The same major place features apply to vowels (V-Place), and like some sonorant consonants, vowels have more than one place feature: all are [Dorsal], but front vowels are also [Coronal, -anterior] and round vowels [Labial].

Finally, laryngeal features distinguish consonants by voicing and the state of the glottis ([spread], [constricted]). The dominated/terminal manner, place, and laryngeal features are often considered binary because phonological patterns refer to their negative or positive value. Further, throughout the phonological hierarchy, a distinction is made between *unmarked defaults* and *marked nondefaults*, a division that derives from frequency and complexity. We return to defaults following the introduction to constraints.

Constraints-based theories

Phonological processes/rules describe phonological alternations, e.g., *take* |tʰeɪk| → [kʰeɪk] (Dorsal/Velar harmony/assimilation). Constraints-based theories seek to motivate the patterns.

Table 24.1 Features and consonants of English

Features	*Consonants*
Manner	
[+consonantal]	p b t d k ɡ m n ŋ f v θ ð s z ʃ ʒ tʃ dʒ l
[–consonantal]	w j ɹ h (ʔ)[a]
[+lateral]	l ɫ
[+nasal]	m n ŋ (ŋ syllable-final only)
[–continuant]	p b t d k ɡ (ʔ)[a] m n ŋ
[+continuant] (& [–sonorant])	f v θ ð s z ʃ ʒ
[–continuant, +continuant]	ʧ ʤ
Place	
Labial	p b m f v (w ɹ)[b]
Labial [+labiodental]	f v
Coronal [+anterior]	t d n θ ð s z l (ɫ)
Coronal [–anterior]	ʃ ʒ ʧ ʤ (j ɹ)
Coronal [+grooved][b]	s z ʃ ʒ ʧ ʤ
Coronal [–grooved]	θ ð (t d n l)
Dorsal	k ɡ ŋ (w j ɫ ɹ)
Labial & Dorsal	w
Coronal & Dorsal	ɫ j ɹ
Labial & Coronal & Dorsal	ɹ (onsets)
Laryngeal	
[+voiced] obstruents	b d ɡ ð v z ʒ ʤ
[–voiced] obstruents	p t k f θ s ʃ ʧ (ʔ)[a]
[+spread glottis]	p^{h} t^{h} k^{h} f θ s ʃ ʧ h
([+constricted glottis])[a]	(ʔ)

Note: Based on Bernhardt and Stemberger (2000, p. 168). Underlined features are unmarked adult defaults.

[a] Glottal stop is non-phonemic.

[b] [grooved] refers to the tongue lengthwise along the midline. The strident quality of sibilants arises by channeling air centrally through a narrow tongue groove.

Optimality Theory is the major constraints-based theory (OT: McCarthy & Prince, 1993; Prince & Smolensky, 1993). OT proposes that potential "outputs" (pronunciations) compete with each other during speech production; being subject to a set of "ranked" constraints, the highest-ranked (most important) or least constrained "wins." Constraints can be negative ("markedness" constraints, prohibiting certain output) or positive ("faithfulness" constraints, requiring survival of certain output). If faithfulness to X is ranked higher than markedness, X will be produced; if markedness is ranked higher, X will not be produced. (Some other element "Y" may be produced, if no constraint prohibits Y.)

Constraints-based theories are related to connectionist models of language processing (Bernhardt & Stemberger, 1998; Bernhardt et al., 2010): elements/units are assumed to have different levels of activation. Elements with low levels of activation are less likely to survive than those with high levels of activation; if element X has insufficient activation, then a high-activation element Y may replace it.

But what are the origins of constraints, rankings, and activation? Frequency and complexity play roles. Frequent and/or less complex elements (in terms of human cognition, anatomy, and physiology) tend to be "unmarked defaults," and less frequent and/or more complex elements, "marked/non-defaults." Cross-linguistically, unmarked defaults are generally: the trochaic foot, the CV syllable, and features of the consonant /t/.

Developmental implications: defaults

In early development, phonological systems may consist primarily of unmarked defaults, sometimes called "favorite sounds" or "sound preferences" in older clinical descriptions (e.g., Weiner, 1979). Although there are cross-linguistic trends, what is marked versus unmarked can differ across languages or speakers because there is a random component to neural organization and development in different speakers, plus anatomical and physiological differences in vocal tracts. Different languages (and even different speakers of the same language) also show differences in the frequency of elements, affecting developmental trends. Knowing about a speaker's language(s) and relative capacities in memory/attention/language processing, auditory/visual perception, anatomy/physiology, and their environment (input) may illuminate sources of their constraints and systemic defaults/nondefaults, and suggest directions for intervention if warranted.

Developmental implications: tier interactions

Output is constrained/facilitated by constraints operating on various levels of hierarchical structure, sometimes independently, and sometimes in interaction with other levels. For example, if a high-ranked markedness constraint prohibits word-initial (WI) clusters, one onset consonant (often the more marked) may fail to surface, e.g., *tray* |ˈtɹeɪ| → [ˈteɪ], even if that segment (|ɹ|) can appear as a WI singleton (*ray* [ˈɹeɪ]). Conversely, constraints on lower units (segments) may affect higher units: e.g., a child may be able to produce a cluster such as [tw] but is still learning to produce [ɹ] across contexts (*[tɹ]). The output will depend on which is more important: /ɹ/ or a cluster. If faithfulness to the complete feature combination for /ɹ/ is higher-ranked than faithfulness to cluster structure, the /ɹ/ or even the whole cluster may fail to appear. A [w] substitution would be faithful to some features of /ɹ/, but be unfavored because it does not have *all* features of the rhotic. The cluster would then be sacrificed. Bernhardt and Stemberger (1998) call this a non-minimal repair, where a constraint is resolved above the level where it could be.

Clinical application

Since 1990, several studies have investigated the application of (constraints-based) nonlinear phonology to phonological intervention for English (e.g., Bernhardt, 1990, 1992; Bernhardt & Major, 2005; Chung et al., 2022; Feehan et al., 2015; Major & Bernhardt, 1998; Von Bremen, 1990). Studies targeted word structure and segments/features in equal or near-equal proportions, and evaluated various interactions of features. Table 24.1 shows the feature-consonant correspondences assumed for these studies, and Table 24.2, elements of word structure.

Children in all studies showed notable treatment effects, and significantly faster gains for word structure (higher level form) than features, and for features higher versus lower in the hierarchy, supporting: (1) the relevance of hierarchical structure; and (2) the importance of addressing word structures separately. Bernhardt and Major (2005) reported better long-term outcomes in language, phonology, and literacy than is typically reported for children with protracted phonological development (PPD).

Constraints-based nonlinear phonological intervention utilizes a child's strengths and needs across the phonological hierarchy (constraint interactions), while taking into account personal and environmental supports for successful outcomes (Bernhardt & Stemberger, 2000). Relative mastery

Table 24.2 Key English word structures for assessment

Syl. per word	*Stress pattern*	*Word shapes*			
		No WF coda No CC	*WF coda, No CC*	*No WF coda WI and/or WM CC*	*WF coda CC*
1	S w[a]	(C)V	(C)VC	CCV(V)	CCVC(C)
2	Sw wS Ss sS	(C)VCV	CVCVC	CCVC(C)V C(C)VCCV	CCVC(C)VC(C) C(C)VCCVC(C) C(C)VC(C)VCC
3	wSw Sww sSw Ssw wwS	(C)VCVCV	(C)VCVCVC	CCVC(C)VC(C)V C(C)VCCVC(C)V C(C)VC(C)VCCV	CCVC(C)VC(C)VC(C) C(C)VCCVC(C)VC(C) C(C)VC(C)VCCVC(C) C(C)VC(C)VC(C)VCC
4	wswS swSw Swsw	(C)VCVCVCV	(C)VCVCVCVC	CCVC(C)VC(C)VC(C)V etc.	CCVC(C)VC(C)VC(C)VC etc.
Any #		With VV	With VV	With CCC and/or VV	With CCC and/or VV

Note. Based on Bernhardt and Stemberger (2000, p. 167). Parentheses indicates optionality. Syl = syllable; C=consonant; V = vowel; WI = word-initial; WM = word-medial; WF = word-final. S = primary stress, s = secondary stress; w = weak or unstressed.

[a] Grammatical morphemes, e.g., "the."

and mismatch patterns for word structures, segments, and their features are examined in multiple ways, with the number and types of analyses reflecting the child's needs:

(1) Elements are evaluated independently (e.g., all WI clusters, all dorsals, all fricatives, etc.).
(2) When particular elements within a category show differences in match proportions (e.g., word-internal or labial codas versus other codas), or mismatch types (e.g., labiodentals |f| > [t], but |v| > [b]), elements are examined in their various interactions (e.g., for codas, in terms of word length, stress or consonant types; for features, in their various combinations, e.g., place-laryngeal, e.g. [Labial] & [+voiced], /b, v, w/; manner-place, e.g. [+continuant] & [Coronal], /s, z, ʃ, ʒ/), etc.
(3) If mismatches for the same element vary across words, *and* there are (C)RAM patterns ([coalescence], reduplication, assimilation, metathesis), segmental features are examined in contiguous and non-contiguous sequences (e.g., Coronal-Labial, /t.m/, /t_p/, /tu/, /s_f/; versus Labial-Coronal, /m.t/, /pi/, /p_t/, /f_s/).

For intervention, both established elements (positive constraints/strengths, which may include nondefaults and defaults) and unestablished or weakly established elements (markedness constraints/needs) are taken into account across the phonological hierarchy. Unlike process or rule-based analyses (which are essentially lists of patterns that accommodate negative constraints), positive constraints (strengths) play an explicit role in the Bernhardt and Stemberger (2000) intervention approach. Established elements typically serve as foundations upon which to address needs (e.g., using strengths in word structure when addressing new segments/features and vice versa; using pronounceable segments as starting points for new ones), particularly when there are factors outside the phonological system (personal/environmental) that may impede successful outcomes. Strengths may be contrasted with needs (e.g., stops/fricatives) in perception and production. Interactions with morphosyntactic, lexical, perceptual, or motor development may be utilized as supports for phonological development, or in order to provide phonological support for development in those areas (following an interactive processing approach, Bernhardt et al., 2010).

Beyond English, intervention case studies have been completed for Canadian French, (Bérubé & Spoor, 2022); Icelandic (Másdóttir & Bernhardt, 2022); and Slovenian (Ozbič & Bernhardt, 2022). In addition, tutorials in English, French, and Spanish, and resources for 18 languages are available at Bernhardt and Stemberger (2015/2022, phonodevelopment.sites.olt.ubc.ca) or for German, in Ullrich (2011). The remainder of the chapter focuses on Kuwaiti Arabic and Mandarin in turn, presenting background on the phonology and its development in each language (in terms of word structure and segments/features), and then outlining clinical applications.

Kuwaiti Arabic

For Arabic, diglossia is an important consideration, i.e., the differences between regional dialects and "standard" Arabic (either Classical or Modern Standard Arabic, MSA). Differences concern, e.g., (1) posterior stops (uvular {q}[2] of MSA is /g/, /ʤ/ or /j/ in Kuwait); and (2) vowels (the root of the word "salt" in MSA is {mlħ}, pronounced [mɪlħ] in Kuwaiti Arabic, etc.

Word structure: Kuwaiti Arabic

Words are typically one to three syllables in length, but can have five or more syllables (especially in borrowings). A foot typically comprises one or two syllables (with a possible extrametrical unstressed syllable). Syllables can be light, heavy, and super-heavy:

1. Light: CV, e.g. /tə/ (feminine present singular prefix).
2. Heavy:
   a. CVC, /ˈsˤəf/ ('classroom'); b. CVV, /liː/ ("mine")
   (Hassan (1950) also includes VC).
3. Super-heavy:
   a. CVCC, /bərd/ ("cold"); b. CVVC, /leiʃ/ ("why").

Stress is predictable and weight-sensitive. Stress falls on:

1. The final super-heavy syllable, e.g., /nas.tə.ˈʕeːn/ ("seek for help"); /jes.tə.ˈquir:/ ("to settle");
2. The penultimate heavy syllable, if the final syllable is not super-heavy, e.g., /ʔəs.ˈtəj.ham/ ("to enquire"); /ju.ˈnaːdi:/ ("calling"); or
3. The antepenult, if neither #1 nor #2 apply, e.g., /ˈʕəl.lə.mɛk/ ("teach you").

Epenthetic schwa is typically unstressed.

Clusters include:

1. Tautosyllabic word-initial (WI) and WM onset sequences (e.g., /dr/ /məˈdrɪsə/), some being morphologically derived, e.g., [hn] ([hnud], plural of /hɪnd/ "man from India"); [χj] ([χjut], plural of /χejt/ "thread").
2. Heterosyllabic word-medial (WM) consonant sequences, e.g., /ʕ.t/ (/ˈzəʕ.tər/ "oregano"; /n.t/ /ˈʤəntˤə/ "handbag"); and
3. Word-final (WF): e.g., /ʃt/, as in /bɪʃt/ "man's robe," /lʧ/, as in /ˈʕɛlʧ/ "gum," some being morphologically derived, e.g., [mʃ] as in [ʔɛmʃ] ("Walk" [imperative]); [b̥t], [jɪb̥t] ("I brought").

Segments and features: Kuwaiti Arabic

Vowels

Like MSA, the Kuwaiti Arabic vowel system has pairs of short and long vowels: /i(:)/, /a(:)/, /u(:)/, plus diphthongs /aj/ and /aw/. Other vowels include diphthong /ej/, [o:] (a variant of /aw/), and epenthetic schwa (often used in clusters, and after a prepausal word-final geminate). Vowels may lower in the context of uvulars, pharyngeals, or glottals, or become advanced in the context of front consonants, giving [ɛ], [ɨ], [æ], or [ʌ].

Consonants

Table 24.3 shows the features and consonants of Kuwaiti Arabic.

Key manner characteristics of Kuwaiti Arabic are:

1. [+nasal]: [ŋ] occurs only before velar stops.
2. [–continuant]: includes emphatics /tˤ/, /dˤ/, (/gˤ/), phonemic /ʔ/, and for some speakers, [q]); /p/ does not occur.
3. [+continuant](&[–sonorant]) fricatives; [–continuant][+continuant] affricates: Fricatives are produced across the vocal tract (except for /v/); affricates are palatoalveolar only (like English). Pharyngeals /ʕ/ and /ħ/ may be approximants in MSA because of lack of turbulence (Bin-Muqbil, 2006) but this needs to be clarified for Kuwaiti Arabic.
4. The rhotic is a trilled /r/.

Table 24.3 Features and consonants of Kuwaiti Arabic

Features	*Consonants*
Manner	
[+ consonantal]	m n ŋ (not word-initially) b t tˤ d dˤ k (kˤ) g (gˤ) {q[a] qˤ}[a] f s sˤ z θ ð ðˤ ʃ ʧ ʤ χ ʁ ħ ʕ r l ʕ
[-consonantal]	j[b] w[b] h ʔ
[+lateral]	l
[+nasal]	m n ŋ (ŋ non-word-initial)
[-continuant] [-nasal]	b t tˤ d dˤ k (kˤ) g (gˤ) {q qˤ)}
[+continuant](and [-sonorant])	f s sˤ z θ ð ðˤ ʃ χ ʁ ħ[b] ʕ[b]
[-continuant]/[+continuant]	ʧ ʤ
Place	
Labial	m b f w
Coronal [+anterior]	n t tˤ d dˤ θ ð ðˤ s sˤ z l r
Coronal [-anterior]	ʃ ʧ ʤ j
Coronal [+grooved]	s sˤ z ʃ ʧ ʤ
Coronal [-grooved]	θ ð ðˤ (plus coronal stops and sonorants)
Dorsal	[+high]: k kˤ g (gˤ) w j (ŋ not WI); [+low] χ ʁ {q qˤ)[c]
Pharyngeal (Guttural/Radical)	χ ʁ ħ ʕ ʔ h (q qˤ)[c]
Laryngeal	
[+voiced] obstruents	b d dˤ g (gˤ) z ð ðˤ ʤ ʁ ʕ
[-voiced]	t tˤ k kˤ (q qˤ) f s sˤ θ ʃ ʧ χ ħ ʔ h
[+spread glottis]	f s sˤ θ ʃ ʧ χ ħ h

Note. Parentheses indicate optionality. Underlined features are unmarked adult defaults.
[a] {q} of Modern Standard Arabic can occur in Kuwaiti Arabic. It may pattern with the other gutturals.
[b] The pharyngeal fricatives may be produced as approximants.
[c] Emphatic consonants may be uvularized ([Dorsal], [–low]) or pharyngealized ([Pharyngeal]/[Guttural]/[Radical]).

Place features [Labial], [Coronal], and [Dorsal] show the following different characteristics from English:

(1) [Labial] does not include */p/ or */v/.
(2) [Coronal] includes emphatics /tˤ/, /dˤ/, /ðˤ/, /sˤ/, and /lˤ/; the emphatics may have either a secondary uvularized ([Dorsal]) or pharyngealized ([Guttural]) feature.
(3) [Dorsal] includes (emphatic /gˤ/) and uvulars ([–high], [–low]) /χ/, /ʁ/, ([q]).
(4) Arabic is described by McCarthy (1994) and Watson (2002) as having a [Pharyngeal] ([Guttural/][Radical]) place node, which groups uvulars /χ, ʁ/, pharyngeals /ħ, ʕ/, and glottals /h, ʔ/.

Laryngeal features, like English, comprise both values of [voiced] for obstruents except for labials (*/p/, */v/). However, aspiration is variable and glottal stop is phonemic.

Acquisition: Kuwaiti Arabic

Word structure

In conversational speech of children aged 1;4–3;7, Alqattan (2015) observed most frequent use of disyllables, followed by trisyllables and monosyllables. Eighty four-year-olds (Ayyad, 2011) showed a word shape match of 90% on a single-word naming task (91 words up to four syllables in length). Mastery was observed for: (1) monosyllables and disyllables with diphthongs/long vowels and codas plus some WM and WF clusters; and (2) multisyllabic word shapes with codas but not clusters.

Segments

Alqattan (2015) and Ayyad et al. (2016) describe consonant acquisition for the same cohorts as noted above. In Alqattan's (2015) study, by 3;7, children produced over half of Kuwaiti Arabic consonants with 75% accuracy: all stops (except for /q/); labial and coronal nasals and glides; /l/; fricatives /z/, /ʃ/, /x/, and /ħ/; emphatics /tˁ/ and /sˁ/. Ayyad et al.'s (2016) four-year-old cohort (on the single-word naming task), had similar results: over 90% of children showed 100% accuracy for stops (except for /q/), labial and coronal nasals and glides, lateral /l/, fricative /f/, and different coronal and pharyngeal fricatives. In both studies, consonants with less marked default features were generally mastered earlier.

Vowel studies remain to be done for Kuwaiti Arabic and expansion of databases is needed for both consonants and word structure.

Clinical application

A tool for nonlinear phonological analysis has supported studies of school-aged children with Down Syndrome (DS: Ayyad et al., 2021; Ayyad & Bernhardt, 2017; 2022) and sensorineural hearing loss (Ayyad & Bernhardt, 2009). Ayyad et al. (2021) report overall consonant and word shape accuracy scores of approximately 50% for six school-aged children with DS (five to 12 years of age). Although their accuracy scores were lower than those of typically developing (TD) four-year-olds, five of the six children and the child with hearing loss were similar to the TD children in showing later development of nondefaults (liquids, fricatives, multisyllabic words, clusters), although one five-year-old with DS showed the opposite pattern: nondefault fricatives and liquids were ahead of stops.

Ayyad et al. (2021) report that place mismatches were most frequent, but consonants often exhibited mismatches affecting more than one feature category (place and manner, e.g., |l| > [g]; place and laryngeal, e.g., |ɡ| > [t]; manner and laryngeal, |ð| > [t], |f| > [b]; or place, manner, and laryngeal, e.g., |b| > [h]; |z| > [k]). Multiple feature category mismatches (non-minimal repairs) have been reported for other children with PPD, e.g., Bernhardt et al. (2015).

Intervention studies applying constraints-based nonlinear theories have yet to be done for Arabic, but as a first step, Ayyad and Bernhardt (2022) propose an intervention plan for the child with DS for whom stops were challenging, adopting principles and strategies of Bernhardt and Stemberger (2000) for English: (1) addressing stops first in strong VC syllables, while avoiding challenging WI-WF sequences across vowels; (2) gradually adding WI and WM stops in longer words.

Mandarin

Mandarin (alternatively Puˇtoˉnghuà, Guóyuˇ, or Huáyuˇ) is spoken by about 800 million people. We use the term Mandarin here, adding location for dialectal considerations.

Word structure: Mandarin

Disyllables are most frequent (He & Li, 1987) but there are also monosyllables and multisyllabic words. Duanmu (2000) argues that the basic syllable is CV(X), i.e., an obligatory onset and nucleus and one (V) or two rime elements (V:, VV, V+ nasal coda). If a syllable has no underlying consonant or glide onset, a default onset is inserted: (1) before high vowels, a homorganic glide, i.e., /i/ → [ji] (alternatively, [ʔʲi]); and (2) elsewhere, [ʔ], [ŋ], [ɣ], or [ɦ]. Duanmu (2000) argues that apparent triphthongs are CVV sequences, with secondary articulation on the consonant (e.g., palatalization, rounding) (i.e., $C^{G}VV$). Consonant sequences occur only word medially (heterosyllabic, e.g., /tia^{HL}n̲s̲i^{HL}r̲t̲i^{H}/ "television").

Mandarin has lexical tone, often transcribed with numbers, although other systems provide more information on tone height. Stressed syllables can have one of four tones: high level [T1, ^{H}]; low-high rising [T2, ^{LH}], high-low falling [T4, ^{HL}]; and [T3], low-falling (^{ML}) in non-final position ($^{L\text{-}ML}$) and low-dipping (mid-low-mid, ^{MLM}) or low-falling (midlow-low, $^{ML\text{-}L}$) in utterance-final position or isolation, especially in Taiwan (Duanmu, 2000). T3 changes to T2 before another T3, and T4 to low-falling after T4 (tone sandhi). A "neutral" tone (^{0}), occurs in unstressed or reduced syllables, and is generally high after T3, and low elsewhere (Duanmu, 2000). The tonal pitch range in Taiwan and Shanghai Mandarin is smaller than in Beijing Mandarin (Chen & Gussenhoven, 2015; Duanmu, 2000; Zhu, 2007).

Syllable nuclei differ in pitch and duration, giving a percept of stress (usually on the first syllable of a disyllabic word, and rightwards in trochaic groupings). Unstressed syllables often show vowel reduction or neutralization in suffixes such as /tsə^{0}/, or /tə^{0}/, and the second syllable of some disyllables.

Segments and features: Mandarin

Vowels

Mandarin has monophthongs, diphthongs, and arguably, triphthongs (but see above). Vowel inventory descriptions differ (Duanmu, 2000; Lee-Kim, 2014; Lin, 2014). Duanmu (2000) proposes five underlying monophthongs /i, y, u, ə, a/, expanded through contextual conditioning, e.g.:

1. Mid vowels: Frontness or rounding can yield [o, ɤ, e, ɛ, ʌ].
2. Low vowels: Relative backness can yield one of [a, ɑ, ɐ, æ].
3. /ɚ/: In Beijing, /ɚ/ varies with [aɹ], suggesting that /ɚ/ is /ə+ɹ/ (Duanmu, 2000).

Lee-Kim (2014) includes "apical vowels," which appear after dental or retroflexed sibilants. However, Duanmu (2000) analyses these as retroflexed syllabic consonants.

For diphthongs, Duanmu (2000) posits four phonemic falling diphthongs /ai/, /əi/, /au/, /əu/, and other vowel sequences that incorporate the contextually conditioned vowels above, e.g., /ou/, /ao/, /ei/ (falling sonority); /ia/, /iɛ/, /ua, /uo/, and /yɛ/ (rising sonority).

Dialectal variants include [i] in Taiwan for Beijing {y} (Duanmu, 2000) and possible reduced diphthong use in Shanghai Mandarin (Ramsay, 1989).

Consonants

Manner categories in Mandarin resemble those of English (see Table 24.4). However, only nasals (/n/, /ŋ/) appear in coda and are often weakly articulated, so that nasality may appear instead on the preceding vowel (Duanmu, 2000). Nasals, /z̩/ and /ɻ̩/ can be syllabic: /z̩/ occurs after dentoalveolars, and /{ɻ̩~ɹ̩}/, after retroflexed consonants.

Table 24.4 Features and consonants of Mandarin

Features	*Consonants*
Manner	
[+consonantal]	p pʰ t tʰ k kʰ m n ŋ f s ʂ ɕ x ʦ ʦʰ tʂ tʂʰ ʨ ʨʰ l ɹ
[–consonantal]	w j
[+sonorant][+cons][–nasal]	l ɹ
[+nasal]	m n ŋ
[–continuant][–nasal]	p pʰ t tʰ k kʰ
[+continuant]–[–sonorant]	f s ʂ ɕ x
[–continuant]–[+continuant]	ʦ ʦʰ tʂ tʂʰ ʨ ʨʰ
Place	
Labial	p pʰ m f w
Coronal [+anterior]	t tʰ n s ʦ ʦʰ l
Coronal [–anterior]	ʂ ɕ tʂ tʂʰ ʨ ʨʰ ɹ j
Coronal [+grooved]	s ʂ ʦ ʦʰ tʂ tʂʰ ɹ
Coronal [–grooved]	t tʰ n ɕ ʨ ʨʰ l j
Dorsal	k kʰ ŋ x w j
Laryngeal	
[–voiced] ([–spread glottis])	p t k ts tʂ ʨ
[–voiced] [+spread glottis]	pʰ tʰ kʰ tsʰ tʂʰ ʨʰ f s ʂ ɕ x

(See also Zhao et al., 2009/2015.)

Unlike English, the laryngeal contrast is based on presence or absence of phonemic aspiration in stops and affricates, although unaspirated stops are sometimes voiced in unstressed syllables (Duanmu, 2000).

Place extends from labial to dorsal, similar to English but with several differences: (1) /w~ʋ/ alternate in Beijing (Duanmu, 2000); (2) anterior coronals /s/ and /ʦ(ʰ)/ are produced dentally; (3) affricates can be alveolar, retroflexed, or alveolopalatal; (4) [-anterior] fricatives/affricates contrast in grooving: [+grooved] retroflexes versus [-grooved] alveolopalatals (i.e., with a flat high tongue body), with some Beijing speakers replacing alveolopalatals with palatalized consonants, e.g., /ɕ~ʦʲ/ (Duanmu, 2000); and (5) the posterior fricative varies: /x~h/.

Taiwan and Shanghai Mandarin may show fewer or more retroflexes than Beijing Mandarin (through hypercorrection). Taiwan Mandarin may also show: (1) vowels for certain syllabic consonants, i.e., [ɯ] for /ʐ̩/, [ɤ] for /ɹ̩/ (Duanmu, 2000); (2) consonant reduction/weakening, except for nasal codas (Duanmu, 2000); and/or (3) neutralization of the velar-alveolar contrast in nasal codas (Zhu, 2007). Shanghai Mandarin speakers may use [h] rather than [x] and more glottal and voiced stops (Chen & Gussenhoven, 2015).

Acquisition: Mandarin

Prosodic structure

CV syllables are common before age three years, both as monosyllabic words and in longer words, e.g., CVCV(CV) (Zhu, 2007). By age four, children appear to have acquired most of the word shapes (Bernhardt et al., 2010). For tones, Zhu (2002) reports error-free production by age two years in a longitudinal study of four children; T1 stabilized from 1;2–1;5, T4 from 1;4–1;7 and T2 and T3, from 1;4.15 to 1;10. However, adult-like values in tonal pitch range and duration may not be established until after age eight (e.g., Tang et al., 2019; Wong, 2012). Further, word stress appears delayed relative to tone (Zhu, 2002).

Vowels

The four children in Zhu's (2002) study acquired most vowels by age two years; [+back] [ɑ] and [u] emerged earliest, and diphthongs, [ei] and [yɛ], latest). Peng and Chen (2020) report: (1) acquisition of monophthongs before diphthongs; and (2) later acquisition of retroflexed vowels and marked /y/. For Shanghai Mandarin vowels, Lai et al. (2011) report that 28 TD four-year-olds had a smaller acoustic vowel space than adult speakers.

Consonants

Zhao et al. (in press) report that children have acquired most of the consonants by 4;6 (some are still mastering more marked liquids, or coronal fricatives/affricates, particularly /s/ and the retroflexes). Earlier-acquired consonants include less complex (more frequent) labial and alveolar stops/nasals; labiodental and velar fricatives /f/ and /x/; and voiceless unaspirated stops. VOT values for aspirated stops may not reach adult-like values until after age six years (Yang, 2018).

Clinical application

A nonlinear phonological scan form (Zhao et al., 2009/2015) has supported analysis and intervention planning for two case studies (Bernhardt & Zhao, 2010; Bernhardt et al., 2022). In addition to the structural and segmental analyses, for Mandarin, it is important to consider the potential dialectal variation.

Bernhardt et al. (2022) present an intervention plan for a three-year-old with severe PPD. His strongest needs for the first period of intervention were for: (1) new word shapes (C)VV and $CVC_{[nasal]}$; and (2) new consonant categories: fricatives/affricates, /l/, and aspirated stops. (C)VV addresses timing units in the rime and vowel quality (vital in a language with CVX syllables), and provides incidental practice with tones. As a second goal, fricatives expand the manner category. For the third goal, another word structure goal, $CVC_{[nasal]}$, further reinforces timing unit faithfulness, and sets up a fourth goal of moving /n/ to onset. As with Arabic, no controlled intervention studies have been conducted, although the case study of Bernhardt and Zhao (2010) did show positive treatment effects from a program focusing on diphthongs, the rhotic, and certain fricatives and affricates.

Conclusion

This chapter presented an overview of constraints-based nonlinear phonology in its clinical application to children with PPD for English, with some preliminary applications to Kuwaiti Arabic and Mandarin. Resources and information are also available for other languages (Bernhardt & Stemberger, 2015/2022; Stemberger & Bernhardt, 2018, 2022).

Some goals and treatment strategies will overlap with those selected in other approaches because of the limited nature of phonological systems, developmental patterns, and treatment options. Clinical judgment is needed to tailor programs for individuals; however, the analysis and treatment strategies derived from constraints-based nonlinear phonology provide a strong framework for analysis and intervention across languages and as theories evolve, and new languages are considered, further opportunities will develop.

Notes

1 Phonemic slashes /_/ indicate broad transcription of adult pronunciations, and square brackets [_] narrower transcriptions of adult and child pronunciations. When presenting adult pronunciations as targets for the child's pronunciation, we follow Rose and Inkelas (2011), using "pipes" |_| for the adult pronunciation; pipes allow portrayal of relevant (narrow) allophonic details that the child may try to match, such as aspiration in English.

2 MSA is represented with {_}, phonemes of dialects with /_/ and narrow transcriptions with [_].

Further reading

Bernhardt, B. M., & Stemberger, J. P. (2020). Phonological development. Research in multilingual and cross-cultural contexts. In F.-F. Li, K. Pollock & R. Gibb (Eds.). *Child Bilingualism and Second Language Learning Bilingual Processing and Acquisition* (pp. 223–247). Philadephia, PA: John Benjamins.

Bérubé, D., & Macleod, A. A. (2022). A comparison of two phonological screening tools for French-speaking children. *International Journal of Speech-Language Pathology, 24*(1), 22–32. https://doi.org/10.1080/17549507.2021.1936174.

Bérubé, D., Bernhardt, B. M., Stemberger, J. P., & Ciocca, V. (2020). Development of singleton consonants in French-speaking children with typical versus protracted phonological development: The influence of word length, word shape and stress. *International Journal of Speech-Language Pathology, 22*(6), 637–647. https://doi.org/10.1080/17549507.2020.1829706.

References

Alqattan, S. (2015). *Early phonological acquisition by Kuwaiti Arabic children* [Unpublished PhD Dissertation], University of Newcastle upon Tyne.

Ayyad, H. (2011). *Phonological development of typically developing Kuwaiti Arabic-speaking preschoolers* [Unpublished PhD Dissertation]. University of British Columbia.

Ayyad, H., & Bernhardt, B. M. (2009/2017). *Kuwaiti Arabic Articulation and Phonology-Test (KAAP-T).* Kuwait University.

Ayyad, H., & Bernhardt, B. M. (2009). Phonological development in Kuwaiti Arabic: A preliminary report. *Clinical Linguistics and Phonetics, 23*(11), 794–807. https://doi.org/10.3109/02699200903236493.

Ayyad, H., & Bernhardt, B. M. (2022). When liquids and fricatives outrank stops: A Kuwaiti Arabic-speaking child with Down syndrome and protracted phonological development. *Clinical Linguistics & Phonetics, 36*(7), 670–682. https://doi.org/10.1080/02699206.2022.2046172.

Ayyad, H. S., Bernhardt, B. M., & Stemberger, J. P. (2016). Kuwaiti Arabic. Acquisition of singleton consonants. *International Journal of Language and Communication Disorders, 51*(5), 531–545. https://doi.org/10.1111/1460-6984.12229.

Ayyad, H., AlBustan, S., & Ayyad, F. (2021). Phonological development in school-aged Kuwaiti Arabic children with Down syndrome: A pilot study. *Journal of Communication Disorders, 93*(3), 106128, 1-15. https://doi.org/10.1016/j.jcomdis.2021.106128

Ayyad, H., Alqattan, S., & Bernhardt, B. M. [in press]. Kuwaiti Arabic speech development. In S. McLeod (Ed.), *Oxford handbook of speech development in languages of the world.* Oxford: Oxford University Press.

Bernhardt, B. (1990). *Application of nonlinear phonological theory to intervention with six phonologically disordered children* [Unpublished PhD Dissertation]. University of British Columbia.

Bernhardt, B. (1992). The application of nonlinear phonological theory to intervention with one phonologically disordered child. *Clinical Linguistics and Phonetics, 6*(4), 283–316. https://doi.org/10.3109/02699209208985537.

Bernhardt, B., & Gilbert, J. (1992). Applying linguistic theory to speech-language pathology: The case for nonlinear phonology. *Clinical Linguistics and Phonetics, 6*(1–2), 123–145. https://doi.org/10.3109/02699209208985523.

Bernhardt, B. M., Liu, C., & Zhao, J. (2022) When in doubt, glottal stop: A Mandarin-speaking three-year-old with protracted phonological development. *Clinical Linguistics & Phonetics, 36*(8), 683-695. https://doi.org/10.1080/02699206.2021.1996632.

Bernhardt, B. M., & Major, E. (2005) [Speech], language and literacy skills three years later: Long-term outcomes of nonlinear phonological intervention *International Journal of Language and Communication Disorders, 40*(1), 1–27. https://doi.org/10.1080/13682820410001686004.

Bernhardt, B. M., Másdóttir, T., Stemberger, J. P., Leonhardt, L., & Hansson, G. O. (2015). Fricative development in Icelandic and English-speaking children with protracted phonological development. *Clinical Linguistics and Phonetics, 29*(8–10), 642–665. https://doi.org/10.3109/02699206.2015.1036463.

Bernhardt, B. M., & Stemberger, J. P. (1998). *Handbook of phonological development: From a nonlinear constraints-based perspective*. San Diego, CA: Academic Press.

Bernhardt, B. M., & Stemberger, J. P. (2000). *Workbook in nonlinear phonology for clinical application*. Austin, TX: Pro-Ed (copyright reverted to authors).

Bernhardt, B. M., & Stemberger, J. P. (2015/2022). *Phonological Development Tools and Cross-Linguistic Phonology Project*. Retrieved from phonodevelopment.sites.olt.ubc.ca.

Bernhardt, B. M., Stemberger, J. P., & Charest, M. (2010a). Speech production models and intervention for speech production impairments in children. *CJASLPA*, *34*(3), 157–167. Retrieved from https://www.cjslpa.ca/detail.php?lang=en&ID=1026

Bernhardt, B. M., & Zhao, J. (2010). Nonlinear phonological analysis in assessment of protracted phonological development in Mandarin. *Canadian Journal of Speech-Language Pathology and Audiology*, *34*(3), 168–180. Retrieved from https://www.cjslpa.ca/detail.php?ID=1027&lang=en.

Bérubé, D., & Spoor, J. (2002). Word structure and consonant interaction in a French-speaking child with protracted phonological development. *Clinical Linguistics and Phonetics*, *36*(8), 696-707. https://doi.org/10.1080/02699206.2021.2019313

Bin-Muqbil, M. S. (2006). *Phonetic and phonological aspects of Arabic emphatics and gutturals* [Unpublished PhD Dissertation]. Madison: University of Wisconsin-Madison.

Chen, Y., & Gussenhoven, C. (2015). Shanghai Chinese. *Journal of the International Phonetic Association*, *45*(3), 321–337. https://doi:10.1017/S0025100315000043t.

Chung, S., Bernhardt, B. M., & Stemberger, J. P. (2022). When codas trump onsets: An English-speaking child with atypical phonological development before and after intervention. *Clinical Linguistics and Phonetics*, *36*(9), 779-792. https://doi.org/10.1080/02699206.2021.2025432.

Clements, G. N., & Keyser, S. J. (1983). *CV phonology*. Cambridge, MA: MIT Press. https://doi.org/10.1080/13682820410001686004.

Duanmu, S. (2000). *The phonology of standard Chinese*. Oxford: Oxford University Press.

Feehan, A., Francis, C., Bernhardt, B. M., & Colozzo, P. (2015). Outcomes of phonological and morphosyntactic intervention for twin boys with protracted speech and language development. *Child Language Teaching and Therapy*, *31*(1), 53–69. https://doi.org/10.1177/0265659014536205.

Goldsmith, J. (1976). *Autosegmental phonology* [PhD Dissertation]. Massachusetts Institute of Technology [New York: Garland Press 1979].

Hassan, T. (1950). *Manahij-l-bahth fi-l-lugha [Research methods in language]*. Kuwait: Ar-risala press.

Hayes, B. (1995). *Metrical stress theory: Principles and case studies*. Chicago, IL: Chicago University Press.

He, K., & Li, D. (1987). *Xiandai HanYu san quian changyong ci biao [Three thousand most commonly used words in modern Chinese]*. Beijing: Shifan Daxue Chubanshe.

Kenstowicz, M. (1994). *Phonology in generative grammar*. Oxford: Blackwell.

Lai, Y., Lin, C.-Y., Bernhardt, B. M., Zhao, J., & Stemberger, J. P. (2011). Acoustic analysis of Mandarin tone in four-year-old typically developing children in Shanghai. *Poster presented at the York Child Phonology Conference*, June 16–17. UK: York.

Lee-Kim, S.-I. (2014). Revisiting Mandarin 'apical vowels': An articulatory and acoustic study. *Journal of the International Phonetic Association*, 44(3), 261–282. https://doi.org/10.1017/S0025100314000267.

Lin, Y.-H. (2014). Segmental phonology. In C.-T. J. Huang, Y.-H. A. Li & A. Simpson (Eds.), *Handbook of Chinese linguistics* (pp. 400–421). Hoboken, NJ: Wiley & Sons.

Major, E., & Bernhardt, B. (1998). Metaphonological skills of children with phonological disorders before and after phonological and metaphonological intervention. *International Journal of Language and Communication Disorders*, *33*(4), 413–444. https://doi.org/10.1080/136828298247712.

Másdóttir, T., & Bernhardt, B. M. (2022). Uncommon timing variation in the speech of an Icelandic-speaking child with protracted phonological development. *Clinical Linguistics & Phonetics*, *36*(9), 806-819. https://doi.org/10.1080/02699206.2021.2011959.

McCarthy, J. J. (1988). Feature geometry and dependency: A review. *Phonetica*, *43*(2–4), 84–108. https://doi.org/10.1159/000261820.

McCarthy, J. J. (1994). The phonetics and phonology of Semitic pharyngeals. In P. Keating (Ed.), *Papers in laboratory phonology III: Phonological structure and phonetic form* (pp. 191–233). Cambridge, MA: Cambridge University Press.

McCarthy, J., & Prince, A. (1993). *Prosodic morphoogy I: Constraint interaction and satisfaction*. Rutgers University Center for Cognitive Science Technical Report 3.

Ozbič, M., & Bernhardt, B. M. (2022). Complexity resolved: Profile of a Slovenian child with protracted phonological development over an intervention period. *Clinical Linguistics & Phonetics*, *36*(9), 765-778. https://doi.org/10.1080/02699206.2021.2010241.

Peng, G., & Chen, F. (2020). Speech development in Mandarin-speaking children. In H. Liu, F. Tsao & P. Li (Eds.), *Speech perception, production and acquisition. Multidisciplinary approaches in Chinese languages* (pp. 219–242). Berlin: Springer. https://doi.org/10.1007/978-981-15-7606-5_12.

Prince, A., & Smolensky, P. (1993). *Optimality theory: Constraint interaction in generative grammar.* Rutgers University Center for Cognitiv Science Technical Report 2.

Ramsay, S. R. (1989). *The languages of China.* Princeton: Princeton University Press.

Rose, Y., & Inkelas, S. (2011). The interpretation of phonological patterns in first language acquisition. In C. J. Ewen, E. Hume, M. van Oostendorp & K. Rice (Eds.), *The Blackwell companion to phonology* (pp. 2414–2438). Hoboken, NJ: Wiley-Blackwell.

Sagey, E. (1986). *The representation of features and relations in non-linear phonology* [PhD Dissertation]. Massachusetts Institute of Technology [New York: Garland Press 1991].

Stemberger, J. P., & Bernhardt, B. M. (2018). Tap and trill clusters in typical and protracted phonological development: Challenging segments in complex phonological environments. Introduction to the special issue. *Clinical Linguistics and Phonetics*, *32*(5–6), 563–575. https://doi.org/10.1080/02699206.2017.1370019

Stemberger, J. P., & Bernhardt, B. M. (2022). Individual profiles in protracted phonological development across languages: Introduction to the special issue. *Clinical Linguistics & Phonetics*, *36(7)*, 597-616. https://doi.org/10.1080/02699206.2022.2057871.

Tang, P., Yuen, I., Xu Rattanasone, N., Gao, L., & Demuth, K. (2019). Acquisition of weak syllables in tonal languages: Acoustic evidence from neutral tone in Mandarin Chinese. *Journal of Child Language*, *46*(1), 24–50. https://doi.org/10.1017/S0305000918000296

Ullrich, A. (2011). *Evidenzbasierte Diagnostik phonologischer Störungen – Entwicklung und Evaluation eines Sprachanalyseverfahrens auf der Basis nichtlinearer phonologischer Theorien. [Evidence-based assessment of phonological disorders – Development and evaluation of speech analysis procedures based on nonlinear phonological theories]* [Unpublished PhD Dissertation]. Cologne: University of Cologne.

Von Bremen, V. (1990). *A nonlinear phonological approach to intervention with severely phonologically disordered twins* [Unpublished MSc Thesis]. University of British Columbia.

Watson, J. (2002). *The phonology and morphology of Arabic.* Oxford: Oxford University Press.

Weiner, F. (1979). *Phonological process analysis.* Baltimore, MD: University Park Press.

Wong, P. (2012). Acoustic characteristics of three-year-olds' correct and incorrect monosyllabic Mandarin lexical tone productions. *Journal of Phonetics*, *40*(1), 141–151. https://doi.org/10.1016/j.wocn.2011.10.005.

Yang, J. (2018). Development of stop consonants in three- to six-year-old Mandarin-speaking children. *Journal of Child Language*, *45*(5), 1091–1115. https://doi.org/10.1017/S0305000918000090.

Zhao, J., Bernhardt, B. M., & Stemberger, J. P. (2009/2015). *Mandarin Phonology Test.* phonodevelopment.sites.olt.ubc.ca/TestMaterials/Mandarin. Retrieved from https://phonodevelopment.sites.olt.ubc.ca/practice-units/mandarin.

Zhu, H. (2002). *Phonological development in specific contexts: Studies of Chinese-speaking children.* Clevedon, UK: Multilingual Matters.

Zhu, H. (2007). Putonghua (Modern Standard Chinese) speech acquisition. In S. McLeod (Ed.), *The international guide to speech acquisition* (pp. 516–527). Clifton Park, NY: Thomson Delmar Learning.

25

BILINGUAL CHILDREN WITH SLI

Theories, research, and future directions

Maria Adelaida Restrepo, Gareth Morgan, and Ekaterina Smyk

Introduction

Bilingualism and specific language impairment (SLI) are at the crossroads of linguistic and psycholinguistic accounts of language. This chapter merges theoretical and research accounts of both areas to explain the limited information available on bilingual children with SLI. The SLI is a developmental language disorder characterized by primary deficits in language, not explained by sensory, gross neurological damage, emotional, or cognitive deficits (Leonard, 1998, 2009). Language difficulties of children with SLI tend to occur on grammatical aspects, although several language aspects can be compromised, such as difficulties in word learning and retrieval, semantic development, and phonological working memory (e.g., Dollaghan & Campbell, 1998; Edwards & Lahey, 1998; Gray, 2003, 2004, 2005). This chapter will discuss how bilingualism interfaces with SLI from the theoretical point of Dynamic Systems Theory (DST; Herdina & Jessner, 2002). We then address theories of SLI from linguistic and processing accounts, and review research evidence of SLI cross-linguistically and from bilingual populations. We conclude with some future directions.

In our work, we use a DST of language, bilingualism, and SLI (Herdina & Jessner, 2002; Kohnert, 2008) because it allows for the interaction of multiple languages, linguistic aspects, and contexts with the different cognitive processes involved in language. Language is a dynamic system; that is, it is a complex system, which is fluid and always changing (Kohnert, 2008). In the context of bilingualism, DST helps us to understand the role of variable linguistic input in different social and cultural contexts, while at the same time acknowledging the interactions across languages and linguistic abilities in terms of language proficiency, and typical or atypical development (Evans & McWhinney, 1999; Herdina & Jessner, 2002; Kohnert, 2008). In DST, language abilities in multilingual children change depending upon the quantity and quality of input needed to induce a change. When the input is strong, language changes can be positive on all the languages that the child speaks, but they can also be negative for one language and positive for the other (Herdina & Jessner, 2002; Kohnert, 2008). The fluid nature of language can respond to change any time there is sufficient input to induce a change. A visit of a family member, schooling in a new language, or new social relationships, for example, can induce change in a child's developing languages. Therefore, DST can account for great variability even in children with similar backgrounds but different language experiences. In addition, using DST we can still examine the processing and linguistic accounts of SLI to help us understand and describe this complex and dynamic system. DST has been used to account for both SLI and bilingualism, and researchers are beginning to use it to explain the two and their interactions (e.g., Kohnert, 2008; Kohnert & Derr, 2004).

 DOI: 10.4324/9781003204213-28

Kohnert (2008) uses DST as one aspect of her theoretical framework, which acknowledges the convergences of several theories: connectionism, social constructivism, DST, general interactive processing, and functionalism. For the purposes of this chapter, we focus on DST and cognitive interactive processes of language to explain some of the phenomena observed in bilingual children with SLI. Nevertheless, we must acknowledge current linguistic theories that attempt to explain the nature of SLI and second language acquisition.

Language knowledge in bilinguals is distributed across the languages they speak in terms of semantic, pragmatic, and grammatical skills (Kohnert, Windsor, & Ebert, 2008; Peña & Kester, 2004). Sequential and simultaneous bilingual children can demonstrate language influences across the different grammars in the languages they acquire. Theories explaining these influences are beyond the scope of this chapter, but we acknowledge that errors, for example, in bilingual discourse can reflect dynamic changes in a language due to transfer from a first language to a second language, from a second language to a first language, or the interlanguage that children develop while acquiring a second language (Gass & Selinker, 2008). Therefore, in addition to SLI characteristics, bilingual children with SLI can have characteristics typical for sequential and simultaneous language learners.

Theoretical accounts of SLI can be categorized in two general domains: linguistic and processing theories (Leonard, 1998; Schwartz, 2009; Ullman & Pierpont, 2005). Linguistic theories hypothesize that SLI deficits are due to limitations in linguistic knowledge, but differ on the locus of the impairment. Processing theories hypothesize that SLI deficits are due to limitations in processing linguistic information, but differ on what specific processes are impaired and whether they are in general domains or specific domains (Schwartz, 2009). To our knowledge, there is limited information on how these theories account for bilingual SLI characteristics and language performance, and thus, research on this population is largely descriptive.

Processing accounts of SLI

Processing accounts can be categorized into two strands, general cognitive processing limitations that affect linguistic and nonlinguistic processes and specific cognitive possessing limitations that affect specific linguistic processes (Leonard, 1998; Schwartz, 2009). In terms of general processing accounts, the primary account of SLI is the Limited Processing Capacity (LPC) Hypothesis; for a review see Leonard (1998, 2009). The LPC hypothesis considers limitations in three different areas: limited space, such as limits in memory capacity; limited attention/energy, such as an inability to complete a task because the energy has already been spent; and limited processing speed, such as an inefficiency to process information fast enough, and thus the information is vulnerable to decay or interference from new incoming information (Leonard, 1998; Schwartz, 2009). More specifically, LPC theory hypothesizes that children with SLI have limitations in working memory capacity (Gutierrez-Clellen, Calderon, & Weismer, 2004; Weismer, 1996; Weismer, Evans, & Hesketh, 1999; Weismer & Hesketh, 1998), which in turn leads to limitations in processing input and output. In this theory, children with SLI present with difficulties processing complex material (Gillam, Cowan, & Marler, 1998). As stimuli become more complex (linguistically, cognitively, or an increase in attention demands) performance deteriorates, especially in comparison to controls. For example, Gillam et al. (1998) found that typical and SLI groups performed similarly on a recall task when audiovisual stimuli were paired with a spoken response. This was an expected effect as visual input is rapidly converted into phonological forms ready for rehearsal, which would be facilitated by the spoken response; however, children with SLI had significantly poorer recall when audiovisual stimuli were paired with a pointing response. The authors do not attribute this difference in performance by children with SLI to any deficits in language, but instead to the cross-modal aspect of the task. In other words, children with SLI were not able to retain the word in memory or use phonological codes, or both when the task demanded cross modal operations like audiovisual stimuli paired with a motor task like pointing.

One criticism of the different LPC hypotheses is that they do not directly address the limitations in the linguistic profile of children with SLI (Schwartz, 2009). This is especially true when discussing those who are bilingual, although correlations have been observed between processing skills and language performance in monolingual populations, such as between processing complex sentences, and phonological memory and vocabulary development (Archibald & Gathercole, 2006; Montgomery, 2003). Further, interpreting research that addresses processing limitations across languages (monolingual vs. bilingual) and across classification (typical vs. atypical) can be complicated because of differential demands in processing across the different groups on similar tasks (Kohnert, Windsor, & Yim, 2006). Using a DST may help researcher to better understand these complex processes in multi-lingual contexts.

The General Slowing Hypothesis (GSH; Kail, 1994), posits that children with SLI demonstrate slower reaction times, lexical access, and learning skills in general. It is particularly applicable to investigate SLI as it uses speed of processing as a method to measure processing capacity and assumes that speed is equal to the amount of work that can be completed in a particular amount of time. Evidence in support of this hypothesis has been reported in slower reaction times or additional time required to complete a task by children with SLI when compared to matched peers, which is consistent with a DST as well (e.g., Hill, 2001; Leonard et al., 2007; Schul, Stiles, Wulfeck, & Townsend, 2004; Windsor & Hwang, 1999). Although children with SLI as a group perform slower than age and language matches, not all children with SLI demonstrate this pattern and both speed and processing skills have been shown to each account for unique variance in language performance (Leonard et al., 2007). The GSH hypothesizes that slower processing skills interfere with processing of complex sentences for example (e.g., Montgomery, 1995), but also with the access of lexical information in tasks such as rapid automatic naming (e.g., Catts et al., 2005), word learning (e.g., Gray, 2004, 2005), and fast mapping (e.g., Gray, 2003). Studies on bilingual SLI in these areas are sparse; however, differences in reaction times in identifying words between typical bilingual Spanish–English children and monolingual English children with language impairments (LI; Windsor & Kohnert, 2004) and in rapid naming (Morgan, Srivastiva, Restrepo, & Auza, 2009) have been found. Such differences can be mistaken as SLI and therefore, research in this area indicates that there is a great need to understand the role of a bilingual's two languages or the acquisition of a second language on the processing skills of typical bilingual children. Competition between languages can account for slower processing times in bilinguals; however, the question remains whether it applies to all fluent bilinguals, to only sequential bilinguals in additive or subtractive language contexts, or to only late sequential bilinguals. In addition, research explaining the relationship of how processing speed affects bilingual children with SLI remains undetermined.

Specific cognitive processing accounts of SLI have hypothesized that a reduction in skills such as phonological working memory (Campbell, Dollaghan, Needleman, & Janosky, 1997; Dollaghan & Campbell, 1998; Gathercole & Baddeley, 1990) or temporal processing (Tallal & Newcombe, 1978) can account for the linguistic difficulties of children with SLI. In the phonological working memory domain, Girabau and Schwartz (2008) tested Spanish–English bilinguals with and without LI on a nonword repetition task; typical bilinguals outperformed bilinguals with LI. An effect of syllable length was observed where performance decreased across both groups as nonwords became longer; however, only six of the 11 typical bilinguals scored below 100% (no less than 95%) syllables correct on all nonwords regardless of length. Bilinguals with LI went from 95% syllables correct for single syllable words to 9% syllables correct for five syllable words. This dramatic decrease in syllable accuracy provides evidence that children with LI have limitations in the amount of information that they can attend to, which in this case supports a deficit in phonological working memory.

Kohnert et al. (2006) measured children who were typically developing monolingual English speakers (EO), typical bilingual Spanish–English speaking children (BI), and monolingual English speaking children with LI (ELI) on the Competing Language Processing Task (CLPT; Gaulin & Campbell, 1994), a measure of verbal working memory capacity, and the nonword repetition task

(NWR), which was developed by Dollaghan and Campbell (1998). They found similar differences to Girabau and Schwartz (2008) on the NWR, where all children showed decreasing accuracy in syllables correct as the nonword length increased; similarly, ELI children showed the most dramatic decrease in accuracy. Kohnert et al. also found that the EO children outperformed ELI children on both tasks, but that BI children did not differ significantly from ELI children on the CLPT. The nonword repetition task, which used nonwords that followed the phonotactics of English (Dollaghan & Campbell, 1998), revealed significant group separation amongst all three groups at the four-syllable nonword level (EO outperformed all groups and BI outperformed the ELI group); however, there was significant group overlap for nonwords with fewer than four syllables. These results provide evidence that children with LI have a reduction in specific skills like verbal working memory and phonological working memory, but that language experience is a mitigating factor when comparing monolinguals and bilinguals.

Gutierrez-Clellen et al. (2004) examined verbal working memory (VWM) in typical bilingual Spanish–English speaking children, typical English-proficient with limited Spanish speaking children and, typical Spanish-proficient with limited English speaking children. English and Spanish versions of the CLPT and Dual Processing Competing Language Test (DPCT) were used to measure VWM in the three groups. Results indicated no differences on measures of VWM between the three groups nor between languages. Conversely, in two experiments Thorn and Gathercole (1999) observed the effect of vocabulary knowledge on phonological short-term memory in French–English bilinguals as compared to their monolingual English and English speaking children learning French as a second language peers. Results indicated a strong relationship between vocabulary knowledge and short-term memory. Multiple regression analyses revealed English vocabulary significantly accounting for 9% of the variance in English nonword repetition performance and French vocabulary significantly accounting for 38% of French NWR; these results support the existence of a language effect in processing measures such as nonword repetition. In terms of processing capacity as a measure by phonological working memory, English speaking children learning French as a second language performed equally on the French nonword repetition task to younger, yet proficient bilingual French–English children matched for performance in French vocabulary. It would be expected that older children (mean age difference of two years six months) would exhibit a larger phonological working memory advantage; however, this finding suggests that despite the age difference, the contribution of language-specific knowledge provides a possible advantage in phonological working memory for the younger proficient bilinguals.

The use of processing measures has been advocated as a tool that is free of language and cultural experience to identify language impairment in language minority populations. Nevertheless, research evidence suggests caution when choosing processing measures for nonmainstream children because these measures contain components that are sensitive to language and cultural experiences. Moreover, norms for such tasks must be validated with bilingual populations.

Linguistic accounts of SLI

Linguistic accounts of SLI share the underlying hypothesis of linguistic knowledge deficits that result in problems with morphosyntax. Although these accounts differ in the assumed locus of deficits, they are centered on domain-specific linguistic knowledge, in contrast with domain-general processing accounts (e.g., Leonard, 1998; Paradis, 2007; van der Lely, 2005).

The Functional Category Deficit Account is based on the concept of acquisition of functional categories, such as determiners, complementizers, and inflections, in typically developing (TD) children. Radford (1988, 1990) has argued that children begin to acquire functional categories around two years of age; thus, the early grammar can be described only in terms of lexical categories. According to this account, children with SLI have greater difficulties with grammatical morphology due to slower development of functional categories. In particular, the grammatical morphemes that appear to be problematic for English-speaking children with SLI are associated with the use of functional categories (e.g., Leonard, Eyer, Bedore, & Grela, 1997). However, the reported differences between children with SLI and MLU-matched children in the use of functional categories relate to the differences in the degree of use (Leonard, 1998).

The functional category deficit account has been extended to studies in other languages. Italian speaking children with SLI are more likely to omit direct object clitics than MLU-matched children (e.g., Leonard, Bortolini, Caselli, McGregor, & Sabbadini, 1992; Leonard, Sabbadini, Volterra, & Leonard, 1988). In contrast with Italian, French speaking children with SLI were reported to use articles to the same extent as MLU-matched children (Le Normand, Leonard, & McGregor, 1993). Omissions and incorrect use of grammatical morphemes were found in Spanish speaking children with SLI (Restrepo, 1998), specifically, articles have been documented as a primary area of difficulty (Anderson & Souto, 2005; Restrepo & Gutierrez-Clellen, 2001). However, studies on Spanish speaking children suggest that grammatical morphemes associated with lexical categories such as the noun plural inflection could also be problematic for children with SLI (Bedore & Leonard, 2001; 2005; Merino, 1983), although the differences are not clinically significant.

The Extended Optional Infinitive Account considers problems with tense-bearing morphology as the source of deficits in children with SLI (Rice & Wexler, 1996; Rice, Wexler, & Cleave, 1995). Wexler (1994) described the Optional Infinitive (OI) stage in early grammar of TD children as a period when the infinitival form of a verb is optionally used instead of the finite form, although children possess the grammatical properties of finiteness. The OI stage was accounted by the Agreement/Tense Omission Model (ATOM; Wexler, Schütze, & Rice, 1998), according to which either agreement and/or tense could be optionally omitted in child grammar. Although, this proposal accounted for instances of missing subject–verb agreement in English, it did not apply to null-subject languages such as Italian or Spanish. To address this issue, Wexler (1998, 2003) proposed the Extended Unique Checking Constrain (EUCC), according to which the OI stage existed in early child grammar only in the non-null subject languages. In particular, in non-null subject languages both the category tense (TNS) and subject agreement (AGRS) have a noninterpretable determiner (D) feature. Grammatical subjects represented as determiner phrases (DP) contain the interpretable D feature, and therefore, the D feature needs to be checked against AGRS and TNS. In null subject languages only TNS has the noninterpretable D feature and, thus, checking is only limited to the TNS, which is not affected in these languages (Leonard, 2009). Wexler's account explains difficulties with function words such as auxiliaries, clitics, and article omissions, but not for their substitutions.

Children with SLI are assumed to have the extended period of the optional infinitive stage (Rice, Wexler, & Cleave, 1995). However, it is not clear how long children with SLI remain in the extended OI stage and what proportion of finite forms indicates the emergence from the OI stage. Because the OI stage is manifested by the omissions of finiteness markings, it is not always evident in English whether the underlying problem refers to the selection of infinitival forms in finite contexts or other factors resulting in omissions of grammatical morphemes. Although cross-linguistic data supported the OI stage in a variety of Romance and Germanic languages (e.g., in French: Paradis & Crago, 2001; in German: Rice, Noll, & Grimm, 1997; in Swedish: Hansson & Nettelbladt, 1995), not all studies are consistent with this account. In particular, Italian and Hebrew speaking children with SLI use the finite forms to the comparable extent as MLU-matched children (e.g., Bortolini & Leonard, 1996; Dromi, Leonard, & Shteiman, 1993). Research with bilingual children with SLI is still needed to account for their variability in the representation of the deficit across languages. For example, how the account handles the use of a place holder article in bilingual children undergoing language loss, or how language influence impacts the types of errors observed in some children (Restrepo, 2003).

The Implicit Grammatical Rule Deficit Account describes the core problem of SLI as a deficit in learning, representation, and/or processing of implicit morphological rules (e.g., Gopnik, 1990;

Ullman & Gopnik, 1999). Originally this account was based on the feature-deficit hypothesis, according to which tense, number, person, case, and gender features are absent in the underlying grammar of children with SLI (Gopnik, 1990). Ullman and Gopnik (1999) suggested the three-level explanation of morphological deficits in SLI: the procedural memory deficit that affects nonlinguistic functions could possibly cause an inability to learn implicit rules; the selection of the appropriate word form relies on conceptual system, which depend on declarative memory; individuals with SLI may employ a compensatory strategy by adding suffix-like endings to forms retrieved by conceptual system.

Two options are available to compensate for the deficit in acquiring morphological rules. The relatively intact lexical memory provides a compensatory way of memorizing the inflected verb forms as unanalyzed lexical items. Taking into account the appropriate age, individuals with SLI could be taught morphological rules. Lexical learning should eventually result in acquiring the inflected forms, especially in English with relatively few inflections; however, this assumption was not supported by data from adults with SLI (Gopnik & Crago, 1991). As pointed out by Leonard (1998), individuals with SLI are characterized by rather inconsistent use of inflections with the same lexical item, which cannot be predicted by this account. Moreover, Swisher, Restrepo, Plante, and Lowell (1995) found that children with SLI made greater gains in generalizing trained bound morpheme to untrained vocabulary item under an implicit-rule learning condition rather than an explicit-rule learning condition. This finding is also inconsistent with the implicit rule deficit account.

Morehead and Ingram (1973) found that children with SLI are limited in the scope of syntactic categories and syntactic rules that can be applied, which is in contrast with the implicit rule deficit account. This finding is supported by studies in other languages and in bilingual SLI children undergoing language loss. In particular, Leonard, Bortolini, Caselli, McGregor, and Sabbadini (1992) found that Italian speaking children with SLI used articles and clitics to a lesser degree than TD MLU-matched children. Restrepo and Gutierrez-Clellen (2001) reported article omissions and gender agreement substitution as the most common types of article errors in Spanish-speaking children with SLI.

Other linguistic accounts assumed that grammatical difficulties in SLI are the result of problems in establishing structural relationships (e.g., Clahsen, Bartke, & Göllner, 1997; Rice & Oetting, 1993; Rothweiler & Clahsen, 1993; van der Lely, 1998). The Missing Agreement Account proposed that children with SLI have difficulties in establishing agreement relations between the two phrase-structure categories (Clahsen, 1989, 1993; Clahsen & Hansen, 1997; Rothweiler & Clahsen, 1993). Although this claim was originally applied to German speaking children, studies on other languages were derivable from this account (Clahsen & Hansen, 1997; Leonard, 1998). According to this approach, the following grammatical areas are problematic for children with SLI: the use of subject–verb agreement (e.g., third person singular in English; number markings on finite verbs in German and Italian), auxiliaries, gender markings on determiners and adjectives, and case markings (in German). In contrast, cross-linguistic data on Italian articles do not seem to support this proposal: clitics and articles are reported to be used with lower percentages by children with SLI, however, when these forms are produced, they show the correct agreement marking in most cases (e.g., Leonard et al., 1992).

Van der Lely and colleagues (e.g., Bishop, Bright, James, Bishop, & van der Lely, 2000; van der Lely, 1994, 1996) proposed that there is a homogeneous subtype of SLI, which is characterized by a representational deficit for dependent relationships. In particular, children with SLI have difficulties forming or understanding structures that mark syntactic dependencies (e.g., subject–verb agreement or a pronoun case marking in English). Marshall and van der Lely (2007) extended this approach as the Computational Grammatical Complexity Hypothesis, according to which the core deficit in the representation of structural linguistic complexity is at the syntactic, morphological, and phonological levels. They argued that because problems in the three levels apply to the realization of tense, it could be a reliable marker of SLI.

In summary, despite differences among linguistic accounts, their proponents argue that individuals with SLI have language difficulties due to limitations in the grammatical knowledge. Although linguistic accounts seem to capture language characteristics of SLI cross-linguistically, not all studies are consistent with their predictions and no single approach seems to account for the wide range of cross-linguistic differences in individuals with SLI (Leonard, 2009). Further, Morgan, Restrepo, and Auza (2009) found that Spanish speaking monolingual children with SLI demonstrated a variable linguistic profile where no single deficit in clitics, subjunctives, articles, or derivational morphemes could be identified as a clinical marker. These results therefore suggest that linguistic accounts often reflect the performance errors that are better explained through processing accounts of SLI. Further, given the variability in the SLI profile in a language such as Spanish, finding a linguistic marker as in English for bilingual SLI may not be a productive endeavor given the variability observe in bilingual and Spanish SLI. This variability may be better understood within DST and cognitive interactive processes (Kohnert, 2008).

Research in bilingual populations with SLI

Despite a growing number of cross-linguistic studies, research on SLI in bilingual populations remains rather limited. Several theoretical issues can be raised with regard to bilingual individuals: the characteristics of dual-language acquisition in individuals with SLI, the linguistic and processing differences between monolingual and bilingual children with SLI, and the specific characteristics of SLI that would be used in assessment and treatment of bilingual populations. One particular phenomenon in bilingual SLI children is the role of the sociolinguistic context in the continued development of the languages the children speak. Bilingual children with SLI who attend programs in which both of the languages are stimulated, also called additive bilingual programs, demonstrate similar characteristics to those of monolingual children and no greater severity in their language (Bruck, 1982). On the other hand, children who are in subtractive language environments, where their native language is not stimulated, are at a great risk of demonstrating native language attrition (Anderson, 2004; Restrepo, 2003). However, it is possible that for some, the second language acquisition process is slowed down. To date, there are very few longitudinal studies that help us understand language acquisition in these children.

Restrepo and Kruth (2000) investigated a grammatical profile of a Spanish–English bilingual child with SLI in comparison with a TD bilingual age-matched child. Using spontaneous language samples in both languages, they found differences in the use of verb forms, tenses, pronouns, and prepositions in English and in the use of definite articles, pronouns, and prepositions in Spanish. Additionally, the language productions of the bilingual child with SLI were characterized by decreased MLU and limited syntactic complexity. The authors argued that although there is no universal marker of SLI in bilingual populations and no single theory could account for a variety of crosslinguistic characteristics, there are qualitative differences in the use of grammatical morphology that are not due to dual-language development. Further, Restrepo (2003) examined the language profiles of two bilingual children with SLI undergoing language loss. The children attended first grade in an English-only educational system and came from homes where they only spoke Spanish. One child demonstrated a decrease in syntactic length and complexity in Spanish, whereas the other child demonstrated an increase in syntactic length, but also an increase in the number of grammatical errors per sentence in Spanish. Both children demonstrated a limited variety of syntactic, morphological, and lexical forms in Spanish. Their English skills on the other hand, while they were highly ungrammatical, they had greater sentence length and complexity than Spanish, their first language. Restrepo's case studies suggest that bilingual children with SLI who live in subtractive language environments are at a great risk of losing grammatical skills in their native language indicating an interaction between linguistic and processing deficits, best explained within a DST.

Research examining sequential bilingual children's second language performance indicates that this language can have some of the same characteristics as monolingual children with LI. In addition, there can be qualitative differences from those of monolingual populations. For example, Jacobson and Schwartz (2005) investigated the English performance in bilingual children with SLI and found that they exhibited past tense difficulties, like monolingual English speaking children do. However, they also found that the pattern of errors differed between typically developing and those with SLI. Children with SLI scored relatively better on irregular verbs and worse on novel verbs; they also exhibited more nonproductive errors such as bare stem verbs. Similarly, some of the characteristics in Restrepo's case studies indicate some errors occur only in bilingual populations like the replacement of the Spanish articles with the English "the" as in "the casa" (the house) or the form "le," which is a clitic, but the form was used as an article in one of the case studies. Both examples indicate that the children were simplifying the article system in Spanish.

These studies suggest that bilingual SLI children presents unique challenges that linguistic and processing accounts of SLI have not considered. Consistent with processing accounts and with the DST, these results are not surprising and indicate that bilingual children with language impairment in subtractive environments demonstrate different language patterns in their native language, while they continue to acquire their second language. These patterns are not predictable yet, until we conduct further longitudinal group studies.

An important issue with language impairment in bilinguals is how we differentiate language impairment from the language performance of second language learners. Paradis and colleagues (Paradis, 2007; Paradis, Crago, & Genesee, 2006; Paradis, Crago, Genesee, & Rice, 2003) investigated whether bilingual French–English speaking children with SLI differed from monolingual age-matched children in each language in acquisition of grammatical morphology. According to the linguistic account, the core deficit of SLI is internal to the linguistic system, and therefore, it was predicted that bilingual children with SLI would not be delayed in comparison with monolingual age-matched children with SLI. Using spontaneous language samples, bilingual children with SLI were compared with monolingual speakers of French and English with and without SLI in the productions of grammatical morphemes that mark tense and nontense features. Results revealed that bilingual and monolingual children with SLI had greater difficulties with tense and nontense morphemes than TD age peers. However, there were no significant differences between bilingual and monolingual SLI groups in the use of grammatical morphemes in either language. Results were consistent with the linguistic account confirming that bilingual children with SLI performed poorly in comparison with TD monolingual children in each language, but to the same extent as monolingual age peers with SLI.

In a subsequent study, Paradis et al. (2006) investigated the use of direct object clitics in French–English bilingual and monolingual children with and without SLI. Additionally, a language-matched TD bilingual group was included to account for any possible acquisition differences between monolingual and bilingual conditions. Results revealed that bilingual children with SLI used object clitics in French to the same extent as the language-matched TD bilingual children, but significantly more often than monolingual French speaking children with SLI. The authors concluded that because bilingual participants were not lagging behind monolingual children with SLI, the difficulties with direct object pronouns were not due to the acquisition of the two languages.

In a more recent study, we examined performance comparing Spanish language skills between monolingual children from Mexico and bilingual children in the United States attending schools in subtractive language environments. Results indicated that the bilingual children shared deficits in the same areas as monolinguals with SLI; however, the bilinguals still outperformed the monolinguals with SLI. In this case, areas that we predicted to be problematic for monolingual Spanish speaking children with SLI also seemed to be difficult for bilinguals living in a subtractive language environment: articles, clitics, subjunctives, derivational morphemes, and rapid naming. These results indicate that norms in bilingual populations are necessary for differential diagnosis of SLI and typical language. To this end, examination of qualitative differences in the native and second language will be helpful.

Linguistic and processing accounts of SLI do not account for the language characteristics of bilingual children with SLI. Nevertheless, these accounts fit within the DST framework of language and bilingualism, which accounts for variability, the competition, and the changes within one child depending on the input and context at any given time. Bilingual children with SLI present with the same linguistic and processing difficulties that monolinguals do. However, bilingual populations in general do not perform like monolingual in some processing skills, such us working memory (Kohnert et al., 2006). Further, bilingual children educated in subtractive language environments are at risk of losing native language skills, which in turn can complicate differential diagnosis. To date, there is no evidence that this is the case for bilingual children with SLI living and educated in additive bilingual environments. In fact, research indicates that bilingual children with SLI perform as well as monolingual children with SLI (Bruck, 1982; Thordardottir, Weismer, & Smith, 1997), which seems to be the case with other populations with language impairment, such as in children with Down Syndrome (Kay-Raining Bird et al., 2005).

Future research needs to describe characteristics in bilingual children with SLI better, and theories must account for these characteristics. Moreover, information on what characteristics of bilingual SLI are universal and those that are language-specific would help in defining the population in general and in understanding the nature of the disorder. This in turn, would lead to better intervention and diagnostic protocols for these children. In addition, intervention research would benefit from examining what skills transfer cross-linguistically and what skills do not. To date, very little research is available to make informed decisions on how to best serve bilingual children with SLI.

Further reading

Andreou, G., & Lemoni, G. (2020). Narrative skills of monolingual and bilingual pre-school and primary school children with developmental language disorder (DLD): A systematic review. *Open Journal of Modern Linguistics, 10*(5), 429–458.

Ruberg, T., Rothweiler, M., Veríssimo, J., & Clahsen, H. (2020). Childhood bilingualism and Specific Language Impairment: A study of the CP-domain in German SLI. *Bilingualism: Language and Cognition, 23*(3), 668–680.

Scherger, A. L. (2022). The role of age and timing in bilingual assessment: Non-word repetition, subject-verb agreement and case marking in L1 and eL2 children with and without SLI. *Clinical Linguistics and Phonetics, 36*(1), 54–74.

References

Anderson, R. T. (2004). First language loss in Spanish-speaking children: Patterns of loss and implications for clinical practice. In B. Goldstein (Ed.), *Bilingual language development & disorders in Spanish-English speakers* (pp. 187–212). Baltimore, MD: Brooks Publishing.

Anderson, R. T., & Souto, S. M. (2005). The use of articles by monolingual Puerto Rican Spanish-speaking children with specific language impairment. *Applied Psycholinguistics, 26*(4), 621–647.

Archibald, L. M. D., & Gathercole, S. E. (2006). Short-term and working memory in specific language impairment. *International Journal of Language and Communication Disorders, 41*(6), 675–693.

Bedore, L., & Leonard, L. (2001). Grammatical morphology deficits in Spanish-speaking children with specific language impairment. *Journal of Speech, Language, and Hearing Research, 44*(4), 905–924.

Bedore, L., & Leonard, L. (2005). Verb inflections and noun phrase morphology in the spontaneous speech of Spanish-speaking children with specific language impairment. *Applied Psycholinguistics, 26*(2), 195–225.

Bishop, B., Bright, P., James, C., Bishop, S., & van der Lely, H. (2000). Grammatical SLI: A distinct subtype of developmental language impairment? *Applied Psycholinguistics, 21*(2), 159–181.

Bortolini, U., & Leonard, L. (1996). Phonology and grammatical morphology in specific language impairment: Accounting for individual variation in English and Italian. *Applied Psycholinguistics, 17*(1), 85–104.

Bruck, M. (1982). Language impaired children's performance in an additive bilingual education program. *Applied Psycholinguistics, 3*(1), 45–60.

Campbell, T., Dollaghan, C., Needleman, H., & Janosky, J. (1997). Reducing bias in language assessment: Processing-dependent measures. *Journal of Speech, Language, and Hearing Research, 40*(3), 519–525.

Catts, H., Adlof, S., Hogan, T., & Ellis Weismer, S. (2005). Are specific language impairment and dyslexia distinct disorders? *Journal of Speech, Language, and Hearing Research, 48*(6), 1378–1396.

Clahsen, H. (1989). The grammatical characterization of developmental dysphasia. *Linguistics, 27*(5), 897–920.

Clahsen, H. (1993). Linguistic perspectives on specific language impairment. Working Papers Series. *Theorie des Lexikons, 37.*

Clahsen, H., & Hansen, D. (1997). The grammatical agreement deficit in Specific Language Impairment: Evidence from therapy experiments. In M. Gopnik (Ed.), *The inheritance and innateness of grammars* (pp. 141–160). Oxford: Oxford University Press.

Clahsen, H., Bartke, S., & Göllner, S. (1997). Formal features in impaired grammars: A comparison of English and German SLI children. *Journal of Neurolinguistics, 10*(2–3), 151–171.

Dollaghan, C., & Campbell, T. F. (1998). Nonword repetition and child language impairment. *Journal of Speech, Language, and Hearing Research, 41*(5), 1136–1146.

Dromi, E., Leonard, L. B., & Shteiman, M. (1993). The grammatical morphology of Hebrew speaking children with specific language impairment: Some competing hypotheses. *Journal of Speech and Hearing Research, 36*(4), 760–771.

Edwards, J., & Lahey, M. (1998). Nonword repetitions of children with specific language impairment: Exploration of some explanations for their inaccuracies. *Applied Psycholinguistics, 19*(2), 279–309.

Evans, J., & McWhinney, B. (1999). Sentence processing strategies in children with expressive and expressive-receptive specific language impairments. *International Journal of Language and Communication Disorders, 34*(2), 117–134.

Gass, S., & Selinker, L. (2008). *Second language acquisition. An introductory course.* New York: Routledge.

Gathercole, S. E., & Baddeley, A. D. (1990). Phonological memory deficits in language disordered children: Is there a causal connection? *Journal of Memory and Language, 29*(3), 336–360.

Gaulin, C., & Campbell, T. (1994). Procedure for assessing verbal working memory in normal school-age children: Some preliminary data. *Perceptual and Motor Skills, 79*(1 Pt 1), 55–64.

Gillam, R., Cowan, N., & Marler, J. (1998). Information processing by school-age children with specific language impairment: Evidence from a modality effect paradigm. *Journal of Speech, Language, and Hearing Research, 41*(4), 913–926.

Girbau, D., & Schwartz, R. G. (2008). Phonological working memory in Spanish–English bilingual children with and without specific language impairment. *Journal of Communication Disorders, 41*(2), 124–145.

Gopnik, M. (1990). Feature blindness: A case study. *Language Acquisition, 1*(2), 139–164.

Gopnik, M., & Crago, M. (1991). Familial aggregation of a developmental language disorder. *Cognition, 39*(1), 1–50.

Gray, S. (2003). Diagnostic accuracy and test-retest reliability of nonword repetition and digit span tasks administered to preschool children with specific language impairment. *Journal of Communication Disorders, 36*(2), 129–151.

Gray, S. (2004). Word learning by preschoolers with specific language impairment predictors and poor learners. *Journal of Speech, Language, and Hearing Research, 47*(5), 1117–1132.

Gray, S. (2005). Word learning by preschoolers with specific language impairment effect of phonological or semantic cues. *Journal of Speech, Language, and Hearing Research, 48*(6), 1452–1467.

Gutierrez-Clellen, V., Calderon, J., & Weismer, S. E. (2004). Verbal working memory in bilingual children. *Journal of Speech and Hearing Research, 47*, 863–876.

Hansson, K., & Nettelbladt, U. (1995). Grammatical characteristics of Swedish children with SLI. *Journal of Speech, Language, and Hearing Research, 38*(3), 589–598.

Herdina, P., & Jessner, U. (2002). *A dynamic model of multilingualism.* Clevedon, UK: Multilingual Matters LTD.

Hill, E. L. (2001). Non-specific nature of specific language impairment: A review of the literature with regard to concomitant motor impairments. *International Journal of Language and Communication Disorders, 36*(2), 149–171.

Jacobson, P. F., & Schwartz, R. G. (2005). English past tense use in bilingual children with language impairment. *American Journal of Speech-Language Pathology, 14*(4), 313–323.

Kail, R. (1994). A method for studying the generalized slowing hypothesis in children with specific language impairment. *Journal of Speech, Language, and Hearing Research, 37*(2), 418.

Kay-Raining Bird, E., Cleave, P., Trureau, N., Thordardottir, E., Sutton, A., & Thorpe, A. (2005). The language abilities of bilingual children with down syndrome. *American Journal of Speech-Language Pathology, 14*(3), 187–199.

Kohnert, K. (2008). *Language disorders in bilingual children and adults.* San Diego: Plural Publishing.

Kohnert, K., & Derr, A. (2004). Language intervention with bilingual children. In B. Goldstein (Ed.), *Bilingual language development and disorders in Spanish-English speakers* (pp. 315–343). Baltimore: Brookes.

Kohnert, K., Windsor, J., & Yim, D. (2006). Do language-based processing tasks separate children with language impairment from typical bilinguals? *Learning Disabilities Research and Practice, 21*(1), 19–29.

Kohnert, K., Windsor, J., & Ebert, K. D. (2008). Primary of "specific" language impairment and children learning a second language. *Brain and Language*, 1–11.

Le Normand, M. T., Leonard, L., & McGregor, K. (1993). A cross-linguistic study of article use by children with specific language impairment. *European Journal of Disorders of Communication, 28*(2), 153–163.

Leonard, L. B. (1998). *Children with specific language impairment*. Cambridge, MA: The MIT Press.

Leonard, L. B. (2009). Crosslinguistic studies of child langauge disorders. In R. G. Schwartz (Ed.), *Handbook of child langauge disorders* (pp. 308–324). New York: Taylor & Francis.

Leonard, L., Bortolini, U., Caselli, M. C., McGregor, K., & Sabbadini, L. (1992a). Morphological deficits in children with specific language impairments: The status of features in underlying grammar. *Language Acquisition, 2*, 151–179.

Leonard, L., Bortolini, U., Caselli, M. C., McGregor, K., & Sabbadini, L. (1992b). Some influences of the grammar of English-and Italian-speaking children with specific language impairment. *Applied Psycholinguistics, 9*, 39–57.

Leonard, L., Eyer, J., Bedore, L., & Grela, B. (1997). Three accounts of the grammatical morpheme difficulties of English-speaking children with specific language impairments. *Journal of Speech, Language, and Hearing Research, 40*(4), 741–753.

Leonard, L. B., Sabbadini, L., Volterra, V., & Leonard, J. S. (1988). Some influences on the grammar of English- and Italian-speaking children with specific language impairment. *Applied Psycholinguistics, 9*(1), 39–57.

Leonard, L. B., Ellis Weismer, S., Miller, C. A., Francis, D. J., Tomblin, J. B., & Kail, R. V. (2007). Speed of processing, working memory, and language impairment in children. *Journal of Speech, Language, and Hearing Research, 50*(2), 408–428.

Marshall, C. R., & van der Lely, H. (2007). Derivational morphology in children with grammatical-specific language impairment. *Clinical Linguistics and Phonetics, 21*(2), 71–91.

Merino, B. (1983). Language development in normal and language handicapped Spanish-speaking children. *Hispanic Journal of Behavioral Sciences, 5*(4), 379–400.

Morehead, D., & Ingram, D. (1973). The development of base syntax in normal and linguistically deviant children. *Journal of Speech, Language, and Hearing Research, 16*(3), 330–352.

Morgan, G., Restrepo, M. A., & Auza, A. (2009). Variability in the grammatical profiles of Spanish-speaking children with specific language impairment. In J. Grinstead (Ed.), *Hispanic child languages: Typical and impaired development.*

Montgomery, J. W. (1995). Sentence comprehension in children with specific language impairment: The role of phonological working memory. *Journal of Speech, Language, and Hearing Research, 38*(1), 187.

Montgomery, J. W. (2003). Working memory and comprehension in children with specific language impairment: What we know so far. *Journal of Communication Disorders, 36*(3), 221–231.

Paradis, J. (2007). Bilingual children with specific language impairment: Theoretical and applied issues. *Applied Psycholinguistics, 28*(3), 551–564.

Paradis, J., & Crago, M. (2001). The morphosyntax of specific language impairment in French: Evidence for an Extended Optional Default account. *Language Acquisition, 9*(4), 269–300.

Paradis, J., Crago, M., Genesee, F., & Rice, M. (2003). Bilingual children with specific language impairment: How do they compare with their monolingual peers? *Journal of Speech, Language, and Hearing Research, 46*, 1–15.

Paradis, J., Crago, M., & Genesee, F. (2006). Domain-specific versus domain-general theories of the deficit in SLI: Object pronoun acquisition by French–English bilingual children. *Language Acquisition, 13/14*, 33–62.

Peña, E., & Kester, E. S. (2004). Semantic development in Spanish-English bilinguals: Theory, assessment, and intervention. In B. Goldstein (Ed.), *Bilingual language development & disorders in Spanish-English speakers* (pp. 105–128). Baltimore, MD: Paul H. Brookes.

Radford, A. (1988). Small children's small clauses. *Transaction of the Philological Society, 86*(1), 1–46.

Radford, A. (1990). *Syntactic theory and the acquisition of English syntax*. Oxford: Blackwell.

Restrepo, M. A. (1998). Identifiers of predominantly Spanish-speaking children with language impairment. *Journal of Speech, Language, and Hearing Research, 41*(6), 1398–1411.

Restrepo, M. A. (2003). Spanish language skills in bilingual children with specific language impairment. In S. Montrul & F. Ordoñez (Eds.), *Linguistic theory and language development in Hispanic languages. Papers from the 5th hispanic linguistics symposium and the 4th conference on the acquisition of Spanish and Portuguese* (pp. 365–374). Summerville: Cascadilla Press.

Restrepo, M. A., & Gutierrez-Clellen, V. F. (2001). Article production in bilingual children with specific language impairment. *Journal of Child Language, 28*(2), 433–452.

Restrepo, M. A., & Kruth, K. (2000). Grammatical characteristics of a bilingual student with specific language impairment. *Journal of Children's Communication Development, 21*, 66–76.

Rice, M., & Oetting, J. (1993). Morphological deficits in children with SLI: Evaluation of number marking and agreement. *Journal of Speech and Hearing Research, 36*(6), 1249–1257.

Rice, M., & Wexler, K. (1996). Toward tense as a clinical marker of specific language impairment in English-speaking children. *Journal of Speech, Language, and Hearing Research, 39*(6), 1239–1257.

Rice, M., Wexler, K., & Cleave, P. (1995). Specific language impairment as a period of extended optional infinitive. *Journal of Speech, Language, and Hearing Research, 38*(4), 850–863.

Rice, M., Noll, R. K., & Grimm, H. (1997). An extended optional infinitive stage in German-speaking children with SLI. *Language Acquisition, 6*(4), 255–296.

Rothweiler, M., & Clahsen, H. (1993). Dissociations in SLI children's inflectional systems: A study of participle inflection and subject-verb-agreement. *Logopedics, Phoniatrics, Vocology, 18*(4), 169–179.

Schul, R., Stiles, J., Wulfeck, B., & Townsend, J. (2004). How 'generalized' is the 'slowed processing'. In SLI? The case of visuospatial attentional orienting. *Neuropsychologia, 42*(5), 661–671.

Schwartz, R. G. (2009). Specific language impairment. In R. G. Schwartz (Ed.), *Handbook of child language disorders* (pp. 3–43). New York: Taylor & Francis.

Swisher, L., Restrepo, M. A., Plante, E., & Lowell, S. (1995). Effects of implicit and explicit "rule" presentation on bound-morpheme generalization in specific language impairment. *Journal of Speech, Language, and Hearing Research, 38*(1), 168–173.

Tallal, P., & Newcombe, F. (1978). Impairment of auditory perception and language comprehension in dyphasia. *Brain and Language, 5*(1), 13–24.

Thordardottir, E. T., Weismer, S. E., & Smith, M. E. (1997). Vocabulary learning in bilingual and monolingual clinical intervention. *Child Language Teaching and Therapy, 13*(3), 215–227.

Thorn, A. S., & Gathercole, S. E. (1999). Language-specific knowledge and short-term memory in bilingual and non-bilingual children. *Quarterly Journal of Experimental Psychology, 52A*(2), 303–324.

Ullman, M. T., & Gopnik, M. (1999). Inflectional morphology in a family with inherited specific language impairment. *Applied Psycholinguistics, 20*(1), 51–117.

Ullman, M. T., & Pierpont, E. (2005). Specific language impairment is not specific to language: The procedural deficit hypothesis. *Cortex, 41*(3), 399–433.

van der Lely, H. (1994). Canonical linking rules: Forward versus reverse linking in normally developing and specifically-language impaired children. *Cognition, 51*(1), 29–72.

van der Lely, H. (1996). Specifically language impaired and normally developing children: Verbal passive vs. adjectival passive interpretation. *Lingua, 98*(4), 243–272.

van der Lely, H. (1998). SLI in children: Movement, economy, and deficits in the computational-syntactic system. *Language Acquisition*, 7(2–4), 161–192.

van der Lely, H. (2005). Domain-specific cognitive systems: Insight from grammatical-SLI. *Trends in Cognitive Sciences, 9*(2), 53–59.

Weismer, S. E. (1996). Capacity limitations in working memory: The impact on lexical and morphological learning by children with language impairment. *Topics in Language Disorders, 17*(1), 33–44.

Weismer, S. E., & Hesketh, L. (1998). The impact of emphatic stress on novel word learning by children with specific language impairment. *Journal of Speech and Hearing Research, 41*(6), 1444–1458.

Weismer, S. E., Evans, J., & Hesketh, L. (1999). An examination of verbal working memory capacity in children with specific language impairment. *Journal of Speech, Language, and Hearing Research, 42*(5), 1249–1260.

Wexler, K. (1994). Optional infinitives, head movement and the economy of derivations. In D. Lightfoot & N. Homstein (Eds.), *Verb movement* (pp. 305–350). Cambridge: Cambridge University Press.

Wexler, K. (1998). Very early parameter setting and the unique checking constraint: A new explanation of the optional infinitive stage. *Lingua, 106*(1–4), 23–79.

Wexler, K. (2003). Lennenberg's dream: Learning, normal language development, and specific language impairment. In Y. Levy & J. Schaeffer (Eds.), *Language competence across populations. Towards a definition of specific language impairment* (pp. 11–62). Mahwah: Erlbaum.

Wexler, K., Schütze, C. T., & Rice, M. (1998). Subject case in children with SLI and unaffected controls: Evidence for the Agr/Tns Omission Model. *Language Acquisition*, 7(2–4), 317–344.

Windsor, J., & Hwang, M. (1999). Testing the generalized slowing hypothesis in specific language impairment. *Journal of Speech, Language, and Hearing Research, 42*(5), 1205–1218.

Windsor, J., & Kohnert, K. (2004). The search for common ground: Part 1. Lexical performance by linguistically diverse learners. *Journal of Speech, Language, and Hearing Research*, 47(4), 877–890.

SECTION III

Acquired disorders

26

APRAXIA OF SPEECH

From psycholinguistic theory to the conceptualization and management of an impairment

Rosemary Varley

Introduction

The processes involved in language and speech production are usually classified into a tripartite division of linguistic encoding, speech control/programming/planning, and motor execution. The parallel division of acquired production disorders into aphasia, apraxia of speech, and dysarthria each align with this sequence of processing phases. This chapter will explore conceptualizations of the processes involved in speech control and their implications for the understanding and management of acquired apraxia of speech (AOS). Both developmental and acquired forms of speech apraxia occur, but this chapter addresses only the acquired form. In acquired AOS, established speech control mechanisms are disrupted by brain injury. These processes sit at the interface between language processing and subsequent phonetic movement execution. They are generally viewed as post-linguistic, where conceptual-semantic and phonological processing have been completed. In standard models, the speaker is seen as successfully activating an abstract phonological representation for a word or phrase. However, this abstract representation cannot drive the muscles of the speech production system. What is needed is a mechanism that converts the abstract representation into a neural code capable of initiating the multiple movements of the articulatory system, all of which must be integrated with each other, and precisely timed and targeted. This mechanism is believed to be impaired in AOS.

AOS is an impairment in speech production that occurs following damage to regions of the language-dominant hemisphere and connected sub-cortical zones that are involved in movement control. Typical sites of damage include left frontal lobe premotor or motor association cortex, and the cortical and sub-cortical areas to which this region is closely interconnected (e.g., basal ganglia and parietal somatosensory cortex) (Basilakos, Rorden, Bonilha, Moser, & Fridriksson, 2015). AOS often co-occurs with aphasia due to the close proximity of these regions to left hemisphere language areas (Conterno, Kümmerer, Dressing, Glauche, Urbach, Weiller, & Rijntjes, 2022), and it only rarely presents as an isolated disorder. Speech output in AOS typically displays inconsistency in articulatory accuracy across utterances, and between the voluntary movements of speech and the involuntary movements of the oral–laryngeal systems that are associated with actions such as chewing, swallowing, and facial expression. AOS is one of a family of apraxic impairments as any motor system that is capable of learned voluntary movement may display apraxic symptoms. For example, limb apraxia impairs volitional movement of the arm and hand; oral apraxia disrupts non-

DOI: 10.4324/9781003204213-30

speech oro-motor movement (Whiteside, Dyson, Cowell, & Varley, 2015). The more a movement is automatic, the more likely it is to be spared in the apraxias. This can be observed within speech production in AOS: sometimes articulatory targets are produced accurately, but on other occasions with errors, and when there are errors, there may be different errors on repeated attempts. In individuals at the mild-moderate end of the severity spectrum, there are islands of fluent, errorless speech, particularly on words and phrases that are used frequently in everyday interactions.

With regard to the differentiation of AOS from aphasic production impairments, this often rests on the striking loss of speech fluency evident in apraxia. The speaker with AOS appears to have retrieved the correct word, but then struggles towards a realization of that word. Sometimes, "struggle and groping" is observed in speech, where there are false starts and multiple attempts to reach an articulatory target. In the process of effortful construction of speech, there are frequent errors that reduce intelligibility. Errors can include substitutions (errors which cross phoneme boundaries), distortions (errors remaining within a phoneme boundary, e.g., affrication on release of a plosive consonant), omissions, and additions, with more errors as word length increases. In addition to these spatial/targeting errors, the temporal basis of speech is altered with prolongation of steady-state components of speech such as vowels, and increased inter-syllabic pauses (Whiteside & Varley, 1998). There is an overall disruption in the prosodic contour of the utterance (Ballard et al., 2016; Varley & Whiteside, 2001). In severe cases, speakers may be virtually nonverbal with only a small inventory of residual utterances (e.g., "yes," "no," "bye"; Varley, Whiteside, Windsor, & Fisher, 2005).

In terms of differentiating AOS from the dysarthrias, a key feature is the inconsistency of movement. In contrast to AOS, speakers with dysarthria have disruptions in the neuromuscular system that implements speech. As a result, speech alterations are typically more consistent, with an absence of islands of fluent production, and impairment of all movements, whether or not they are volitional or automatic. Furthermore, movement difficulties are observed in non-speech activities such as eating and drinking. However, although speech-language pathology employs this tripartite categorization of production disorders into aphasia, apraxia, and dysarthria, clinical diagnosis is often not clear-cut. One reason for diagnostic uncertainty is that the neural systems engaged in speech and language processing are distributed across multiple brains sites and are tightly interconnected. Following damage caused by a stroke (or other form of brain injury), a lesion may extend over the substrates of more than one processing system and disrupt the interconnectivity of the speech/language network. As a result, an individual is faced with multiple processing disruptions and displays signs from more than one category of impairment.

A second reason for diagnostic complexity is that the theoretical models underpinning our conceptualisation of speech and language production remain a subject for debate. Although many influential psycholinguistic models identify a set of relatively independent or autonomous steps in production (e.g., Levelt, 1989), the nature of representations and the extent of interactions between phases are not fully understood (Smith, 2006). Indeed, the tripartite division of production disorders into aphasia, AOS, and dysarthria is influenced by these multi-stage models of language processing, and in turn reciprocally reinforces the three-stage model. The next section will explore the influence of a standard approach to speech control on the conceptualization and management of AOS. It suggests that at the interface between completed linguistic processing and speech planning, an abstract phonological representation for a word or phrase is mapped to its individual phonemes. In turn, these phonemes activate matching phonetic plans for segments, with these plans containing the necessary spatial and temporal coordinates to direct movement of the articulators.

Segments and AOS: a generative approach

A standard approach to speech control claims that most speech output – words and phrases – are assembled from more basic subcomponents on each occasion of use. This type of approach is influenced by generative linguistic traditions (Chomsky & Halle, 1968). By this view, each time a speaker says a word, and even a frequent word such as *tomorrow*, the various subcomponents of the word, such as individual segments, are activated and combined in the correct order to produce a cohesive syllable/word. These models are often described as elegant or parsimonious in that only a small number of representations are stored in memory (such as the various vowels and consonants of a language, or an even smaller set comprising the distinctive features that signal meaning contrasts in a language such as [+/-VOICE] in English). From these subcomponents, potentially infinite outputs can be generated. Hence words such as *to* and *more* can be built out of the very same subcomponents that were the source of *tomorrow*. However, although modest in memory costs, this type of process requires a large computational mechanism that operates in real time to select and assign segments to their position in the word, as well as maintaining (or buffering) intermediate products of assembly while remaining elements of the word are processed. Because of this buffering demand, longer words might be more prone to errors than shorter ones. An early development of such assembly models was the Slots and Fillers model of Shattuck-Hufnagel (1979). In this influential model, the process of speech control was seen as involving the generation of the skeleton of the word from its phonological representation, with various "slots" for the onset, nucleus, etc., and a parallel but independent activation of its matching segments ("fillers"). In a separate processing stage, each segment is mapped to the appropriate slot in the developing syllable.

The evidence in support of this approach comes from the errors of healthy speakers. In particular, transposition (or exchange or switch) errors such as *tog and froad* for *frog and toad*, where the onsets of two syllables have switched, indicate that at some phase in the speech production process segments appear to be individually represented and assigned. In the terms of Shattuck-Hufnagel's Slots and Fillers model, the pre-vocalic onsets of the nouns have been mapped to the wrong syllable slot. An assumption made in such models is that this (mis-) mapping occurs in the conversion from the abstract phonological representation to a motoric phonetic representation. However, notice that the exchange error has occurred between the two syllable onsets and across word boundaries. This is typical in transposition errors, and exchanges within a syllable (e.g., changing *cat* to *tac*) are rare. Dell (1988) proposed that the between-syllable constraint on exchange errors occurs because there are separate representations for phonemes depending on their syllable position. Hence for English, /t/ would have two independent representations: one for syllable initial and one for final position. By contrast, /h/would have a single representation as it only occurs in a syllable initial position. The error of *cat* to *tac* would not occur as, following the activation of the phonological representation, the subsequent segmental activation would involve only /k _ / (initial), but not /_ k/ (final). In an exchange error, /k _ / might be assigned to another initial slot, but it is barred from entering a syllable final slot. This is a neat solution, but notice it proliferates demands on memory storage and begins to compromise the economy of segmental assembly models. Furthermore, it blurs the distinction between slots and their fillers as slot information is now intrinsic to the segment/filler representation.

Although transposition errors provide a window on some phase of the speech production process, it is not clear that it is at the phonology-phonetic interface. For example, exchanges might occur post-phonetic encoding, and due to interference between elements held in a speech output buffer while other words in a phrase are selected. Such an account would be consistent with the cross-syllable/cross-word preponderance of such errors. Furthermore, there is a surprising absence of such errors in the speech of young children or in the output of people with various neurogenic speech and language disorders (Stemberger, 1989; Varley & Whiteside, 2001). One would predict that a young child learning to use a segmental assembly mechanism would make many errors of segmental assignment. However, transposition errors appear in child speech at around the ages of six to seven, and at the same time that literacy develops. Similarly, we might expect "transpositional aphasia" to have been described. However, in impaired speech it is possible to observe many substitution errors, perseverations, deletions, and contextually motivated errors such as assimilation and dissimilation, but exchange errors are uncommon. It may well be that a key factor in exchange errors is the simultaneous activation of large amounts of phonetic-phonological information: that is, all elements of the developing phrase are highly activated and therefore potentially in competition with each other. In the case of speech and language pathology (and early child language), less linguistic information is active and, as result, there is less competing activation and fewer exchange errors.

It appears very obvious that words are made up of individual segments and that *cat* is produced from the concatenation of /k/, /a/, and /t/. However, this is a metalinguistic, conscious insight into the automatic and unconscious processes involved in speech control, and this insight is not shared by all speakers. People who have never learned to read (not because of dyslexia, but because of limited access to formal education) do not share the notion that a spoken word consists of a string of segments (de Santos et al., 2004; Morias, Cary, Alegria, & Berterlson, 1979). Similarly individuals who have learned only a logographic writing system such as Chinese have difficulty making correct decisions when asked "What word do you get if you add [tʃ] to the end of the word *purr*?" (Read, Zhang, Nie, & Ding, 1986). Furthermore, the segmental judgments of speakers (or more importantly, readers and writers) of languages with alphabetic spelling systems do not always reflect phonetic realities. For example, many will judge that *apple* contains four or five sounds, and that there are five vowels in spoken English. It is clear that such decisions regarding segmental composition are based upon knowledge of the orthography of the language, and these conscious judgments may provide little insight into the unconscious or implicit mechanisms of speech control. Knowledge of an orthographic writing system might introduce bias into perceptions of the compositionality of words.

The generative approach to speech control has exerted a strong influence on the conceptualization and management of AOS to the extent that it might be termed a standard or traditional view. The impairment has been seen as a post-lexical disorder in which there is failure in activating segmental movement plans that match to phonological representations. In addition, the capacity to combine individual segments to form cohesive syllables is also thought to be impaired (e.g., Darley, Aronson, & Brown, 1975). Such characterizations are entirely consistent with the observed surface behavior in AOS. The speaker struggles and gropes for articulatory positions, suggesting a loss of the spatial coordinates and temporal parameters for speech. Short-term maintenance or buffering resources may be limited and rapidly overloaded by processing demands, resulting in greater difficulty as word length increases (Ballard et al., 2016).

This traditional view of AOS as a segmental access and assembly deficit led to the development of highly principled therapies for the impairment that aim to re-build or re-activate segment plans for speech. Typically, they involve presentation of multisensory information as to the starting point of an articulatory gesture. A clinician might use diagrams, mirrors, or signs as cues. More recently, technology such as electropalatography (EPG), ultrasound, or electromagnetic articulography (EMA) is available in well-resourced research laboratories (although rarely in standard clinical settings) that provide information both on the starting point, trajectory, and the dynamics of an articulatory movement (Wambaugh, 2020). Sound production therapy is initially directed to more visible speech gestures such as bilabials and other anterior articulatory gestures. Once the patient has acquired a basic repertoire of gestures, the patterns are combined with the aim of practising the production of cohesive syllables. For example, as a first step /m/ might be differentiated from /f/, and then both combined with vowels at the periphery of the vowel space, such as /i, ɑ, u/. Often the lexical status of the resulting syllable (i.e., real or non-word, or if a real word, its functional value), is not seen as important as the therapy is directed at reactivating a retrieval/assembly mechanism that builds syllables from segments and, consistent with a three-stage model, is independent from prior linguistic processing. The evidence for the effectiveness of such interventions suggests that typical outcomes might be improved performance on trained syllables, but often disappointing evidence for the generalization of improvements to untrained items or to more spontaneous speech (Ballard, Wambaugh, Duffy, Layfield, Maas, Mauszycki, & McNeil, 2015; Wambaugh, 2020). This is a particular problem if non-words are the primary content of therapy as there would be no functional gain for the patient in everyday communicative settings.

There are many reasons why an intervention may have limited outcomes. More often than not therapies are administered at too low a dose to stimulate reorganisation of a damaged neurocognitive system (Varley, 2011). Some impairments might be intractable because they result from damage to a mechanism that is very narrowly localized within the brain. If the system is not distributed across neural sites then, in the event of damage to the processing hub, there is less potential for re-routing of information through undamaged components. However, another reason might be that the underlying theory of a disorder is not fully correct. If we modify the theory and motivate new therapies, then the treatment outcomes might improve. In the following section, I explore an alternative view of the mechanisms of speech control and how it might inform a different approach to the management of AOS.

Usage-based approaches and AOS

Levelt (1992) identifies a "paradox" that lies at the heart of segmental assembly models of speech production, such as the Slots and Fillers model:

> In fact, the frame-filling notion seems quite paradoxical. Why would a speaker go to the trouble of first generating an empty skeleton for the word, and then filling it with segments? In some way or another both must proceed from a stored phonological representation, the word's phonological code in the lexicon. Isn't it wasteful of processing resources to pull these apart first, and then to combine them again (on the risk of creating a slip).
>
> *(Levelt, 1992, p. 10)*

To resolve this paradox, Levelt proposed the existence of a "syllabary" – a store of phonetic plans for frequently-used syllables. The notion of storage of larger chunks of phonetic information is consistent with the observation of islands of fluent and accurate speech in AOS (and also in aphasic impairments, Bruns et al., 2019). For example, it is difficult to argue that the segmental plan for /s/ is impaired when it is produced accurately in the word *sorry*, although with an error in *soda*. Typically, the residual utterances produced by speakers with AOS are of relatively high-usage frequency (Varley et al., 2005). However, and in contrast to Levelt's proposal, once usage frequency determines the route to speech encoding, there is no necessary reason to restrict its influence to a unit of preordained size – such as a syllable. If a sequence of linguistic units regularly co-occurs, then associative bonds can form between its sub-elements, creating a cohesive chunk (a gestalt or schema) that can be stored in memory for future use. By this account, complete phonetic plans could be established for whole utterances so long as they are of high usage frequency. Examples might be phrases such as *I don't know*, *where's the* _ (Conklin & Schmidt, 2012). One possible objection to the claim for memory storage of phonetic plans for whole words and phrases might be that it creates overwhelming demands on long-term memory. Levelt (1989) suggests that the productive vocabulary for adults might be around 30,000 words (and this estimate might be doubled or trebled for bilingual and trilingual speakers). Notice that we are comfortable with the idea that vocabulary in the form of abstract phonological representations is stored in the lexicon, and it might be inefficient to store both phonological and phonetic representations in memory. One justification for storage of more abstract representations of word forms is that syllables and words are not produced in an invariant fashion but may vary in relation to surrounding context or speech style. For example, the point of palatal contact for /k/ varies depending on the following vowel: contrast its location in *kitten*, versus *cat*. However, this allophonic variation may not need to be specified in a phonetic plan as it might simply result from the dynamics and inertia inherent of the articulators.

The notion of a motor schema is well-established in other forms of skilled movement control, where the sub-components of a complex movement are chained together – consider, for example, expertise in playing a piece of music, or in sport – movements such as a golf swing or a backhand shot in tennis. A more everyday example would be the actions involved in tying shoelaces: once this complex action is learned, the motor schema has a beginning and an end point, but there are no obvious segments within the sequence. Notice that this account also provides a means to distinguish the learner or novice (or impaired speaker) from an expert. Neurotypical speakers (sometimes labelled "normal" or "healthy") are experts, while people with AOS have, a result of a brain lesion, lost that expertise and may fall back on compensatory mechanisms in order to produce speech.

This usage-based account simplifies the process of speech control: for output that is frequent, processing proceeds from activation in long-term memory of a stored phonetic plan for the whole word/utterance (Bybee, 2007). However, activation from stored gestalts cannot be the whole story in speech control as the speaker also needs resources to deal with novel or rarely-used forms. In this case, some generative/assembly work will be needed, although it might not involve segment-by-segment assembly. Existing stored representations, with the support of buffering resources, might be "cut-and-pasted" to form novel outputs. The different processing mechanisms involved in production of high- or low-frequency forms may leave subtle traces in the surface characteristics of words. For example, Gahl (2008) reports that homophone pairs, such as *time* and *thyme*, display durational differences with the lower frequency form (*thyme*) being of longer duration than its high-frequency twin (see also Levelt & Wheeldon, 1994). The shorter duration of the high-frequency twin results from consolidation and compression in long-term storage. The differences between high- and low-frequency forms, and entirely novel output, will also extend to the neural substrates underpinning in their production (Guenther, 2006). The process of learning a new word will place greater demands on somatosensory and auditory feedback (and consequently temporal and parietal cortex) to ensure a close match between the intended target and the developing motor plan. However, once the output is learned and consolidated, there is diminished need for feedback, and production can proceed from activation of the stored motor plan.

The demand for new word learning will differ across the lifespan. New words are constantly entering a language, and an individual might be exposed to a new language at any point in her/his life. The demand for a mechanism to deal with novel outputs is at its highest at the period of peak vocabulary acquisition, typically in childhood and adolescence where there is fast-mapping between the auditory representation of a new heard word and a developing motor plan (Bloom, 2000). Word learning continues throughout the lifespan, although the efficiency of the mechanisms that support mapping from auditory representation to motor plans, and the plasticity within the articulatory system to acquire new motor patterns may reduce with age (Crompton, 1981). For example, in learning a further language in adulthood, the degree of accentedness in a new language increases with age because the patterns of existing language(s) constrain new articulatory targets (Piske, MacKay, & Flege, 2001).

A usage-based approach has implications for both the conceptualization and management of AOS. Within the parameters of this approach, AOS might be seen as graded damage to the established store of word and phrase phonetic plans. In milder cases, the disruption may be evident only on lower frequency words. However, with more extensive damage, there would be a continuum of retrieval failure. In the most severe cases, only a small inventory of high-frequency forms remains accessible. In the face of activation/retrieval failure, the speaker with AOS might attempt to fill an utterance gap through building an output representation "on the fly," using the same mechanisms that are employed by neurotypical speakers in new word learning. Many of the characteristics that are observed in the surface behavior of speakers with AOS such as segmental omissions, distortions, and errors, groping for articulatory gestures, prosodic abnormalities, and reduced gestural overlap (Whiteside & Varley, 1998) might stem from the challenging computational task of online control of speech production. Note that fluent speech is fast – produced at around four to six syllables per second. The production system involves multiple sub-systems whose activity needs to be constrained and coordinated. Keller (1987) suggests that control of 60 muscle groups is required. Furthermore, the speaker with AOS is not in the same position as a child during the period of maximal vocabulary acquisition. The speaker with AOS is generally an older adult and many of the mechanisms that are necessary for fast-mapping from auditory representations to motor systems, and subsequent refinements of motor plans in response to auditory and somatosensory feedback, are likely to have undergone some age-related decline. Further, the lesions that cause AOS rarely disrupt only one processing mechanism. Recall that AOS usually co-occurs with aphasia, and auditory processing and interconnectivity between temporal and frontal cortex can also be impaired. The fundamental interconnectedness of input and output mechanisms and the likelihood of disturbed dynamics of activation across a distributed network means that there is no guarantee that the auditory and auditory-to-motor transcoding systems necessary for creating new phonetic representations are available to the speaker with AOS. This results in inadequate compensation in all but a small number of speakers with AOS (Varley, Whiteside, Hammill, & Cooper, 2006), and resultant error-filled speech output.

Implications for treatment of AOS

As well as developing theory of the processes involved in speech control, and the underlying impairment in AOS, a usage-based approach can offer insights into the management of the disorder. First, it allows a conceptual framework for traditional sound production therapies. At their core, sound production interventions are directed at the compensatory mechanisms utilized by a speaker in the face of failure to activate a motor plan. They involve maximizing auditory (listen), visual (articulograms, modelling articulatory gestures), and somatosensory (heightening awareness of articulatory postures) feedback in order to create new or reactivate established articulatory plans. However, an important issue is whether individual articulatory gestures need to be rebuilt if these same gestures are produced accurately in residual output at least some of the time. An important activity for a clinician is to note what is present and error-free in speech output, as well as to record errors and structures than are error prone.

An alternative management approach, motivated by the claim of stored phonetic plans for higher frequency words and phrases, is to consolidate residual word and utterance motor plans, and then use them to extend the speech repertoire of the person with AOS. This strategy was first described by Square-Storer (1989). She outlined a key word technique that starts with a word that remains accessible (perhaps a higher-frequency form) and then using that as a base to re-access/re-build related word forms. For example, if *yes* is produced fluently, can the multisyllable form *yesterday* be re-established? Rather than using non-words and articulatory exercises, the content of therapy is real lexical items, ideally of relatively high-usage frequency and therefore also of likely high functional value. A particular advantage of such an approach is that most individuals with AOS also have aphasic impairments. Therapies that use meaningful stimuli are thus likely to target underpinning linguistic processing as well as disruptions of speech control. In a randomized trial with a relatively large sample of participations with AOS – and all with some degree of comorbid aphasia – we explored the outcomes of computer therapy that primed real words through auditory and visual stimulation, before they were produced both at a single word level and by insertion into high-frequency sentence stems (e.g., *Where is* ___; *It is* ___). As a group, participants made modest gains in word production, with those receiving the highest therapy dose achieving the greatest gains (Varley, Cowell, Dyson, Inglis, Roper, & Whiteside, 2016).

Summary and conclusions

In this chapter, I have described two broad approaches to the processes that are involved in speech control. One focuses on assembly of speech output from subcomponent units each time they are used. The second, a usage-based account, proposes that complete motor plans for high-frequency words and utterances are stored, while the production of low-frequency or entirely novel words is likely to involve some online computational processing. The latter approach is sometimes termed a dual-route model as it proposes two pathways in speech processing. The two routes involve, at least to some degree, different computations and neural substrates.

Theoretical debates – in this case between a generative/speech assembly versus a usage-based account – may appear dry and remote, particularly to the student or novice reader. However, in an applied field such as speech and language pathology, the theory one adopts informs assessment and management practice. For example, should the clinician document residual speech, or conduct detailed error analysis? Segmental assembly models motivate one approach to therapy, such as sound production therapy with a focus on the precision and timing of articulatory gestures, while usage-based models suggest directing intervention at whole words and phrases, and perhaps starting from residual utterances. Clinicians have to evaluate different theoretical and therapeutic options and provide a principled case for the strategies they adopt. An individual who displays strong ability to transcode from auditory input to speech output (typically assessed with non-word repetition tasks in clinics), might be a better candidate for sound production therapy than somebody with a small repertoire of residual utterances, and poor auditory perceptual ability.

The inter-relationship between psycholinguistic theory (and evidence) and the applied field of speech/language pathology is often distant and, typically, with a time-lag between domains. Although usage-based approaches in mainstream psycholinguistics have been an influential theme for around 20 years, their impact on pathology has been rather limited. An exchange of ideas and data between fields is an advantage to both disciplines and the relationship should not be uni-directional. Evidence from pathology can be used to inform normative processing models, as is the case of lexical errors from aphasic anomia in structuring of models of word-finding. With regard to speech production and AOS, the relationship has been more remote. For example, the scarcity of exchange/transposition errors in pathology represents an important strand of (negative) evidence that might influence segmental assembly models of speech production. In the reverse direction, innovations in psycholinguistic theory suggest new avenues in the management of complex impairments of speech and language processing. The need for interdisciplinary exchange is clear.

Further reading

Ballard, K., Wambaugh, J., Duffy, J., Layfield, C., Maas, E., Mauszycki, S., & McNeil, M. R. (2015). Treatment for acquired apraxia of speech: A systematic review of intervention research between 2004 and 2012. *American Journal of Speech-Language Pathology, 24*(2), 316–337. https://doi.org/10.1044/2015_AJSLP-14-0118.

Forum on apraxia of speech. (2001). *Aphasiology, 15*(1), 39–84.

Guenther, F. H. (2006). Cortical interactions underlying the production of speech sounds. *Journal of Communication Disorders, 39*(5), 350–365.

References

Ballard, K., Wambaugh, J., Duffy, J., Layfield, C., Maas, E., Mauszycki, S., & McNeil, M. R. (2015). Treatment for acquired apraxia of speech: A systematic review of intervention research between 2004 and 2012. *American Journal of Speech-Language Pathology, 24*(2), 316–337. https://doi.org/10.1044/2015_AJSLP-14-0118.

Ballard, K. J., Azizi, L., Duffy, J. R., McNeil, M. R., Halaki, M., O'Dwyer, N., … Robin, D. A. (2016). A predictive model for diagnosing stroke-related apraxia of speech. *Neuropsychologia, 81*, 129–139.

Basilakos, A., Rorden, C., Bonilha, L., Moser, D., & Fridriksson, J. (2015). Patterns of poststroke brain damage that predict speech production errors in apraxia of speech and aphasia dissociate. *Stroke, 46*(6), 1561–1566. https://doi.org/10.1161/STROKEAHA.115.009211.

Bloom, P. (2000). *How children learn the meaning of words*. Cambridge, MA: Bradford Books.

Bruns, C., Varley, R., Zimmerer, V. C., Carragher, M., Brekelmans, G., & Beeke, S. (2019). "I don't know": A usage-based approach to familiar collocations in non-fluent aphasia. *Aphasiology, 33*(2), 140–162. https://doi.org/10.1080/02687038.2018.1535692.

Bybee, J. (2007). *Frequency of use and the organisation of language*. Oxford: OUP.

Chomsky, N., & Halle, M. (1968). *The sound pattern of English*. New York: Harper and Row.

Conklin, K., & Schmitt, N. (2012). The processing of formulaic language. *Annual Review of Applied Linguistics, 32*, 45–61. https://doi.org/10.1017/S0267190512000074.

Conterno, M., Kümmerer, D., Dressing, A., Glauche, V., Urbach, H., Weiller, C., & Rijntjes, M. (2022). Speech apraxia and oral apraxia: Association or dissociation? A multivariate lesion–symptom mapping study in acute stroke patients. *Experimental Brain Research, 240*(1), 39–51. https://doi.org/10.1007/s00221-021-06224-3.

Crompton, A. (1981). Syllables and segments in speech production. In A. Cutler (Ed.), *Slips of the tongue and language production* (pp. 109–162). Berlin: Mouton.

Darley, F., Aronson, A., & Brown, J. (1975). *Motor speech disorders*. Philadelphia, PA: W.B. Saunders.

de Santos Loureiro, C., Braga, L. W., Souza Ldo, N., Filho, G. N., Queiroz, E., & Dellatolas, G. (2004). Degree of illiteracy and phonological and metaphonological skills in unschooled adults. *Brain and Language, 89*(3), 499–502.

Dell, G. (1988). The retrieval of phonological forms in production: Test of predictions from a connectionist model. *Journal of Memory and Language, 27*(2), 124–142.

Gahl, S. (2008). *Time* and *thyme* are not homophones: The effect of lemma frequency on word durations in spontaneous speech. *Language, 84*(3), 474–496. https://doi.org/10.1353/lan.0.0035.

Guenther, F. H. (2006). Cortical interactions underlying the production of speech sounds. *Journal of Communication Disorders, 39*(5), 350–365.

Keller, E. (1987). The cortical representations of motor processes of speech. In E. Keller & M. Gopnik (Eds.), *Motor and sensory processes of language* (pp. 125–162). Hillsdale, NJ: Lawrence Erlbaum Associates Inc.

Levelt, W. J. M. (1989). *Speaking: From intention to articulation*. Cambridge, MA: MIT Press.

Levelt, W. J. M. (1992). Accessing words in speech production: Stages, processes and representations. *Cognition, 42*(1–3), 1–22. https://doi.org/10.1016/0010-0277(92)90038-j.

Levelt, W. J. M., & Wheeldon, L. (1994). Do speakers have access to a mental syllabary? *Cognition, 50*(1–3), 239–269.

Morais, J., Cary, L., Alegria, J., & Bertelson, P. (1979). Does awareness of speech as a sequence of phones arise spontaneously? *Cognition*, 7(4), 323–331. https://doi.org/10.1016/0010-0277(79)90020-9.

Piske, T., MacKay, I. R. A., & Flege, J. E. (2001). Factors affecting degree of foreign accent in an L2: A review. *Journal of Phonetics, 29*(2), 191–215.

Read, C., Zhang, Y.-F., Nie, H.-Y., & Ding, B.-Q. (1986). The ability to manipulate speech sounds depends on knowing alphabetic writing. *Cognition, 24*(1–2), 31–44. https://doi.org/10.1016/0010-0277(86)90003-X.

Shattuck-Hufnagel, S. (1979). Speech errors as evidence for a serial-ordering mechanism in sentence production. In W. E. Cooper & E. C. T. Walker (Eds.), *Sentence processing: Psycholinguistic studies presented to Merrill Garrett* (pp. 295–342). Hillsdale, NJ: Lawrence Erlbaum.

Smith, A. (2006). Speech motor development: Integrating muscles, movements and linguistic units. *Journal of Communication Disorders, 39*(5), 331–349.

Square-Storer, P. (1989). Traditional therapies for apraxia of speech reviewed and rationalized. In P. Square-Storer (Ed.), *Acquired apraxia of speech in adults*. Hove: Lawrence Erlbaum Associates Ltd.

Stemberger, J. P. (1989). Speech errors in early child language production. *Journal of Memory and Language, 28*(2), 164–188.

Varley, R. (2011). Rethinking aphasia therapy: A neuroscience perspective. *International Journal of Speech-Language Pathology, 13*(1), 11–20. https://doi.org/10.3109/17549507.2010.497561.

Varley, R., Cowell, P. E., Dyson, L., Inglis, L., Roper, A., & Whiteside, S. P. (2016). Self-administered computer therapy for apraxia of speech: Two-period randomized control trial with crossover. *Stroke, 47*(3), 822–828. https://doi.org/10.1161/STROKEAHA.115.011939.

Varley, R., Whiteside, S., Hammill, C., & Cooper, K. (2006). Phases in speech encoding and foreign accent syndrome. *Journal of Neurolinguistics, 19*(5), 356–369.

Varley, R. A., & Whiteside, S. P. (2001). What is the underlying impairment in acquired apraxia of speech? *Aphasiology, 15*(1), 39–49.

Varley, R., Whiteside, S. P., Windsor, F., & Fisher, H. (2005). Moving up from the segment: A comment on Aichert and Ziegler's syllable frequency and syllable structure in apraxia of speech. *Brain and Language, 96*(2), 235–239.

Wambaugh, J. L. (2020). An expanding apraxia of speech (AOS) treatment evidence base: An update of recent developments. *Aphasiology*. https://doi.org/10.1080/02687038.2020.1732289.

Whiteside, S. P., Dyson, L., Cowell, P. E., & Varley, R. A. (2015). The relationship between apraxia of speech and oral apraxia: Association or dissociation? *Archives of Clinical Neuropsychology, 30*(7), 670–682. https://doi.org/10.1093/arclin/acv051.

Whiteside, S. P., & Varley, R. A. (1998). A reconceptualisation of apraxia of speech: A synthesis of evidence. *Cortex, 34*(2), 221–231.

27

THE ROLE OF MEMORY AND ATTENTION IN APHASIC LANGUAGE PERFORMANCE

Malcolm McNeil, William Hula, and Jee Eun Sung

Introduction

There is a scientific paradigm (Kuhn, 1962) within which research in aphasia is conducted. This paradigm encompasses the tacit assumptions about the underlying nature of the disorder (aphasia in this case) and in general dictates the kind of the research questions and methods used for answering them that is acceptably conducted by its practitioners. The paradigm is determined by the majority of the scientists working in the discipline. Although there is the possibility of coexisting paradigms for the clinical practice in aphasia on the one hand and theory-driven investigation of aphasia on the other, the practice of science in most Western cultures dictates coherence between them and the theoretical perspective typically holds more capital than the clinical one. That is, because it is generally believed that theory is the guiding principle for practice, the theoretical paradigm typically has a strong and perhaps dominating influence on the clinical paradigm. Such is the case with clinical aphasiology. This theoretical paradigm may be best characterized as the centers and pathways paradigm and is a direct descendent of the Wernicke/Lichtheim model of aphasia (Eggert, 1977). It is based on the notion that there are language centers in the brain that house specific linguistic rules and representations and that these centers are connected to one another by direct pathways. To illustrate, within this centers and pathways conceptualization of aphasia, the arcuate fasciculus pathway connects the posterior temporal lobe (putative) language comprehension center (Wernicke's area) to the inferior and posterior two-thirds of the third frontal convolution (putative) speech production center (Broca's Area). These centers and this specific pathway allow the association of representations and the performance of specific linguistic computations and language tasks (e.g., speech repetition in this instance). The aphasia classification system adhered to by the majority of aphasiologists best represents this scientific paradigm and is firmly grounded in this "anatomical connectionist" (not to be confused with "computational connectionist") models of aphasia. Within this model of aphasia, damage to a specific center (e.g., Wernicke's area) or a specific pathway (e.g., the arcuate fasciculus) will yield a specific pattern of language (Wernicke's Aphasia) or modality (repetition deficit in "Conduction Aphasia") deficit respectively, which corresponds to a "classical" type or category of aphasia (Geschwind, 1965a, 1965b; Goodglass, Kaplan, & Barresi, 2001; Kertesz, 1979). In general, this model of aphasic deficits, and the adherents of its derived classification system have tended to view aphasia as a loss of representations subserving specific language functions due to the damaged language center or the damaged or disconnected pathway. In its strongest formulations, it is assumed that the rules and the representations have either been deleted from the patient's repertoire or become permanently inaccessible because of a structural

 DOI: 10.4324/9781003204213-31

lesion in the relevant neural substrates responsible for the language computation or association. This assumption is reflected in definitions of aphasia as a "loss" of language (Benson, 1979), and in some formal theories and hypotheses proposed to account for specific signs and symptoms of aphasia such as the "trace deletion hypothesis" of Grodzinsky (2000), which was proposed to account for the failure of specific syntactic operations. Proponents of the centers and pathways model have tended to emphasize the differences among persons with aphasia by dividing them into the model-derived behavioral categories arranged along modality and psycholinguistic dimensions.

There is another view of the underlying mechanisms of aphasia held by a relatively small minority of aphasiologists. This view holds that some other part of the cognitive apparatus (e.g., attention or memory) may serve as an explanatory mechanism. This view of aphasia has been described to be in opposition to the classical anatomical connectionist view. For example, a view of aphasia that incorporates attention as an important construct tends to have more in common with accounts that emphasize the commonality of impairments among persons with aphasia. This view regards aphasia as a disorder of performance in which representations are not lost, but access to representations or moment-to-moment failures to map obligatory components of the language system (the assembly of representations) is impaired. This view of language and aphasia suggests that components of language (e.g., phonology, morphology, syntax) are always the product of online computations involving much smaller units of information and complex mapping processes among them. From this perspective it follows that a failure of the processes used to build the relevant products can account for the observed linguistic disorders. Processing models of language such as that proposed by Saffran, Schwartz, and Marin (1980) and computational models such as that of Martin, Dell, Saffran, and Schwartz (1994) have provided converging evidence for some of the hypothesized mechanisms underlying the observed pathologies of language and have highlighted some of the processes for the online construction of representations. Process and computational models of language pathologies are generally favored by the research community and the rather simplistic "loss" view of language is infrequently adhered to by aphasia researchers. Nevertheless, the "loss" view of aphasia permeates the nonaphasiologists' views of aphasia and is with very rare exception, held among health care professionals outside of the aphasia research community (Craven & Hirnle, 2009). It also is the norm among rehabilitation specialists, including those charged with the treatment of aphasia. As summarized by Hula and McNeil (2008), it is recognized that one consequence of assuming that linguistic units are deleted or made permanently unavailable is that treatment is then directed toward the restoration of those units with the intent of replacing the lost components. Additionally, this position has promoted diagnostic tools that have focused on quantifying how much or what specific representations are left intact. This has led clinicians to attempt to assay vocabulary (e.g., the number of words within specific word classes), or determine those specific phonemes, derivational morphemes, syntactic structures, or semantic categories that remain in the patient's repertoire. These assumptions have given rise to aphasia treatment as "teaching"; as one might structure linguistic experience for first language acquisition or as one would systematically expose a person to a second language by providing them the specific representations (e.g., the phonology or the lexical forms) and rules (e.g., the morphologic and syntactic structures; pragmatic or situational contextual rules) for assembly and usage. This type of treatment is frequently administered in a didactic format. However, the alternative view that language representations are preserved in aphasia and that aphasic language performance is due to an impaired processing mechanism suggests that specific representations, rules, or language content may not be the most appropriate targets for rehabilitation. Instead, the underlying processing deficits might be used to organize the content of treatment, and measurements of the impaired process(es) might become primary or intermediate outcome targets.

Consistent with the view of aphasia that holds that the language representations and the rules used for their assembly are fundamentally intact in persons with aphasia is the claim that the cognitive support system necessary for "doing" language or building the representations and forming the necessary mappings among components of the linguistic system is responsible for the impaired products. Variants of this view have been discussed as "processing" or "access" impairments, and have been explored within a number of psychological constructs, but most frequently and productively as "memory" and "attention."

While strong assumptions about the localization of the brain lesion underlying aphasia types are frequently made from the centers and pathways model (Weems & Reggia, 2007), the alternative "processing" approaches have tended to minimize the connections between specific aphasic symptoms and circumscribed lesion sites and have emphasized both the similarities between persons with aphasia and the variability within them according to both internal and external factors. The writings of Freud (1953), Marie (1906), and Head (1926; reviewed by: Caplan, 1987; Darley, 1982; Schuell, Jenkins, & Jimenez-Pabon, 1964) emphasized the unidimensionality of the disorder. These early aphasiologists have provided an important historical background for theories that are consistent with the view of aphasia as a disorder that affects language-specific cognitive operations but is itself not a primary disorder of language; a perspective that underlies a memorial, attentional, or impaired processing view of aphasia. In the processing view, the elemental language representations and the algorithms used for their construction are proposed to be essentially intact. Again, this is differentiated from primary language differences or impairments such as that seen in second language learners or individuals who have not yet acquired the rules and representations due to maturation, social/cultural deprivation, or with severe cognitive impairments as may occur in some persons with autism or mental retardation.

Motivating arguments for a processing view of aphasia

An alternative to the centers and pathways view and definition of aphasia has been proposed because there are a number of observations about aphasia that suggest fundamentally preserved linguistics (both linguistic rules and representations) as well as preserved processing capacities that are adequate for successful language functioning in the presence of the observed language impairments. Several indirect sources of evidence have been proposed to support the notion and that a source for the "breakdown" in language performance must be explained by the cognitive mechanisms involved in building the representations and not the loss of any of the building blocks themselves. Additionally, these mechanisms cannot involve a permanent or static impairment in the ability to enlist the cognitive mechanisms necessary for accomplishing the construction of the linguistic representations. A search for the source of these impaired cognitive mechanisms has taken a variety of forms including the description and experimental manipulation of behavioral patterns of performance (Hageman & Folkstad, 1986; Hageman, McNeil, Rucci-Zimmer, & Cariski, 1982; McNeil, Hageman, & Matthews, 2005) as well as anatomical (Nelson, Reuter-Lorenz, Persson, Sylvester, & Jonides, 2009; Thompson-Schill, Bedny, & Goldberg, 2005; Thompson-Schill et al., 2002) and physiological indices (King & Kutas, 1998; Peach, Rubin, & Newhoff, 1994). In support of their proposal that aphasia is the result of impairments in the underlying cognitive apparatus that supports language (the ability to allocate attentional or processing resources supporting language in this specific instance), McNeil and colleagues (McNeil, 1982, 1988; McNeil & Kimelman, 1986; McNeil, Odell, & Tseng, 1991) appealed to several phenomena that are inconsistent with the centers and pathways paradigm. They observed that aphasia affects all domains (phonology, morphology, syntax, semantics) and modalities of language (see Darley, 1982 for review). McNeil et al. (1991), in particular, took issue with the idea that damage to specific linguistic operations (e.g., coindexing of pronouns) could account for aphasic performance, and furthermore challenged the empirical bases of single- and double-dissociations (Odell, Hashi, Miller, & McNeil, 1995), which constitute much of the evidence for such arguments. They proposed that the broad impairments typically observed in aphasia can only be accounted for by a "superordinate mechanism [that] is shared by linguistic processing units" (McNeil et al., 1991, p. 28). Results showing that the centers and pathways derived aphasia categories are not reliable predictors of the syntactic comprehension of different sentence types (e.g., Caplan, Waters, & Hildebrandt, 1997) are consistent with this view.

Second, a variety of linguistic and nonlinguistic factors, such as word stress (Kimelman & McNeil, 1987; Pashek & Brookshire, 1982), phonemic, semantic, and phrase cueing (Podraza & Darley, 1977), perceptual redundancy of visual naming stimuli (Benton, Smith, & Lang, 1972; Bisiach, 1966), and rate of presentation of auditory stimuli (Gardner, Albert, & Weintraub, 1975; Weidner & Lasky, 1976) can stimulate correct or improved language performance in persons with aphasia (for review, see Darley, 1976, 1982; Duffy & Coelho, 2001). More recently, repetitive transcranial magnetic stimulation to the right-hemisphere homologue of Broca's area was claimed to improve naming in some persons with aphasia in the absence of other treatment (Naeser et al., 2005). This stimulability of aphasic persons for correct or improved performance in the absence of specific linguistic information can only be explained by a disorder of processing language in which the fundamental rules and representations are preserved.

McNeil (1982, 1983, 1988) and McNeil et al. (1991) also noted that persons with aphasia are highly variable in their performance and that this variability cannot be accounted for by a loss of representations or functions. The specific kind of variability to which they refer is the tendency of persons with aphasia to respond differently to the same stimulus under the same contextual conditions on repeated presentations over very short periods of time such as days, minutes, or even seconds. The recognition of this sort of variability is not new and evidence for it can be found prominently in the work of Kreindler and Fradis (1968), who concluded that variability was fundamental to the disorder. More recent work has documented substantial variability of performance over brief periods of time on the same or similar items on a variety of task such as auditory comprehension and naming performance. With regard to auditory comprehension, it has been demonstrated that persons with aphasia can vary widely in their performance across homogeneous items (McNeil & Hageman, 1979; McNeil, Odell, & Campbell, 1982) but with sufficient numbers of homogeneous stimuli, reliable patterns of variability can be captured (Hageman et al., 1982). Furthermore, this variability is not limited to the moment-to-moment fluctuations of performance. In one naming study (Freed, Marshall, & Chulantseff, 1996), five individuals with mild to moderate aphasia were presented with 100 pictures five times over five consecutive days. Across individuals, 10–38% of the pictures elicited correct responses on some administrations with incorrect responses on one or more others. On average, across subjects, approximately 23% of the pictures were named with inconsistent correctness/incorrectness over the five sessions. Other studies have produced similar results supporting the conclusion that, despite relatively consistent overall or averaged error rates on repeated trials of the same stimuli, success or failure at naming a particular item in one instance is not an especially reliable predictor of performance on that item on a subsequent occasion (Crisman, 1971; Howard, Patterson, Franklin, Morton, & Orchard-Lisle, 1984). More recently, Caplan, Waters, DeDe, Michaud, and Reddy (2007) appealed to the notion of processing resources to account for the prominent variability they observed in sentence comprehension in a large group of unselected individuals with aphasia.

One explanation for the large moment-to-moment or repeated trial variability across all tasks in persons with aphasia could be that individuals have a number of ways to solve linguistic computational requirements and that there is a great deal of flexibility in compensation or strategy selections. However, this does not explain why individuals would routinely select suboptimal solutions, either consciously or unconsciously. Ultimately, the underlying mechanisms that account for this within-task variability are not consistent with a "loss" of linguistic representations, rules, or to the cognitive apparatus used for processing language. That persons with aphasia are variable has received increasing support (Caplan et al., 2007; Crisman, 1971; Freed et al., 1996; Howard et al., 1984; Kreindler & Fradis, 1968) since early suggestions that variability should play an important role in the understanding of the underlying mechanisms in aphasia (McNeil, 1982). Linguistic variability was viewed by Kolk (2007) as a "hallmark of aphasic behavior." Indeed, Kolk proposed, as others had before him (McNeil, 1982, 1988), that an interaction between the language and an executive system would be required to account for this variability. Additionally, he proposed that a processing cost account was necessary to explain aphasic variability in syntactic processing. We extend this necessity to all linguistic domains and processing modalities.

A fourth argument marshaled by McNeil (1982, 1988) in favor of aphasia as a performance deficit concerns the fact that aphasia can be transient. Ictal and post-ictal aphasia has been reported in patients with epilepsy (Hamilton & Matthews, 1979; Lebrun, 1994; Lecours & Joanette, 1980; Linebaugh, Coakley, Arrigan, & Racy, 1979) with return to normal linguistic and cognitive status surrounding the episode. Aphasia is not an uncommon sign, with rapidly resolving or intermittent appearance with transient ischemic attacks (Mlcoch & Metter, 2001) and other neurological conditions (Kaminski, Hlavin, Likavec, & Schmidley, 1992; Rahimi & Poorkay, 2000).

Finally, McNeil (1982, 1988) suggested that the qualitative similarity of language performance in normal and aphasic individuals provides evidence that aphasia is best considered a disorder in the efficiency with which language is constructed or representations are built rather than one in which linguistic rules or representations are lost or permanently inaccessible. The idea that aphasic language performance represents a low end on a continuum shared with normal performance is not a new realization and was embraced by earlier aphasiologists (e.g., Freud, 1953). A number of empirical studies have demonstrated that persons with aphasia and normal individuals produce similar patterns of responses on a variety of language comprehension (Bates, Friederici, & Wulfeck, 1987; Brookshire & Nicholas, 1980, 1984; Dick et al., 2001; Hageman, 1980; Kilborn, 1991; McNeil et al., 1982; Miyake, Carpenter, & Just, 1994; Nicholas & Brookshire, 1986; Shewan, 1976; Shewan & Canter, 1971), language production (Ernest-Baron, Brookshire, & Nicholas, 1987; Schwartz, Saffran, Bloch, & Dell, 1994; Silkes, McNeil, & Drton, 2004), and grammaticality judgment (Bates et al., 1994; Blackwell & Bates, 1995; Wilson, Saygin, Schleicher, Dick, & Bates, 2003) tasks. These patterns have been realized when the normal individuals are stressed by time pressure, task complexity, or competing tasks. The relevance of these observations and the normal-to-aphasic continuum (also called the "continuity hypothesis") for understanding the nature of aphasic language impairment is that a structural lesion or an impaired linguistic system is not necessary to produce linguistic behaviors indistinguishable from those that characterize and define aphasia. Further, the cognitive conditions under which these patterns can be elicited may provide models for testing mechanisms underlying specific aphasic behaviors as well as for assessing diagnostic and treatment methods.

If not a disorder of the linguistic units, what then?

The role of memory in aphasic language deficits

Aphasia is typically defined as a "language disorder" or more rarely as a disorder that affects language (McNeil & Pratt, 2001). Linguistic constructs are used for its description and linguistic theory is applied as explanation for the behaviors observed. Indeed, aphasia is a disorder that affects language-specific behavior and is separated from its clinical neighbors by the presence of these disorders in the context of other intact cognitive functions such as procedural memory, affective and personality characteristics, perception, visual–spatial abilities, movement or motor abilities, or general world knowledge. Aphasia can coexist with disorders in these other domains of knowledge or processing; however, its diagnosis requires strong evidence that it cannot be accounted for by impairments of affect, movement, musical or artistic ability, or by primary impairments of memory. However, memory (in addition to attention and other conceptualizations of executive functions, discussed below) is always utilized for the activation of language representations, the application of linguistic rules and for the necessary integration of the many products derived from the multiple linguistic components of language construction. Therefore, deficits in the storage of linguistic information for comprehension and the retrieval of information for production define aphasia and are, by their very nature, impairments of memory for linguistic information. The centers and pathways paradigm requires acceptance of the proposition that the deficits are not within the operations of the memory system per se, but rather within the linguistic computations. This is required because it is assumed that memorial systems are general purpose processing devices that serve all cognitive systems and would, if impaired, obligatorily affect nonlinguistic cognitive operations as well as linguistic ones. The argument is that aphasia is not a disorder of memory (or attention), because these other domains of cognition (e.g., perception, motor, visual–spatial, nonlinguistic reasoning, etc.), are by definition excluded in aphasia. However, impairments of these cognitive functions could subtend the impairments within the language-specific domain in persons with aphasia if linguistic-specific memory and attention systems existed and if they could be differentially or selectively impaired. This proposition is certainly consistent with many models of linguistic processing that are integrated within the constructs of memory and attention (e.g., Baddeley's working memory model, discussed later in this chapter).

Several theories of memory have been proposed that account for many aspects of language performance (e.g., Gibson, 1998; Gibson & Pearlmutter, 2000) and for those behaviors that characterize aphasia (e.g., Martin & Saffran, 1997). There is in fact a relatively long history of research into impaired memory systems in aphasia. One review of this research (McNeil, 1988) concluded that long-term memory (LTM; either episodic or semantic) was unrelated to the language impairments in aphasia; at least in the sense that persons with aphasia do not "forget" how to do things that they knew pre-morbidly (fix a motor, make a bed, drive a car, or bake a cake) and they do not forget world events, people that they know or how to get from point A to point B, or what they comprehended minutes or hours before. One source of evidence supporting this later claim comes from the work on immediate and delayed story retelling. Bayles, Boone, Tomoeda, Slauson, and Kaszniak (1989), for example, demonstrated that persons with aphasia performed similarly to normal elderly individuals, and significantly better than individuals with mild Alzheimer's disease (AD) on a story retelling following a 60-minute filled delay. While the amount of information retold in the immediate condition by persons with both aphasia and AD can be expected to vary considerably across individuals (and to correlate highly with the overall severity of their comprehension deficits in the persons with aphasia), the story information that was comprehended and stored by the persons with aphasia, unlike that also initially comprehended by the persons with AD, was clearly held in LTM by whatever mechanisms that were available (e.g., rehearsal, chunking strategies, association with LTM, etc.). Additionally, they were accessible for recall without substantive decrement (not greater than normal-nonimpaired individuals).

Such preservation of performance is not the case with short-term memory (STM) as measured by span tasks (Adamovich, 1978; Albert, 1976; Cermak & Moreines, 1976; Cermak & Tarlow, 1978; Flowers, 1975; Swinney & Taylor, 1971). Indeed, a review of the STM literature suggests that span is always impaired in large, unselected groups of persons with aphasia compared to nonbrain damaged control groups and in most studies yields language spans of approximately 50% ($\pm$ 30%; or approximately 3.5, $\pm$ 1) of the normal control population (7, $\pm$ 2; or approximately 30% of the normal span) regardless of language task. Furthermore, span tasks do not appear to separate populations by aphasia type, even when the recall tasks are optimized to detect the suspected underlying grammatical (Broca) versus semantic (Wernicke) deficit (Caramazza, Zurif, & Gardner, 1978). They also do not separate normal from aphasic performance by the serial exhaustive versus self-terminating type of search (Warren, Hubbard, & Knox, 1977) or by the presence or absence of top-down strategies used for aiding STM (Lubinski & Chapey, 1978).

However, STM has been recognized as being only one integrally linked component of the memory system when engaged for language processing. An important development in the identification of independent components within the memory system was provided by Baddeley and Hitch (1974) as a working memory (WM) system. This model was later elaborated by Baddeley

(1986, 1993), and Baddeley and Logie (1999), among many others, and it has had a large and enduring impact on models of linguistic processing. It was originally proposed to contain two independent and cognitively autonomous systems: a "phonological loop," concerned with maintenance and processing of acoustic and verbal information, and the "visuospatial sketchpad," which supports the same functions for nonlinguistic visual and spatial information (Baddeley, 1986). The activities of these two components were proposed to be regulated and coordinated by a "central executive." This phonological loop was proposed as a STM or "storage" system within which linguistic processing or a computation (work) is performed. The STM buffer is limited in the quantity of information that it can hold and the time-course over which the work of the computation can occur. The central executive system is responsible for supplying the necessary attention or effort for both the computations and maintenance of information within the STM buffer as well as the other necessary information processing operations (e.g., goal maintenance, response selection, etc.) required for linguistic comprehension and production. Critically, the STM, as well as the computational part of the model, require access to, and continuous support from the attentional component of the central executive. Failure or degraded performance on tasks considered to be valid measures of WM can occur because of a failure of any of the three components of the model. Importantly, the computations as well as the STM system are considered by the current authors to be relatively fixed properties of the architecture and have person-specific defined capacity limitations. However, the central executive component of the WM system is viewed as a resource that can be variably and proportionally allocated in service of the processing/computations and the storage components of the WM system. As such, in our view, it is only this component of the WM system that has the potential to account for the phenomena described above that the centers and pathways account cannot. Nonetheless, the study of, and identified impairment of WM has become synonymous with impairments of any component of the model. Within this frame of reference, an impairment of WM does not separate which component(s) of the model are impaired. This lack of specificity has not only confused the assignment of impairment within the functional architecture, but it has diminished the search for the underlying impairment in persons performing pathologically on tests of WM. Importantly, this conflation has been well recognized by Baddeley and colleagues and has received substantial experimental and theoretical attention by many cognitive scientists (e.g., Cowan, 1995, 1999; Engle, Kane, & Tuholski, 1999; Shah & Miyake, 1999).

It is important to discuss WM in the context of a chapter focused primarily on attention and aphasia. The popularity of WM models, the important role that the central executive is believed to play in the overall success of the models, and the conflation of the three elements of the WM models requires consideration. Considerable work on attention and resource allocation has been conducted within the WM framework as well outside of it. The remainder of this discussion will focus on the role of the attentional system (controlled and automatic) in language processing and its potential as a viable account for the phenomenology of aphasia.

Working memory, attention, and resource allocation

Several WM models subsequent to Baddeley and colleagues have developed the notion of the central executive by employing "capacity" or "resource" concepts from the attentional literature. Just and Carpenter (1992, p. 124), for example, described this component of the model as "an energy source," which was analogous to Kahneman's (1973) attention resource capacity and they placed their theory in the tradition of Kahneman's work. They defined WM capacity as the activation available for supporting either of the two functions (storage and processing). They suggested that a unitary pool of resources is engaged in both language computations and in the maintenance of information used for the computation and for the storage of their products.

Such a line of research arguing that there is a single pool of resources utilized for all verbally mediated tasks predicts that there should be a trading relationship (though not necessarily an equivalent cost between components) between storage and computation when the overall task demands are high enough to exceed the individuals' available resources (Just & Carpenter, 1992; King & Just, 1991; MacDonald, Just, & Carpenter, 1992; Miyake et al., 1994). One way in which this trading relationship has been demonstrated in the context of sentence comprehension is by means of reading span tasks (Daneman & Carpenter, 1980). This specific task requires participants to read sentences and at the same time remember the final word from each sentence presented within a given set. Listening span versions of the task also have been developed (e.g., Gaulin & Campbell, 1994; Tompkins, Bloise, Timko, & Baumgaertner, 1994) and unlike their reading counterparts, have received at least basic psychometric development. According to Just and Carpenter (1992), some individuals may have greater total capacity and/or use their available resources more efficiently. These persons are expected to score high on WM span tasks and demonstrate better performance on a variety of sentence processing measures. Conversely, individuals who have lower total capacity or who use WM resources less efficiently should score lower in WM span tasks and have slower and/or less accurate performance in sentence processing.

If WM impairment is a strong determinant of language performance in aphasia, then WM span measures should correlate with performance on standardized aphasia tests. Caspari, Parkinson, LaPointe, and Katz (1998) found a high correlation (r = .79) between listening span and performance on the Western Aphasia Battery (WAB; Kertesz, 1982) among 22 individuals with aphasia. Sung and colleagues (2009) recently found similar correlations in a group of 20 persons with aphasia between listening span and performance on the Porch Index of Communicative Ability (PICA; Porch, 2001; r = .70) and a computerized version (CRTT) of the Revised Token Test (McNeil & Prescott, 1978; r = .60). However, Caspari et al. (1998) and Sung et al. (2009) both noted that the strong correlations between the WM measures used and language performance in aphasia could be interpreted as evidence that both are general measures of the severity of language impairment. Nonetheless, the fact that the requirements among the correlated language tasks (overall scores on the CRTT, PICA, and WAB) and the WM tasks (a visual recognition version by Caspari et al. and the auditory version of the Daneman and Carpenter task by Sung et al.) vary considerably in both linguistic computational requirements and STM span requirements, leaves open the strong possibility that there may be a common underlying source for the shared variance in the third component of the WM model; the attentional or resource requirements. While this hypothesis has received experimental attention with normal nonaphasic populations (e.g., Engle, Tuholski, Laughlin, & Conway, 1999) it has not been investigated within the same pool of persons with aphasia, using the same measures of language computation, STM and attention; a test that appears necessary to evaluate the interrelationships and unique contributions of the three components of the WM model to the underlying abilities/impairments.

Another prediction relative to aphasia that is consistent with the WM model and with the normal → aphasia continuum (the continuity hypothesis) is that if comprehension deficits in persons with aphasia are the result of reduced resource availability, normal individuals should also perform similarly when operating with reduced available resources. Miyake et al. (1994) presented sentences of varying complexity to normal individuals under time pressure using a rapid serial visual processing procedure. They found that the ordering of sentence types by difficulty was similar to that previously observed in individuals with aphasia. The ordinal ranking of the sentences was derived empirically from previous studies of sentence comprehension in persons with aphasia (Caplan, Baker, & Dehaut, 1985; Naeser et al., 1987), and the ranking agreed with a complexity metric based on the dichotomous sentence characteristics of three versus two thematic roles for a single verb, two versus one verbs present in a sentence, and noncanonical versus canonical order of thematic roles. Furthermore, as predicted by the WM capacity model, linguistic complexity interacted with both speed and subjects grouped by WM span (although there was no three-way interaction that would also be predicted by the model). In both cases, greater WM limitations were associated with larger decrements on complex than on simpler sentences. This study also reported performance in the normal lower WM group operating under capacity limitation that was similar to the persons with aphasia. The low WM group showed over-additive impairments on the more complex sentences as was shown by the group with aphasia. Based on this finding, Miyake et al. argued that the over-additive effect on the more complex sentences for the group with aphasia was not due to specific linguistic impairments for selected syntactic structures because the same pattern was also elicited by the normal individuals with lower WM performance. The authors also speculated that these differences could be due to randomness inherent in the comprehension system, individual differences in the efficiency of certain processes, or differences in preferred strategies for adapting to a heavy resource load.

Berndt, Mitchum, and Wayland (1997) examined the capacity hypothesis in relation to two linguistically based hypotheses of aphasic comprehension; the trace deletion hypothesis and the hypothesis that agrammatic aphasia causes selective difficulty processing grammatical morphemes. They administered a sentence-picture matching task to ten persons with aphasia, five of whom were classified by the Western Aphasia Battery as having Broca's aphasia and five who were classified as anomic. The results failed to provide support for the trace deletion hypothesis, which predicts above chance performance on active and subject relative sentences and chance performance on passives and object relatives. Four of the five participants with Broca's aphasia performed above chance on both active and passive sentences, while the one subject who showed the predicted pattern on actives and passives performed at chance on both subject relative and object relative sentences. The results also failed to support the grammatical morpheme hypothesis, which predicts that active and subject relative sentences should be similarly well understood, with passive and object relative sentences showing a similar degree of increased difficulty. When the performance of the five persons labeled as Broca's was examined together, active and passive sentences were equally easy to understand, with subject relative sentences being harder and object relative sentences being the most difficult to understand. These results were interpreted as support for the capacity theory. In analyzing the performance of all 10 participants together, the ordinal pattern of sentence difficulty across types was the pattern predicted by capacity theory. In other words, performance degradation was most evident in all individuals with aphasia regardless of the type of aphasia; especially when the two complexity factors of sentence length and syntactic structure were combined.

As mentioned above, the most common model of WM assumes a single, shared pool of processing resources for the phonological loop. However, debate about single versus multiple pools of attentional resources has a long history (Friedman & Polson, 1981; Gopher, Brickner, & Navon, 1982; Kahneman, 1973; Wickens, 1980, 1984) but a more limited one in terms of verbal WM. Caplan and Waters proposed that WM resources are fractionated into at least two parts (Caplan & Waters, 1995, 1996; Waters & Caplan, 1996a, 1996b, 2004). They differentiated the interpretive language processing characterized by initial, first-pass, unconscious, obligatory processing from the post-interpretive processing that is conscious, controlled, and verbally mediated (Caplan & Waters, 1999; Waters & Caplan, 2004). They argued that traditional verbal WM span tasks, which rely on post-interpretive processing, only predict performance on tasks that also require post-interpretive processing; but not on tasks that rely heavily on interpretive processing such as automatic syntactic parsing. Additionally, they argued that the single capacity theory necessarily predicts interactions between effects of WM capacity and syntactic complexity, and many studies have failed to find such interactions. They further argued that where interactions have been found, they were due to the number of propositions contained in a sentence, a factor they relegate to post-interpretive processing.

In order to further assess the single versus multiple WM resource hypothesis, Caplan and Waters (1996) administered a sentence comprehension task to a group of ten persons with aphasia carefully chosen to have performance above chance but below ceiling on semantically reversible, syntactically complex sentences. Sentence types were systematically varied in terms of syntactic complexity (canonicity) and number of propositions, and were presented in single and dual-task conditions. In the dual-task conditions, subjects had to continuously repeat a random digit string with a length equal to their digit span and their digit span minus one while comprehending the sentence. They were instructed to give primary emphasis to the digit task when it was present. Analyses of sentence comprehension showed reliable effects of both canonicity and number of propositions, but no effect of digit load or an interaction. In analyzing digit recall, main effects of both sentence type and number of digits were found, but without a significant interaction. A finer-grained analysis separating out the effects of canonicity and propositional load revealed a null effect of canonicity and a positive effect of propositional load on digit recall. Caplan and Waters interpreted these results as evidence for the separation of resources dedicated to syntactic processing from those available to other kinds of language processing. However, without demonstrating a bidirectional trading effect, it is very difficult to invoke a "resource" explanation for the findings rather than a simple interference effect, or a number of other explanations.

Some proponents of the single capacity hypothesis have responded to the criticism outlined above by noting the problems inherent in using null findings as support for a theoretical position, especially when the effect in question involves interactions that may be difficult to detect (Miyake, Emerson, & Friedman, 1999). Others have suggested that a single language resource capacity could account for null effects of digit load on processing of complex syntax by highlighting the distinction between encoding and storage processes (Bates, Dick, & Wulfeck, 1999; Dick et al., 2001). They propose that some task manipulations may primarily affect encoding (e.g., time pressure or noise masking) while others may primarily affect maintenance (e.g., digit load), and that processing of low frequency word orders, for example, may be vulnerable only to the former while inflectional morphology may be affected by both.

Also relevant to this discussion of resource capacity limitations as an explanatory construct in aphasia are theories and models that directly relate resources and processing speed. Haarmann and Kolk (1991) hypothesized that sentence comprehension deficits in aphasia could be due to a reduction in the resources deployed per unit time to drive the computations responsible for parsing syntax. They further proposed that this reduction in resources was compatible with either slow activation or rapid decay of critical sentence elements. Haarmann and Kolk conducted a syntactic priming experiment to test these two hypotheses against each other and also a third alternative; that the size of aphasic individuals' processing buffer is reduced. The results supported the slow-activation hypothesis: participants with aphasia demonstrated significant priming only in the longest prime-target stimulus onset asynchrony (SOA) condition, whereas an age-matched control group showed priming effects across the entire range of SOAs tested (300–1100 ms). The authors argued that the participants with aphasia had not lost their syntactic knowledge, but rather that their comprehension deficits were due to processing inefficiency rendering them unable to perform linguistic computations within a necessary time frame. While the methods of their study were novel, their interpretation of the results as a slowed processing mechanism underlying the comprehension impairments in individuals with aphasia is not unique (Blanchard & Prescott, 1980; Blumstein, Katz, Goodglass, Shrier, & Dworetsky, 1985; Campbell & McNeil, 1985; Salvatore, 1974; Weidner & Lasky, 1976) and is consistent with a reduced availability of resources account as demonstrated using the psychological refractory period experimental method (Hula & McNeil, 2008; Hula, McNeil, & Sung, 2007).

A number of other studies have been carried out to address the issue of whether the phenomenology of aphasia can be accounted for by a failure of an attentional/resource allocation system (Arvedson & McNeil, 1987; Erickson, Goldinger, & LaPointe, 1996; LaPointe & Erickson, 1991; Murray, 2000; Murray, Holland, & Beeson, 1997b; Murray, Holland, & Beeson, 1998; Slansky & McNeil, 1997; Tseng, McNeil, & Milenkovic, 1993). These studies have generally adopted the strategy of manipulating the presence, priority, or difficulty of competing language or nonlanguage tasks. One consistent finding from these studies is that the language performance in persons with aphasia is more vulnerable to the introduction of a competing task than language performance in normal individuals (Arvedson, 1986; Murray, 2000; Murray, Holland, & Beeson, 1997a; Murray, Holland, & Beeson, 1997c; Murray et al., 1998). Unfortunately, such single-to-dual task comparisons are difficult to interpret within the context of resource theory, and although this finding is consistent with the notion that individuals with aphasia have impairments of attentional resource allocation, it is amenable to other interpretations as well, including (but not limited to) a fundamental capacity reduction. Other studies that have held the dual-task requirements constant have found that individuals with aphasia are less responsive than normal individuals to task manipulations that putatively affect task priority or allocation ratio. For example, Tseng et al. (1993) asked normal and persons with aphasia to monitor word strings for semantic and phonological targets, and found that, while normal individuals showed expected increases in reaction time (RT) associated with decreases in target frequency, participants with aphasia showed no effects of target frequency on RT or accuracy. Slansky and McNeil (1997) obtained similar findings when manipulating the linguistic stress of category decision and lexical decision stimuli presented in a sentence context. These findings suggest that individuals with aphasia may be impaired in their ability to accurately evaluate task demands, and/or to appropriately mobilize resources to maximize performance in meeting those demands. The former possibility is consistent with other studies demonstrating that ratings of task difficulty by individuals with aphasia do not correlate well with their reaction times, in contrast to nonbrain-injured persons' ratings (Clark & Robin, 1995; Murray et al., 1997a).

One problem that has plagued much (though not all) of the literature on attentional explanations for aphasia is a tendency toward vague usage of resource terminology. While Kahneman (1973) and Navon and Gopher (1979, 1980) were quite specific in describing theoretical distinctions critical to resource theory (e.g., processing resources vs. processing structures, concurrence costs vs. interference costs, task difficulty vs. task demand, data limits vs. resource limits), many aphasiologists who have employed both resource theory and linguistic (primarily syntax) theory as motivating constructs have often conflated them or ignored them altogether. Part of this tendency toward vague usage of the term resource may be due to their use of Baddeley's working memory model as a motivating construct. While this model has been elaborated by Baddeley (1993, 1996, 1998) and many others since its original formulation, it remains rather nonspecific in its employment of the concept of the "central executive" and related concepts such as "controlled attention," "resources," and "capacity" as employed by many users. Fortunately, many researchers have recognized the construct's over-simplification and evidence has been assembled supporting the validity for its fractionation (cf. Fournier, Larigauderie, & Gaonac'h, 2004; Fournier-Vicente, Larigauderie, & Gaonac'h, 2008; Kane & Engle, 2003; Miyake et al., 2000). For example, Kane and Engle (2003) demonstrated the differential demands of "goal maintenance" relative to those of "task switching" in the Stroop task. Fournier et al. (2004) identified such general functions as "coordination" among constituents, "inhibition," and "long-term memory retrieval" (similar to Miyake et al., 2000) as relevant components of the attentional/central executive. Fournier and colleagues argued for six separable functions of the central executive component of the WM model (verbal storage-and-processing coordination, visuospatial storage-and-processing coordination, dual-task coordination, strategic retrieval, selective attention, and shifting). Using a group of 180 young college students, these researchers demonstrated that, through confirmatory factor analysis, five of the six functions were related but distinguishable from one another. Importantly for this discussion, these investigators measured selective attention for linguistic information with the naming Stroop task; a task closely tied by these and other authors to the construct of inhibition.

It is reasonable to suggest that since persons with aphasia have a language problem, any appropriate test of attention in this population might require its assessment using nonlinguistic stimuli. However, if one source of executive resources is specialized for linguistic processing, as proposed by the WM model and supported by a sizable experimental literature as discussed above, then the use of nonlinguistic tasks would not provide the appropriate test of or insight into a resource account as a mechanism subtending the observed language impairment. Alternatively, if one used an attentional task that requires language processing, any observed impairments could not be unambiguously attributed to the attentional demands of the task and would lead to the inevitable equivocal interpretation that the impairment was as likely derived from impairments in linguistic computations as from the attentional component of the task. The Stroop task offers one potential method for resolving this situation.

Stroop and Stroop-like tasks

Without doubt, the Stroop task is the most frequently studied attention paradigm in existence and it is clear why it is considered the "gold standard" of attentional measures (MacLeod, 1992). Review articles (e.g., Jensen & Rohwer, 1966; MacLeod, 1991) have catalogued hundreds of Stroop-like tasks and perhaps thousands of studies investigating an incredible array of variables involved in their performance. The original Stroop task (Stroop, 1935) involved rapidly naming the color of the ink for a printed color word with colored ink under two conditions; where the ink is either congruent with color word (e.g., the word "red" printed in red ink) or incongruent (e.g., the word "red" printed in blue ink) with it compared to a neutral condition (e.g., naming a color patch or reading the color word in traditional black ink). The ubiquitous and robust effect reveal that naming the ink color in the incongruent condition is more difficult (produces long reaction times and creates more errors) than the neutral condition. Conversely, naming the ink color in the congruent condition is often facilitative (produces shorter reaction times and less errors) compared to the relevant neutral condition. The incongruent result is considered to be an "interference" effect and is generally considered to be due to the required inhibition of the "automatic" activation of the word compared to the "controlled" processing required to name the color. Stroop task variants have been used to investigate attentional functions/impairments in persons with aphasia, though perhaps surprisingly infrequently given their acceptance and popularity in general psychology.

The first "Stroop" task used to investigate aphasia appears to have been conducted by Cohen, Meier, and Schulze (1983). They examined a version of the Stroop task (three-color, three-choice button response instead of the traditional oral naming task) and a nonlinguistic (three-position parallel line identification, three-choice button response) task in two groups with aphasia (21 persons with Broca aphasia, ten with Wernicke aphasia) and two groups of brain damaged persons without aphasia (15 with right hemisphere damage and 15 with diffuse brain damage) that when combined, formed the control group. The results revealed that the nonlinguistic task was responded to significantly faster than the linguistic task for all groups with no difference between groups for the nonlinguistic task or the congruent condition of linguistic task. The persons with aphasia showed significantly less interference than the control group on the linguistic incongruent condition. Further, the severity of aphasia, as indexed by the number of errors on an unspecified version of a "token test," correlated negatively ($r = -.42$) with the size of the interference effect, whereas age, time post onset and score on the Trail Making test correlated poorly ($r = .10$–$.18$) with the interference effect. The conclusion was that persons with aphasia showed less Stroop interference than the other brain damaged control participants. Whether this means that they did not have automatic access to the word meaning, which is believed to create the interference, or whether they had superior inhibitory processes for the automatic color word was not discussed. No distinctions in performance were discussed relative to the two groups with aphasia; a finding that could inform the debate about preserved automatic processing in persons with Wernicke's aphasia and its impairment in Broca's aphasia (Blumstein, Milberg, & Shrier, 1982).

Revonsuo (1995) appears to have been the first to observe the expected Stroop interference and facilitative effects (reduced reaction times for the congruent condition – e.g., word "red" in red ink relative to the control condition) in a person with aphasia. These effects paralleled the control participant's patterns and exceeded them in the magnitude of the total Stroop effect (the difference between the RTs in the congruent and incongruent word conditions).

Ansaldo, Arguin, and Lecours (2002) used a nonlinguistic "orientation" Stroop task to investigate the hemispheric lateralization of language recovery in a single participant described as having "severe Broca's aphasia" (p. 287). While the results for the congruent and incongruent conditions were not reported relative to a control condition (the traditional comparison for determining the interference and facilitation effects), reaction times were longer and error rates higher in the incongruent condition relative to the congruent condition on four separate occasions over a 12-month recovery period. While no test–retest reliability was established for this task, there was considerable variability in reaction times across the four measurements.

Finally, Wiener, Connor, and Obler (2004) administered a computerized manual-response numerical version of the Stroop task to five individuals with Wernicke's aphasia and 12 nonbrain-injured controls. The results indicated a significantly larger interference effect for the group with aphasia relative to the control group. The facilitation effect and error rates were not significantly different between the groups. They also reported a significant and large negative correlation ($r = -.91$) between the interference effect and Token Test (from the Neurosensory Center Comprehensive Examination for Aphasia; Spreen and Benton, 1969) score; indicating that the larger the Stroop interference effect, the lower the auditory comprehension test score. A non-significant correlation between the interference effect size and the Complex Ideational Material subtest from the Boston Diagnostic Examination for Aphasia (Goodglass & Kaplan, 1983) also was reported. The authors interpreted these results as support for their hypothesis that persons with Wernicke's aphasia have a deficit of inhibition at the lexical/semantic level of language processing.

Although the total number of individuals with aphasia that has been assessed with a Stroop-like task is small, several tentative conclusions seem warranted from the data presented thus far. First, persons with aphasia can perform the Stroop and Stroop-like tasks, even persons with very severe aphasia as evidenced by very low error rates. Second, while brain damaged participants can be expected to have slowed reaction times relative to normal controls, a generalized cognitive slowing does seem to account for the differential pattern of findings across the studies. Third, the presence and degree of interference revealed by the incongruent task relative to a legitimate control condition has varied across studies. The largest study (Cohen et al., 1983) showed no interference effects, suggesting either impaired access to word meanings or a hyper-normal inhibition mechanism. The Wiener et al. (2004) study reported an abnormally large interference effect, suggesting an impaired inhibitory mechanism. Differences in participants and tasks are likely sources for these differences across the two studies. Fourth, interference effects have been demonstrated in both linguistic and nonlinguistic tasks and failures to find differences have also been reported. Fifth, the size of the interference effects shown in the persons with aphasia, regardless of the comparisons with control populations, correlates significantly and negatively with Token Test-like tasks and this is present in the absence of such correlations on other linguistic and nonlinguistic tasks.

Summary

The dominant view of aphasia held by the overwhelming majority of researchers, aphasia clinicians, and related healthcare professionals is that it is a language disorder that conforms to a neurological centers and pathways model. The model makes specific predictions about lesioned neural centers and pathways that yield to "classical" types of aphasia. Nearly blind adherence to this view of aphasia has perpetuated the notion that refined linguistic description, tied to increasing specificity of lesion localization has the power to explain the phenomenology of aphasia and make relevant predictions about the underlying mechanisms, potential for recovery, and its most appropriate treatment. We have attempted to review some of the observed phenomena that are incompatible with such a view and have also argued that this view of aphasia has diminished the search for the cognitive mechanisms that subtend the observed language impairments that define the condition.

There are a relatively small, but perhaps growing number of aphasia researchers that have recognized that the cognitive apparatus required for "doing" language may be the source for the observed linguistic behavior in persons with aphasia and that an exploration of these mechanisms may offer explanation and prediction that the traditional view cannot. A focus on WM as a construct has been helpful to the challenge of the traditional and accepted paradigm. That is, the WM model focused on the separation and individual contributions of STM and executive attention as critical components of language processing, in addition to the specific linguistic computational task requirements that is the exclusive domain of the traditional paradigm. We have attempted to argue that the most parsimonious account for the disparate phenomena of aphasia is an impairment of a language dedicated (executive) attentional system, with secondary, rather than primary impairments of the linguistic computational or STM component of the WM system.

A brief review of the dual task aphasia literature has revealed consistent findings of impairments in language processing (though not always restricted to the linguistic domain) that are not easily reconciled with simple linguistic explanations but that are compatible with attentional/resource impairments. Further, while dual-task methods have shed light on the nature of the attentional mechanisms, the methods are difficult to implement and they have not found their way into the armamentaria of clinical aphasiologists.

A review of the known studies that have used a Stroop task to investigate attentional mechanisms and impairments in persons with aphasia yielded only two group investigations and the results were contradictory. Although Stroop and Stroop-like task(s) are technically also dual tasks, there is an extensive knowledge base about them, and they appear to be relatively easy to implement into language assessment procedures that extend beyond the traditional word naming task. This method may provide a platform for evaluating attention-related facilitative, inhibitory and goal maintenance abilities, and impairments in persons with aphasia on a person-by-person basis; all cognitive mechanisms that have been implicated as sources for their linguistic impairments.

Further reading

Dresang, H. C., Hula, W. D., Yeh, F. C., Warren, T., & Dickey, M. W. (2021). White-matter neuroanatomical predictors of aphasic verb retrieval. *Brain Connectivity, 11*(4), 319–330.

Hickok, G. (2022). The dual stream model of speech and language processing. *Handbook of Clinical Neurology, 185*, 57–69.

Hula, W. D., Panesar, S., Gravier, M. L., Yeh, F. C., Dresang, H. C., Dickey, M. W., & Fernandez-Miranda, J. C. (2020). Structural white matter connectometry of word production in aphasia: An observational study. *Brain, 143*(8), 2532–2544,

Wong, W. S. W., & Law, S. P. (2022). Relationship between cognitive functions and multilevel language processing: Data from Chinese speakers with aphasia and implications. *Journal of Speech, Language, and Hearing Research, 65*(3), 1128–1144.

References

Adamovich, B. L. (1978). A comparison of the process of memory and perception between aphasic and non-brain-injured adults. *Clinical Aphasiology, 8*, 327.

Albert, M. L. (1976). Short-term memory and Aphasia. *Brain and Language, 3*(1), 28–33.

Ansaldo, A. I., Arguin, M., & Lecours, A. R. (2002). Initial right hemisphere take-over and subsequent bilateral participation during recovery from aphasia. *Aphasiology, 16*(3), 287–304.

Arvedson, J. C. (1986). Effect of lexical decisions on auditory semantic judgments using divided attention in adults with left and right hemisphere damage. Unpublished doctoral dissertation, University of Wisconsin-Madison.

Arvedson, J. C., & McNeil, M. R. (1987). Accuracy and response times for semantic judgments and lexical decisions with left and right hemisphere lesions. *Clinical Aphasiology, 17*, 188–200.

Baddeley, A. D. (1986). *Working memory*. Oxford: Clarendon.

Baddeley, A. D. (1993). Working memory or working attention. In A. D. Baddeley & L. Weiskrantz (Eds.), *Attention: Selection, awareness and control: A tribute to Donald Broadbent* (pp. 152–170). Oxford: Oxford University Press.

Baddeley, A. D. (1996). Exploring the central executive. *Quarterly Journal of Experimental Psychology, 49A*, 5–28.

Baddeley, A. D. (1998). The central executive: A concept and some misconceptions. *Journal of the International Neuropsychological Society, 4*(5), 523–528.

Baddeley, A. D., & Hitch, G. J. (1974). Working memory. In G. H. Bower (Ed.), *Psychology of learning and motivation: Advances in research and theory* (pp. 47–89). New York: Academic Press.

Baddeley, A. D., & Logie, R. H. (1999). Working memory: The multiple-component model. In A. Miyake & P. Shah (Eds.), *Models of working memory: Mechanisms of active maintenance and executive control* (pp. 28–61). Cambridge: Cambridge University Press.

Bates, E., Devescovi, A., Dronkers, N., Pizzamiglio, L., Wulfeck, B., Hernandez, A. … Marangolo, P. (1994). Grammatical deficits in patients without agrammatism: Sentence interpretation under stress in English and Italian. Abstracts from the Academy of Aphasia 1994 annual meeting [Special issue]. *Brain and Language, 47*, 400–402.

Bates, E., Dick, F., & Wulfeck, B. (1999). Not so fast: Domain-general factors can account for selective deficits in grammatical processing. *Behavioral and Brain Sciences, 22*(1), 96–97.

Bates, E., Friederici, A., & Wulfeck, B. (1987). Comprehension in aphasia: A cross-linguistic study. *Brain and Language, 32*(1), 19–67.

Bayles, K. A., Boone, D. R., Tomoeda, C. K., Slauson, T. J., & Kaszniak, A. W. (1989). Differentiating Alzheimer's patients from normal elderly and stroke patients with aphasia. *Journal of Speech and Hearing Disorders, 54*(1), 74–87.

Benson, D. F. (1979). *Aphasia, alexia, and agraphia*. New York: Churchill Livingstone.

Benton, A. L., Smith, K. C., & Lang, M. (1972). Stimulus characteristics and object naming in aphasic patients. *Journal of Communication Disorders, 5*(1), 19–24.

Berndt, R. S., Mitchum, C. C., & Wayland, S. (1997). Patterns of sentence comprehension in aphasia: A consideration of three hypotheses. *Brain and Language, 60*(2), 197–221.

Bisiach, E. (1966). Perceptual factors in the pathogenesis of anomia. *Cortex, 2*(1), 90–95.

Blackwell, A., & Bates, E. (1995). Inducing agrammatic profiles in normals: Evidence for the selective vulnerability of morphology under cognitive resource limitation. *Journal of Cognitive Neuroscience, 7*(2), 228–257.

Blanchard, S. L., & Prescott, T. E. (1980). The effects of temporal expansion upon auditory comprehension in aphasic adults. *British Journal of Disorders of Communication, 15*(2), 115–127.

Blumstein, S. E., Katz, B., Goodglass, H., Shrier, R., & Dworetsky, B. (1985). The effects of slowed speech on auditory comprehension in aphasia. *Brain and Language, 24*(2), 246–265.

Blumstein, S. E., Milberg, W., & Shrier, R. (1982). Semantic processing in aphasia: Evidence from an auditory lexical decision task. *Brain and Language, 17*(2), 301–315.

Botvinick, M., Nystrom, L. E., Fissell, K., Carter, C. S., & Cohen, J. D. (1999). Conflict monitoring versus selection-for-action in anterior cingulate cortex. *Nature, 402*(6758), 179–181.

Brookshire, R. H., & Nicholas, L. E. (1980). Verification of active and passive sentences by aphasic and nonaphasic subjects. *Journal of Speech and Hearing Research, 23*(4), 878–893.

Brookshire, R. H., & Nicholas, L. E. (1984). Comprehension of directly and nondirectly stated main ideas and details in discourse by brain-damaged and non-brain-damaged listeners. *Brain and Language, 21*(1), 21–36.

Campbell, T. F., & McNeil, M. R. (1985). Effects of presentation rate and divided attention on auditory comprehension in children with acquired language disorder. *Journal of Speech and Hearing Research, 28*(4), 513–520.

Caplan, D. (1987). *Neurolinguistics and linguistic aphasiology*. Cambridge, MA: Cambridge University Press.

Caplan, D., Baker, C., & Dehaut, F. (1985). Syntactic determinants of sentence comprehension in aphasia. *Cognition, 21*(2), 117–175.

Caplan, D., Waters, G., Dede, G., Michaud, J., & Reddy, A. (2007). A study of syntactic processing in aphasia I: Behavioral (psycholinguistic) aspects. *Brain and Language, 101*(2), 103–150.

Caplan, D., & Waters, G. S. (1995). Aphasic disorders of syntactic comprehension and working memory capacity. *Cognitive Neuropsychology, 12*(6), 637–649.

Caplan, D., & Waters, G. S. (1996). Syntactic processing in sentence comprehension under dual-task conditions in aphasic patients. *Language and Cognitive Processes, 11*(5), 525–551.

Caplan, D., & Waters, G. S. (1999). Verbal working memory and sentence comprehension. *Behavioral and Brain Sciences, 22*(1), 77–126.

Caplan, D., Waters, G. S., & Hildebrandt, N. (1997). Determinants of sentence comprehension in aphasic sentence-picture matching tasks. *Journal of Speech, Language, and Hearing Research, 40*(3), 542–555.

Caramazza, A., Zurif, E. B., & Gardner, H. (1978). Sentence memory in aphasia. *Neuropschologia, 16*(6), 661–669.

Caspari, I., Parkinson, S. R., LaPointe, L. L., & Katz, R. C. (1998). Working memory and aphasia. *Brain and Cognition, 37*(2), 205–223.
Cermak, L. S., & Moreines, J. (1976). Verbal retention deficits in aphasic and amnestic patients. *Brain and Language, 3*(1), 16–27.
Cermak, L. S., & Tarlow, S. (1978). Aphasic and amnesic patients' verbal vs. nonverbal retentive abilities. *Cortex, 16*(1), 32–40.
Chmiel, N. (1984). Phonological recoding for reading: The effect of concurrent articulation in a Stroop task. *British Journal of Psychology, 75*(2), 213–220.
Clark, H. M., & Robin, D. A. (1995). Sense of effort during a lexical decision task: Resource allocation deficits following brain damage. *American Journal of Speech-Language Pathology, 4*(4), 143–147.
Cohen, R., Meier, E., & Schulze, U. (1983). Spontanes Lesen aphasischer Patienten entgegen der Instruktion? (Stroop-Test). *Nervenarzt, 54*(6), 299–303.
Cowan, N. (1995). *Attention and memory: An integrated framework*. New York: Oxford University Press.
Cowan, N. (1999). An embedded-processes model of working memory. In A. Miyake & P. Shah (Eds.), *Models of working memory and executive control* (pp. 62–101). Cambridge: Cambridge University Press.
Craven, R. R., & Hirnle, C. J. (Eds.). (2009). *Fundamentals of nursing: Human health and function*. Philadelphia, PA: Lippincott, Williams, & Wilkins.
Crisman, L. G. (1971). Response variability in naming behavior of aphasic patients. Unpublished master's thesis, University of Pittsburgh.
Daneman, M. A., & Carpenter, P. A. (1980). Individual differences in working memory and reading. *Journal of Verbal Learning and Verbal Behavior, 19*(4), 450–466.
Darley, F. L. (1976). Maximizing input to the aphasic patient: A review of research. *Clinical Aphasiology, 6*, 1–21.
Darley, F. L. (1982). *Aphasia*. Philadelphia, PA: W.B. Saunders.
Dick, F., Bates, E., Wulfeck, B., Utman, J. A., Dronkers, N., & Gernsbacher, M. A. (2001). Language deficits, localization, and grammar: Evidence for a distributive model of language breakdown in aphasic patients and neurologically intact individuals. *Psychological Review, 108*(4), 759–788.
Duffy, J. R., & Coelho, C. A. (2001). Schuell's stimulation approach to rehabilitation. In R. Chapey (Ed.), *Language intervention strategies in aphasia and related neurogenic communication disorders* (4th ed., pp. 341–382). Baltimore, MD: Lippincott Williams & Wilkins.
Eggert, G. H. (1977). *Wernicke's works on aphasia: A sourcebook and review*. The Hague: Mouton.
Engle, R. W., Kane, M. J., & Tuholski, S. W. (1999). Individual differences in working memory capacity and what they tell us about controlled attention, general fluid intelligence, and functions of the prefrontal cortex. In A. Miyake & P. Shah (Eds.), *Models of working memory and executive control* (pp. 102–134). Cambridge, MA: Cambridge University Press.
Engle, R. W., Tuholski, S. W., Laughlin, J. E., & Conway, A. R. A. (1999). Working memory, short-term memory, and general fluid intelligence: A latent variable approach. *Journal of Experimental Psychology: General, 128*(3), 309–331.
Erickson, R. J., Goldinger, S. D., & LaPointe, L. L. (1996). Auditory vigilance in aphasic individuals: Detecting nonlinguistic stimuli with full or divided attention. *Brain and Cognition, 30*(2), 244–253.
Ernest-Baron, C. R., Brookshire, R. H., & Nicholas, L. E. (1987). Story structure and retelling of narratives by aphasic and non-brain-damaged adults. *Journal of Speech and Hearing Research, 30*(1), 44–49.
Flowers, C. R. (1975). Proactive interference in short-term recall by aphasic, brain-damaged nonaphasic and normal subjects. *Neuropsychologia, 13*(1), 59–68.
Fournier, S., Larigauderie, P., & Gaonac'h, D. (2004). Exploring how the central executive works: A search for independent components. *Psychologica Belgica, 44*(3), 159–188.
Fournier-Vicente, S., Larigauderie, P., & Gaonac'h, D. (2008). More dissociations and interactions within central executive functioning: A comprehensive latent-variable analysis. *Acta Psychologica, 129*(1), 32–48.
Freed, D. B., Marshall, R. C., & Chulantseff, E. A. (1996). Picture naming variability: A methodological consideration of inconsistent naming responses in fluent and nonfluent aphasia. *Clinical Aphasiology, 26*, 193–205.
Freud, S. (1953). *On aphasia*. New York: International Universities Press, Inc. (originally published in German, 1891).
Friedman, A., & Polson, M. C. (1981). Hemispheres as independent resource systems: Limited-capacity processing and cerebral specialization. *Journal of Experimental Psychology: Human Perception and Performance, 7*(5), 1031–1058.
Gardner, H., Albert, M. L., & Weintraub, S. (1975). Comprehending a word: The influence of speed and redundancy on auditory comprehension in aphasia. *Cortex, 11*(2), 155–162.
Gaulin, C. A., & Campbell, T. F. (1994). Procedure for assessing verbal working memory in normal school-age children: Some preliminary data. *Perceptual and Motor Skills, 79*(1 Pt 1), 55–64.
Geschwind, N. (1965a). Disconnexion syndromes in animals and man. Part I. *Brain, 88*(2), 237–294.
Geschwind, N. (1965b). Disconnexion syndromes in animals and man. Part II. *Brain, 88*(3), 585–644.

Gibson, E. (1998). Linguistic complexity: Locality of syntactic dependencies. *Cognition, 68*(1), 1–76.
Gibson, E., & Pearlmutter, N. J. (2000). Distinguishing serial and parallel parsing. *Journal of Psycholinguistic Research, 29*(2), 231–240.
Golden, C. J. (1976). Identification of brain disorders by the Stroop color and word test. *Journal of Clinical Psychology, 32*(3), 654–658.
Goodglass, H., & Kaplan, E. (1983). *The assessment of aphasia and related disorders* (2nd ed.). Philadelphia, PA: Lea & Febiger.
Goodglass, H., Kaplan, E., & Barresi, B. (2001). *The assessment of aphasia and related disorders* (3rd ed.). Baltimore, MD: Lippincott, Williams, & Wilkins.
Gopher, D., Brickner, M., & Navon, D. (1982). Different difficulty manipulations interact differently with task emphasis: Evidence for multiple resources. *Journal of Experimental Psychology: Human Perception and Performance, 8*(1), 146–157.
Grodzinsky, Y. (2000). The neurology of syntax. *Behavioral and Brain Sciences, 23*(1), 1–71.
Haarmann, H. J., & Kolk, H. H. J. (1991). Syntactic priming in Broca's aphasics: Evidence for slow activation. *Aphasiology, 5*(3), 247–263.
Hageman, C. F. (1980). Attentional mechanisms underlying patterns of auditory comprehension brain-damaged aphasic, non-aphasic, and normal listeners. Unpublished doctoral dissertation, University of Colorado.
Hageman, C. F., & Folkstad, A. (1986). Performance of aphasic listeners on an expanded revised token test subtest presented verbally and nonverbally. *Clinical Aphasiology, 16*, 226–233.
Hageman, C. F., McNeil, M. R., Rucci-Zimmer, S., & Cariski, D. M. (1982). The reliability of patterns of auditory processing deficits: Evidence from the revised Token Test. *Clinical Aphasiology, 12*, 230–234.
Hamilton, N. G., & Matthews, T. (1979). Aphasia: The sole manifestation of focal status epilepticus. *Neurology, 29*(5), 745–748.
Head, H. (1926). *Aphasia and kindred disorders* (Vol. I, II). London: Cambridge University Press.
Howard, D., Patterson, K., Franklin, S., Morton, J., & Orchard-Lisle, V. (1984). Variability and consistency in naming by aphasic patients. *Advances in Neurology, 42*, 263–276.
Hula, W. D., & McNeil, M. R. (2008). Models of attention and dual-task performance as explanatory constructs in aphasia. *Seminars in Speech and Language, 29*(3), 169–187.
Hula, W. D., McNeil, M. R., & Sung, J. E. (2007). Is there an impairment of language-specific processing in aphasia? *Brain and Language, 103*(1–2), 240–241.
Jensen, A. R., & Rohwer, W. D. (1966). The Stroop color-word test: A review. *Acta Psychologica, 25*(1), 36–93.
Just, M. A., & Carpenter, P. A. (1992). A capacity theory of comprehension: Individual differences in working memory. *Psychological Review, 99*(1), 122–149.
Kahneman, D. (1973). *Attention and effort*. Englewood Cliffs, NJ: Prentice-Hall.
Kaminski, H. J., Hlavin, M. L., Likavec, M., & Schmidley, J. W. (1992). Transient neurologic deficit caused by chronic subdural hematoma. *American Journal of Medicine, 92*(6), 698–700.
Kane, M. J., & Engle, R. W. (2003). Working-memory capacity and the control of attention: The contributions of goal neglect, response competition, and task set to Stroop interference. *Journal of Experimental Psychology: General, 132*(1), 47–70.
Kertesz, A. (1979). *Aphasia and associated disorders*. New York: Grune & Stratton.
Kertesz, A. (1982). *Western aphasia battery*. New York: Grune & Stratton.
Kilborn, K. (1991). Selective impairment of grammatical morphology due to induced stress in normal listeners: Implications for aphasia. *Brain and Language, 41*(2), 275–288.
Kimelman, M. D. Z., & McNeil, M. R. (1987). An investigation of emphatic stress comprehension in adult aphasia. *Journal of Speech, Language, and Hearing Research, 30*(3), 295–300.
King, J., & Just, M. A. (1991). Individual differences in syntactic processing: The role of working memory. *Journal of Memory and Language, 30*(5), 580–602.
King, J. W., & Kutas, M. (1998). Neural plasticity in the dynamics of human visual word recognition. *Neuroscience Letters, 244*(2), 61–64.
Kolk, H. (2007). Variability is the hallmark of aphasic behaviour: Grammatical behaviour is no exception. *Brain and Language, 101*(2), 99–102.
Kreindler, A., & Fradis, A. (1968). *Performances in aphasia: A neurodynamical diagnostic and psychological study*. Paris: Gauthier-Villars.
Kuhn, T. S. (1962). *The structure of scientific revolutions*. Chicago, IL: University of Chicago Press.
LaPointe, L. L., & Erickson, R. J. (1991). Auditory vigilance during divided task attention in aphasic individuals. *Aphasiology, 5*(6), 511–520.
Larson, M. J., Kaufman, D. A. S., & Perlstein, W. M. (2009). Neural time course of conflict adaptation effects on the Stroop task. *Neuropsychologia, 47*(3), 663–670.
Lebrun, Y. (1994). Ictal verbal behaviour: A review. *Seizur, 3*(1), 45–54.

Lecours, A. R., & Joanette, Y. (1980). Linguistic and other psychological aspects of paroxysmal aphasia. *Brain and Language*, *10*(1), 1–23.
Linebaugh, C. W., Coakley, A. S., Arrigan, A. F., & Racy, A. (1979). Epileptogenic aphasia. *Clinical Aphasiology*, *9*, 70–78.
Lubinski, R., & Chapey, R. (1978). Constructive recall strategies in adult aphasia. *Clinical Aphasiology*, *18*, 338–350.
MacDonald, M. C., Just, M. A., & Carpenter, P. A. (1992). Working memory constraints on the processing of syntactic ambiguity. *Cognitive Psychology*, *24*(1), 56–98.
MacLeod, C. M. (1991). Half a century of research on the Stroop effect: An integrative review. *Psychological Bulletin*, *109*(2), 163–203.
MacLeod, C. M. (1992). The Stroop task: The "gold standard" of attentional measures. *Journal of Experimental Psychology: General*, *121*(1), 12–14.
Marie, P. (1906). Revision de la question de l'aphasie: La troisieme circonvolution forntale gauche ne joue aucun role speciale dans la function du langage. *Seminars in Medicine*, *26*, 241–247.
Martin, N., Dell, G. S., Saffran, E. M., & Schwartz, M. F. (1994). Origins of paraphasias in deep dysphasia: Testing the consequences of a decay impairment to an interactive spreading activation model of lexical retrieval. *Brain and Language*, *47*(4), 609–660.
Martin, N., & Saffran, E. M. (1997). Language and auditory-verbal short-term memory impairments: Evidence for common underlying processes. *Cognitive Neuropsychology*, *14*(5), 641–682.
McNeil, M. R. (1982). The nature of aphasia in adults. In N. J. Lass, L. V. McReynolds, J. L. Northern, & D. E. Yoder (Eds.), *Speech, language, and hearing (Vol. II): Pathologies of speech and language* (pp. 692–740). Philadelphia, PA: Saunders.
McNeil, M. R. (1983). Aphasia: Neurological considerations. *Topics in Language Disorders*, *3*(4), 1–19.
McNeil, M. R. (1988). Aphasia in the adult. In N. J. Lass, L. V. McReynolds, J. Northern, & D. E. Yoder (Eds.), *Handbook of speech-language pathology and audiology* (pp. 738–786). Toronto: D.C. Becker, Inc.
McNeil, M. R., & Hageman, C. F. (1979). Auditory processing deficits in aphasia evidenced on the revised Token Test: Incidence and prediction of across subtest and across item within subtest patterns. *Clinical Aphasiology*, *9*, 47–69.
McNeil, M. R., Hageman, C. F., & Matthews, C. T. (2005). Auditory processing deficits in aphasia evidenced on the revised Token Test: Incidence and prediction of across subtest and across item within subtest patterns. *Aphasiology*, *19*(2), 179–198.
McNeil, M. R., & Kimelman, M. D. Z. (1986). Toward an integrative information-processing structure of auditory comprehension and processing in adult aphasia. *Seminars in Speech and Language*, 7(2), 123–146.
McNeil, M. R., Odell, K. H., & Campbell, T. F. (1982). The frequency and amplitude of fluctuating auditory processing in aphasic and nonaphasic brain-damaged persons. *Clinical Aphasiology*, *12*, 220–229.
McNeil, M. R., Odell, K. H., & Tseng, C. H. (1991). Toward the integration of resource allocation into a general theory of aphasia. *Clinical Aphasiology*, *21*, 21–39.
McNeil, M. R., & Pratt, S. R. (2001). Defining aphasia: Some theoretical and clinical implications of operating from a formal definition. *Aphasiology*, *15*(10–11), 901–911.
McNeil, M. R., & Prescott, T. E. (1978). *Revised token test*. Austin, TX: Pro-Ed.
Miyake, A., Carpenter, P. A., & Just, M. A. (1994). A capacity approach to syntactic comprehension disorders: Making normal adults perform like aphasic patients. *Cognitive Neuropsychology*, *11*(6), 671–717.
Miyake, A., Emerson, M. J., & Friedman, N. P. (1999). Good interactions are hard to find. *Behavioral and Brain Sciences*, *22*(1), 108–109.
Miyake, A., Friedman, N. P., Emerson, M. J., Witzki, A. H., Howerter, A., & Wager, T. D. (2000). The unity and diversity of executive functions and their contributions to complex "frontal lobe" tasks: A latent variable analysis. *Cognitive Psychology*, *41*(1), 49–100.
Mlcoch, A. G., & Metter, E. J. (2001). Medical aspects of stroke rehabilitation. In R. Chapey (Ed.), *Language intervention strategies in aphasia and related neurogenic communication disorders* (pp. 37–54). Baltimore, MD: Lippincott Williams & Wilkins.
Murray, L. L. (2000). The effects of varying attentional demands on the word retrieval skills of adults with aphasia, right hemisphere brain damage, or no brain damage. *Brain and Language*, *72*(1), 40–72.
Murray, L. L., Holland, A. L., & Beeson, P. M. (1997a). Accuracy monitoring and task demand evaluation in aphasia. *Aphasiology*, *11*(4–5), 401–414.
Murray, L. L., Holland, A. L., & Beeson, P. M. (1997b). Auditory processing in individuals with mild aphasia: A study of resource allocation. *Journal of Speech, Language, and Hearing Research*, *40*(4), 792–808.
Murray, L. L., Holland, A. L., & Beeson, P. M. (1997c). Grammaticality judgments of mildly aphasic individuals under dual-task conditions. *Aphasiology*, *11*(10), 993–1016.
Murray, L. L., Holland, A. L., & Beeson, P. M. (1998). Spoken language of individuals with mild fluent aphasia under focused and divided-attention conditions. *Journal of Speech, Language, and Hearing Research*, *41*(1), 213–227.

Naeser, M. A., Martin, P. I., Nicholas, M., Baker, E. H., Seekins, H., Kobayashi, M., … Pascual-Leone, A. (2005). Improved picture naming in chronic aphasia after TMS to part of right Broca's area: An open-protocol study. *Brain and Language*, *93*(1), 95–105.

Naeser, M. A., Mazurski, P., Goodglass, H., Peraino, M., Laughlin, S., & Leaper, W. C. (1987). Auditory syntactic comprehension in nine aphasia groups (with CT scans) and children: Differences in degree but not order of difficulty observed. *Cortex*, *23*(3), 359–380.

Navon, D., & Gopher, D. (1979). On the economy of the human-processing system. *Psychological Review*, *86*(3), 214–255.

Navon, D., & Gopher, D. (1980). Task difficulty, resources, and dual-task performance. In R. S. Nickerson (Ed.), *Attention and performance* (pp. 297–315). Hillsdale, NJ: Erlbaum.

Nelson, J. K., Reuter-Lorenz, P. A., Persson, J., Sylvester, C. Y., & Jonides, J. (2009). Mapping interference resolution across task domains: A shared control process in left inferior frontal gyrus. *Brain Research*, *1256*, 92–100.

Nicholas, L. E., & Brookshire, R. H. (1986). Consistency of the effects of rate of speech on brain-damaged adults' comprehension of narrative discourse. *Journal of Speech and Hearing Research*, *29*(4), 462–470.

Odell, K. H., Hashi, M., Miller, S. B., & McNeil, M. R. (1995). A critical look at the notion of selective impairment. *Clinical Aphasiology*, *23*, 1–8.

Pashek, G. V., & Brookshire, R. H. (1982). Effects of rate of speech and linguistic stress on auditory paragraph comprehension of aphasic individuals. *Journal of Speech and Hearing Research*, *25*(3), 377–383.

Peach, R. K., Rubin, S. S., & Newhoff, M. (1994). A topographic event-related potential analysis of the attention deficit for auditory processing in aphasia. *Clinical Aphasiology*, *24*, 81–96.

Perret, E. (1974). The left frontal lobe of man and the suppression of habitual responses in verbal categorical behavior. *Neuropsychologia*, *12*(3), 323–330.

Podraza, B. L., & Darley, F. L. (1977). Effect of auditory prestimulation on naming in aphasia. *Journal of Speech and Hearing Research*, *20*(4), 669–683.

Porch, B. (2001). *Porch index of communicative ability*. Albuquerque, NM: PICA Programs.

Rahimi, A. R., & Poorkay, M. (2000). Subdural hematomas and isolated transient aphasia. *Journal of the American Medical Directors Association*, *1*(3), 129–131.

Revonsou, A. (1995). Words interact with colors in a globally aphasic patient: Evidence from a stroop-like task. *Cortex*, *31*(2), 377–386.

Saffran, E. M., Schwartz, M. F., & Marin, O. S. M. (1980). Evidence from aphasia: Isolating the components of a word production model. In B. Butterworth (Ed.), *Language production* (pp. 221–240). London: Academic Press.

Salvatore, A. (1974). An investigation of the effects of pause duration on sentence comprehension by aphasic subjects. Unpublished doctoral dissertation, University of Pittsburgh.

Schuell, H., Jenkins, J. J., & Jimenez-Pabon, E. (1964). *Aphasia in adults: Diagnosis, prognosis, and treatment*. New York: Harper and Row.

Schwartz, M. F., Saffran, E. M., Bloch, D. E., & Dell, G. S. (1994). Disordered speech production in aphasic and normal speakers. *Brain and Language*, *47*(1), 52–88.

Shah, P., & Miyake, A. (1999). Models of working memory: An introduction. In A. Miyake & P. Shah (Eds.), *Models of working memory: Mechanisms of active maintenance and executive control* (pp. 1–28). Cambridge: Cambridge University Press.

Shewan, C. M. (1976). Error patterns in auditory comprehension of adult aphasics. *Cortex*, *12*(4), 325–336.

Shewan, C. M., & Canter, G. J. (1971). Effects of vocabulary, syntax, and sentence length on auditory comprehension in aphasic patients. *Cortex*, *7*(3), 209–226.

Silkes, J., McNeil, M. R., & Drton, M. (2004). Simulation of aphasic naming performance in non-brain-damaged adults. *Journal of Speech, Language, and Hearing Research*, *47*(3), 610–623.

Slansky, B. L., & McNeil, M. R. (1997). Resource allocation in auditory processing of emphatically stressed stimuli in aphasia. *Aphasiology*, *11*(4–5), 461–472.

Spreen, O., & Benton, A. L. (1969). *Neurosensory center comprehensive examination for aphasia*. Victoria: University of Victoria, Department of Psychology, Neuropsychology Laboratory.

Stroop, J. R. (1935). Studies of interference in serial verbal reactions. *Journal and Experimental Psychology*, *6*(6), 643–662.

Stuss, D. T., Floden, D., Alexander, M. P., Levine, B., & Katz, D. (2001). Stroop performance in focal lesion patients: Dissociation of processes and frontal lobe lesion location. *Neuropsychologia*, *39*(8), 771–786.

Sung, J. E., McNeil, M. R., Pratt, S. R., Dickey, M. W., Hula, W. D., Szuminsky, N. J., & Doyle, P. J. (2009). Verbal working memory and its relationship to sentence-level reading and listening comprehension in persons with aphasia. *Aphasiology*, *23*(7–8), 1040–1052.

Swinney, D. A., & Taylor, O. L. (1971). Short-term memory recognition search in aphasics. *Journal and Speech and Hearing Research*, *14*(3), 578–588.

Thompson-Schill, S. L., Bedny, M., & Goldberg, R. F. (2005). The frontal lobes and the regulation of mental activity. *Current Opinion in Neurobiology, 15*(2), 219–224.

Thompson-Schill, S. L., Jonides, J., Marshuetz, C., Smith, E. E., D'Esposito, M., Kan, I. P., ... Swick, D. (2002). Effects of frontal lobe damage on interference effects in working memory. *Cognitive, Affective, and Behavioral Neuroscience, 2*(2), 109–120.

Tompkins, C. A., Bloise, C. G. R., Timko, M. L., & Baumgaertner, A. (1994). Working memory and inference revision in brain-damaged and normally aging adults. *Journal of Speech and Hearing Research, 37*(4), 896–912.

Tseng, C.-H., McNeil, M. R., & Milenkovic, P. (1993). An investigation of attention allocation deficits in aphasia. *Brain and Language, 45*(2), 276–296.

Warren, R. L., Hubbard, D. J., & Knox, A. W. (1977). Short-term memory scan in normal individuals and individuals with aphasia. *Journal of Speech and Hearing Research, 20*(3), 497–509.

Waters, G. S., & Caplan, D. (1996a). Processing resource capacity and the comprehension of garden path sentences. *Memory and Cognition, 24*(3), 342–355.

Waters, G. S., & Caplan, D. (1996b). The capacity theory of sentence comprehension: Critique of just and carpenter (1992). *Psychologica, 103*(4), 761–772.

Waters, G. S., & Caplan, D. (2004). Verbal working memory and on-line syntactic processing: Evidence from self-paced listening. *Quarterly Journal of Experimental Psychology, 57A*(1), 129–163.

Weems, S. A., & Reggia, J. A. (2007). Simulating single word processing in the classic aphasia syndromes based on the Wernicke–Lichtheim–Geschwind theory. *Brain and Language, 98*(3), 291–309.

Weidner, W. E., & Lasky, E. Z. (1976). The interaction of rate and complexity of stimulus on the performance of adult aphasic subjects. *Brain and Language, 3*(1), 34–40.

West, R. (2003). Neural correlates of cognitive control and conflict detection in the Stroop and digit-location tasks. *Neuropsychologia, 41*(8), 1122–1135.

West, R., & Alain, C. (2000). Effect of task context and fluctuations of attention on neural activity supporting performance of the Stroop task. *Brain Research, 873*(1), 102–111.

Wickens, C. D. (1980). The structure of attentional resources. In R. S. Nickerson (Ed.), *Attention and performance VIII* (pp. 239–258). Hillsdale, NJ: Erlbaum.

Wickens, C. D. (1984). Processing resources in attention. In R. Parasuraman & D. R. Davies (Eds.), *Varieties of attention* (pp. 63–102). New York: Academic Press.

Wiener, D. A., Connor, L. T., & Obler, L. K. (2004). Inhibition and auditory comprehension in Wernicke's aphasia. *Aphasiology, 18*(5–7), 599–609.

Wilson, S. M., Saygin, A. P., Schleicher, E., Dick, F., & Bates, E. (2003). Grammaticality judgment under non-optimal processing conditions: Deficits observed in normal participants resemble those observed in aphasic patients. Abstracts from the Academy of Aphasia [Special Issue]. *Brain and Language, 87*(1), 67–68.

28

REMEDIATION OF THEORY OF MIND IMPAIRMENTS IN ADULTS WITH ACQUIRED BRAIN INJURY

Kristine Lundgren and Hiram Brownell[1]

Introduction

Successful communication relies on conversational partners having access to each other's thoughts and feelings. This interpersonal understanding, often labeled Theory of Mind (ToM) goes well beyond competence with words and sentences to include individuals' representations of the world that can at times conflict with objective truth (e.g., Dennett, 1978; Leslie, 1987; Premack & Woodruff, 1978). Consider the following vignette to illustrate how consideration of people's beliefs provides a powerful framework for analyzing communication. While at work, Jim spends 45 minutes in his office playing video games with his officemate and, as a result, is late for a meeting. The coworkers at the meeting who have no direct access to the reason for Jim's arriving late will have incorrect or incomplete first-order beliefs about the situation. Jim could decide to tell the coworkers the literal truth (that he lost track of time while playing video games). Alternatively, he could lie to them by saying that he was delayed due to a lengthy email from an important client. Use of intentional deception rests on a speaker's (Jim's) second-order beliefs, i.e., what he knows about the listeners' (co-workers') beliefs: Jim can attempt a deceptive lie only if he believes his listeners do not know the truth. Finally, on returning to his office after the meeting, Jim might use the same untrue statement (that he was late due to a client email) to get a laugh out of his officemate. Jim's second-order belief about his officemate's mental state suggests an ironic or humorous intent in making this comment. ToM is a broad construct. It relates to a range of notions from pragmatics and discourse, such as the importance of shared knowledge between participants in a conversation (e.g., "common ground," Clark & Marshall, 1981) or Grice's conversational postulates (e.g., supplying an appropriate but not excessive amount of information, Grice, 1975).

ToM impairments characterize disparate populations without aphasia including individuals with autism spectrum disorders, with right hemisphere disorder (RHD) due to stroke, and Traumatic Brain Injury (TBI) (Baron-Cohen, Leslie, & Frith, 1985; Bibby & McDonald, 2005; Happé, Brownell, & Winner, 1999; Shamay-Tsoory, Tomer, Berger, & Aharon-Peretz, 2005; Balaban, Friedmann, & Ziv, 2016; Balaban, Biran, & Sacher, 2019). In this chapter, we describe a treatment approach for ToM impairments designed for use with individuals with RHD or with TBI. In our previous chapter describing this treatment (Lundgren & Brownell, 2011), we reported results from a person with RHD due to stroke. Here, we summarize results obtained with two persons with RHD due to stroke and three with TBI as offering "proof of concept": evidence that the basic approach can work and merits development. Our extension to persons with TBI reflects an addi-

 DOI: 10.4324/9781003204213-32

tional societal need: TBI is an epidemic in the United States with an estimated 1.7 million people sustaining an injury annually (Faul, Xu, Wald, & Coronado, 2010).

A number of experimental paradigms and assessments have been used to study ToM, ranging from story comprehension (Dodell-Feder, Lincoln, Coulson, & Hooker, 2013) to having people infer emotions from partial facial expressions (Baron-Cohen, Wheelwright, Hill, Raste, & Plumb, 2001). One common paradigm is the false belief task based on the notion that different people can have conflicting beliefs about the world, some of which must be false (Leslie, 1987). False belief scenarios, similar to the vignette presented above, typically involve characters whose distinct – and possibly conflicting – beliefs must be remembered and compared. In addition, characters may lose or gain perceptual access to true information independently of one another as events unfold. The attraction of the false belief task stems from the explicit role of conflicting beliefs, with obvious relevance to deception and irony. In addition, classic work by Zaitchik (1990) manipulated the structure of a false belief task to distinguish the ability to reason about mental states from the ability to reason about equally complex non-mentalist false representations such as outdated photographs. Imaging studies with non-injured adults indicate a mentalizing network that includes prefrontal regions as well as temporal-parietal regions (Van Overwalle & Vandekerckhove, 2013), and evidence that ToM activation can, with careful experimental design, be distinguished from that associated with executive function (Saxe & Kanwisher, 2003; Saxe, Schulz, & Liang, 2006).

The complexity of false belief tasks raises several issues in the context of brain injured individuals. The false belief paradigm places demands on attention and executive function more broadly, which can make distinguishing impairments in ToM from those in other domains problematic. Stuss, Gallop, and Alexander (2001) looked at the contributions of attention, visual perception, reversal learning, and memory to patients' ToM following frontal lesions due to stroke. Tompkins and her colleagues (Tompkins, Scharp, Fassbinder, Meigh, & Armstrong, 2008) compared the performance of patients with RHD on standard second-order belief scenarios presented auditorily to carefully constructed, equivalent passages that did not require theory of mind processing. Tompkins et al.'s conclusion was that controlling the complexity of required processing eliminated any selective theory of mind impairment in persons with RHD. The same concern applies to work with individuals with TBI.

The relevance of executive function for the TBI population is similarly based on the prevalence of frontal and, in addition, prefrontal system involvement. Focal contusions occur at characteristic locations due to the shape of the skull and typical direction of brain movement within the skull. These areas of damage usually include frontal regions among others, and their impact is often amplified by disconnection due to widespread diffuse axonal shearing (e.g., Cicerone, Levin, Malec, Stuss, & Whyte, 2006). The overlap between ToM and other cognitive domains presents a theoretical and practical challenge for treatment programs, as will be discussed below. Even if ToM processing can be isolated in non-brain-injured adults (e.g., Saxe et al., 2006), the cognitive impairments associated with TBI and RHD often include executive dysfunction, which may impact ToM assessment or treatment (Schneider, Lam, Baykiss, & Dux, 2012).

Despite the evidence suggesting that social cognition is often impaired following TBI and RHD, there are just a handful of studies that have explored the treatment of these impairments following acquired brain injury (Blake, Frymark, & Venedictov, 2013; Cassel, McDonald, Kelly, & Togher, 2019). This is in stark contrast to the treatment of social cognition, particularly ToM impairments in a number of other diagnostic groups. In their systematic review, Vass and colleagues, for example, describe seven different intervention approaches to treat ToM in individuals diagnosed with schizophrenia (Vass, Fekete, Simon, & Simon, 2018).

In this chapter we begin to address this gap in remediation options for ToM impairment appropriate for people who have experienced significant impairment due to either stroke or TBI. We describe an approach to treating ToM impairments and present promising evidence that ToM treatment is associated with gains beyond what could be expected in terms of overall recovery across cognitive domains. Then, we consider ToM treatment in the context of executive function impairments. That is, we offer two working hypotheses: (1) ToM can be improved with practice, and (2) ToM can, in practical terms, be distinguished from other cognitive domains such as visuospatial processing and executive function, even if many individuals can benefit from treatment that targets both domains. To anticipate our findings, the first hypothesis is well supported. Evidence bearing on the second hypothesis varies with the domain: visuospatial processing appears to be distinct from ToM, while support for the separation of ToM from executive function is intriguing but less clear cut.

Theory of Mind training protocol

One foundation for ToM is shared perceptual access to relevant information. For example, a typical standard false belief task uses two characters whose perceptual access to on object's changed location (or the contents of a box) differs. For purposes of reminding a person with TBI about the importance of shared knowledge, a visually based paradigm is an obvious choice. In our work, different people are portrayed as being in the same or different rooms in a cut-away diagram of a house (see Figure 28.1).

Another foundation of our ToM training is to make explicit and concrete the relevant facts underlying conflicting beliefs so that an individual can see and review them. Explicit provision of essential links in a task has worked in other domains. Wellman et al. (2002) used thought bubbles (balloons used to convey thoughts of cartoon characters) to help autistic children perform ToM tasks with greater success: beliefs represented in thought balloons become just another sentence describing something about the world. In addition, memory demands are reduced because the visual display is present. A similar approach has been used successfully with participants with brain injury due to right hemisphere stroke or TBI: in a pair of studies, a metaphor training protocol used circles with line segments to represent the semantic features that are or are not shared across word concepts (Brownell et al., 2013; Lundgren et al., 2011).

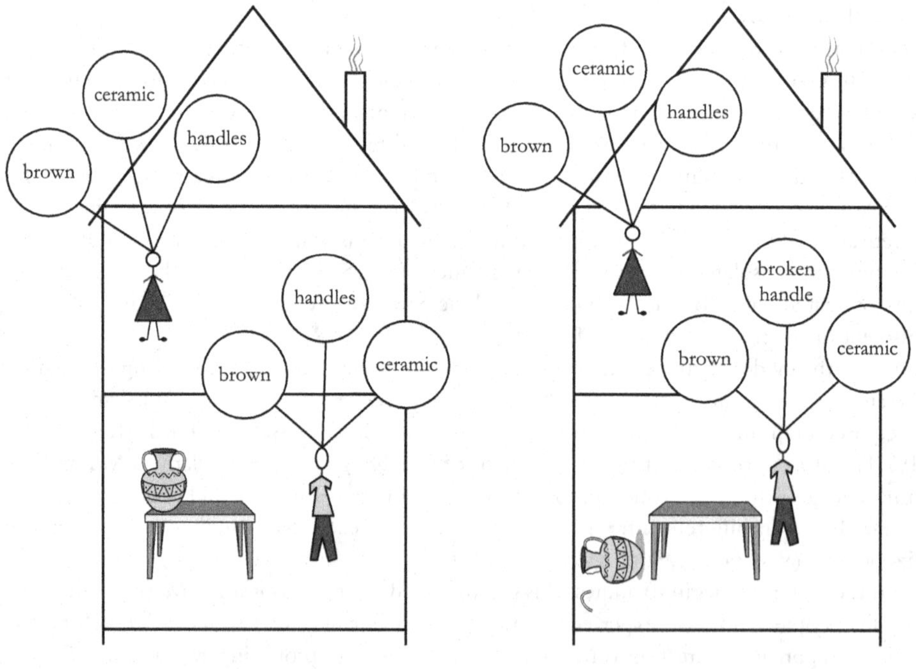

Figure 28.1 Multilevel home.

The training tasks, which are grouped into phases, are ordered to move a patient along a conceptually and empirically defined performance continuum from easier to more difficult. Also, some tasks build directly on other tasks, as detailed below. The protocol begins with a "Warm-Up Phase," which is then followed by Phase I and II. On the basis of testing completed to date, we know that Phase I and II, which both involve first-order belief, are relatively easy and should be presented first in order to engage patients. Phase III and IV, which involve second-order belief, require more effort and call on a number of skills that are often at risk in brain-injured individuals. Phase III and IV are roughly comparable to each other in difficulty except that Phase IV requires additional processing of motivation in one of the characters. While the ordering of difficulty of Phase III and IV varies across participants, these two tasks were the most difficult of the program. The training program is designed to provide multiple opportunities for the participant to practice, correct, and learn skills necessary to progress from one phase of the training program to another.

Warm up phase: generating words

Overview. The participant is provided multiple items in each of three tasks in order to practice generating associations for printed and pictured nouns. Five trials of ten items each are presented to the participant for each task.

Scoring. The warm-up phase is not scored.

Phase I

Overview. During Phase I the participant is asked to help tell a number of stories. Each story involves two characters: Alice and Greg, living in a multilevel home (see Figure 28.1). The participant is told that both Alice and Greg have thoughts about what is happening in each story. Sometimes the characters' thoughts stay the same over several turns of events, and sometimes their thoughts change. The participant is instructed to observe each situation to help decide when the characters' thought change and when their thoughts do not. (This phase and later phases include multiple tasks and a variety of situations.)

Scoring. Responses to each task are scored as correct (1 point), delayed correct (.5), or incorrect (0). A participant can progress to the next task after receiving 90% accuracy on five trials of ten items or 100% accuracy on three trials of ten items.

Phase II

Overview. During Phase II, the participant is asked to help tell a number of stories. Each story involves two characters: Alice and Greg, living in a multilevel home. The participant is told that both Alice and Greg have thoughts about what is happening in each story. Sometimes each character's thoughts will stay the same over several turns of events, and sometimes their thoughts will change. In addition, in some stories one character will know something that the other character does not know. This knowledge will alter one character's thoughts but not the other's. The participant is instructed to observe each situation to help decide when the characters' thoughts change and when their thoughts do not.

Scoring. Responses to each task are scored as correct (1 point), delayed correct (.5), or incorrect (0). A participant can progress to the next task after receiving 90% accuracy on five trials of ten items or 100% accuracy on three trials of ten items.

Phase III

Overview. During Phase III, the participant is asked to help tell a number of stories. Each story involves two characters: Alice and Greg, living in a multilevel home (see Figure 28.1). The participant is told that both Alice and Greg have thoughts about what is happening in each story. Sometimes each character's thoughts will stay the same over several turns of events, and sometimes their thoughts will change. In addition, in some stories one character will know something that the other character does not know, and in some stories one of the characters will lie to the other character. This knowledge or lack of knowledge will alter one character's thoughts but not the others. The participant is instructed to observe each situation to help decide when the characters' thoughts change and when their thoughts do not.

Scoring. Responses to this task are scored as correct (1 point), delayed correct (.5), or incorrect (0). A participant can progress to the next task after receiving 90% accuracy on five trials of ten items or 100% accuracy on three trials of ten items.

Phase IV

Overview. During Phase IV, the participant is asked to help tell a number of stories. Each story involves two characters: Alice and Greg living in a multilevel home. The participant is told that both Alice and Greg have thoughts about what is happening in each story. Sometimes each character's thoughts will stay the same over several turns of events, and sometimes their thoughts will change. In addition, in some stories one character will know something that the other character does not know, and in some stories one of the characters will play a joke on the other character. This knowledge or lack of knowledge will alter one character's thoughts but not the others. The participant is instructed to observe each situation to help decide when the characters' thoughts change and when their thoughts do not.

Scoring. Responses to each task are scored as correct (1 point), delayed correct (.5), or incorrect (0). A participant can progress to the next task after receiving 90% accuracy on five trials of ten items or 100% accuracy on three trials of ten items.

Measuring Theory of Mind: the Cartoon Interpretation scale

ToM performance is based on a cartoon interpretation task (Lundgren & Brownell, 2011). The cartoons were selected from Gary Larson's *The Far Side* (Larson, 2003) whose humor often relies on first- or second-order beliefs. A participant is asked to identify salient features in the picture, read the caption, and, finally, describe what most people would find amusing. It is less important that the participant judge the cartoon to be funny, but that the participant understand what most people would identify as being humorous. A 0–6 scale (see below) for scoring quality of Cartoon Interpretations is used to evaluate the individual's performance (inter-rater reliability = 90%, Lundgren, Brownell, Cayer-Meade, Spitzer, 2007a). We identified many suitable Far Side cartoons, which allowed assessment without repeating the same test items over and over. For our demonstration studies, interpretations were recorded for later transcription and scoring (refer to Table 28.1 for scoring criteria). Three judges rated each interpretation and resolved any discrepancies via discussion.

Measuring visuo-spatial ability

We included another dependent measure to provide a control for non-specific recovery of function that was not directly related to the treatment target: a short form of the Benton Judgments of Line Orientation Task that tapped visuospatial ability (Qualls, Bliwise, & Stringer, 2000). A line segment at an angle to a horizontal reference line is presented briefly and then removed from view. The participant then selects a line segment with a matching orientation from an array. Any change in line orientation score should be, by hypothesis, unrelated to starting ToM training or practice with cartoon interpretation.

Table 28.1 Scoring criteria

Score	*Description*
6	Complete and appropriate, identifies the second-order belief/mental state of the character(s).
5	Complete and appropriate, identifies the first-order belief/mental state of the character(s).
4	Complete and appropriate, identifies the mental state of the character(s) but (a) delayed (>5 seconds before response initiation), (b) may contain self-corrections, or false starts but eventually gets to the correct response, or (c) may include some tangential comments and/or personalization.
3	Provides a mental state term relevant to the cartoon but inaccurate (i.e., wrong mental state, mental state of self rather than the character/wrong character) identification of the mental state.
2	Mentions oddness or incongruity of elements.
1	Indicates elements of understanding the incongruous nature of the critical elements of the cartoon and may describe the physical details in the picture, but does not identify the mental state of the character(s).
0	No response, "I don't know," or completely off topic comments such as unrelated, personalized associations tangential to the cartoon.

Separating ToM from non-specific recovery of function

We used variants of multiple baselines, single subject experimental designs which are most useful at early stages of program development to provide empirical support for treatment efficacy on a case-by-case basis (e.g., Barlow, Nock, & Herson, 2009). These designs can accommodate differences across participants who often progress through program stages at different rates and, in addition, allow within-subject comparisons of alternative treatments, as will be discussed below. However, single subject designs entail substantially greater expense per participant because several baseline sessions prior to starting treatment for comparisons needed to gauge confounding factors such as practice effects, spontaneous recovery, and psychological benefits of extended social contact. The single subject design studies reported below (See Table 28.2) typically had ten baseline assessment sessions prior to the start of treatment, which lasted usually approximately ten sessions, and, finally, another approximately ten post-training sessions. Most important from a practical perspective is that all of these individuals completed the protocol with all of the pre- and post-training sessions without any trouble, which suggests that people with brain injury are willing to stay with the program for multiple sessions extending over many weeks. Once a treatment approach has been shown effective, of course, the inefficiencies associated with repeated baseline and post-training assessments can be eliminated.

In what follows we treat Cartoon Interpretation and Benton Line Orientation scores as interval level measurement for practical reasons. This assumption is important to note in that measurement issues render exact numerical values for effect size and other statistical calculations tentative. Also, our analyses consider the different observations from a single individual as statistically independent (i.e., as if they came from different people). The compelling advantage of this approach consists of the insights and suggestions to be corroborated in future investigations.

We start with demonstrations of selective training effects: that a participant's performance on ToM can improve while performance in a different domain, visuospatial ability does not. We report results from two male participants who had sustained RHD due to a middle cerebral artery stroke several years prior to treatment and from two male participants with moderate to severe TBI sustained at least two years prior. (Later, we report results from a fifth man who had sustained a moderate TBI to explore the possible separation of executive function from ToM.) The procedures

Table 28.2 Results of treatment

Case	*Gender*	*Age*	*Education*	*Time Post Injury*	*Effect Size (d) Theory of Mind: Cartoon Interpretation*	*Number Baseline Sessions/Number Training Sessions/ Number Post Training Sessions*	*Effect Size (d) Comparison Benton: RHD 0, TBI 01, TBI 02 Paced Serial Addition Task: TBI 03*
RHD 0	male	60	18 years	20 years	+1.68*	10/5/10	+0.64*
RHD 1	male	60	12 years	6 years	+3.86*	11/9/9	+0.44*
TBI 1	male	58	16 years	2 years	+5.10*	10/10/10	-0.34*
TBI 2	male	27	14 years	3 years	+5.58*	10/10/10	-.0.95*
TBI 03	male	24	13 years	1 year	+0.78** +2.45***	See Figure 28.2	+8.42** +1.15***

*(Mean PostToM Training – Mean Baseline)/SDBaseline
**(Mean Post APT Training – Mean Baseline 1)/SDBaseline 1
***(Mean PostToM Training – Mean Baseline 2)/SDBaseline 2

and results for the three TBI cases are reported in detail in Lundgren and Brownell (2015). The results for the two persons with RHD were summarized in Lundgren, Brownell, Cayer-Meade, and Spitzer (2007a, 2007b). Table 28.1 provides summary information for all five cases.

Training effect size can be expressed using Cohen's d defined as d = (Mean Post-treatment – Mean Pre-treatment Baseline) / SD Pre-treatment Baseline, calculated using raw scores. (Note that the mean Post-treatment was calculated using only observations after treatment had stopped. Lundgren and Brownell (2015) instead calculated Cohen's d values including assessments conducted concurrently with treatment in addition to assessments conducted after training had ceased.) Effect sizes for single subject investigations are hard to interpret without context provided by other treatment studies in the same domain. Beeson and Robey (2006; Robey, Schultz, Crawford, & Sinner, 1999) have suggested the following benchmarks for single subject studies of aphasia treatments: small = 2.6, medium = 3.9, and large = 5.8. These guidelines are quite different from those often cited for group studies, for which a Cohen's d of .8 or higher is considered "large." The ToM gains shown in Table 28.2 are medium to large for some individuals. Together with the smaller and even slightly negative changes in Benton Line Orientation scores, these results suggest that the participants responded well to the treatment and, typically, showed substantially greater gains in ToM than in untreated visuospatial ability.

Less clear from these results is whether simply practice with our assessment tool for ToM, Cartoon Interpretation, contributed to these gains. Lundgren and Brownell (2015) also report hypothesis testing results for TBI 01 and TBI 02 based on a simulation/bootstrapping procedure developed by Borckardt et al. (2008) that effectively separates the training effect (pre- versus post-initiation of training performance) from any steady trend over all sessions and provides a significance test that is immune to problems with the error term used for conventional tests of statistical significance in single subject designs. For both TBI 01 and TBI 02, the effect of training on Cartoon assessment was significant, $p = .03$, which supports the existence effect of treatment that is distinct from widespread improvement due to practice.

The role of executive function

There exists an array of treatment options for executive function. We have used a modified version of a well-established protocol: the Attention Processing Training Program (APT) (Sohlberg &

Mateer, 1987; 2011). This is a multilevel treatment program that targets selective, sustained, divided and alternating attention along a hierarchical continuum of easiest to most difficult. Early versions of the APT have been shown to be effective in the treatment of attention deficits in adults with traumatic brain injury (Neimann, Ruff, & Baser, 1990; Parks & Ingles, 2001). Our modifications to Sohlberg and Mateer's APT-1 protocol included reducing the number of sessions required to ten, while retaining the multilevel focus and the hierarchy of presentation. Exercises included all five levels of attention: focused, sustained, selective, alternating, and divided.

Measuring executive function

Our assessment measure to monitor change in performance is the Paced Serial Addition Task (PASAT) that requires sustained attention and working memory (Gronwall, 1977). In PASAT, the participant listens to single digits presented every three seconds on an audio CD. (There is also a two-second version that can be used with less impaired individuals.) The task is to add the two last digits heard and to report the sum. For example, if the first two digits were six and seven, the patient would respond "thirteen"; if the third digit was four, the patient would then respond "eleven," and so on. The maximum score is 60 (based on 61 presented digits). PASAT scores provide a measure of attention performance that served as a comparison for ToM performance. While PASAT performance is sensitive to practice effects, these are described as greatest in the first few administrations (Tombaugh, 2006).

Separating ToM from executive function

This single subject design entailed administration of both the Attention Process Training (APT-1, Sohlberg & Mateer, 1987) and the ToM training to the same individual to evaluate (1) the role of practice as well as non-specific improvement, (2) whether improvement can be attributed specifically to either APT or ToM treatment, and (3) carryover between APT and ToM such that training in one domain improves performance in the other domain. The Line Orientation Task was replaced by the PASAT, which requires working memory and sustained and divided attention (Gronwall, 1977).

The two training programs were administered sequentially to improve their separation. We began with the APT rather than the ToM because the APT is an established, effective program that would very likely produce improvement at least in executive function. Placing the ToM training after APT presents a very conservative test of treating ToM: any remediation impact of executive function on ToM (that is, any overlap between executive function and ToM) would most likely diminish the potential for further improvement linked to ToM training over and above gains achieved from attention training. Again, the APT-1 is closer to current clinical practice. Our question is whether ToM training adds any benefit.

By necessity, we used a more complex design that included a temporal lag between the two training protocols. After a series of seven Baseline sessions, TBI 03 received APT training, followed by a second set of baseline sessions without training and, then, received ToM training. To complete the study, there were seven additional sessions without any training.

Pretraining Baseline 1 Probes (Sessions 1–7, three per week for approximately 2.5 weeks). Each session included Cartoon Interpretation and PASAT assessments (seven data points for each dependent measure).

APT Training and Probes (Sessions 8–17, three per week for approximately 3.5 weeks during APT-1). Each training session included ToM or APT-1 training plus assessment of Cartoon Interpretation and PASAT tasks (ten data points for each dependent measure).

Post APT training Baseline 2 Probes (Sessions 18–31, three per week). Each session included Cartoon Interpretation and PASAT (14 data points for each dependent measure), without any training.

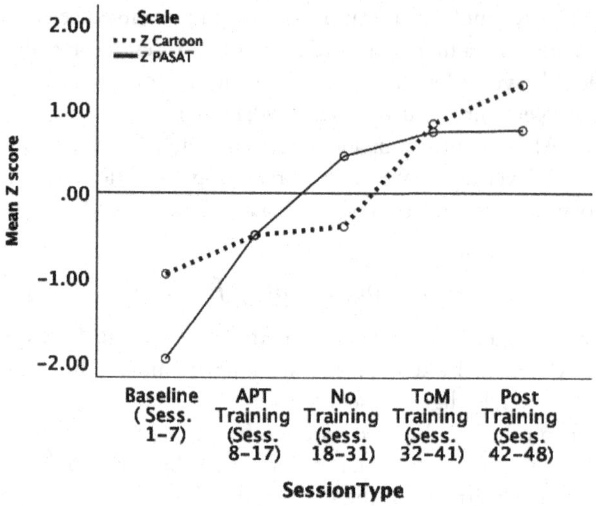

Figure 28.2 Cartoon Interpretation and Paced Serial Addition Task performance.

ToM Training and Probes (Sessions 32-–41, three per week). Each session included ToM training plus assessment of Cartoon Interpretation and PASAT tasks (ten data points for each dependent measure).

Post ToM Training Phase Probes (Sessions 42-–48, three per week). Each session included Cartoon Interpretation and PASAT tasks (seven data points for each dependent measure), without any training.

Figure 28.2 summarizes TBI 03's scores for PASAT and Cartoon Interpretation averaged across the sessions within each study stage. Prior to averaging, PASAT and Cartoon interpretation scores were converted to z score form to facilitate presentation in a single graph. Looking first at the PASAT scores, one sees a strong effect of APT training from Baseline 1 to the interval between training programs, as confirmed by the extremely large effect size shown in Table 28.1. This striking improvement, however, levels off and is not greatly affected by ToM training, as shown by the comparison by the interval between training programs (Baseline 2) and the post-training sessions. Examination of the Cartoon performance suggests some improvement that coincides with attention training, i.e., the improvement between Baseline 1 and the Baseline 2, which suggests some overlap in cognitive skills. However, there is another strong improvement shown by difference between Baseline 2 and the final sessions after all training had ceased: the ToM training has additional value for Cartoon interpretation that does not extend to PASAT. Note too that Lundgren and Brownell (2015) present statistical support for a separation among practice effects, ToM training, and APT.

Conclusions and next steps

These preliminary results strongly suggest that ToM can and should be treated in persons with acquired brain injury who are beyond the first months of recovery: we have shown gains in a task –cartoon interpretation – that rests on understanding other people's feelings and beliefs. That improvement on its own is important and justifies further study. With respect to the theoretical status of the ToM treatment, preliminary evidence suggests the improvement is distinct from any very general, domain-general recovery of function because visuo-spatial ability did not improve.

Our results add to the evidence for effective treatment of executive function deficits. The effect size was very large. The strength of the improvement linked to attention training is encouraging and has obvious clinical relevance: executive dysfunction is a broad impairment that can limit performance in all sorts of tasks, including some requiring ToM, especially second order beliefs.

Executive function and ToM appear to dissociate in some respects. APT, presented first, showed a more pronounced change in attention performance than in ToM performance. Some improvement in ToM tied to APT is not surprising in that we have developed a ToM treatment that requires executive function. We anticipate that our ToM training program – if presented first or presented on its own – would improve attention performance (e.g., PASAT) as well as improving Cartoon interpretation. That overlap suggests an efficient therapeutic approach and reinforces the need for empirical evaluation to document the areas of overlap and non-overlap.

A related issue that we have not addressed here concerns the separation between assessment and treatment. Repeated assessments using Cartoon Interpretation or the Paced Serial Addition Task might by themselves – with no explicit treatment – lead to improved performance. Baseline performance assessed over several sessions prior to initiation of treatment provided a reasonable basis for comparison; however, our assessments shared elements with the training programs, which makes any separation all the more striking. Other modes of assessment, such as the Reading the Mind in the Eyes test for ToM (Baron-Cohen et al., 2001) or other executive function batteries (e.g., Delis, Kaplan, & Kramer, 2001) might provide alternatives with less overlap with the training programs per se.

Finally, complete success of any treatment approach, such as outlined in this chapter, will rest on improved quality of life in addition to improved test performance.

Note

1 Both authors contributed equally to the writing of this chapter.

Further reading

Di Tella, M., Ardito, R. B., Dutto, F., & Adenzato, M. (2020). On the (lack of) association between theory of mind and executive functions: A study in a non-clinical adult sample. *Scientific Reports, 10*(1), 1–9.

Ruitenberg, M. F., Santens, P., & Notebaert, W. (2020). Cognitive and affective theory of mind in healthy aging. *Experimental Aging Research, 46*(5), 382–395.

Yi, Z., Zhao, P., Zhang, H., Shi, Y., Shi, H., Zhong, J., & Pan, P. (2020). Theory of mind in Alzheimer's disease and amnestic mild cognitive impairment: A meta-analysis. *Neurological Sciences, 41*(5), 1027–1039.

References

Balaban, N., Biran, M., & Sacher, Y. (2019). Theory of mind and referring expressions after traumatic Brain Injury. *Aphasiology, 33*(11), 1319–1347. https://doi.org/10.1080/02687038.2019.1637812.

Balaban, N., Friedmann, N., & Ziv, M. (2016). Theory of mind impairment after right-hemisphere damage. *Aphasiology, 30*(12), 1399–1423. https://doi.org/10.1080/02687038.2015.1137275.

Barlow, D., Nock, M., & Herson, M. (2009). *Single case experimental designs: Strategies for studying behavior for change* (3rd ed.). London: Pearson.

Baron-Cohen, S., Leslie, A. M., & Frith, U. (1985). Does the autistic child have a "theory of mind"? *Journal of Cognition, 21*(1), 3746.

Baron-Cohen, S., Wheelwright, S., Hill, J., Raste, Y., & Plumb, I. (2001). The "reading the mind in the eyes" test revised version: A study with normal adults, and adults with Asperger syndrome or high-functioning autism. *Journal of Child Psychology and Psychiatry, and Allied Disciplines, 42*(2), 241–251.

Beeson, P. M., & Robey, R. R. (2006). Evaluating single subject treatment research: Lessons from the aphasia literature. *Neuropsychological Review, 16*, 161169.

Bibby, H., & McDonald, S. (2005). Theory of mind after traumatic brain injury. *Neuropsychologia, 43*(1), 99–114.

Blake, M. L., Frymark, T., & Venedictov, R. (2013). An evidence-based systematic review on communication treatments for individuals with right hemisphere brain damage. *American Journal of Speech-Language Pathology, 22*(1), 146–160. https://doi.org/10.1044/1058-0360(2012/12-0021).

Borckardt, J. J., Nash, M. R., Murphy, M. D., Moore, M., Shaw, D., & O'Neil, P. (2008). Clinical practice as natural laboratory for psychotherapy research: A guide to case based timeseries analysis. *Journal of American Psychologist, 63*(2), 7793.

Brownell, H., Lundgren, K., Cayer-Meade, C., Milione, J., Katz, D., & Kearns, K. (2013). Treatment of metaphor interpretation subsequent to traumatic brain injury. *Journal of Head Trauma Rehabilitation, 28*(6), 446–452.

Cassel, A., McDonald, S., Kelly, M., & Togher, L. (2016). Learning from the minds of others: A review of social cognition treatments and their relevance to traumatic brain injury, Neuropsychological. *Rehabilitation, 29*(1), 22–25. Retrieved from https://doi-org.libproxy.uncg.edu/10.1080/09602011.2016.1257435.

Cicerone, K., Levin, H., Malec, J., Stuss, D., & Whyte, J. (2006). Cognitive rehabilitation interventions for executive function: Moving from bench to bedside inpatients with traumatic brain injury. *Journal of Cognitive Neuroscience, 18*(7), 1212–1222.

Clark, H. H., & Marshall, C. (1981). Definite reference and mutual knowledge. In A. K. Joshi, B. L. Webber, & I. A. Sag (Eds.), *Elements of discourse understanding* (pp. 10–63). Cambridge: Cambridge University Press.

Delis, D. C., Kaplan, E., & Kramer, J. H. (2001). *Delis-Kaplan executive function system (D-KEFS).* San Antonio, TX: The Psychological Corporation.

Dennett, D. (1978). Beliefs about beliefs. *Behavioral and Brain Sciences, 1*(4), 568–570.

Dodell-Feder, D., Lincoln, S. H., Coulson, J. P., & Hooker, C. I. (2013). Using fiction to assess mental state understanding: A new task for assessing theory of mind in adults. *PLOS ONE, 8*(11), e81279. https://doi.org/10.1371/journal.pone.0081279.

Faul, M., Xu, L., Wald, M. M., & Coronado, V. G. (2010). *Traumatic brain injury in the United States: Emergency department visits, hospitalizations, and deaths.* Atlanta, GA: Centers for Disease Control and Prevention, National Center for Injury Prevention and Control. http://www.cdc.gov/traumaticbraininjury/statistics.html.

Grice, H. P. (1975). The logic of conversation. In P. Cole, & J. L. Morgan. (Eds.), *Syntax and Semantics, Vol. 3: Speech acts* (pp. 41–58). New York: Seminar Press.

Gronwall, D. M. (1977). Paced auditory serial-addition task: A measure of recovery from concussion. *Perceptual and Motor Skills, 44*(2), 367–373. https://doi.org/10.2466/pms.1977.44.2.367.

Happé, F., Brownell, H., & Winner, E. (1999). Acquired "theory of mind" impairments following stroke. *Cognition, 70*(3), 211–240.

Larson, G. (2003). *The complete far side 1980–1994.* Kansas City, MO: Andrews McMeel Publishing Inc.

Leslie, A. M. (1987). Pretense and representation: The origins of "theory of mind". *Psychological Review, 94*(4), 412–426.

Lundgren, K., & Brownell, H. (2011). Theory of mind training following acquired brain damage. In J. Guendouzi, F. Loncke, & M. J. Williams (Eds.), *Handbook of psycholinguistics & cognitive processing: Perspectives in communication disorders* (pp. 579–602). London: Psychology Press.

Lundgren, K., & Brownell, H. (2015). Selective training in theory of mind in traumatic brain injury: A series of single subject treatment studies. *Open Behavioral Science Journal, 9*, 1–11.

Lundgren, K., Brownell, H., Cayer-Meade, C., Milione, J., & Kearns, K. (2011). Treating metaphor comprehension deficits subsequent to right hemisphere brain damage: Preliminary results. *Aphasiology, 25*(4), 456–475.

Lundgren, K., Brownell, H., Cayer-Meade, C., & Spitzer, J. (2007a). Theory of mind training following right hemisphere brain damage. Poster presentation at the annual convention of the American Speech-Language Hearing Association, Boston, MA.

Lundgren, K., Brownell, H., Cayer-Meade, C., & Spitzer, J. (2007b). Training theory of mind following right hemisphere damage: A pilot study. *Journal of Brain and Language, 103*(1–2), 209–210.

Niemann, H., Ruff, R. M., & Baser, C. A. (1990). Computer-assisted attention retraining in head-injured individuals: A controlled efficacy study of an outpatient program. *Journal of Consulting and Clinical Psychology, 58*(6), 811–817. https://doi.org/10.1037/0022-006X.58.6.811.

Parks, N., & Ingles, J. L. (2001). Effectiveness of attention rehabilitation after an acquired brain injury: A metaanalysis. *Journal of Neuropsychology, 15*, 199.

Premack, D., & Woodruff, G. (1978). Does the chimpanzee have a theory of mind? *Behavioral and Brain Sciences, 1*(4), 515–526.

Qualls, C. E., Bliwise, N. G., & Stringer, A. Y. (2000). Short forms of Benton judgment of line orientation test: Development and psychometric properties. *Archives of Clinical Neuropsychology, 15*(2), 159–163.

Robey, R. R., Schultz, M. C., Crawford, A. B., & Sinner, C. A. (1999). Single subject clinical outcome research: Design, data, effect sizes, and analyses. *Aphasiology, 13*(6), 445–473.

Saxe, R., & Kanwisher, N. (2003). People thinking about people: The role of the temporo-parietal junction in "theory of mind". *NeuroImage, 19*(4), 1835–1842.

Saxe, R., Schulz, L. E., & Jiang, Y. V. (2006). Reading minds versus following rules: Dissociating theory of mind from executive control in the brain. *Society for Neuroscience, 1*(34), 284298.

Schneider, D., Lam, R., Bayliss, A. R., & Dux, P. E. (2012). Cognitive load disrupts implicit theory-of-mind processing. *Psychological Science*, *23*, 843–847.

Shamay-Tsoory, S. G., Tomer, R., Berger, B. D., & Aharon-Peretz, J. (2005). Impaired affective 'theory of mind' is associated with right ventromedial prefrontal damage. *Cognitive and Behavioral Neurology*, *18*(1), 55–67.

Sohlberg, M. M., & Mateer, C. A. (1987). Effectiveness of an attention training program. *Journal of Clinical and Experimental Neuropsychology*, *9*(2), 117–130.

Sohlberg, M. M., & Mateer, C. A. (2011). *Attention process training III*. Youngsville, NC: Lash & Associates.

Stuss, D., Gallup, G., & Alexander, M. (2001). The frontal lobes are necessary for "theory of mind". *Annual Review of Psychology*, *53*, 401433.

Tombaugh, T. N. (2006). A comprehensive review of the paced auditory serial addition test (PASAT). *Archives of Clinical Neuropsychology*, *21*(1), 5376.

Tompkins, C. A., Scharp, V. L., Fassbinder, W., Meigh, K. M., & Armstrong, E. M. (2008). A different story on "theory of mind" deficit in adults with right hemisphere brain damage. *Aphasiology*, *22*(1), 4261.

Van Overwalle, F., & Vandekerckhove, M. (2013). Implicit and explicit social mentalizing: Dual processes driven by a shared neural network. *Frontiers in Human Neuroscience*, 7(560). https://doi.org/10.3389/fnhum.2013.00560.

Vass, E., Fekete, Z., Simon, V., & Simon, L. (2018). Interventions for the treatment of theory of mind deficits in schizophrenia: Systematic literature review. *Psychiatry Research*, *267*, 37–47.

Wellman, H. M., Baron-Cohen, S., Caswell, R., Gomez, J. C., Swettenham, J., Toyer, E., & Lagattuta, K. (2002). Thought-bubbles help children with autism acquire an alternative to a theory of mind. *Autism*, *6*(4), 343–363.

Zaitchik, D. (1990). When representations conflict with reality: The preschooler's problem with false beliefs and "false" photographs. *Cognition*, *35*(1), 41–68. https://doi.org/10.1016/0010-0277(90)90036-j.

29

BREAKDOWN OF SEMANTICS IN APHASIA AND DEMENTIA

A role for attention?

John Shelley-Tremblay

Introduction

In Chapter 10 of this volume, we reviewed the semantic memory system and suggested that an understanding of semantic memory may help us to understand the nature of language breakdown in several disorders that involve difficulties with communication. In this chapter, I address two of the most diagnosed disorders of adulthood, aphasia, and Alzheimer's dementia (AD), and examine how problems with semantic memory may be contributing to clinical communication problems. I try to provide support for the hypothesis that what is going on in both disorders may be partially explained not only by problems with the representation of semantic information but also by problems with the allocation of attention to the concepts.

I begin with a brief presentation of a center-surround model (CSM) to account for the attentional selection of semantic concepts, followed by some evidence about the nature of the language disturbance in aphasia, and whether or not it can be classified as semantic. I then discuss how the CSM may be used to explain aphasic language behavior. Since the publication of the first edition of the book, several important studies have emerged to reinforce the functional importance of the CSM and attentional modulation of semantic access in general. I have added some of the studies from my lab, as well as included a new discussion of internally directed attention and working memory. Following the review of the issues in aphasia, we will continue with a discussion on the nature of the semantic deficit in AD. We end by reviewing some event-related potential studies of AD and propose that these results can also be partially explained by the action of an attentional center-surround mechanism.

An attentional center-surround model

Dagenbach and Carr (1994) proposed a model where individuals would facilitate access to word meanings in semantic memory by directing their attention selectively to different parts of their spreading activation network. The attentional center-surround theory draws on the work of Hubel and Weisel (1962) on the structure and function of visual interneurons. In summary, it is established that the action of one visual interneuron inhibits that of its neighbors that fall along a sort of inhibitory border (surround). At the cytoarchitectural level, this border seems to be comprised of microcolumns of like-functioning neurons. These functional groups are structured to amplify the summed activity of their own group and dampen the activity of neighboring groups. Those neurons falling within the center of the structural group and the edge of its surround may

DOI: 10.4324/9781003204213-33

not be inhibited, or even mildly facilitated, while those neurons slightly farther away, but falling on the border of this surround, may be dampened. Neurons beyond the center-surround field should not be directly affected but may be indirectly affected by the action of a mutually connected interneuron.

Dagenbach, Carr, and Wilhelmsen (1989) first proposed a CSM as a possible mechanism to explain unexpected results in a masked behavioral semantic priming paradigm. Subjects were required to make lexical decisions to targets following masked primes, and their performance varied as a function of the threshold setting task used. In the key condition, participants performed a semantic similarity judgment task in the threshold setting phase, which lead to related words being responded to less quickly than words from an unrelated baseline condition. This finding lead Carr and Dagenbach (1990) to replicate and extend these findings using both semantic and repetition priming in the same task. In the first phase of this study, subjects made either detection or semantic similarity judgments under the assumption that the latter would encourage subjects to continue to use primarily semantic information to complete the lexical decision task in phase two. The prediction was that when subjects encountered a masked prime it would produce relatively little activation, and they would subsequently focus their attention on the prime. This attentional allocation would take the form of increased activation for the weak prime, in conjunction with a decrement in activation for associated words (CSM). Results indicated that subjects in the semantic decision condition showed facilitation for responses to repeats and inhibition for semantic associates. I shall attempt to present a case that this type of mechanism may play a role in the language problems seen in aphasia and AD.

Since the time of the first edition of this book, much research in this area has been completed, and the notion of directing attention to internal representations has been more fully explored. Generally, while selective attention has been thought to deal with the selection of a subset of possible external stimuli for further processing, the notion of directed attention has come to refer to the allocation of attentional resources to internal representations. This work has become an important part of the discussion around working memory and also the concept of the default mode network (DMN) within cognitive neuroscience. The seminal worker in working memory, Baddeley (2010) defines working memory as "the system or systems that are assumed to be necessary to keep things in mind while performing complex tasks such as reasoning, comprehension, and learning." Critical to the operation of working memory is the central executive, part of the system that directed the operations of other aspects of working memory. Critical to this review, Cowan (2005) suggested that the central executive serves to determine the focus of an internal, attentional spotlight on relevant aspects of long-term memory. This notion is illustrated in Figure 29.1.

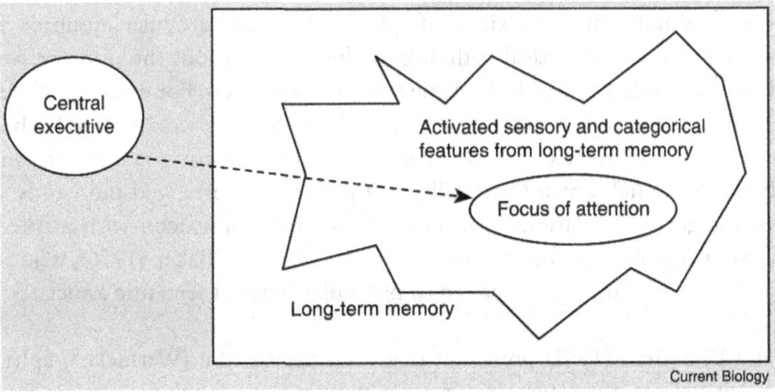

Figure 29.1. Diagrammatic representation of the role of the central executive in focusing attention in long term memory. From Cowan (2005).

Within cognitive neuroscience, the DMN has become an increasingly important concept, with numerous studies showing that alternations to the DMN are associated with dementia and other disorders that affect communication (Badhwar et al., 2017). The DMN. As described by pioneering researcher Marcus Raichle "consists of discrete, bilateral and symmetrical cortical areas, in the medial and lateral parietal, medial prefrontal, and medial and lateral temporal cortices of the human, nonhuman primate, cat, and rodent brains" (Raichle, 2015). The default mode network reliably decreases its activity when compared with activity during relaxed non-task states. It is the network of connected brain regions that are active when individuals are engaged in self-directed cognition about their own thoughts and memories. Badhwar and colleagues performed a meta-analysis with 34 studies and 1363 participants that found consistent alterations in the connectivity of the DMN, over and above alterations of other brain networks.

Aphasia

Many individuals suffering from brain damage can be classified as aphasic. A common symptom associated with many subtypes of aphasia is semantic paraphasia and related paralexias. There exists some debate about the nature of this semantic deficit, with some researchers arguing for a qualitative difference in aphasic semantic processing (Zurif et al., 1974) that manifests itself as a disorganization of the structure of the semantic store (Goodglass & Baker, 1976). The other position views the semantic difficulties exhibited by aphasics as quantitatively different from people without aphasia (Chenery et al., 1990; Milberg & Blumstein, 1981).

Blumstein, Milberg, and Shrier (1982) performed a study using a variety of aphasic patients with naming and comprehension deficits ranging from moderate to severe, as assessed by performance on the Token Test, and multiple confrontation naming tasks. However, these same patients showed evidence of semantic priming for semantic level relation judgments, regardless of the level of severity of their naming deficits. These authors interpreted this striking dissociation of explicit and implicit processes as evidence that the lexicon of even profound aphasics is intact, but that conscious access to that lexicon is impaired. Other studies were conducted (Zurif et al., 1974) that were designed to measure the intactness of aphasics semantic lexicon. Wernicke's and Broca's aphasics and normal controls were presented with triplets of words and the task of grouping them according to "what goes best together." The words varied along multiple semantic dimensions, including human-nonhuman, male-female, and so on. The individuals without the disorder and Broca's aphasics clustered according to category or functional relationship. Wernicke's aphasics showed no systematic pattern of grouping. These results were taken as evidence that the structure of the lexicon is significantly affected in Wernicke's aphasics.

In a related experiment, Fromkin (unpublished) used a hierarchical grouping technique to test the degree of cohesion in the lexicon of aphasics. For this particular group of patients with language disorders due to subcortical pathology, individuals without the disorder were found to place related words together in much the same way across subjects. For example, if presented with the triplet "husband, chair, wife," individuals without the disorder would place husband and wife together over 85% of the time, and move chair to join the category of furniture and its associates. Aphasics showed much greater variability in the way they arranged the words, often ignoring traditional category boundaries, confirming the notion of a lexicon with marked differences from normal. Similar conclusions were drawn by Goodglass and Baker (1976), who required that aphasics judge whether a target word paired to particular types of semantic associates were related to each other.

Milberg and Blumstein (1981) point out that even though the (Wernicke's) aphasics demonstrated significant deficits, there may be alternate explanations for their poor performance. One such explanation is that these subjects have an intact lexicon, but that they cannot consciously access that lexicon to the degree that individuals without the disorder can. In addition, all of the above tasks required the overt classification of words into overtly demarcated lexical categories. A failure to complete this kind of task along normal parameters could reflect the altered operation of classification mechanisms, or of any number of metalinguistic processes.

Chenery et al. (1990) sought to replicate and extend these results by carrying out further behavioral semantic priming studies. Their studies classified aphasics as low comprehension (LC) or high comprehension (HC) based on their performance above or below 50% on the Neurosensory Center Comprehensive Examination for Aphasics (NCCEA). These subjects were matched with normal and nonaphasic brain injured controls. The subjects were required to complete the RT task to targets preceded by nonwords, real word unrelated primes, real word functionally associated primes, and real word superordinate categorically related primes. They were required to listen to pairs of words and make a lexical decision about the target. In a secondary task, the subjects were required to judge the pictures of the target stimuli according to their relatedness to real word targets from the lexical decision stimulus set. Subjects were also asked to name the target during this phase of the experiment.

The results of this experiment were complex: (1) All brain damaged patients showed slowed reaction times compared to individuals without the disorder; (2) marked differences appeared in the ability of LC aphasics to perform accurate semantic judgments, as compared to normal and HC controls; (3) normal and HC controls showed normal semantic facilitation of RT, regardless of accuracy rate of their responses; but (4) LC aphasics showed a pattern of results in their association judgments contingent upon their ability to name the targets, but performed equivalently (even slightly better than nonaphasic brain damaged controls) to HC aphasics. In particular, LCs showed no difficulty with one task that HC and individuals without the disorder did have trouble with. When asked to respond to stimuli that seemed to be related by means of a super-ordinate category, LC subjects showed no slowing in reaction, while individuals without the disorder did. This suggests LC subjects, who did not have access to the normal judgment mechanisms, were left with simple association mediated by spreading activation (Meyer & Schvaneveldt, 1971).

It appears that LC aphasics can make relatedness judgments, but that they may use different, more simplified strategies than individuals without the disorder and less impaired aphasics. Chenery et al. (1990) explain that LC aphasics "base their relatedness decisions on a global comparison of perceived referential similarity." For example, a response linking "chair" to "knife" or "fence" to "sheep" would tend to suggest a global comparison of referential similarity rather than a conscious, critical evaluation of shared features. Luria explains this phenomenon by hypothesizing that when effected by a lesion the cerebral cortex has its inhibitory mechanisms disrupted, and therefore has trouble distinguishing important connections from less important connections, and therefore that a more relevant feature will fail to override irrelevant or more abstract features.

Relationship to the center-surround model (CSM)

Chiarello (1985) proposed a model of left (LH) and right hemisphere (RH) language function that ascribes different levels of automaticity and control in lexical access to each hemisphere. Specifically, she showed that priming based on phonological relatedness was equal between the hemispheres, but that priming was greater for categorically and associatively related words in the LH, and orthographically similar words produced greater priming in the RH. This suggests significantly different approaches to lexical access between hemispheres. It may be that the differences seen in aphasic relationship judgment tasks, and similarly, in semantic paraphasias, are due to the continued functioning of automatic processes in intact RH structures. Some of the representational lexicon may indeed be intact in aphasics, but the processes available for the inspection and manipulation of that lexicon are largely those found in normal RH language operation.

Recently, researchers have begun to propose mechanisms for how the left hemisphere uses attention to achieve selective activation and inhibition of the lexicon (Barnhardt et al., 1996;

Burgess & Simpson, 1988). It may be that anomias due to competition between related targets, and accompanying paraphasia can best be ascribed to the failure of an attentional inhibition mechanism found primarily in the left hemisphere, in the case of language. Building on the model of the attentional center-surround mechanism of Dagenbach and Carr (1994) described above, Barnhardt et al. (1996) sought to directly test the prediction that synonyms would be facilitated while associated would be inhibited for weakly represented words. After learning a list of rare words to criterion (50% recall), subjects performed a lexical decision task with the newly learned rare words as primes. When targets were weakly associatively related to the primes lexical decisions were speeded only for correctly recalled words. But following synonyms of the rare word responses were speeded regardless of their being remembered or not remembered. They interpreted this finding to support a model in which very closely related words have a facilitatory relationship, due to their proximity in semantic space. On the other hand, those words that are weakly associated are inhibited so as to better differentiate them from the weakly associated concept. Unrelated words would fall beyond the edge of this "surround" mechanism, and hence would be unaffected.

This is particularly relevant to the current review in that Chenery et al. (1990) suggest that aphasics may base their semantic decisions more heavily on postlexical information, because normal, controlled lexical strategies are less available. If this is true, then perhaps other disorders involving a disruption of language will evidence a relatively normal semantic network but show evidence of a reliance on postlexical processes as a means of compensatory mechanism. It is proposed next that at least the earlier stages of AD provide an example of such a situation, and that the operation of the CSM mechanism has been the source of some of the disparate results obtained thus far.

In the last few years, research from our laboratory, as well as others, has provided direct support for the operation of an attentional CSM in the brain. Deacon, Shelley-Tremblay, & Ritter (2013) performed an experiment to explicitly test the hypothesis that the CSM would operate differently in the left and right cerebral hemispheres. In this study low levels of activation were created by having subjects learn the meanings of novel, real but very rare English words to a recall criterion of 50%. Participants who attained this approximate criterion level of performance were subsequently included in a semantic priming task, during which ERPs were recorded. Primes were the newly learned rare words, and targets were either synonyms, non-synonymously related words, or unrelated words. All stimuli were presented to the RVF/LH (right visual field/left hemisphere) or the LVF/RH (left visual field/right hemisphere). Under RVF/LH stimulation the newly learned word primes produced facilitation on N400 for synonym targets, and inhibition for related targets. No differences were observed under LVF/RH stimulation. The LH thus, supports a CSM, whereby a synonym in the center of attention, focused on the newly learned word, is facilitated, whereas a related word in the surround is inhibited. The data are consistent with the notion that semantic memory is subserved by a spreading activation system in the LH. Also consistent with our view, there was no evidence of spreading activation in the RH. These authors speculate that the adult right hemisphere may require more learning than the LH in order to demonstrate evidence of meaning acquisition.

A more recent ERP study from our laboratory also supports the idea of a CSM in operation for attentional selection in semantic processing, but not for newly learned words (Shelley-Tremblay et al., 2019). This study reports the results of two neurophysiological experiments using a forced-choice recognition task built from the stimuli of the Word Memory Test and Medical Symptom Validity Test as well as a new linguistically informed stimulus set. Participant volunteers were instructed either to do their best or to feign cognitive impairment consistent with a mild traumatic brain injury while their brain activity was monitored using event-related potentials (ERP). Experiment 1 varied instructions across individuals, whereas Experiment 2 varied instructions within individuals. The target brain component was a positive deflection indicating stimulus recognition that occurs approximately 300 ms after exposure to a stimulus (i.e., the P300). Multimodal comparison (P300 amplitude to behavioral accuracy) allowed the detection of feigned cognitive

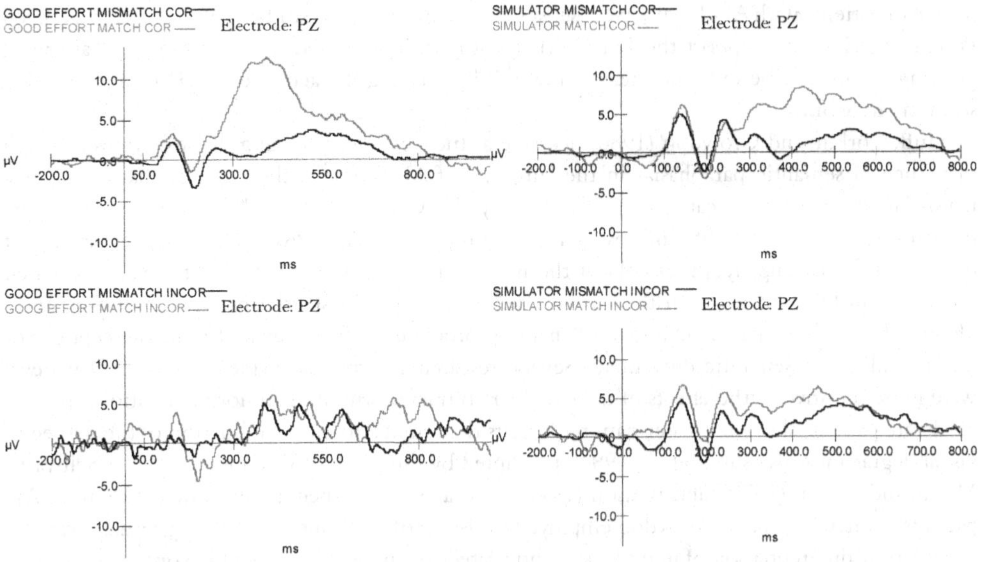

Figure 29.2 Grand average waveforms for P3 for Malingering and Full Effort groups, showing the effects of behavioral response accuracy. Shelley-Tremblay, J. F., Eyer, J. C., & Hill, B. D. (2019). A Laboratory Word Memory Test Analogue Differentiates Intentional Feigning from True Responding Using the P300 Event-Related Potential. *Brain Sciences*, 9(5), 109. https://doi.org/10.3390/brainsci9050109. Reprinted by permission of the authors.

impairment. Results indicate that, for correct responses, P300s were equivalent for the simulated malingering and good effort conditions. However, for incorrect responses, feigned impairment produced reliable but significantly reduced P300 amplitudes.

Germain to the CSM, we found that when participants directed attention to concepts that they were specifically trying to get incorrect on the behavioral task, their reduced behavioral accuracy was accompanied by a reduction in P300 amplitude. This can be seen by comparing the top graph on the left in Figure 29.2 with the top graph on the right. This finding was replicated in a second experiment that presented the stimuli in a within-subjects manner and controlled for true forgetting. We interpret this finding as evidence of attention dependent inhibition of semantic activation. The CSM in this case would act to reduce competition between the actually correct item and the new incorrect response that participants need to make in order to successfully malinger.

Alzheimer's dementia (AD)

It is well agreed upon that a high percentage of dementia patients suffer from a decline in language that appears to be correlated with the severity of their impairment in memory and cognitive functioning (Bayles & Tomoeda, 1983; Heilman & Valenstein, 1993). What is unclear is the precise nature of this language impairment. In light of the prevalence and severity of AD, it is important to attempt to understand as much as possible about the nature of the language disturbance, and also to attempt to create theories that can explain how the general decline in cognitive functioning interacts with the language problems.

First, articles arguing that there is a true degradation of the semantic lexical network itself will be discussed, followed by studies advocating for a disruption in the organization of the semantic system that may not imply any loss of content. It is suggested that the center-surround mechanism introduced earlier may reside primarily in the LH, and may contribute to the disordered performance of patients with AD. Finally, we discuss several neuroimaging studies utilizing Event-Related Potentials (ERPs) to support the LH CSM hypothesis. It is argued that the disparate pattern of priming results may be explained reasonably well by positing the action of a CSM on a degraded semantic network.

Huff, Corkin, and Growdon (1986) describe a study of object naming that examines the high incidence of semantic paraphasias in the language of AD. These authors report that of the five major language function categories measured by the Western Aphasia Battery, naming was the most severely impaired ability in those persons with probable AD (PAD). The study reportedly set out to test competing hypothesis about the nature of the naming deficit: (1) the naming deficit reflects an inability to establish the correct "set" in a naming task (the proper category is never identified, or cannot be maintained); (2) naming problems reflect impaired visual perception; or (3) an underlying semantic decrement. Several researchers provided evidence that PAD patients were more sensitive to the effects of degraded, or abstracted stimuli than normal controls, and that moderate patients showed greater naming deficits than mild patients as a function of the degree of visual degradation (Kirshner et al., 1984). Prompted by the work of Warrington (1975), Schwartz, Marin, and Saffran (1979), and Benson (1979), who all showed specific semantic problems in AD patients, Huff, Corkin and Growdon employed measures of confrontation naming, visual form discrimination, differentiation of items by semantic category, and lexical-semantic word retrieval tasks.

Using the Battig and Montague (1969) norms, the authors prepared a list of common words and their frequent associates, as well as a group of line drawings depicting the associates, for example: corn, bus, drill, and pants. In the first experiment, subjects with PAD performed dramatically worse on a word fluency test with category names as prompts (52.6 for individuals without the disorder, 23.9 for PAD). When the authors used form discrimination scores as the covariant, and naming ability as the dependant variable, differences in naming ability were highly significant. The authors suggest that this is strong evidence that impaired confrontation naming is independent of any visual processing decline. In a second experiment, the authors provided evidence that while AD patients were able to reject incorrect category designations on a category recognition test, they were impaired in rejecting incorrect names from within the same category. This was accomplished by using the same stimuli in two separate tasks. First, subjects were shown an item (in picture, and later in word form) and asked if it was a kind of "X," like a vegetable, vehicle, tool, or clothing. Then subjects were shown the same items as stimuli, but asked, "Is this called an 'X'?" where X was either the correct name or a foil from the same category.

Several aspects are remarkable in this study, the first of which is that subjects' results on a category fluency task were the same regardless of dementia severity. Many authors have made the point that, similarly to aphasia, the semantic difficulties associated with dementia seem to show distinctive patterns based on severity (Nicholas et al., 1996). Second, in contrast to Huff et al. (1986), they showed that subjects' difficulty with naming at the moderate stages of AD and beyond may be exacerbated by, if not largely due to, failure to get a clean perceptual activation of concepts as a result of perceptual impairment. This is particularly germane to an abstract debate such as this one, in that it reminds us to keep lower level deficits in mind at all times when trying to interpret cognitive level ones.

The previous study was not alone in finding evidence for semantic degeneration in PAD with pictorial stimuli. Margolin, Pate, and Friedrich (1996) employed a priming task with combinations of visually presented word targets and pictorial primes in the form of line drawings. The subjects experienced one of four types of trials: (1) identity, where prime and target represented the same semantic information (picture of dog-word dog); (2) semantically related, in which prime and target were exemplars from within the same category; (3) nonrelated, where prime and target were from different categories with no obvious relationship; and (4) nonsense, where the prime was a nonobject shape. As an aside, the study could be criticized for not adequately controlling possible aspects of the prime-target relationship. For example, the authors list the example of bed-dog as being "unrelated," when both often have four legs. It would perhaps be better if they referred to this category of relationship as "noncategorically related."

The results of their first experiment were partitioned according to subject type, with normal elderly, very mild PAD, and mild PAD showing some differences. First, it must be noted that these authors failed to achieve significant semantic priming in the normal and very mild PAD groups, so all of their findings must be interpreted with caution. Margolin et al. (1996) did find a significant amount of identity priming in the individuals without the disorder and very mild PAD patients, but no effect of identity priming in mild PAD. They interpreted this to signify a serious deterioration in the semantic network, even relatively early in the disease course. Specifically, when pictures were used as primes, the mild PAD subjects showed significantly slower reaction times compared to nonsense primes. These authors ask us to imagine a semantic network that has been degraded such that normal spreading activation may occur automatically (Meyer & Schvaneveldt, 1971), but inhibition is faulty.

In this conceptualization, semantically related information actually served to inhibit processing for mild PADs, possibly because the eroded category boundaries allow for multiple exemplars to become activated, but with no reliable way of determining the correct target. If this were so, then the delayed RT may reflect the use of postlexical processes to try to sharpen the distinction between concepts—a process that would normally happen automatically. It is also possible that the CSM becomes activated at inappropriate times in AD patients because words that are normally strongly represented are difficult to access or have damaged representations. If this is the case, then the identity primes that would normally produce facilitation may be treated as associates, because the degraded semantic network may result in increased semantic distances between normally close concepts. As reviewed above, concepts that fall outside of the immediate surround of the currently activated representation may be inhibited to reduce noise in the recognition process.

Their second experiment, using word-word pairs, produced initially unintuitive results. As would be expected, RTs slowed as a function of subject group, with mild PAD being the slowest. Similarly, word primes were faster than non-word across the board. However, significant priming was produced by both identical and semantically related words in the mild PAD group only, but neither type of prime was effective for individuals without the disorder and very mild PAD groups. This phenomenon, termed "hyperpriming" has been seen in tasks involving degraded stimuli.

Margolin et al. (1996) attempt to form a connection between visually degraded stimuli, and possible internal degradation of the semantic network. This idea explains how mild AD subjects could initially appear to be more "sensitive" to the relationships between words than individuals without the disorder. While responding more slowly overall, mild AD subjects may benefit from information that individuals without the disorder would not; individuals without the disorder may perceive this information but their system has already made the necessary lexical selection by the time the additional information reaches their decision mechanism. They refer to this idea as a "cognitive crutch." Alternately, it may not be a question of time-to-decision being effected directly by AD, but perhaps the threshold for decision is higher, and semantic relatedness decisions not much utilized in individuals without the disorder becomes needed in the lexical selection process of ADs.

On the other hand, a more parsimonious explanation for this effect can be seen if we interpret Margolin et al.'s (1996) results in light of Huff et al.'s (1986) finding that the quality of the perceptual information available to the AD subject is significantly degraded as their disease progresses. The blurring, addition of noise, or attention fluctuations, or reduction in contrast and luminance done experimentally by some authors (Schvaneveldt & Meyer, 1976; Stanovich & West, 1983) may happen internally in more severe AD patients. It does not follow that we must look to a detriment in the content of the patient's semantic network at all; instead, we may postulate that an intact network is receiving an inferior quality of information from perception. In summary, these authors findings are consistent with the proposition that more detailed semantic information is eroded first, thereby blurring distinctions within categories, then progressing to a pervasive difficulty that is reflected in anomia. It is not clear, as they claim, that this pattern necessarily reflects information loss within the semantic network.

Goldstein, Green, Presley, and Green (1992) performed a study consistent with the notion of a semantic processing deficit in PAD. Their patients were classified as having a verbal, visual, or global type of dementia. This subdivision is not typically observed in studies of the language of dementia, may prove to be as important as subtyping based on severity. Shuttleworth and Huber (1988) stated that:

> Attempting to average patient scores may tend to confuse rather than to clarify the nature of their naming disorder. In fact, at any given time, there may well be several possible anomic syndromes in DAT, varying over a continuum from mostly verbal to mostly visual.
>
> *(Shuttleworth & Huber, 1988, p. 309)*

This statement is compatible with the distinction cited previously by Huff et al. (1986) in which patients' difficulties with word naming tasks could be due to the poor quality of their perceptual input. Subjects were presented with a group of normed line drawings selected from the Boston Naming Task (BNT; Van Gorp et al., 1986) that were grouped according to two variables: complexity and frequency (high and low levels for both). Subjects were to name the pictures as quickly as possible.

The results of this study indicated that there was no difference in naming performance between any AD group and individuals without the disorder for high frequency words. This may be related to the findings cited earlier that mild AD patients were highly accurate at simple tasks with common English words. However, in the low frequency word condition, individuals without the disorder were significantly better at naming than all AD subtypes. These results were taken to signify the presence of a semantic deficit in AD. The authors found support for their subtyping system because their visual-type AD patients showed more visually based errors, and their semantic subtype patients showed more semantic errors, according to the Bayles and Tomoeda (1983) coding scheme. This scheme has face validity in that errors that resemble surface alexias, such as mistaking "dog" for "log" are seen as visually based, while mistaking "dog" for "cat" would be a semantic error, like that seen in deep dyslexia. In conclusion, this paper showed classic effects of frequency in naming for AD, such that low frequency words were harder to name. However, this paper is open to the criticism that no semantic content deficit is necessary to account for these findings; a lexical access problem could just as well be the culprit.

One possible explanation of PAD patients' poor language performance relates to their primary short-term memory deficit. While short-term memory is usually assessed for episodic memory, as in the Weschler Memory Scale story memory task, there may be an equivalent decline in semantic memory. One author, Kopelman (1986) explored the relationship between global memory loss and semantic decline. Subjects included normal controls, depressed patients, Korsakoff's amnesiacs, and mildly demented PAD patients. These people were told to repeat eight sentences exactly as they were read to them, with the sentences falling into four types: two semantically/syntactically normal (The team of workers built the bridge), four syntactically legal/semantically aberrant (Colorless green ideas sleep furiously), one semantically reversible, and one random word string.

Results showed that all subjects were able to recall the normal sentences without difficulty, and that all subjects experienced a drop in recall for the anomalous sentences. However, PAD subjects scored more than three times worse than individuals without the disorder and clinical controls on the semantically anomalous sentences. The explanation offered for this phenomenon is that Alzheimer's patients rely more heavily on semantic cues in the verbal environment as a way of compensating for their semantic difficulties. This is germane both to the claims of postlexical dependence cited above, as well as to the auditory ERP studies discussed below. In an analysis of error types made by all subjects, it was found that PAD patients made a large proportion of "normalizing" semantic errors, suggesting that semantic processors were functioning enough to automatically regularize semantically anomalous sentences. This performance was drastically limited by impaired verbal short-term memory. The conclusion of this author is that the presence of a semantic deficit is indicated, but that it must be viewed in interaction with the inability to maintain internal semantic mediation for any length of time.

Several studies emphasize the nature of the language deficit in AD is not in the content of the semantic network, but in its organization, or in impaired access to this network. Similarly, they point out that methodological errors may lead to erroneous conclusions. The first of these papers (Nicholas et al., 1996) investigated the nature of naming errors produced in response to Boston Naming Test stimuli using an experimental scoring system. This system divides error types into misperceptions and nonmisperceptions. The misperceptions were excluded from the analysis, and included responses like, "Some kind of bottle," for whistle, or "Needle to give a shot," for dart. This might appear to create a bias in the results right away, creating a percentage error analysis in favor of non-PAD controls. In actuality, older controls produced more errors overall (218) than mild (130) and moderate PAD (206) subjects. Similarly, blind raters judged the number of misperception errors to be greater in older controls (19) than in mild AD patients (13). Moderate AD patients did produce the most misperception errors (38).

An analysis of the remaining errors was completed in which new, blind raters with significant experience in the field of dementia rated each response according to its degree of semantic relatedness to the target. It was found that no significant differences existed between groups in the degree of semantic relatedness of their single word errors. It seems as if PAD patients, even moderate ones, are no "more wrong" than normal controls. For multiword responses, a significant effect of group was obtained, but the significantly highest group was the mild AD, not the moderate AD. In fact, Moderate PAD patients and older controls performed equivalently in this regard. This study did find significant evidence of gross naming defects, prior to semantic cuing, in AD subjects, but the further analysis of these errors is incompatible with a semantic deterioration hypothesis. The authors suggest that much of the evidence showing that a specific semantic deficit exists in AD may be an artifact of the dichotomous nature of the testing tasks imposed by researchers.

Particularly relevant to this question is the research report of Bayles, Tomoeda, and Rein (1996) who state that their results failed to confirm a performance pattern consistent with semantic memory loss theory. Their study exposed subjects (PAD and matched controls) to sentences of six or nine syllables that were meaningful, improbable, or meaningless. For all subjects, meaningless nine syllable sentences were significantly more difficult to remember correctly. For mild PAD subjects, nine syllable improbable phrases were more difficult than nine syllable meaningful and six syllable improbable phrases. The results were similar for moderate AD patients. In general, the effect of stimulus meaningfulness did not diminish as a function of disease severity, as would be the case if a pure semantic loss theory were true. It is argued that semantic information is not lost, but that for mild and moderate PAD patients it becomes difficult to work with this information, and to make fine grained distinctions between semantic exemplars. This inability to discriminate is consistent with the working hypothesis of this review that AD involves the abnormal action of a CSM that would ordinarily function to aid in fine comparisons by boosting signal to noise ratios for semantic decisions.

Grober, Buschke, Kawas, and Fuld (1985) explored the loss of semantic attributes that is said to occur in dementia. These authors also view the deterioration in language ability that accompanies dementia as being due to a problem with semantic organization more than of a loss of semantic organization. They performed three experiments attempting to demonstrate that under certain conditions, the semantic content of their concepts was relatively well preserved. The first study assessed the extent to which attributes have been eroded from common words like "airplane" and "car."

In selecting this kind of task, Grober et al. (1985) make an assumption that may not be well founded, namely that one can assess the intactness of a concept's representation by examining the number of appropriate associates that the subject judges to be related to it. This technique may be susceptible to the intrusion of nonsemantic attributes, such as mere frequency of association, as well as post semantic processes, such as attentional mediation. This problem is addressed somewhat in their second and third experiments.

Experiment one asked subjects to complete a checklist that contained words that were closely related to, or foils to, a common English word. Subjects were normal controls, those with MID, PAD, normal pressure hydrocephalus, or dementia of a mixed etiology. Normal subjects were 98% accurate at identifying the words that had been previously determined to be highly related to the target. Remarkably, the demented subjects were 95% accurate on the same task. It appears as if even moderately demented subjects (as assessed by the Blessed Mental Status Test) knew what words "go with" another common English word, at this basic level. In experiment two, subjects were presented a target word and a dichotomous forced choice task with a related word and a foil. Again, there was no significant difference between individuals without the disorder and subjects with dementia. This surprising lack of deficit can be contrasted with the results of experiment three. Experiment three provided subjects with a list of words related to a target by various degrees and had them rank order these words according to degree of relation. Here, persons with dementia had great difficulty.

In experiments one and two, demented subjects were equally as likely to miss a highly related word as they were to miss a distant associate. Combined with experiment three, these results suggest that a significant amount of semantic information (if not 95%) is intact in the patient group, but that it is difficult for the subjects to differentiate its relative importance. Grober et al. (1985) cite the work of Smith and Medin (1981) as a framework to interpret these results. Smith and Medin describe semantic networks in terms of weights on the links between concepts, such that a normal semantic network would contain a high value for the link between "dog" and "cat," but a lower weight for "dog" and "dish." This type of theory is also compatible with parallel distributed processing models of cognition, which have the advantage of a structure that is analogous to actual neural structures. It may be that if the neurochemical milieu of the cortex is compromised by plaques and abnormal transmitter levels, this would appear as an equalizing of the strengths of associations.

As an analogy, imagine an ice cube tray with different amounts of water in each compartment. This tray becomes old and cracked from freezing and warming, and develops cracks in its structure, thereby permitting the gradual flow of water from section to section. If this analogy is extended, it would follow that structural changes would result in changes in semantic informational content (water level changes). This may be helpful in reconciling the dichotomy that exists between the "structure" and "content" theorists, in that what begins as a structural problem directly effects content. It is important not to allow ourselves to slip backward to the 1950s and view human memory as a "warehouse," but instead to realize that information concepts are represented by distinctive patterns of neurochemical activity.

Much evidence has been accumulated both for and against a semantic loss theory of language deterioration in AD. One way to reconcile these accounts is to posit that semantic information is actually not lost but appears as if it is lost on many of the classic tests of confrontation naming, and other explicit measures. In addition to overt responses, ERPs may offer converging evidence about the functioning of semantic processes in AD, and allow us to make some guesses about the underlying neural substrates that may accompany the language deficits.

Event-related potentials (ERPS) in the study of Alzheimer's disease

ERPs reflect the action of populations of synchronously firing neurons that are continuously recorded, and then averaged according to the occurrence of time-locked stimuli. One ERP, the N400, has been shown to reliably covary with the magnitude of semantic discrepancy between a target word and its preceding prime (Holcomb, 1993; see Kutas & Van Petten, 1994 for a review; Otten et al., 1993). The amplitude of the N400 decreases with word frequency, repetition, orthographic, phonological, and most commonly, with semantic priming (Ganis et al., 1996). The N400 may be particularly well-suited to probe the nature of the language deficit in AD because it can provide evidence for intact semantic processing, if it exists, even in patients who may have difficulty with an overt response. The N400 has also been shown to be strongly correlated with paper-and-pencil measures of semantic knowledge, such as the Dementia Rating Scale (Ford et al., 2001). In the case of AD patients, who are often confused and significantly slowed during task administration, it may be a more sensitive tool than RT for demonstrating a differential response to primed and unprimed targets.

Only a handful of studies thus far have employed the N400 in a semantic priming task with an AD population (Castañeda et al., 1997; Ford et al., 2001; Hamberger et al., 1995; Revonsuo et al., 1998; Schwartz et al., 1996). Of these studies, some have reported reduced or non-existent N400 priming, while others have reported normal priming (Ford et al., 2001; Hamberger et al., 1995; Schwartz et al., 1996). While all these studies used AD patients who were mild to moderate in disease severity, and long SOAs (1000 msec or more), many other factors differ among them. While some use auditorily presented category names as primes, others use pictures, and still others use words. I propose that the large discrepancy in the results of these studies may best be explained by differences in materials, specifically the semantic distance between the prime and target and the amount of context provided in single stimulus versus sentence priming paradigms.

Hamberger et al. (1995) presented AD patients and normal elderly controls with sentences that had either congruent or incongruent final words in a variation of the first N400 studies performed by Kutas and Hillyard (1980). They found that while the controls showed evidence of reduced efficiency of semantic processing in the form of smaller and later N400 priming effects, the AD group, surprisingly showed no evidence of a smaller N400 effect than younger adults. The N400 response (not the effect produced by subtracting primed from unprimed waves) for unprimed words was larger for AD patients than age-matched controls, which may indicate that in the absence of facilitating context, AD patients have greater difficulty in accessing the word's meaning. The presence of significant priming, coupled with the long SOA, could suggest the action of the type of "crutch" mechanism discussed above in behavioral studies.

To my knowledge, the only other studies to report significant N400 priming in AD patients were both reported by Ford et al. (1996, 2001), and Schwartz et al. (1996). Ford et al. (1996) used similar sentences to Hamberger et al. (1995) as primes, but presented them in the auditory modality in an attempt to reduce the confounding influence of education level and reading ability that may have influenced the above results. They found that the N400 priming effect was significantly smaller for AD patients than for elderly controls, but that it was still significant in a pair-wise comparison for the AD group. An inspection of their waves reveals that the amplitude of this effect is about half of that seen in elderly controls, and about one-quarter of the amplitude of young adults' N400 effect.

Interestingly, these authors also reported that when all subjects were required to engage in a phoneme monitoring task that was designed to draw their attention away from actively processing the meaning of the task, their N400 amplitudes did not decrease. This would seem to indicate that even AD patients can perform automatic semantic analysis on sentence level stimuli, or perhaps only lexical analysis on each item in the sentence without concomitant integration. Unfortunately, the phoneme task may not have imposed a very high attentional load on the subjects, and so the common criticism of attention switching between tasks raised in Holender's (1986) criticism of automatic semantic processing studies may be leveled against this study as well, and leaves the implications of this finding unclear.

The next study to test AD patients using the N400 was Schwartz et al. (1996) who used auditorily presented category names as primes, and visually presented words that were judged to be either related or unrelated to these categories as targets. The category names were either superordinate (living, non-living), ordinate (animal, musical instrument, etc.), or subordinate (land animals, wind instruments, etc.). In addition to demonstrating N400 priming in AD patients, this study had the goal of showing that N400 priming effect amplitude would be sensitive to the degree of category constraint imposed by the level of the category name. Behavioral studies had indicated a deficit in lower level category priming for AD patients with relatively normal superordinate level priming. While the category level manipulation was for the most part successful, with N400 amplitude inversely related to specificity, AD patients did not show significant N400 priming at any level. This study can be criticized for failing to report, and most likely to control for the associative strength of the primes and targets adequately. This may be important, because the lower level category primes may not have effectively limited the set size for semantic search, but may have produced smaller N400 effects simply because they were less associated to the targets.

Castañeda et al. (1997) used pictures of common objects and animals as stimuli, with related primes defined as pictures belonging to the same category, and unrelated primes being from different categories. The subjects performed a category discrimination task. As in the previous study, the level of association was not strictly controlled for. These authors also found no significant N400 priming but performed an additional comparison to illuminate the nature of their N400 effect. AD patients had the same N400 response to congruent trials as individuals without the disorder, but the N400 for incongruent trials was significantly more positive. Two explanations are offered for this result, one that supposes that the N400 is an indicator of lexical level activation (Deacon et al., 2004; Kutas & Hillyard, 1984) and a second that supposes that it indexes postlexical processes (Hagoort et al., 1996; Halgren et al., 1990). Because the preponderance of evidence to date argues for the first interpretation, we will discuss this option more thoroughly (Deacon & Shelley-Tremblay, 2000).

Castañeda et al. (1997) suggest that this finding tells us that less priming is produced by incongruent stimuli, "since the amount of negativity should be inversely related to the amount of contextual preactivation." A normal congruent response combined with a diminished incongruent response again could suggest that while abnormal activation often occurs, subjects are able to benefit enough from the presence of congruent information (priming) to effectively over-come some of the processing deficit. This should not be possible if the semantic representations were truly impaired. Instead, a degradation of the associative links may occur that results in a shifting of the semantic space. This is consistent with Castañeda et al.'s (1997) comment that AD is known as a "neocortical disconnection syndrome," in which the associative network is deteriorated perhaps due to the accumulation of neurofibrillary plaques and tangles.

Revonsuo et al. (1998) reported greatly diminished N400 responses for AD patients compared to controls in a spoken sentence priming paradigm. However, they included an analysis of another ERP component, the phonological mismatch negativity, which is purported to be a measure of early lexical selection. For this component, peaking at about 300 msec, AD patients showed normal responses. Analyses of congruent and incongruent words were also carried out separately in this study and indicated that while congruous responses were equivalent between the mild AD patients and elderly controls, the incongruent responses were greatly reduced. Revonsuo et al. suggest that their study, which uses spoken sentences as well, supports the position of a relatively well-preserved lexicon.

The most recent study to test the effects of priming on N400 in AD is Ford et al. (2001). Unlike Revonsuo et al. (1998) and Castañeda et al. (1997), they reported significant N400 priming effects for AD patients. Their stimuli deserve special notice, as they are a (serendipitously) critical test of a CSM account of semantic priming in AD. While most of the ERP studies cited here used stimuli with varying degrees of associative strength and found reduced or eliminated N400 effects in AD, these authors defined their congruent condition as a picture prime, followed a word that named the picture. This is effectively a synonym. Their incongruent condition was defined simply as a word, from the same category that did not name the picture. Common words that are categorically related are likely to share at least some features, and will often be associatively related. Thus, this study provides an approximate test of the Barnhardt et al. (1996) behavioral study described above that used synonyms and associates. As in Barnhardt et al. (1996), the present study showed facilitation for synonyms, and a lack of priming for associates.

Ford et al. (2001) offer that their results are evidence of spared semantic knowledge in AD, and I tend to agree. To this could be added the idea that under conditions where individuals have difficulty accessing the semantic representation, then a normally adaptive signal-to-noise enhancement mechanism may serve to interfere with normal processing. Further studies should be conducted to test for the action of an inhibitory CSM using ERPs in both normal and AD populations. Preliminary data from my own study suggests that such a mechanism is in effect, and that it is localized to the LH. If such a mechanism were operating in AD, then it could help to understand the seemingly discordant body of research.

An obvious problem for this hypothesis is the finding of normal priming in the studies using auditory and visual sentences as primes. For these studies, the CSM may activate, but its effects are reduced by the build-up of evidence from the sentence. To say that the N400 is sensitive to the accumulation of the rich sources of evidence in a sentence does not necessitate that it is indexing a postlexical integrative process. Instead, as suggested by Deacon (personal communication), the semantic information gleaned from each word in the sentence may act to reset the level of activation in the target word's representation before its meaning is processed. Thus, the AD patient may benefit greatly from context, because they must in order to approach normal performance to any degree, but still battle against a normally beneficial center-surround mechanism.

Summary of clinical evidence

We have reviewed evidence that a CSM may be at work in both aphasia, and AD. In aphasia, the CSM that normally facilitates word recognition and subsequent naming may go awry when confronted with a damaged LH. The preserved priming seen in some studies of aphasics was suggested to be due in part to the intact functioning of the RH that, when unchecked by the LH, may contribute to semantic paraphasias. In AD, it has been suggested that priming should be found when (1) there is a high degree of semantic support, in the form of sentence context; and/or (2) when the prime and target are synonymous, and thus cannot activate the CSM. What remains to be discussed is the final topic outlined in the introduction; namely, how can we conceptualize the format of the semantic system in a way that is compatible with evidence from the study of the functional anatomy and physiology of the brain? If we are to posit the action of a general cognitive mechanism, such as the CSM, in modulating semantic processing in AD, then we must at least attempt to specify in what format the information is likely to be stored in cortex.

Further reading

Bayles, K., Kim, E., Azuma, T., Chapman, S., Cleary, S., Hopper, T., et al. (2005). Developing evidence-based practice guidelines for speech-language pathologists serving individuals with Alzheimer's dementia. *Journal of Medical Speech-Language Pathology*, *13*(4), xiii–xxv.

Bayles, K., & Tomoeda, C. (2007). *Cognitive-communication disorders of dementia*. San Diego, CA: Plural Publishing.

Mathalon, D., Roach, B., & Ford, J. (2010). Automatic semantic priming abnormalities in schizophrenia. *International Journal of Psychophysiology*, *75*(2), 157–166.

References

Baddeley, A. (2010). Working memory. *Current Biology*, *20*(4), R136–R140. https://doi.org/10.1016/j.cub.2009.12.014.

Badhwar, A., Tam, A., Dansereau, C., Orban, P., Hoffstaedter, F., & Bellec, P. (2017). Resting-state network dysfunction in Alzheimer's disease: A systematic review and meta-analysis. *Alzheimer's and Dementia: Diagnosis, Assessment and Disease Monitoring, 8*, 73–85. https://doi.org/10.1016/j.dadm.2017.03.007.
Barnhardt, T. M., Glisky, E. L., Polster, M. R., & Elam, L. (1996). Inhibition of associates and activation of synonyms in the rare-word paradigm: Further evidence for a center–Surround mechanism. *Memory and Cognition, 24*(1), 60–69.
Battig, W. F., & Montague, W. E. (1969). Category norms of verbal items in 56 categories a replication and extension of the Connecticut category norms. *Journal of Experimental Psychology, 80*(3, Pt.2), 1–46. https://doi.org/10.1037/h0027577.
Bayles, K. A., & Tomoeda, C. K. (1983). Confrontation naming impairment in dementia. *Brain and Language, 19*(1), 98–114. https://doi.org/10.1016/0093-934X(83)90057-3.
Bayles, K. A., Tomoeda, C. K., & Rein, J. A. (1996). Phrase repetition in Alzheimer's disease: Effect of meaning and length. *Brain and Language, 54*(2), 246–261. https://doi.org/10.1006/brln.1996.0074.
Benson, D. F. (1979). *8*—Neurologic Correlates of Anomia[1]. Research for this chapter was supported by the Medical Research Service of the Veterans Administration and by Grant NS06209 from the National Institutes of Health to Boston University. In H. Whitaker & H. A. Whitaker (Eds.), *Studies in neurolinguistics* (pp. 293–328). Cambridge, MA: Academic Press. https://doi.org/10.1016/B978-0-12-746304-9.50015-X.
Blumstein, S. E., Milberg, W., & Shrier, R. (1982). Semantic processing in aphasia: Evidence from an auditory lexical decision task. *Brain and Language, 17*(2), 301–315. https://doi.org/10.1016/0093-934X(82)90023-2.
Burgess, C., & Simpson, G. B. (1988). Cerebral hemispheric mechanisms in the retrieval of ambiguous word meanings. *Brain and Language, 33*(1), 86–103. https://doi.org/10.1016/0093-934X(88)90056-9.
Carr, T. H., & Dagenbach, D. (1990). Semantic priming and repetition priming from masked words: Evidence for a center-surround attentional mechanism in perceptual recognition. *Journal of Experimental Psychology. Learning, Memory, and Cognition, 16*(2), 341–350.
Castañeda, M., Ostrosky-Solis, F., Pérez, M., Bobes, M. A., & Rangel, L. E. (1997). ERP assessment of semantic memory in Alzheimer's disease. *International Journal of Psychophysiology, 27*(3), 201–214. https://doi.org/10.1016/S0167-8760(97)00064-0.
Chenery, H. J., Ingram, J. C. L., & Murdoch, B. E. (1990). Automatic and volitional semantic processing in aphasia. *Brain and Language, 38*(2), 215–232. https://doi.org/10.1016/0093-934X(90)90112-T.
Chiarello, C. (1985). Hemisphere dynamics in lexical access: Automatic and controlled priming. *Brain and Language, 26*(1), 146–172. https://doi.org/10.1016/0093-934X(85)90034-3.
Cowan, N. (2005). *Working memory capacity*. Hove: Psychology Press. Retrieved from https://scholar.google.com/scholar_lookup?title=working%20memory%20capacity&publication_year=2005&author=n.%20cowan
Dagenbach, D., & Carr, T. H. (1994). Inhibitory processes in perceptual recognition: Evidence for a center-surround attentional mechanism. In *Inhibitory processes in attention, memory, and language* (pp. 327–357). Cambridge, MA: Academic Press.
Dagenbach, D., Carr, T. H., & Wilhelmsen, A. (1989). Task-induced strategies and near-threshold priming: Conscious influences on unconscious perception. *Journal of Memory and Language, 28*(4), 412–443.
Deacon, D., Dynowska, A., Ritter, W., & Grose-Fifer, J. (2004). Repetition and semantic priming of nonwords: Implications for theories of N400 and word recognition. *Psychophysiology, 41*(1), 60–74. https://doi.org/10.1111/1469-8986.00120.
Deacon, D., & Shelley-Tremblay, J. (2000). How automatically is meaning accessed: A review of the effects of attention on semantic processing. *Frontiers in Bioscience: A Journal and Virtual Library, 5*, E82–E94. https://doi.org/10.2741/deacon.
Deacon, D., Shelley-Tremblay, J. F., & Ritter, W. (2013). Electrophysiological evidence for the action of a center-surround mechanism on semantic processing in the left hemisphere. *Frontiers in Cognitive Science, 4*, 936. https://doi.org/10.3389/fpsyg.2013.00936.
Ford, J. M., Askari, N., Mathalon, D. H., Menon, V., Gabrieli, J. D., Tinklenberg, J. R., & Yesavage, J. (2001). Event-related brain potential evidence of spared knowledge in Alzheimer's disease. *Psychology and Aging, 16*(1), 161–176. https://doi.org/10.1037/0882-7974.16.1.161.
Ford, J. M., Woodward, S. H., Sullivan, E. V., Isaacks, B. G., Tinklenberg, J. R., Yesavage, J. A., & Roth, W. T. (1996). N400 evidence of abnormal responses to speech in Alzheimer's disease. *Electroencephalography and Clinical Neurophysiology, 99*(3), 235–246. https://doi.org/10.1016/0013-4694(96)95049-x.
Ganis, G., Kutas, M., & Sereno, M. I. (1996). The search for "common sense": An electrophysiological study of the comprehension of words and pictures in reading. *Journal of Cognitive Neuroscience, 8*(2), 89–106. https://doi.org/10.1162/jocn.1996.8.2.89.
Goldstein, F. C., Green, J., Presley, R., & Green, R. C. (1992). Dysnomia in Alzheimer's disease: An evaluation of neurobehavioral subtypes. *Brain and Language, 43*(2), 308–322. https://doi.org/10.1016/0093-934x(92)90132-x.

Goodglass, H., & Baker, E. (1976). Semantic field, naming, and auditory comprehension in aphasia. *Brain and Language*, *3*(3), 359–374. https://doi.org/10.1016/0093-934x(76)90032-8.

Grober, E., Buschke, H., Kawas, C., & Fuld, P. (1985). Impaired ranking of semantic attributes in dementia. *Brain and Language*, *26*(2), 276–286. https://doi.org/10.1016/0093-934x(85)90043-4.

Hagoort, P., Brown, C. M., & Swaab, T.Y. (1996). Lexical—Semantic event-related potential effects in patients with left hemisphere lesions and aphasia, and patients with right hemisphere lesions without aphasia. *Brain*, *119*(2), 627–649. https://doi.org/10.1093/brain/119.2.627.

Halgren, E., Scheibel, A. B., & Weschler, A. F. (1990). Insights from evoked potentials into the neuropsychological mechanisms of reading. In *Neurobiology of higher cognitive function* (pp. 103–150). New York: Guilford Press.

Hamberger, M. J., Friedman, D., Ritter, W., & Rosen, J. (1995). Event-related potential and behavioral correlates of semantic processing in Alzheimer's patients and normal controls. *Brain and Language*, *48*(1), 33–68. https://doi.org/10.1006/brln.1995.1002.

Heilman, K., & Valenstein, E. (Eds.). (1993). *Clinical neuropsychology* (3rd ed.). Oxford: Oxford University Press.

Holcomb, P. J. (1993). Semantic priming and stimulus degradation: Implications for the role of the N400 in language processing. *Psychophysiology*, *30*(1), 47–61.

Holender, D. (1986). Semantic activation without conscious identification in dichotic listening, parafoveal vision, and visual masking: A survey and appraisal. *Behavioral and Brain Sciences*, *9*(1), 1–66. https://doi.org/10.1017/S0140525X00021269.

Hubel, D. H., & Wiesel, T. N. (1962). Receptive fields, binocular interaction and functional architecture in the cat's visual cortex. *Journal of Physiology*, *160*(1), 106–154. https://doi.org/10.1113/jphysiol.1962.sp006837.

Huff, F. J., Corkin, S., & Growdon, J. H. (1986). Semantic impairment and anomia in Alzheimer's disease. *Brain and Language*, *28*(2), 235–249. https://doi.org/10.1016/0093-934x(86)90103-3.

Kirshner, H. S., Webb, W. G., & Kelly, M. P. (1984). The naming disorder of dementia. *Neuropsychologia*, *22*(1), 23–30. https://doi.org/10.1016/0028-3932(84)90004-6.

Kopelman, M. D. (1986). Recall of anomalous sentences in dementia and amnesia. *Brain and Language*, *29*(1), 154–170. https://doi.org/10.1016/0093-934x(86)90040-4.

Kutas, M., & Hillyard, S. A. (1980). Event-related brain potentials to semantically inappropriate and surprisingly large words. *Biological Psychology*, *11*(2), 99–116. https://doi.org/10.1016/0301-0511(80)90046-0.

Kutas, M., & Hillyard, S. A. (1984). Event-related brain potentials (ERPs) elicited by novel stimuli during sentence processing. *Annals of the New York Academy of Sciences*, *425*, 236–241. https://doi.org/10.1111/j.1749-6632.1984.tb23540.x.

Kutas, M., & Van Petten, C. K. (1994). Psycholinguistics electrified: Event-related brain potential investigations. In *Handbook of psycholinguistics* (pp. 83–143). Cambridge, MA: Academic Press.

Margolin, D. I., Pate, D. S., & Friedrich, F. J. (1996). Lexical priming by pictures and words in normal aging and in dementia of the Alzheimer's type. *Brain and Language*, *54*(2), 275–301. https://doi.org/10.1006/brln.1996.0076.

Meyer, D. E., & Schvaneveldt, R. W. (1971). Facilitation in recognizing pairs of words: Evidence of a dependence between retrieval operations. *Journal of Experimental Psychology*, *90*(2), 227–234. https://doi.org/10.1037/h0031564.

Milberg, W., & Blumstein, S. E. (1981). Lexical decision and aphasia: Evidence for semantic processing. *Brain and Language*, *14*(2), 371–385. https://doi.org/10.1016/0093-934x(81)90086-9.

Nicholas, M., Obler, L. K., Au, R., & Albert, M. L. (1996). On the nature of naming errors in aging and dementia: A study of semantic relatedness. *Brain and Language*, *54*(2), 184–195. https://doi.org/10.1006/brln.1996.0070.

Otten, L. J., Rugg, M. D., & Doyle, M. C. (1993). Modulation of event-related potentials by word repetition: The role of visual selective attention. *Psychophysiology*, *30*(6), 559–571. https://doi.org/10.1111/j.1469-8986.1993.tb02082.x.

Raichle, M. E. (2015). The Brain's default mode network. *Annual Review of Neuroscience*, *38*(1), 433–447. https://doi.org/10.1146/annurev-neuro-071013-014030.

Revonsuo, A., Portin, R., Juottonen, K., & Rinne, J. O. (1998). Semantic processing of spoken words in Alzheimer's disease: An electrophysiological study. *Journal of Cognitive Neuroscience*, *10*(3), 408–420. https://doi.org/10.1162/089892998562726.

Schvaneveldt, R. W., & Meyer, D. E. (1976). Lexical ambiguity, semantic context, and visual word recognition. *Journal of Experimental Psychology Human Perception and Performance*, *2*(2), 243–256. https://doi.org/10.1037//0096-1523.2.2.243.

Schwartz, M. F., Marin, O. S., & Saffran, E. M. (1979). Dissociations of language function in dementia: A case study. *Brain and Language*, 7(3), 277–306. https://doi.org/10.1016/0093-934x(79)90024-5.

Schwartz, T. J., Kutas, M., Butters, N., Paulsen, J. S., & Salmon, D. P. (1996). Electrophysiological insights into the nature of the semantic deficit in Alzheimer's disease. *Neuropsychologia, 34*(8), 827–841. https://doi.org/10.1016/0028-3932(95)00164-6.

Shelley-Tremblay, J. F., Eyer, J. C., & Hill, B. D. (2019). A laboratory word memory Test analogue differentiates intentional feigning from true responding using the P300 event-related potential. *Brain Sciences, 9*(5), 109. https://doi.org/10.3390/brainsci9050109.

Shuttleworth, E. C., & Huber, S. J. (1988). A longitudinal study of the naming disorder of dementia of the Alzheimer type. *Neuropsychiatry, Neuropsychology, and Behavioral Neurology, 1*(4), 267–282.

Smith, E. E., & Medin, D. L. (1981). *Categories and concepts*. Cambridge, MA: Harvard University Press.

Stanovich, K. E., & West, R. F. (1983). On priming by a sentence context. *Journal of Experimental Psychology: General, 112*(1), 1–36. https://doi.org/10.1037//0096-3445.112.1.1.

Van Gorp, W. G., Satz, P., Kiersch, M. E., & Henry, R. (1986). Normative data on the Boston Naming Test for a group of normal older adults. *Journal of Clinical and Experimental Neuropsychology, 8*(6), 702–705. https://doi.org/10.1080/01688638608405189.

Warrington, E. K. (1975). The selective impairment of semantic memory. *Quarterly Journal of Experimental Psychology, 27*(4), 635–657. https://doi.org/10.1080/14640747508400525.

Zurif, E. B., Caramazza, A., Myerson, R., & Galvin, J. (1974). Semantic feature representations for normal and aphasic language. *Brain and Language, 1*(2), 167–187.

30

NEUROLINGUISTIC AND NEUROCOGNITIVE CONSIDERATIONS OF LANGUAGE ORGANIZATION AND PROCESSING IN MULTILINGUAL INDIVIDUALS

José G. Centeno

Introduction

As the world steadily ages, an anticipated increase in aging-related cardiovascular complications, including strokes, is estimated to translate into a markedly higher prevalence of post-stroke disabilities in older populations, including language impairments or aphasia (Dickey et al., 2010). Bilingual and multilingual individuals (speakers of two or more languages, respectively) will be prominently represented in geriatric aphasia caseloads across the world as the migration-driven growth in multiethnic populations continues to expand language coexistence globally (Centeno et al., 2020). While there are about 7,151 languages spoken in a world scenario of 195 recognized countries (Eberhard et al., 2022; World Atlas, 2022), language diversity in many world regions has exponentially increased from the continuous increase in international migration (International Organization for Migration, 2019). The expanding numbers of bilingual and multilingual older adults with post-stroke aphasia in neurorehabilitation services worldwide may exhibit diverse patterns of language impairment. They may show the same extent of impairment in both languages after the brain insult (parallel recovery pattern) or a variety of language restitution profiles in which there is uneven recovery of the two languages (nonparallel or differential recovery patterns) (Kuzmina et al., 2019; Lerman et al., 2020; Paradis, 2004).

Efforts to explicate the neurological underpinnings of multilingual aphasia heterogeneity has generated valuable grounds to illuminate neurolinguistic (brain-language) and neurocognitive (brain-cognition) connections in the multilingual brain. These theoretical claims have relied on evidence from unimpaired and clinical multilingual speakers that links language representation (organization) and processing (operations and interactions) in the multilingual brain with language-cognition interconnections in individual bilingual development and skills (Centeno, 2007a; Del Maschio & Abutalebi, 2019; Kuzmina et al., 2019; Peñaloza & Kiran, 2019). While research initially aimed to elucidate whether the bilingual brain is organized differently from the monolingual brain, investigations gradually shifted their focus to explore whether neural organization for

DOI: 10.4324/9781003204213-34

the first (L1) language is similar to or contrasts with that for the second (L2) language, whether some important factors in bilingual development, such as age of L2 acquisition and L2 proficiency, have an effect on neural distribution, and the extent typical expressive demands in bilingual speakers (i.e., language mixing, selection, and translation) interconnect multilingualism, cognition, and neural substrates in the multilingual brain (Claussenius-Kalman et al., 2021; DeLuca et al., 2020; Goral et al., 2002; Mooijman et al., 2022).

In this chapter, we will provide an overview of the experimental trajectory in the research to address the preceding queries and highlight the merits, limitations, and trends in the reported evidence on the interconnections among language, cognition, and brain that impact language representation and processing in the multilingual brain. Throughout our discussion, the terms bilingual and multilingual will be used interchangeably as the multilingual post-stroke population with aphasia includes bilingual and multilingual speakers.

We start with important information on multilingualism relevant to the understanding of the studies and theoretical constructs discussed in the chapter and follow with a summary of investigations that have generated valuable evidential and theoretical foundations to explain cerebral language organization and processing in multiple language users. We will end with future directions in this research and its possible clinical implications.

Acquisitional, communicative, and cognitive factors in neurolinguistic and neurocognitive research with multilingual speakers

Language representation and processing in multilingual speakers, be it bilingual or multilingual learners, represent complex individual trajectories of language exposure, communication contexts, and cognitive engagement that, shaped by personal life circumstances and learning aptitudes, impact brain function and structure (Centeno, 2007a, b; Claussenius-Kalman et al., 2021; DeLuca et al., 2020; López et al., 2021; Luk & Rothman, 2022). Contemporary neurolinguistic and neurocognitive approaches to multilingualism call for a broad intersectional perspective that intertwines personal psycholinguistic expertise with the social and communicative ecosystem of individual multilingual learners to drive neural language organization and processing in the multilingual brain (Claussenius-Kalman et al., 2021; López et al., 2021).

Bilingual acquisition and linguistic proficiency are highly variable personal processes. Multiple terms have been proposed to describe the numerous bilingual learning contexts associated with the considerable heterogeneity in dual-language abilities among bilingual speakers (see Austin, Blume, & Sánchez, 2015; Centeno, 2007a). In general, bilingual communication environments and their learners may be classified as simultaneous or sequential (successive). Simultaneous bilinguals refer to young language learners regularly exposed to two languages since a very early age whereas sequential bilinguals are introduced to L2 later in childhood often when they start school onwards (Centeno, 2007a; Kuzmina et al., 2019). In both acquisitional contexts, mastery in each language and engagement of supporting cognitive operations depend on individual communication demands, personal social histories, and language learning aptitudes throughout life. While individual communication environments drive exposure and practice in L1 and L2 and recruitment of executive functions (e.g. attention, selection, inhibition, etc.) along the oral-literate-metalinguistic continuum of language experiences (Bialystok, 2001; Bialystok & Barac, 2013; DeLuca et al., 2020), each bilingual learner's sociocultural and educational history (e.g., acculturation, socioeconomic contexts, and schooling) and personal attributes (e.g., motivation, language learning capacity) shape neurocognitive engagement in very personal experience-based directions (Bialystok & Barac, 2013; Centeno, 2007a, b; Claussenius-Kalman et al., 2021; DeLuca et al., 2020; López et al., 2021).

Age of acquisition additionally has been implicated in bilingual development and linguistic mastery. Maturational age-related constraints in bilingual development were initially described as a time-restricted critical period for language development that lasted from birth to puberty, reflecting progressive lateralization of cerebral language sites (see Centeno, 2007a; Li, 2013, for review). However, the evidence for child and adult L2 learners suggest a more flexible maturational situation. While most research suggests that younger learners have better results than older learners, it also shows less rigid time-windows for L2 acquisition that may extend beyond puberty. Some postpubertal L2 learners may show L2 native-like performance in several linguistic areas, such as grammaticality judgment and pronunciation (Johnson & Newport, 1989; Yavaş, 1996). Age-related acquisitional restrictions may thus be viewed as a gradual decrease in cerebral plasticity resulting in separate sensitive periods or multiple critical periods for different linguistic skills (Johnson & Newport, 1989; Li, 2013).

Expressive demands in bilingual communication similarly have cognitive implications. Multiple language users routinely have to monitor their communication contexts in order to inhibit and/or activate one or several of their languages and language-specific resources for appropriate language retrieval and choice during conversation. Particularly, cognitive accounts, grounded in the recruitment of executive functions (i.e., monitoring, attention, inhibition, and selection), have been proposed to explain how translation, language mixing, or switching (using both languages in the same utterance either as a lexical item [mixing] or a longer syntactic structure [switching]), and language selection may have individual neural implications based on each multilingual speaker's communicative history (Ansaldo & Marcotte, 2007; Claussenius-Kalman et al., 2021; Dash et al., 2020; Del Maschio & Abutalebi, 2019; DeLuca et al., 2020; Green, 2005; Paradis, 2004).

Hence, understanding the interconnections among language, cognition, and brain participating in language organization and processing in multilingual speakers requires knowledge about the complex interactions in linguistic experiences, communication contexts, age of acquisition, and cognitive demands for each language as shaped by each individual bilingual learner's life trajectory. Given the different language modalities (i.e., reading, listening, writing, and speaking), the different linguistic levels (i.e., vocabulary, sentence comprehension and production, etc.), and the different contexts of language use (i.e., formal [academic/literary] vs. informal [social/conversational]), etc.), linguistic processing and outcomes in each language would depend on the extent of input and practice each bilingual person has had in each language in the preceding domains (modality, skill, and context) throughout life (Centeno, 2007a, b; Claussenius-Kalman et al., 2021; DeLuca et al, 2020; López et al., 2021).

Neurological bases of language representation and processing in multilingual speakers

Understanding the neural sites and processes participating in language lateralization (specific hemisphere) and localization (specific hemispheric site) in the bilingual brain has been possible through the insights provided by the symptomatology of aphasia cases and experimental results from laterality studies, electro-cortical stimulation investigations, and neuroimaging research. Exhaustive reviews of the available evidence and theoretical proposals have been published (e.g., Abutalebi et al., 2005; Hull & Vaid, 2005; Goral et al., 2002; Paradis, 2004; Vaid, 2018). In this section, we provide an overview of the evolution of this research and summarize important clinical and experimental evidence to highlight merits, limitations, and trends in the reported data.

Interest in the study of brain-language relationships dates back to the mid-18th century. At that time, phrenologists, such as Gall and Sperzheim, claimed that human moral, intellectual, and spiritual faculties were stored in discrete brain organs, whose individual sizes reflected the extent of activity in the organ and, in turn, the size of the skull area just above the organ. Speech abilities, according to phrenologists, were in the frontal lobe, just above the eye socket (Code, 2022). Next, Broca's and Wernicke's careful analysis of aphasic symptoms paved the way to view language abilities and complex thinking as being associated with specific brain convolutions. Specifically, Broca identified the inferior frontal convolution as the area responsible to articulate language. Wernicke suggested that the posterior part of the first temporal gyrus was the site for the sensory image of words or language comprehension. Wernicke additionally provided a theoretical framework consisting of motor and sensory speech areas, interconnected by fibers, to account for many aphasic symptoms (see Code, 2022; Ijalba et al., 2004, for historical discussion).

The multilingual European context in which these early discussions on brain-language relationships were taking place soon provided the clinical cases that stimulated thinking about language localization in the bilingual and multilingual brain. Reacting to claims suggesting separate cerebral areas for the languages known by a bilingual, Albert Pitres (as cited in Abutalebi et al., 2005; Ijalba et al., 2004) proposed that it would be very unlikely for lesions to affect all of the proposed independent cerebral centers (sensory centers [for auditory and visual images] and motor centers [for graphic and phonetic images]) for each language. Rather, an initial disruption after the stroke would affect all of the language centers followed by a gradual recovery of both comprehension and expression in the most familiar language (known as Pitres' principle to language restitution).

In the following sections, we turn to the clinical and experimental evidence that has shaped the ongoing discussion on language localization and processing in the brain of multiple language users.

Clinical evidence

Aphasia cases of bilingual and multilingual speakers have provided symptomatology to generate accounts on the possible neuroanatomical sites and processing determinants for language localization in bilingual individuals. As mentioned earlier, post-stroke aphasia profiles include diverse patterns of language impairment that encompass parallel and differential recovery patterns (Kuzmina et al., 2019). Such clinical variability in language restitution prompted multiple explanatory claims.

Although parallel language restitution has been interpreted in terms of damage in overlapping processing sites for both L1 and L2 (Peñaloza & Kiran, 2019), several earlier proposals attempted to account for the differential recovery of a stronger post-stroke language. These proposals included the language most familiar to the patient at the time of the stroke (Pitres' principle), discussed above; the language first acquired because it involves the oldest memories, most resistant to impairment (Ribot's principle), the language associated with the strongest affective experiences (Minkowski's account), and the language most useful to the patient at the time of the cerebral insult (Goldstein's account) (Paradis, 2004). Very often, however, clinical literature on multilingual aphasia reports single cases of unusual symptomatology (Goral et al., 2002; Kuzmina et al., 2019). Meta-analytic data suggest that the languages known by a multilingual speaker premorbidly are recovered proportionally to their pre-stroke proficiency. While early high-proficiency bilingual speakers (bilingually proficient individuals who acquired their two languages since a young age) show comparable post-stroke performance in both languages, late high-L1 proficiency bilingual speakers (individuals who acquired their L2 after seven years of age) exhibit better post-stroke L1 performance relative to their L2 (Kuzmina et al., 2019).

Crossed aphasia in multilingual speakers (aphasia resulting from damage in the right hemisphere, the non-dominant hemisphere for language) has similarly provided observational grounds for speculation. Prompted by a tendency to report unusual bilingual aphasia patients in the literature, as mentioned above, some early cases suggested a possible higher incidence of crossed aphasia in multiple language users hence encouraging the claim of right-sided language processing in these speakers. However, the overwhelming occurrence of aphasia in multilingual individuals after left-sided lesions strongly supports the left hemisphere to be dominant for both languages (Goral et al., 2002).

More recently, differential language loss or recovery in bilingual persons with aphasia has been described in terms of language representations or neurocognitive operations. The representational account posits that selective language impairments reflect damage to specialized neural networks for each language which may be housed in the same or different areas of the left or right hemisphere (Vaid, 2018). Neurocognitive accounts suggest that procedural-declarative memory processes or cognitive control mechanisms are involved in nonparallel language restitution. Paradis (2004) advances the notion that language recovery in bilingual individuals with aphasia appears to depend on the possible interaction between each bilingual speaker's acquisitional context (simultaneous vs. sequential bilingualism) and its concomitant memory strategies. A first language or two simultaneously learned languages since a young age, mostly in informal communication environments, rely on implicit/procedural memory strategies, dependent on subcortical neural regions. Languages successively learned later in life, often in structured instructional contexts, rely on declarative/explicit memory strategies (emphasizing metalinguistic knowledge), housed in cortical areas. Thus, in this perspective, nonparallel recovery may reflect the neurofunctional modularity (separation) of the languages known by the multilingual speaker; the language recovered in a nonparallel pattern would reflect the interplay of acquisitional factors, procedural/declarative memory traces affected, and the extent of subcortical-cortical damage (see also Ullman, 2001). Additionally, an influential proposal in aphasia research by Green (2005) and Green and Abutalebi (2008) supports that the parallel-differential variability in aphasia symptomatology in multilingual speakers may depend on the extent of damage in the cortical-subcortical connectivity regulating the executive control mechanisms that selectively activate or inhibit the bilingual language system.

Hence, clinical evidence has provided important information on the heterogeneity and complexity in the language recovery patterns in multilingual language users with aphasia that has served to formulate theoretical accounts on the multilingual brain. Recent meta-analytic evidence of published clinical cases highlights that the interaction of age of acquisition, frequency of use, and proficiency plays an important role in post-stroke language recovery. There is comparable recovery in both L1 and L2 when both languages are learned early and used regularly in life contrary to better recovery of L1 when L2 was learned later and not used very frequently; frequency of use, particularly through education, can enhance proficiency with favorable impact on language recovery (Kuzmina et al., 2019).

Experimental data, based on the assessment of brain activity in bilingual speakers, have yielded critical complementary data on the inter- and intra-hemispheric processing sites and the possible variables impacting neural language distribution in bilingual individuals. Though there are numerous techniques to study brain-language relationships (see Abutalebi et al., 2005; Vaid, 2018), we provide an overview of frequently used methodology to study cerebral language representation and processing in multilingual individuals, particularly laterality measures and electrophysiological and neuroimaging research.

Laterality studies

Hemispheric language processing has been examined using the presentation of auditory (dichotic listening) or visual stimuli (tachitoscopic viewing). These techniques rely on the contralateral (opposite side) sensory organization of the brain. For example, auditory or visual stimuli presented to the left ear or left visual field will be processed in the right hemisphere. By assessing processing differences between stimuli presented contralaterally or ipsilaterally (same side), for example, in terms of stimulus recognition speed, researchers may gauge the extent of specific hemispheric involvement. For monolinguals, a right ear advantage (REA) or right visual field advantage (RFVA) generally are reported for verbal information (i.e., words, syllables, etc.) thus suggesting faster language recognition when linguistic items arrive in the left hemisphere auditorily or visually, respectively (Vaid, 2018).

Extensive reviews of the laterality evidence revealed no difference between L1 and L2 or between bilinguals and monolinguals for left hemispheric language localization (Goral et al., 2002; Hull & Vaid, 2005; Vaid, 2018). Some studies suggest the possibility of bilateral hemispheric representation in early simultaneous bilinguals, apparently due to semantic (meaning-based) processing compared to syntactic (form-based) processing in late, sequential bilinguals. Yet, some methodological issues, concerning language pairs examined, limited bilingualism history of the participants, linguistic level studied (e.g., words vs. sentences), and so forth, raise interpretive issues about this research (see Hull & Vaid, 2005; Vaid, 2018, for discussion). Current findings, however, overwhelmingly support the dominant role of the left hemisphere in language representation for both monolingual and bilingual persons and for both languages known by the bilingual speaker, including the possibility of bilateral involvement in early stages of bilingualism (Goral et al., 2002; Vaid, 2018).

Hence, laterality measures have shed light into interhemispheric language organization. For intrahemispheric localization and processing, electrophysiological and neuroimaging studies have yielded important evidence, as summarized next.

Electro-cortical stimulation investigations

The study of language organization in the bilingual brain was stimulated by the use of electro-cortical stimulation to map out cortical language areas in epileptic patients undergoing surgical removal of epileptogenic brain sites. This technique applies electricity to cortical language sites thus causing temporary aphasia when the electrical current briefly inhibits the stimulated area from functioning. Identification of the cerebral language regions before surgery prevents them from damage during the surgical intervention. Because the brain has no pain receptors, testing language functions under cortical stimulation can be carried out in the conscious patient once the craniotomy has exposed the target brain areas and the patient is fully awake (Lucas et al., 2004).

Ojemann and Whitaker (1978) and Rapport et al. (1983) conducted the first electro-cortical studies on bilingual and multilingual individuals, respectively. Based on naming tasks, results suggested that naming could be impaired in either language in some cortical sites, could be more impaired in one language than in the other in other areas, or could be simultaneously impaired in both languages in other areas. The regions of language disruption, however, were not the same for all the bilingual or multilingual speakers tested. Essential areas for naming in the later-acquired, less-fluent language were more dispersed than those areas in the earlier-acquired, more-fluent language. All of the naming regions detected were within the frontal and temporoparietal cortex (Ojemann, 1991; Ojemann & Whitaker, 1978).

Later cortical mapping studies further highlight the variability in language localization in bilingual persons. For example, Roux and Trémoulet (2002) investigated 12 French-speaking bilinguals of various L2 backgrounds on three different tasks (counting, naming, and reading) in each language. These patients were classified in terms of age of acquisition and proficiency as early-acquisition/high-proficiency, late-acquisition/high-proficiency, and late-acquisition/low-proficiency. The age of seven years was chosen as the cutoff date to identify a patient as early or late L2 learner. Results showed a heterogenous localization pattern with five patients having overlapping language regions (for all language tasks) and the remaining seven patients having at least one area that was language-specific and, sometimes, task-specific. In terms of age of acquisition and proficiency, results similarly differed among participants. The authors found that three out of four early bilinguals exhibited naming difficulty in one language under electrical stimulation, which suggests separate foci. Regarding proficiency level, only one patient demonstrated more cortical sites dedicated to the less fluent language. Like earlier studies, all language areas were found in the temporoparietal regions and in frontal regions of the brain.

Lucas et al. (2004) set out to examine language representation in 22 bilingual patients by assessing naming. They aimed to answer whether multiple languages are functionally separated within the brain, whether these languages are similarly organized, and whether language organization in bilingual individuals mirror that in monolingual individuals. The authors found that the most common pattern of language representation in bilingual speakers was one of discrete language-specific sites (either for L1 or L2) co-existing with shared (S) sites. However, eight patients had no S sites.

The number of essential sites for L1, L2, and S did not differ thus suggesting a similar extent of site distribution. Neither L1 or L2 proficiency scores predicted the number of L1, L2, or S regions. In terms of anatomical distribution, the L2-specific sites were located exclusively in the posterior temporal and parietal regions, whereas the L1-specific sites and S could be found throughout the mapped regions. When comparing language areas in both monolingual and bilingual brains, L1 representation was indistinguishable hence suggesting that L2 acquisition does not alter L1 organization. However, L2 sites were distributed differently from L1 sites in the bilingual brain, clustered around the receptive language areas and in significantly smaller proportions of L2 sites relative to language sites in monolinguals. This finding led the authors to argue that, once cortical regions are dedicated to L1 processing, they may inhibit the establishment of new language sites (for L2) in their vicinity.

The preceding studies advance the descriptive symptomatology reported by clinical cases and laterality studies. Specifically, there seems to be left-hemispheric representational dominance for both languages whose individual distribution may depend on age of acquisition, proficiency, and linguistic task. The evidence generated by electro-cortical research, however, is largely variable and based on the assessment of naming skills. It also is limited by the extent and site of the craniotomy. Stimulation only is applied on the surface of the exposed areas in the left hemisphere, a frequent site of epileptic foci. Therefore, we do not know about the patterns of language organization in the areas deeper in the brain, beyond the craniotomy, or in the nondominant right hemisphere (see Goral et al., 2002; Vaid, 2018, for discussion).

Evoked response potential measures

Evoked response potential (ERP) studies measure the normal electrical activity that takes place in the brain under the effect of specific and controlled sensory stimulation. In this technique, signal averaging is employed to extract stimulus-relevant ERP activity from non-stimulus related background signals. The resulting ERP, representing a summation and average of the activity of multiple neurons, allow researchers to infer the extent and timing of neuronal activation upon a presented task (Hull & Vaid, 2005). This unobtrusive technique only employs electrodes on the participant's scalp thus allowing the examination of real-time (online) brain activity while, for example, the person is engaged in a reading or listening task.

ERP measures of both semantic and syntactic processing support the role of age of L2 acquisition and proficiency in neural language organization in bilinguals. Late and fluent (high-proficiency) bilinguals and monolinguals show similar left hemispheric patterns of language organization whereas early and nonfluent (low-proficiency) bilinguals tend to be less lateralized, demonstrating more bilateral involvement, consistent with the laterality findings reported above. For example, Meuter et al. (1987) assessed the ERP (N400 effect) responses of French-English bilingual speakers to semantically congruent and incongruent sentences. A response approximately 400ms after presentation of an incongruent sentence suggests the participant has recognized the anomaly. Meuter et al. (1987) found larger ERP effects for left parietal areas in late French-English bilinguals reading semantically incongruent sentences, particularly in their L2 (English) hence supporting more L2-related brain activity. Likewise, ERP measures in late bilingual and monolingual participants detecting semantic anomalies (Weber-Fox & Neville, 2001) and late fluent and nonfluent bilinguals processing syntactic violations (Friederici et al., 2002) further supported that late, fluent L2 learners show lateralization patterns similar to those in monolingual persons. Indeed, exhaustive meta-analysis of laterality, in which fluent bilingual persons are subdivided by age of acquisition, robustly reveal that late bilinguals are more left-hemisphere dominant relative to early bilingual language users, who show more bilateral hemispheric participation overall (Hull & Vaid, 2005).

ERP evidence, however, warrants caution in view of the small data sets reported and the need for further research along different lines. Specifically, ERP data would be enhanced by examining multilingual speakers from a larger group of contrasting language pairs (i.e., inflectionally rich [Spanish] vs. inflectionally limited [English], alphabetic [Spanish] vs. ideographic scripts [Chinese], etc.) in a larger variety of semantic and syntactic tasks in the various language modalities (see also Hull & Vaid, 2005; Goral et al., 2002).

Neuroimaging research

Advances in neuroimaging techniques, particularly positron emission tomography (PET) and functional magnetic resonance imaging (fMRI) have contributed to the study of intra-hemispheric language organization in bilingual speakers (Abutalebi et al., 2005; Cargnelutti et al., 2019). These hemodynamic techniques are based on the changes in regional cerebral blood flow (rCBF) resulting from synaptic activity. As neuronal functioning increases, this physiological event results in increased metabolic rate and rCBF. Hence, both PET and fMRI allow us to capture in vivo images of brain functioning as neuronal activation, in response to the online (real-time) execution of a cognitive task, results in changes in local cerebral blood flow and concomitant metabolic activity (Dougherty et al., 2004)

Neuroimaging investigations of the multilingual brain have examined both production (e.g., word repetition and word generation) and comprehension abilities (e.g., grammatical and semantic judgment) as well as language selection and translation in bilingual speakers (see Abutalebi et al., 2005, for exhaustive review). Language imaging research assessing production areas in bilingual and multilingual individuals suggest a dominant pattern of left-sided language organization in the multilingual brain similar to that reported for monolingual persons, namely, the most brain activation occurs in the left perisylvian area, accompanied by lesser activation in some regions away from the left perisylvian area and in some regions of the right hemisphere (Abutalebi et al., 2005; Vaid, 2018). Yet, the distribution of language foci in the multilingual brain appears to primarily include overlapping language-processing sites, whose distribution may depend on certain variables, such as language proficiency, age of acquisition, and language exposure.

Regarding proficiency, early evidence from PET studies by Klein et al. (1994, 1995) suggested that late, fluent English-French bilinguals engaged very similar areas of the left frontal lobe during word repetition and word generation tasks (e.g., rhyming, synonyms, and translation) in each language. Based on a word generation activity administered to trilinguals, Yetkin et al. (1996) provided fMRI results that supported a widespread organization of the foci for the less-fluent language, actively involving the left prefrontal cortex. Hence, high proficiency may result in a tighter left-sided representational frontal area for lexical foci.

In terms of age of acquisition, Kim et al. (1997) conducted fMRI scannings of early and late bilingual speakers of different language backgrounds as they silently produced sentences in each language. In Broca's area, patterns of brain activity included common areas of activation, if the languages were learned early, and segregated areas, if L2 was learned late, at a mean age of 11.2 years for the participants. In Wernicke's area, there was minimal or no separation of foci for both early and late bilinguals. However, Chee et al. (1999) found considerable left-sided activation involving minimal differences in the fMRI readings of early and late Mandarin-English bilingual speakers of similar fluency levels in a stem-based word completion task. Likewise, in another study controlling the degree of proficiency, Illes et al. (1999) showed that high fluency may be associated with common left-hemisphere language foci independent of age of acquisition, as supported by fMRI patterns of early and late fluent English-Spanish bilinguals performing semantic judgment tasks. Substantial activation was observed in the left inferior frontal gyrus in the participants with minimal activation in homologous right-sided sites in a few participants. Thus, proficiency, rather than age, appears to be critical in the distribution of language foci (high proficiency/common sites) in the dominant left hemisphere, as supported by different bilingual groups (Mandarin-English and English-Spanish) and different tasks (word completion and semantic decision).

Environmental language exposure seems to be an additional variable. Perani et al. (2003) examined fMRI imaging in early, fluent Spanish-Catalan bilingual speakers who were dominant in either Spanish or Catalan, and who lived in a Catalan environment. Perani and colleagues found that the dominant language (which coincided with the L1 in these bilingual individuals) engaged fewer cerebral areas in a word generation task. Additionally, for speakers producing words in the language with the least daily exposure, namely, Spanish in the Catalan-dominant bilingual cohort, there was more widespread brain activation (in the left dorsolateral frontal region) when these speakers generated words in Spanish, relative to Spanish-dominant bilingual speakers generating words in Catalan, the language of the community. Hence, according to these findings, the brain engages fewer neural networks when processing the dominant language or the more frequently used language.

Imaging studies examining cerebral foci for comprehension in bilingual speakers further support the important role of proficiency in language localization. Perani et al. (1996) investigated PET activation in late, low-proficiency Italian-English bilingual participants while listening to stories in each language. Results showed minimal overlap for the two languages; for L1 (Italian), activation was concentrated in the left perisylvian regions with participation of some homologous right-sided areas, and for the low-proficient language (L2, English), activation was considerably more reduced in both left and right hemispheres, mainly involving the temporal area. In contrast, for both early and late high-proficiency bilingual participants of Spanish-Catalan and Italian-English backgrounds, respectively, Perani et al. (1998) found a different PET pattern. Both groups listened to stories in each language. The Italian-English group listened to a story in an additional unknown language (Japanese). Activation showed in similar left temporal regions for both languages in both groups and, only for the late bilinguals, in the unknown language. Activation also included some right areas for both languages in both groups.

Support to the critical role of fluency in language organization comes from studies of bilingual speakers of languages of contrasting orthographies such as English (alphabetic orthography) and Mandarin (ideographic orthography). Chee et al. (1999) examined fMRI scannings of early, high-fluency English-Mandarin bilingual speakers in a printed sentence comprehension task to assess sentence meaning. The investigators found a similar brain activation pattern for both languages involving an extensive portion of the left fronto-temporal region and, to a lesser extent, bilateral parieto-occipital areas.

Despite left-sided dominance, the preceding evidence, nonetheless, suggests the possible recruitment of the right hemisphere in language processing in cases of low L2 proficiency. Similarly, based on fMRI readings, Dehaene and colleagues (1997) found that late, low-proficiency French-English bilingual persons engaged a considerably larger portion of the left frontal area when listening to stories in L1 (French) relative to a much larger right-sided fronto-temporal participation in their less-fluent L2 (English). Interestingly, Dehaene et al.'s findings suggested that, while L1 is localized in the left frontal lobe, there was large intersubject variability for the organization of the less-fluent L2, involving both left and right frontal and temporal areas and, in some participants, an exclusive right-sided activation pattern.

In sum, the preceding findings suggest that, regardless of acquisition age, high proficiency may be associated with left-sided overlapping of L1 and L2 in the perisylvian region for both aural and written comprehension. Right-sided involvement seems to be related to low L2 proficiency. Recent meta-analytic evidence of fMRI and PET research expanded these findings by highlighting that L2 representation was wider than that associated with L1, particularly in late bilingual speakers, because L2 processing engaged a larger control network (Cargnelutti et al., 2019).

Translation and language switching and selection, two typical expressive routines in bilingual speakers, have also been examined using neuroimaging tools for their valuable insights into language representation in the bilingual brain (Ansaldo & Marcotte, 2007; Paradis, 2004). For example, Price et al. (1999) used PET to explore neural activation during word reading and word translation in late, fluent German-English bilinguals. Results showed contrasting PET patterns for both tasks. For reading, considerable activity was seen in the left Broca's area and bilateral supramarginal gyri. For translation, extensive engagement outside the typical left perisylvian language zone, including bilateral subcortical regions, was observed. The authors claim that activation differences may be related to mapping orthography to phonology (reading) and semantic processing (translation). Hernández et al. (2001) found active participation of the left dorsolateral prefrontal cortex when examining language switching in early, high-proficiency Spanish-English speakers, based on fMRI readings. Further, Rodriguez-Fornells et al.'s (2002) ERP and fMRI data suggested considerable involvement of the left anterior prefrontal region when early, high-proficiency Catalan-Spanish bilingual individuals had to inhibit either language for target language selection in a lexical access task.

The three preceding studies provide evidence on translation, language switching, and language selection that supports the participation of different neural areas for contrasting tasks (reading vs. translation) and the dominant role of the left hemisphere across linguistic tasks in both languages. Consistent with the neuroimaging studies discussed earlier, findings from these studies underscore the control requirements in situations of considerable expressive demands. Recruitment of a wide cortical-subcortical network, including regions outside the classical perisylvian language area, increase when the bilingual language system requires high control to synergize language processing and executive functions in the regulation of language production by the bilingual speaker (Centeno et al., 2022; Del Maschio & Abutalebi, 2019; Mooijman et al., 2022).

Future directions

The preceding overview provided a brief snapshot of valuable research to explicate language representation and processing in the bilingual brain that can assist in the understanding of the variability in bilingual aphasia profiles. While the evidence is far from conclusive, findings support the robust role of the language-dominant left hemisphere in bilingual speakers, particularly in its perisylvian regions, just like in monolinguals; the possible recruitment of the right hemisphere in early stages of bilingualism and in low L2 proficiency, and the high incidence of overlapping L1-L2 sites over separate sites for each language in cases of high proficiency. Acquisition age, frequency of use, and proficiency seem to interact to facilitate post-stroke recovery. Evidence on special expressive demands in bilingual speakers, particularly translation and language switching and selection, while further supporting the role of left-sided neural foci in language representation and executive function in bilingual communication, has highlighted the engagement of a wide cortico-subcortical network beyond the classical perisylvian language region in the synergized language retrieval and control required for language production by bilingual speakers.

Evidence is still emerging. Gaps in the research need to be addressed. Much research focuses on naming and the spoken modality and uses a small number of contrasting language pairs. Also, because the experienced-based linguistic and cognitive variability resulting from the personal life histories of each multilingual language user may have individual neurolinguistic and neurocognitive implications, studies must carefully acknowledge individual trajectories in premorbid bilingual acquisition, communication, and expressive abilities in the research participants. Considerable research in multilingual persons includes minimal information on the bilingualism history of the participants. Both individual and group data analyses are valuable. Knowledge of the dynamic language-cognition interactions throughout the individual lives of bilingual speakers should guide participant selection, experimental task design and administration, and data interpretation to generate robust insights on the impact of linguistic and cognitive practices on the function and structure of the bilingual brain, especially for its clinical implications. Applying neurocognitive accounts of bilingualism has shown great promise to stimulate post-stroke neural reorganization in bilingual speakers with aphasia (Ansaldo & Marcotte, 2007; Centeno et al., 2022; Dash et al.,

2020; Gray & Kiran, 2019). The exponential growth of multilingual speakers across the world warrant sound neuroscientific explications to interpret their clinical language symptomatology and create optimal experienced-based personalized aphasia intervention services (Centeno & Higby, 2022).

Further reading

Cattaneo, G., Costa, A., Gironell, A., & Calabria, M. (2020). On the specificity of bilingual language control: A study with Parkinson's disease patients. *Bilingualism: Language and Cognition, 23*(3), 570–578.

Lerman, A., Goral, M., & Obler, L. K. (2020). The complex relationship between pre-stroke and post-stroke language abilities in multilingual individuals with aphasia. *Aphasiology, 34*(11), 1319–1340.

Peñaloza, C., Barrett, K., & Kiran, S. (2020). The influence of prestroke proficiency on poststroke lexical-semantic performance in bilingual aphasia. *Aphasiology, 34*(10), 1223–1240.

References

Abutalebi, J., Cappa, S. F., & Perani, D. (2005). What can functional neuroimaging tell us about the bilingual brain. In J. F. Kroll & A. M. B. de Groot (Eds.), *Handbook of bilingualism: Psycholinguistic approaches* (pp. 497–515). Oxford: Oxford University Press.

Ansaldo, A. I., & Marcotte, K. (2007). Language switching in the context of Spanish-English bilingual aphasia. In J. G. Centeno, R. T. Anderson, & L. K. Obler (Eds.), *Communication disorders in Spanish speakers: Theoretical, research, and clinical aspects* (pp. 214–230). Clevedon, UK: Multilingual Matters.

Austin, J., Blume, M., & Sánchez, L. (2015). *Bilingualism in the Spanish-speaking world: Linguistic and cognitive perspectives*. Cambridge: Cambridge University Press.

Bialystok, E. (2001). *Bilingualism in development: Language, literacy, and cognition*. Cambridge: Cambridge University Press.

Bialystok, E., & Barac, R. (2013). Cognitive effects. In F. Grosjean & P. Li (Eds.), *The psycholinguistics of bilingualism* (pp. 145–167). West Sussex, UK: Wiley-Blackwell.

Cargnelutti, E., Tomasino, B., & Fabbron, F. (2019). Language brain representation in bilinguals with different age of appropriation and proficiency of second language: A meta-analysis of functional imaging studies. *Frontiers in Human Neuroscience, 13*, 154. https://doi.org/10.3389/fnhum.2019.00154.

Centeno, J. G. (2007a). Bilingual development and communication: Implications for clinical language studies. In J. G. Centeno, R. T. Anderson & L. K. Obler (Eds.), *Communication disorders in Spanish speakers: Theoretical, research, and clinical aspects* (pp. 46–56). Clevedon, UK: Multilingual Matters.

Centeno, J. G. (2007b). Considerations for an ethnopsycholinguistic framework for aphasia intervention with bilingual speakers. In A. Ardila & E. Ramos (Eds.), *Speech and Language disorders in bilingual adults* (pp. 195–212). New York, NY: Nova Science.

Centeno, J. G., Ghazi-Saidi, L., & Ansaldo, A. I. (2022). Aphasia management in ethnoracially diverse multilingual populations. In I. Papathanasiou & P. Coppens (Eds.), *Aphasia and related neurogenic communication disorders* (3rd ed., pp. 379–402). Jones and Bartlett Learning.

Centeno, J. G., & Higby, E. (2022). Strategizing for neuroscientifically-sound socially-responsive aphasia management in multilingual ethnogeriatric stroke services [Manuscript in preparation].

Centeno, J. G., Kiran, S., & Armstrong, E. (2020). Editorial: Aphasia management in growing multiethnic populations. *Aphasiology, 34*(11), 1314–1318. https://doi.org/10.1080/02687038.2020.1781420.

Chee, M. W., Tan, E. W., & Thiel, T. (1999). Mandarin and English single word processing studied with functional magnetic resonance imaging. *Journal of Neuroscience, 19*(8), 3050–3056. https://doi.org/10.1523/JNEUROSCI.19-08-03050.1999.

Chee, M., Caplan, D., Soon, C. S., Sriram, N., Tan, E. W., Thiel, T., & Weekes, B. (1999). Processing of visually presented sentences in Mandarin and English studied with fMRI. *Neuron, 23*(1), 127–137. https://doi.org/10.1016/S0896-6273(00)80759-X.

Claussenius-Kalman, H., Hernandez, A. E., & Li, P. (2021). Expertise, ecosystem, and emergentism: Dynamic developmental bilingualism. *Brain and Language, 222*, 105013. https://doi.org/10.1016/j.bandl.2021.105013.

Code, C. (2022). Significant landmarks in the history of aphasia and its therapy. In I. Papathanasiou & P. Coppens (Eds.), *Aphasia and related neurogenic communication disorders* (3rd ed., pp. 15–38). Burlington, MA: Jones and Bartlett Learning.

Dash, T., Masson-Trottier, M., & Ansaldo, A. I. (2020). Efficiency of attentional processes in bilingual speakers with aphasia. *Aphasiology, 34*(11), 1–25. https://doi.org/10.1080/02687038.2020.1719970.

Dehaene, S., Dupoux, E., Mehler, J., Cohen, L., Paulesu, E., Perani, D., … Le Bihan, D. (1997). Anatomical variability in the cortical representation of first and second languages. *NeuroReport, 8*(17), 3809–3815. https://doi.org/10.1097/00001756-199712010-00030.

Del Maschio, N., & Abutalebi, J. (2019). Language organization in the bilingual and multilingual brain. In J. W. Schwieter (Ed.), *The handbook of the neuroscience of multilingualism* (pp. 199–213). Chichester: John Wiley and Sons.

DeLuca, V., Segaert, K., Mazaheri, A., & Krott, A. (2020). Understanding bilingual brain function and structure changes? U bet! A unified bilingual experience trajectory model. *Journal of Neurolinguistics, 56*, 100930. https://doi.org/10.1016/j.jneuroling.2020.100930.

Dickey, L., Kagan, A., Lindsay, M. P., Fang, J., Rowland, A., & Black, S. (2010). Incidence and profile of inpatient stroke-induced aphasia in Ontario, Canada. *Archives of Physical Medicine and Rehabilitation, 91*(2), 196–202. https://doi.org/10.1016/j.apmr.2009.09.020.

Dougherty, D. D., Rauch, S. L., & Rosenbaum, J. F. (Eds.). (2004). *Essentials of neuroimaging for clinical practice*. Washington, DC: American Psychiatric Publishing.

Eberhard, D. M., Simons, G. F., & Fennig, C. D. (Eds.). (2022). *Ethnologue: Languages of the world* (25th ed.). Dallas: TX: SIL International.

Friederici, A., Steinhauer, K., & Pfeifer, E. (2002). Brain signatures of artificial language processing: Evidence challenging the critical period hypothesis. *Proceedings of the National Academy of Sciences, 99*(1), 529–534. https://doi.org/10.1073/pnas.012611199.

Goral, M., Levy, E., & Obler, L. K. (2002). Neurolinguistic aspects of bilingualism. *International Journal of Bilingualism, 6*(4), 411–440. https://doi.org/10.1177/13670069020060040301.

Gray, T., & Kiran, S. (2019). The effect of task complexity on linguistic and non-linguistic control mechanisms in bilingual aphasia. *Bilingualism: Language and Cognition, 22*(2), 266–284. https://doi.org/10.1017/S1366728917000712.

Green, D. (2005). The neurocognition of recovery patterns in bilingual aphasics. In J. F. Kroll & A. M. B. de Groot (Eds.), *Handbook of bilingualism: Psycholinguistic approaches* (pp. 516–530). Oxford: Oxford University Press.

Green, D., & Abutalebi, J. (2008). Understanding the link between bilingual aphasia and language control. *Journal of Neurolinguistics, 21*(6), 558–576. https://doi.org/10.1016/j.jneuroling.2008.01.002.

Grosjean, F. (2004). Studying bilinguals: Methodological and conceptual issues. In T. K. Bhatia & W. C. Ritchie (Eds.), *The handbook of bilingualism* (pp. 32–63). Oxford: Blackwell.

Hernández, A., Dapretto, M., Mazziotta, J., & Bookheimer, S. (2001). Language switching and language representation in Spanish-English bilinguals: An fMRI study. *Neuroimage, 14*(2), 510–520. https://doi.org/10.1006/nimg.2001.0810.

Hull, R., & Vaid, J. (2005). Clearing the cobwebs from the study of the bilingual brain: Converging evidence from laterality and electrophysiological research. In J. F. Kroll & A. M. B. de Groot (Eds.), *Handbook of bilingualism: Psycholinguistic approaches* (pp. 480–496). Oxford: Oxford University Press.

Ijalba, E., Obler, L. K., & Chengappa, S. (2004). Bilingual aphasia. In T. K. Bhatia & W. C. Ritchie (Eds.), *The handbook of bilingualism* (pp. 32–63). Oxford: Blackwell.

Illes, J., Francis, W., Desmond, J., Gabrieli, J., Glover, G., Poldrack, R., … Wagner, A. D. (1999). Convergent cortical representation of semantic processing in bilinguals. *Brain and Language, 70*(3), 347–363. https://doi.org/10.1006/brln.1999.2186.

International Organization for Migration. (2019). World migration report 2020. wmr_2020.pdf(iom.int).

Johnson, J. S., & Newport, E. L. (1989). Critical periods effects in second language learning: The influence of maturational state on the acquisition of English as a second language. *Cognitive Psychology, 21*(1), 60–99. https://doi.org/10.1016/0010-0285(89)90003-0.

Kim, K. H. S., Relkin, N. R., Lee, K. M., & Hirsch, J. (1997). Distinct cortical areas associated with native and second languages. *Nature, 388*(6638), 171–174. https://doi.org/10.1038/40623.

Klein, D., Milner, B., Zatorre, R., Meyer, E., & Evans, A. (1995). The neural substrates underlying word generation: A bilingual functional-imaging study. *Proceedings of the National Academy of Sciences of the UnitedStates of America, 92*(7), 2899–2903. https://doi.org/10.1073/pnas.92.7.2899.

Klein, D., Zatorre, R., Milner, B., Meyer, E., & Evans, A. (1994). Left putaminal activation when speaking a second language: Evidence from PET. *NeuroReport, 5*(17), 2295–2297. https://doi.org/10.1097/00001756-199411000-00022.

Kuzmina, E., Goral, M., Norvik, M., & Weekes, B. (2019). What influences language impairment in bilingual aphasia? A meta-analytic review. *Frontiers in Psychology, 10*, Article 445. https://doi.org/10.3389/fpsyg.2019.00445.

Lerman, A., Goral, M., & Obler, L. K. (2020). The complex relationship between pre-stroke and poststroke language abilities in multilingual individuals with aphasia. *Aphasiology, 34*(11), 1319–1340. https://doi.org/10.1080/02687038.2019.1673303.

Li, P. (2013). Successive language acquisition. In F. Grosjean & P. Li (Eds.), *The psycholinguistics of bilingualism* (pp. 145–167). West Sussex, UK: Wiley-Blackwell.

López, B. G., Luque, A., & Piña-Watson, B. (2021). Context, intersectionality, and resilience: Moving toward a more holistic study of bilingualism in cognitive science. *Cultural Diversity and Ethnic Minority Psychology*. https://doi.org/10.1037/cdp0000472.

Lucas, T. H., McKhann, G. M., & Ojemann, G. A. (2004). Functional separation of languages in the bilingual brain: A comparison of electrical stimulation language mapping in 25 bilingual patients and 117 monolingual control patients. *Journal of Neurologicalsurgery*, *101*(3), 449–457. https://doi.org/10.3171/jns.2004.101.3.0449.

Luk, G., & Rothman, J. (2022). Experience-based individual differences modulate language, mind, and brain outcomes in multilinguals. *Brain and Language*, *228*, 105107. https://doi.org/10.1016/j.bandl.2022.105107.

Marian, V. (2018). Bilingual research methods. In J. Altarriba & R. R. Heredia (Eds.), *An introduction to bilingualism: Principles and processes* (pp. 12–36). New York, NY: Routledge.

Meuter, R., Donald, M., & Ardal, S. (1987). A comparison of first- and second-langauge ERPs in bilinguals. *Electroencephalography and Clinical Neurophysiology*, *40*, 412–416.

Mooijman, S., Schoonen, R., Roelofs, A., & Ruiter, M. B. (2022). Executive control in bilingual aphasia: A systematic review. *Bilingualism: Language and Cognition*, *25*(1), 13–28. https://doi.org/10.1017/S136672892100047X.

Ojemann, G. A. (1991). Cortical organization of language. *Journal of Neuroscience*, *11*(8), 2281–2287. https://doi.org/10.1523/JNEUROSCI.11-08-02281.1991.

Ojemann, G. A., & Whitaker, H. (1978). The bilingual brain. *Archives of Neurology*, *35*(7), 409–412. https://doi:10.1001/archneur.1978.00500310011002.

Paradis, M. (1997). The cognitive neuropsychology of bilingualism. In A. M. B. De Groot & J. J. Kroll (Eds.), *Tutorials in bilingualism: Psyholinguistic perspectives* (pp. 331–354). Mahwah, NJ: Lawrence Erlbaum.

Paradis, M. (2004). *A neurolinguistic theory of bilingualism*. Philadelphia, PA: John Benjamins.

Peñaloza, C., & Kiran, S. (2019). Recovery and rehabilitation patterns in bilingual and multilingual aphasia. In J. W. Schwieter (Ed.), *The handbook of the neuroscience of multilingualism* (pp. 553–571). Chichester: John Wiley and Sons.

Perani, D., Abutalebi, J., Paulesu, E., Brambati, S., Scifo, P., Cappa, S. F., & Fazio, F. (2003). The role of age of acquisition and language usage in early, high-proficient bilinguals: An fMRI study during verbal fluency. *Human Brain Mapping*, *19*(3), 179–182. https://doi.org/10.1002/hbm.10110.

Perani, D., Dehaene, S., Grassi, F., Cohen, L., Cappa, S. F., Dupoux, E., … Mehler, J. (1996). Brain processing of native and foreign languages. *NeuroReport*, 7(15–17), 2439–2444. https://doi.org/10.1097/00001756-199611040-00007.

Perani, D., Paulesu, E., Sebastian Galles, N., Dupoux, E., Dehaene, S., Bettinerdi, V., Cappa, S. F., Fazio, F., & Mehler, J. (1998). The bilingual brain: Proficiency and age of acquisition of the second language. *Brain*, *121*(10), 1841–1852. https://doi.org/10.1093/brain/121.10.1841.

Price, C. J., Green, D. W., & von Studnitz, R. (1999). A functional imaging study of translation and language switching. *Brain*, *122*(12), 2221–2235. https://doi.org/10.1093/brain/122.12.2221.

Rapport, R. L., Tan, C. T., & Whitaker, H. (1983). Language function and dysfunction among Chinese- and English-speaking polyglots: Cortical stimulation, Wada testing, and clinical studies. *Brain and Language*, *18*(2), 342–366. https://doi.org/10.1016/0093-934X(83)90024-X.

Rodriguez-Fornells, A., Rotte, M., Heinze, H. J., Nősselt, T., & Münte, T. F. (2002). Brain potential and functional MRI evidence for how to handle two languages with one brain. *Nature*, *415*(6875), 1026–1029. https://doi.org/10.1038/4151026a.

Roux, F. E., & Trémoulet, M. (2002). Organization of language areas in bilingual patients: A cortical stimulation study. *Journal of Neurosurgey*, *97*(4), 857–864. https://doi.org/10.3171/jns.2002.97.4.0857.

Ullman, M. T. (2001). The neural basis of lexicon and grammar in first and second language: The declarative/procedural model. *Bilingualism: Language and Cognition*, *4*(2), 105–122. https://doi.org/10.1017/S1366728901000220.

Vaid, J. (2018). The bilingual brain revisited: What is right and what is left? In J. Altarriba & R. R. Heredia (Eds.), *An introduction to bilingualism: Principles and processes* (pp. 139–156). New York, NY: Routledge.

Weber-Fox, C., & Neville, H. J. (2001). Sensitive periods differentiate processing of open- and closed-class words: An ERP study of bilinguals. *Journal of Speech, Language, and Hearing Research*, *44*(6), 1338–1353. https://doi.org/10.1044/1092-4388(2001/104).

World Atlas. (2022). *How many countries are there in the world?* Retrieved from www.worldatlas.com.

Yavaş, M. (1996). Differences in voice onset time in early and late Spanish-English bilinguals. In J. Jensen & A. Roca (Eds.), *Spanish in contact: Issues in bilingualism* (pp. 131–141). Sommerville, MA: Cascadilla Press.

Yetkin, O., Yetzkin, F. Z., Haughton, V., & Cox, R. W. (1996). Use of functional MR to map language in multilingual volunteers. *American Journal of Neuroradiology*, 17(3), 473–477.

SECTION IV

Language and other modalities

31
GESTURES AND GROWTH POINTS IN LANGUAGE DISORDERS

David McNeill and Susan Duncan

Introduction

Gestures shed light on thinking-for-(and while)-speaking. They do this because they are components of speaking, not accompaniments but actually integral parts of it. Much evidence supports this idea, but its full implications have not always been recognized. Consider modular-style modeling of the relationship between gesture and speech, for example, De Ruiter (2000) and Kita and Özyürek (2003), based on the theory of speech production in Levelt (1989). Modular theory and its spin-offs are incompatible, we have argued, with the facts of integration of gesture into speaking (McNeill, 2000; McNeill & Duncan, 2000). Such models require a fundamental separation of speech and gesture; the "modules" exchange signals but cannot combine into a unit. The growth point (GP) hypothesis, which we describe here, is designed in contrast to explicate the integral linkage of gesture and speech in natural language production. In a GP, speaking and gesture are never separated, and do not occupy different brain processes that must in turn then be linked (cf. the brain model, below). A key insight is that speech on the one hand and gesture (or, more broadly speaking, global-imagistic thinking), on the other, jointly forming a GP, bring together semiotically opposite modes of cognition at the same moment. This opposition, and the processes that speakers undergo to resolve it, propels thought and speech forward. Semiotic contrasts are a key component in the dynamic dimension of language. It is in this mechanism that we seek insights into language disorders. We explore four situations—disfluent (agrammatic) aphasia, Down syndrome (DS), Williams syndrome (WS), and autism. Each can be seen to stem from a breakdown, interruption, or inaccessibility of a different part of the GP, and from a disturbance of the dynamic dimension of language in general. Considered together, they manifest—by interruption—aspects of the processes of thinking-for/while-speaking itself. In this chapter we do not attempt to review the field of gesture studies, the psycholinguistics of speech production, or language disorders, but we do provide a brief exposition of the GP hypothesis and spell out some implications of a new paradigm in which language and cognition are embodied (cf. Johnson, 1987) and dynamic, and show how a theory within this paradigm, the GP theory, leads to new insights into four language disorders.

The growth point

The GP is so named because it is a distillation of a growth process—an ontogenetic-like process but vastly sped up and made functional in online thinking-for-speaking. While we are not addressing language acquisition as such, we regard it as a general model of cognitive change valid across

DOI: 10.4324/9781003204213-36

many time scales. According to this framework, the GP is the initial unit of thinking-for/while-speaking (from Slobin, 1987, elaborated to include thinking online, during speech) out of which a dynamic process of utterance-level and discourse-level organization emerges. Imagery and spoken form are mutually influencing. It is not that imagery is the input to spoken form or spoken form is the input to imagery. The GP is fundamentally both. The following exposition of the GP covers essential points for the purpose of elucidating language abnormalities. More thorough presentations are in McNeill (2005), McNeill and Duncan (2000), and, with a language origins slant, in McNeill, Duncan, Cole, Gallagher, and Bertenthal (2008).

A minimal unit of imagery-language dialectic

The GP is an irreducible, "minimal unit" of imagery-language code combination. It is the smallest packet of an idea unit encompassing the unlike semiotic modes of imagery and linguistic encoding. A GP is empirically recoverable, inferred from speech-gesture synchrony and co-expressiveness. Even when the information (the "semantic content") in speech and gesture is similar, it is formed according to contrasting semiotic modes. Simultaneous unlike modes create instability. Instability fuels thinking-for-speaking as it seeks resolution (McNeill & Duncan, 2000). The result is an idea unit in which holistic imagery and discrete code are combined, and this drives thinking-for/while-speaking.

Example

The temporal and semantic synchronies represented in Figure 31.1 imply a GP built on the idea of rising interiority. We infer the simultaneous presence of the idea of ascent inside the pipe in two unlike semiotic modes. The speaker was describing a cartoon episode in which one character (a cat named Sylvester) tries to reach another character (a bird named Tweety) by climbing up inside a drain-pipe. The speaker is saying, "and he tries going up thróugh it this time," with the gesture occurring during the boldfaced portion (the illustration captures the moment when the speaker says the vowel of "thróugh"). Co-expressively with "up" her hand rose upward and co-expressively

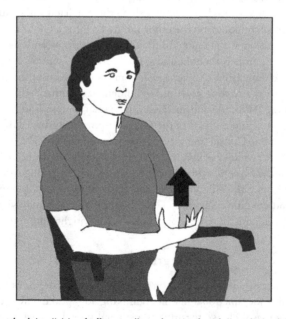

Figure 31.1 Gesture embodying "rising hollowness" synchronized with "up thróugh."

with "thróugh" her fingers spread outward to create an interior space. These took place together, and were synchronized with the entirety of "up thróugh," the linguistic package that carries the same meanings.

The GP pairs linguistic segments with a uniquely gestural way of packaging meaning—something like "rising hollowness," which does not exist as a semantic package of English at all. Speech and gesture, at the moment of their synchronization, were co-expressive, yet embodied this shared idea in contrasting semiotic modes. The very fact that there is a shared reference to the character's climbing up inside the pipe makes clear that it is being represented by the speaker simultaneously in two ways—analytic/combinatoric in speech and global/synthetic in gesture.

And context

An important point is that we can fully understand what motivates any gesture-speech combination only with reference to how a GP relates to its context of occurrence. The GP-to-context relationship is mutually constitutive. The GP is a point of differentiation from the context, what Vygotsky termed a "psychological predicate." The speaker shapes her representation of the context, or "field of oppositions," to make this differentiation possible. A robust phenomenon is that the gesture form and its timing with speech embody just those features that differentiate the psychological predicate in a context that is at least partly the speaker's own creation. In the "up through" example, interiority is newsworthy in a field of oppositions concerning Ways of Getting at Tweety By Climbing Up A Pipe; a previous description had been that it was on the outside, now it is on the inside (see McNeill, 2005, pp. 108–112).

The catchment

The effective contextual background can often be discovered by finding the catchment(s) of which a target gesture is a part. Catchments are when space, trajectory, hand shapes, and so on, recur in two or more (not necessarily consecutive) gestures. The recurring imagery embodies the discourse theme (the metaphor relates to the geophysical domain, referring to the land area—"the theme"—that drains—"the significant oppositions"—into a body of water—"the GP"). For both climbing up the outside and climbing up the inside of the pipe the same space and trajectory occurred (iconically depicting Sylvester's entrance at the bottom of the pipe)—verbally, too, the full expression, "he goes up thróugh it this time," indexes the catchment theme in that the inside ascent was a recurrent attempt. Newsworthy content appears as a modification of the catchment, relating itself to the theme while also adding new contrast. For the inside ascent the speaker's hand rose at the lower periphery, as before, but now also created the open space seen in Figure 31.1—not only a shape change but also, to the up-the-pipe theme, adding the newsworthy content that it was on the inside this time. Jointly with co-expressive "thróugh," prosodic emphasis also highlighting interiority, the gesture was part of a fresh psychological predicate in this context.

Catchments, if they are present or absent and if present how they are formed, and what restrictions if any they impose on potential discourse themes (cf. Furuyama and Sekine, 2007), are important variables that we can conceptualize systematically by applying the GP theory to the three language disorders. We are unaware of other approaches that frame these questions.

Unpacking the growth point (GP)

Unpacking is the process that creates the structures with which to stabilize the combination of unlike cognitive modes in the GP. It is "unpacking" the GP into a grammatical construction (or viable approximation thereto) that preserves the core significance of the GP while cradling it in a stable grammatical format. Achieving this often takes additional meaning formulation. The process is regulated by the speaker's linguistic intuitions—called intuitions-1 (a sense of well-formedness and contextual appropriateness of the linked semantic frame). The construction also supplies a "stop-order" for the impulse to change initiated by the imagery-linguistic code instability. In Figure 31.1, "up thróugh" is analytic: up-ness and interiority are separated and combined grammatically. The linguistic encoding has meaning because it combines meaningful parts. The synchronous gestural image embodies similar information without combining separately meaningful parts—"Sylvester as rising hollowness"; the gesture's parts are meaningful only because of the gesture as a whole. Unpacking resolves the tension of the semiotic modes. The full construction, "(he) goes up thróugh it this time," its co-expressive elements exactly synchronizing with the gesture stroke, preserves the GP, does not dim the highlighted interiority, and adds indexing of the catchment value—that it was a second ascent—which was also in the gesture.

At times, of course, unpacking fails. A construction may not be found; or one is found but its semantic pattern conflicts with the GP on some dimension; or the conflict is with the field of oppositions, the context of the GP. It is important to keep these possibilities in mind, for they appear in different language disorders. To illustrate one case, not a chronic disorder but a momentary interruption of normally fluent speech, we offer an example from a paper by Dray (Dray & McNeill, 1990)—the "nurturing" example: a speaker (having a conversation with a friend) was attempting to convey a delicately nuanced idea that a third person she was describing was given to performing nurturing acts, but these good deeds were also intrusive, cloying, and unwelcome. Initial false starts were based on the use of "nurture" as a transitive verb (she would "nurture" someone) and were repeatedly rejected as inappropriate. Ultimately the right construction was found. The field of oppositions was initially something like, Things This Woman Would Do, and "nurture" was an appropriate significant opposition. The direct object construction the speaker first attempted ("she's ... she's nu-uh") means that, roughly, the woman described has a direct transformative impact via nurturing on the recipient of her action. However, this meaning distorted the idea the speaker intended to convey—an oblique reference that separated effect from act. A slight updating of the field of oppositions to something like Otiose Things This Woman Would Do yielded the final construction, which could differentiate it appropriately with a meaning of doing something without implying transformative efficacy ("she's done this nurturing thing"). This example illustrates a subtle but far from uncommon occurrence of GP differentiation, context shaping, and unpacking going awry.

Further comments

Some additional comments to fill out the GP picture:

- First, the following question may come to mind: if gesture is "part of language," how could it and language be "semiotically unalike"? We admit a certain polysemy in the word "language." When we say gesture is part of language, we mean language in the sense of Saussure's language. When we say that gesture contrasts to language, we mean it in the sense of langue. We are analyzing parole/speaking but we believe in a way broader than this concept is usually understood (Saussure himself, in his recently discovered notes, seems to have had the aim of combining parole and langue—here we rely on Harris's (2003) interpretation).
- By "gesture" most centrally we mean a kind of semiosis that is both "global" and "synthetic." By "global" we mean that the significance of the gesture's parts (= the hands/fingers/trajec tory/space/orientation/ movement details of it) is dependent upon the meaning of the gesture as a whole. The parts do not have their own separate meanings, and the meaning of the whole is not composed out of the parts; rather, meaning moves downward, whole to parts. This is the reverse of the linguistic semiotic mode, where the meaning of the whole is composed of the parts, which, for this to work, must have their own separate meanings. By "syn-

thetic" we mean that the gesture has a meaning as a whole that may be analytically separated into different linguistic segments in the speech counterpart.

- Another contrast is that gestures (and imagery more broadly) lack so-called duality of patterning. The form of the gesture-signifier is a nonarbitrary product of the signified content (including, via metaphor, abstract "nonimagistic" meanings), so its form doesn't need or get its own level of structure (= "patterning" in the Hockett, 1960 phraseology). Speech again contrasts: it has this duality of patterning—meaning and sound are each structured by schemes at their own levels, and are paired arbitrarily.
- This has to do with the role of convention and where it intrudes. There are conventions of good-form for speech, but none for gesture (apart from the well-known emblem vocabularies in every culture; also general kinesic conventions for how much space you can use, whether you can enter the space of an interlocutor with a gesture, and the many kinds of metaphor that constrain forms in their gesture versions. These, however, are not specific gesture conventions in parallel with the sound-system conventions of speech).
- Even constructions, like "up through it," while they are macro-units, don't negate the possibility of decomposing them into separately meaningful subunits (up, through, it). Also, the meaning of "up through it," as a construction, is still something traceable to lexical atoms. The gesture, on the other hand, does not admit any decomposition, since there are no subunits with independent meanings, no repeatable significances to the outspread fingers, upward palm, and motion upward (arguably, there is upward motion and it independently means upward, but there are exceptions to this seeming transparency as well, gestures where up-down signifies the vertical dimension as a whole, and up actually means down in some cases). Significance exists only in the whole gesture. Also, we think the gesture is more a unified whole than just the combination of up and through. We have tried to convey the unification with the expression "rising hollowness" but whatever the phrase, the gesture has interiority, entity, and upward motion in one undecomposable symbolic form.
- In a GP, then, two semiotic modes, contrasting in the ways listed above, combine to embody the same underlying idea. The instability of having one idea in two "unlike" modes fuels thought and is the dynamic dimension of language viewed psycholinguistically.
- In the verbal modality, as in the manual modality, the meaning of the first part ("up" or the spread fingers) remains, as Quaeghebeur (personal communication, 2008) wrote, "alive," "present," or "active" while the second part is being produced ("thróugh" or the upward movement). There is this kind of continuation in both cases, but the explanation differs—a construction in the verbal case; a global image in the gesture case. The continuities differ as well—sequential in the linguistic form, simultaneous in the gesture. Between the two means of attaining continuation the difference comes down to whether symbolic actions are organized by syntactic patterns or by imagery.

Four language disorders

We now make use of the GP hypothesis to elucidate aspects of four forms of language disorder. The four are disfluent (agrammatic) aphasia, DS, WS, and autism. To develop our analyses, we begin by proposing the necessary aspects of a brain model.

A brain model

Based on what we currently understand of gesture-speech semiosis a neurogesture system involves both the right and left sides of the brain in a choreographed operation with the following parts (see McNeill, 2005, for supporting references). The left posterior temporal speech region of Wernicke's area supplies categorical content, not only for comprehension but for the creative production of verbal thought. This content becomes available to the right hemisphere, which seems particularly adept at creating imagery and to capture discourse content. The right hemisphere must also play a role in the creation of GPs. This is plausible since GPs depend on the differentiation of newsworthy content from context and require the simultaneous presence of linguistic categorical content and imagery, both of which seem to be activated in the right hemisphere. The frontal cortex may also play a role in constructing fields of oppositions and psychological predicates, and supply these contrasts to the right hemisphere, there to be embodied in GPs. Underlying the rhythmicity of speech "pulses" (cf. Duncan, 2006) and interactional entrainment (cf. Gill, 2007) we assume a continuous circulation of cerebellum inputs or feedback. Finally, the right hemisphere and the prefrontal cortex are almost certainly involved in metaphor. The results of processing (right hemisphere, left posterior hemisphere, frontal cortex, cerebellum) converge on the left anterior hemisphere, specifically Broca's area, and the circuits specialized there for action orchestration (cf. McNeill et al., 2008, for a brain mechanism, "Mead's Loop," to account for how GP units orchestrate/synchronize movements of the articulators, manual and vocal). Broca's area may also be the location of two other aspects of the imagery-language dialectic—the generation of further meanings in constructions and their semantic frames, and intuitions of formal completeness to provide "stop orders" to this dialectic. All of these—left, right, cerebellar, frontal—thus may be called language areas of the brain.

The language centers of the brain have classically been regarded as just two, Wernicke's and Broca's areas, but if we are on the right track in our sketch of a brain model, contextual background information must be present to activate the broader spectrum of brain regions that the model describes. Typical item-recognition and production tests, inspired by modular-type conceptions in which language is regarded as encapsulated, would not tap these other brain regions but discourse, conversation, play, work, and the exigencies of language in daily life would.

Disfluent (agrammatic) aphasia

The "verb problem" in Broca's aphasia is the tendency to omit or nominalize verbs in utterances (Miceli, Silveri, Villa, & Caramazza, 1984; Zingester & Berndt, 1990). On the assumption that verbs are the core syntactic constituents of utterances, this symptom has been studied and interpreted by some as evidence in support of a neurologically grounded grammar "module." However, depending upon discourse context, verb salience varies within-language and across languages, depending on facts about verb behavior in each language. Conceptualized in the GP framework, Broca's aphasia arises from a more or less severe disruption of the unpacking cycle, but the GP itself (formed, we hypothesize, by the uninjured right hemisphere with inputs from the prefrontal cortex and the posterior left hemisphere language area) is unimpaired. A Broca's aphasic speaker differentiates psychological predicates in reasonably constituted fields of oppositions, but is unable to unpack the GP. The following excerpt (Duncan & Pedelty, 2007, p. 271) is a person with Broca aphasia's description of Sylvester trying to reach Tweety by climbing the drainpipe and the sequel in which Tweety drops a bowling ball into it. There are only two identifiable verbs, "is" and "shows." In contrast, six noun tokens were uttered generally clearly and forcefully (Table 31.1).

The speaker performed two well-synchronized, co-expressive gestures. With speech they constituted a likely (repeated) psychological predicate:

[a- and down] [(pause) t- d- down (breath)]

(Boldface font indicates a gesture "stroke." This is the meaningful phase of a gesture. Brackets indicate the larger gesture phrase. This is the period including preparation before and retraction after the stroke.) The strokes in this instance were downward thrusts of the right hand synchronized closely with the two occurrences of the co-expressive path particle, "down," the second stammered. Figure 31.2 illustrates these downward strokes.

Table 31.1 Agrammatic aphasic's description of a cartoon event

(1) the (pause) vlk- (pause) uh (breath) bird? (pause) and c- (breath) cat
(2) (pause) and uh (breath) ss- uh (pause) she ss- (breath) (pause) apartment
(3) and uh- (pause) the (pause) uh (pause) old (pause) my (breath) ss- uh (pause) woman (pause)
(4) and uh (pause) she ss- (pause) like (pause) uh ae- f- f-fas-t (breath)
(5) cat (pause) and uh (pause) bird is-ss-ss (pause) (breath)
(6) I uh (pause)
(7) (breath) sh-sho- shows t- (pause)
(8) a- an' down (pause) t- d- down (breath)

Source: Transcription from Duncan and Pedelty (2007, p. 271).

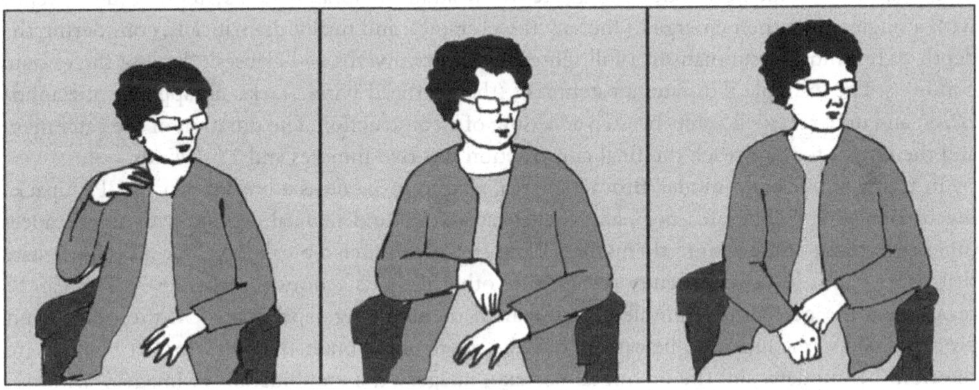

Figure 31.2 Gesture by a disfluent (agrammatic) speaker timed with (a) and (b) "an' down," and (c) "t- d- down."

In the context of the cartoon story that we, as observers, independently recognize, plus her own fragments of speech in advance of the two instantiations of the gesture, we can identify the gesture plus the synchronous particle, "down," as the single piece of newsworthy information in the excerpt. The speech–gesture pairings thus suggest an intact GP (repeated). Equally important, no verbs occur at all as the linguistic components of the GPs and the verbs that did occur were utterly non-news-worthy; one a copula coupling nothing, the other "shows" showing nothing.

This lack of participation by verbs may be no accident. Duncan and Pedelty propose that in English and some other languages (they refer to Chinese as well), "sentential main verbs are often not the information-loaded, discourse-focal utterance constituents that our usual ways of thinking about them would suggest" (Duncan & Pedelty, 2007, p. 280). The omission or nominalization of verbs in Broca's aphasic speech (whatever the role of their internal semantic complexity in causing an absence from picture-naming and other nondiscourse tasks) is also a predictable result of how GPs embody newsworthy content in the context of speaking. Verb absence would accordingly be, at best, ambiguous evidence for support of modular brain models of language.

Verb absence in Broca's discourse (as opposed to naming) can be explained by a lack of ready access to constructions. In normal speech, noninformation-laden verbs enter utterances riding on these kinds of structures. Nonetheless, agrammatic speakers can formulate and differentiate contexts to obtain GPs. Thus, our first illustration of language abnormality demonstrates a separation of GP formation and unpacking, normally two seamlessly fused (while analytically distinct) steps of utterance formation.

The lack of construction-access in Broca's aphasia, nonetheless, is far from absolute. With time and catchment support constructions can be accessed by even highly agrammatic aphasic speakers. A case described in McNeill (2005, p. 217) demonstrates the phenomenon: a patient began his description with single nouns but after more than two minutes of gradual expansion, accompanied by appropriate spatial gesture mappings, came out eventually with a two-clause, embedded sentence including appropriate verbs—slow speech indeed but far from "agrammatic." Figure 31.3 depicts the stages in this gradual unpacking.

The speaker begins by referring to a trolley as the "el," which is the local way of referring to Chicago's elevated train system. The important feature of the example is his repeated indicating of the upper gesture space—first raising his left arm at the elbow, and then lifting his arm overhead. This recurrent indexing is a source of gestural cohesion. Verbally, speech was initially limited to just "el" (with and without an article). Then it expanded to "on the tracks" (which, like the trolley wires in the cartoon episode he was describing, are overhead in an elevated train system). A full sentence with a single clause then emerged ("he saw the el train"), and finally, dramatically, considering the depth of his initial agrammatism, a full sentence with two verbs and clauses ("he saw the el train comin' "). The example illustrates a catchment (the overhead wires/tracks, no apparent metaphoricity) and under its spell a step-by-step accessing of a construction. The duration of the catchment and the time it took to reach the final construction was two minutes and 17 seconds.

In terms of our brain model, Broca's aphasia, true to its name, is a breakdown of GP unpacking in Broca's area. The area normally orchestrates vocal and manual actions with significances other than those of the actions themselves. Consistent with such a breakdown, recent reports state that Broca's aphasics have difficulty recognizing other people's actions (Fadiga, 2007). This can be regarded as the perceptual equivalent of impaired orchestrating capabilities. On the other hand, processes said in the model to be carried out elsewhere in the brain, the posterior left hemisphere, the right hemisphere, and the prefrontal cortex—imagery, the combination of imagery with linguistically encoded categories, and the relating of all this to tailor-made fields of oppositions, as well as prosodic emphasis on the linguistic realization (cf. Goodglass, 1993)—appear intact, evi-

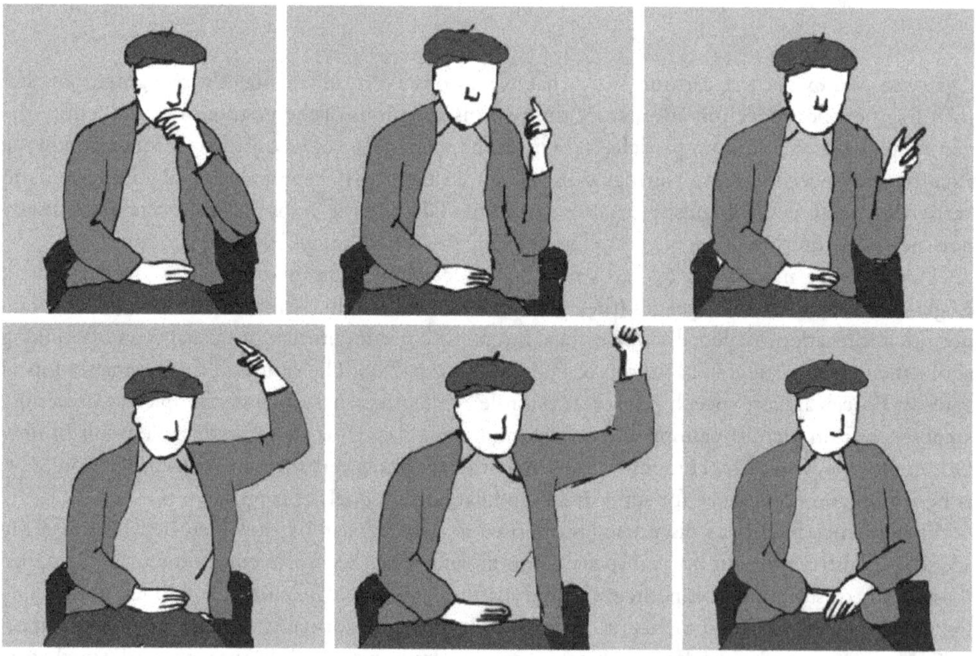

Figure 31.3 Catchment from a disfluent (agrammatic) speaker made of repeated gestures in upper space.

denced in the continuing ability by agrammatic speakers to synchronize co-expressive speech and gesture, and to differentiate contextually newsworthy information with them.

Down syndrome

Down syndrome is characterized by a linguistic disability beyond what an also-present cognitive disability would predict. The DS children lag in language but are relatively spared in visuospatial and visuomotor abilities (Stefanini, Caselli, & Volterra, 2007). It is not surprising therefore that DS children show a "gesture advantage" (also called gesture enhancement)—a preference for and receptivity to gesture over vocal speech, a phenomenon first noted by Abrahamsen, Cavallo, and McCluer (1985) with taught signs and words. A gesture advantage has also been observed with spontaneous gestures during naming tests in recent studies at the Institute of Cognitive Science and Technology (ISTC), in Rome, part of the CNR. However, in this situation, unlike Abrahamsen et al.'s (1985) findings with signs, DS children do not show gesture enhancement at the one-word stage; enhancement emerges only after the children reach the two-word threshold. DS, the ISTC finds, display a significantly smaller repertoire of representational gestures but produce them with a frequency equaling that of typically developing (TD) children (Stefanini et al., 2007). In picture naming, DS gestures are semantically related to meaning in the picture, and so can convey information even if there is nothing corresponding to them in speech. These "unimodal" messages suggest a mode of information processing fundamentally unlike that of the typical GP. Ultimately, according to Abrahamsen et al. (1985), the gesture advantage weakens and disappears with the emergence of syntax. So it is a transient phenomenon of development, emerging earlier with taught signs than with spontaneous gestures, and eventually disappearing or reducing in size with the establishment of some kind of syntax.

Typically developing children also show a gesture advantage at early ages, but with two crucial differences: unlike DS, the gestures of TD combine with words to encode semantic relations, whereas for DS the word-gesture combinations tend to be redundant. Secondly, the gesture advantage with TD occurs before the two-word threshold, and in fact, reliably predicts when and with what semantic relations this threshold will be crossed (Butcher & Goldin-Meadow, 2000; Goldin-Meadow & Butcher, 2003). These differences, when examined, shed light on the nature of the DS linguistic deficit itself.

What is impressive about DS, revealed by work at the Rome Institute, is that DS gestures are often "unimodal," as noted, and, further, when they occur with speech they are mostly semantically redundant with the accompanying speech. What does this imply for GPs? The chart in Figure 31.4, from Iverson, Longobardi, and Caselli (2003), shows that the predominant gesture-speech combination in DS (white bars) is "equivalent" ("redundant"), in contrast to TD (dark bars). Volterra, Caselli, Capirici, and Pizzuto (2005, p. 29) say of this:

> [w]hen children with DS combined gestures and words, they did so primarily in an informationally redundant fashion. The vast majority of combinations produced by these children were in fact equivalent combinations in which the two representational elements referred to the same referent and conveyed the same meaning (e.g., headshake for no = "no"). In TD, on the other hand, early speech-gesture combinations are "complementary" (partially redundant gesture and speech referring to the same object but different aspects of it, which DS also create, though far less than "equivalent") and "supplementary" (nonredundant, gesture and speech referring to different entities in some kind of semantic relation, like POINT AT CHAIR + "daddy" = "daddy's chair," possessive, which DS create virtually not at all).

Goldin-Meadow and Butcher (2003), with TD children, classified the semantic relationships in speech and gesture combinations, and found that speech-gesture combinations foreshadowed the

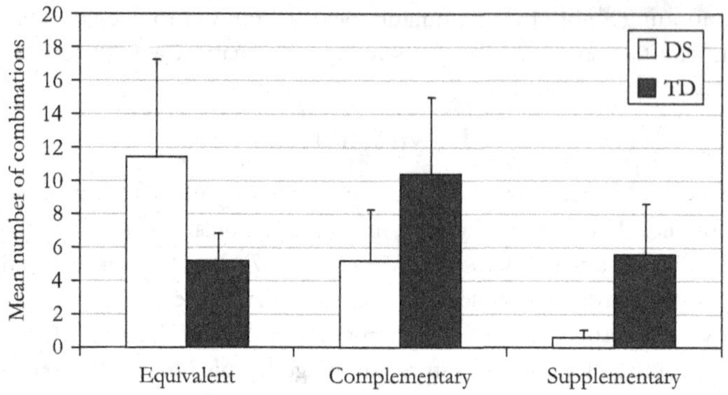

Figure 31.4 Information conveyed in gesture plus word combinations by Down syndrome and mental age matched typically developing children (Iverson, J. M., Longobardi, E., and Caselli, M. C. International Journal of Language and Communicative Disorders, 38, 179–197, 2003. With permission.)

child's first word-word combinations, these appearing a few weeks later with the same semantic relationships. A child who pointed at an object and said "go" would, a couple of weeks later, produce word-word combinations with "go" plus object names. The early gesture-word combinations cover a range of semantic relations: "open" + points at drawer, "out" + holds up toy bag, "hot" + points at furnace, "no" + points at box, "monster" + two vertical palms spread apart (= big; Goldin-Meadow & Butcher, 2003, Table 31.3). Kelly (2006) observed an earlier step, in which the first pairings involve gestures and speech that denote the same elements; it is only slightly later that different speech and gesture elements synchronize to form the semantic units described by Goldin-Meadow and Butcher (2003).

Thus, TD children begin with a gesture advantage, first with redundant gestures and speech, then with semantic combinations of gesture and speech fore-shadowing the same semantic combinations a few weeks later in speech-speech. DS in contrast appear to take only the first step. Even their "complementary" gesture-speech combinations are a species of redundant combination. It is only "supplementary" combinations that combine semantic elements into structures that foreshadow combinations of words, and DS lack these almost totally.

To understand these differences in GP terms, we note that redundancy and the exclusion of semantic connections between gesture and speech suggest that DS GPs, in whatever form they exist, are narrowly constrained. The opposition of semiotic modes within these narrow limits would give them little traction. The type of example in Figure 31.1, in which the underlying idea of Sylvester moving up inside a pipe is symbolized in two semiotically opposite forms, may be beyond their reach. Imagining them recounting this episode, they may say "pipe" and gesture its shape; or "sidewalk" (where Sylvester paced before going up the pipe) and gesture a flat surface; or "ball" and make a circle; but not "rising hollowness" or even "down" if, as we suppose, the Figure 31.2 aphasic speaker was differentiating the idea of downward force in a context of things that Tweety and Sylvester were doing. In DS, this apparent narrowness in turn could impact the dependence of the GP on fields of oppositions. DS GPs, redundantly welded, would differentiate only equally narrow contexts where synonymy of gesture and speech is meaningful. Verbalized thought, for DS, would then be confined in at least two ways—GPs with little dynamic push, and contexts cramped to make minimal differentiation significant: in this way coming up short on the dynamic dimension of language. Their dynamic shortfall joins the deficits on the static dimension of factual linguistic competence (where naming and syntactic deficits are noted). The aphasic speaker who after two arduous minutes reached a two-clause, embedded sentence was sustained throughout by his spatially configured catchment (observable in gesture), and this kind of achievement, and any benefit of catchment formations in general, may be largely out of reach for a DS speaker. Finally, a lack of GP semiotic opposition could impair the unpacking step, limiting access to constructions, even if they have been acquired. So the picture is of limited GP potential, lessened dynamism of thinking-for/while-speaking, limited contextual scope, and limited potential to form gestural (catchment) discourse segments. Bellugi, Wang, and Jernigan (1994) describe older DS responses to vocabulary tests as often involving perseverations or category errors (e.g., "horsie, dog, ice cream" to one picture), which also seem to be manifestations of cognitive narrowness.

Given that DS speakers have comparatively good visuo-spatial and visuo-motor cognition, the shortcomings we describe refer specifically to GP formation. Our suggestion is that DS start out with gestures preferentially. In this they are not unlike TD children in the second year. But they differ in that, when they add speech, the speech-gesture combinations are redundant, totally, or partially. As such, speech-gesture combinations fail to carry the DS over the language threshold. So if normal development involves certain types of gesture-speech combinations as way stations toward language, DS development seems excessively stuck at the level of redundant gestures. It is telling that the gestures they do produce, after considerable experience, are also not ones likely to foster semiotic oppositions with linguistic encodings. Volterra et al. (2005) offer an interesting suggestion: children with DS may be able to make use of actions produced in the context of object-related activities and social routines as communicative gestures. Once this happens, they may begin to develop relatively large repertoires of gestures and make enhanced use of gesture to compensate for poor productive language. (p. 32)

These kinds of compensatory gestures are the not co-equal participants with encoded language with which to create the semiotic oppositions a GP demands; in fact, such gestures are substitutes, and doubly so—not only for deficient language, but also for deficient gestures (cf. Chan & Iacono, 2001).

Williams syndrome

Williams syndrome (WS) is often pictured as the mirror image of DS. WS children have cognitive deficits, IQs in the 50–70 range, yet seem to have greater language skills than the cognitive deficits would predict. They are also highly socially engaged, musical, and lively. Social engagement and musicality we think are the keys to their language as well.

WS poses an interesting challenge to the GP theory: how, given the theory, can language go beyond cognition's offerings? The seeming sparing of language has made WS the poster child of purported language modules. However, from a nonmodular, GP perspective, another interpretation seems possible. We shall answer the challenge in the following way. Although it may seem perverse to refer to better-than-predicted language as a "disorder" we shall in fact conclude that, in the WS case, good language arises from disruption of the GP, namely a disconnect between the social framing of thinking-for-speaking, of which WS clearly are capable, and what Vygotsky (1987) termed "pure thought." Gesture mimicry and other forms of "mind-merging" (Franklin, 2007; Kimbara, 2006, 2007; McNeill et al., 2010) participate in constructing social interactions (Kimbara, 2006), and we believe that WS children have similar capabilities. In effect, WS speakers maintain the connection of idea units, GPs, to the social context of speaking, via what is sometimes called hypersociability (Bellugi, Lichtenberger, Mills, Galaburda, & Korenberg, 1999), creating joint GPs with interlocutors (as unimpaired speakers also do), but are unable to shape thought outside the social fabric, and this is their disorder. Vygotsky visualized thought and speech as overlapping circles, one for thought, one for speech, and the overlap was inner speech; the GP is a theory about this overlap, and what we propose for WS is truncation or inaccessibility of the thought circle from the overlap. An important factor in this flattening could be a WS weakness at global organization in the visual domain (Bellugi et al., 1999). If WS are unable to create visual global wholes they would gain little from the global-synthetic imagery created in GPs as part of the speaking process. The result leaves little room for the GP to shape cognition—the reverse of trying to explain how cognition affects language: it is cognition in WS that is not shaped by the ongoing thinking-for-speaking process.

If this is on the right track, WS is thus a disorder of the dynamic dimension of language par excellence. Language is weak at shaping cognition, while it retains what is also usually integrated with thought, the social-interactive fabric. There is a distinctive gesture profile of WS (Bello et al., 2004), in which only certain kinds of imagery take part: iconic gestures and a plenitude of socially constituted "emblems," if available in the culture, both of which are engaged in social interactions, but also an absence of gesture metaphor with metadiscourse resonances. An interpretation of WS in terms of our proposed brain model is far from certain, and we do not attempt it, other than to suggest that among the unique qualities of WS, GP formation is an energetic rhythmicity that can underlie both their fluency of speaking as well as the other quality of the syndrome, musicality. The role of the cerebellum in organizing rhythmic pulses of speech (Duncan, 2006) is echoed by the discovery of hyperdevelopment of the cerebellar vermis of WS. The vermis is thought to play a role in human rhythmic sense and movement (Schmitt, Eliez, Warsofsky, Bellugi, & Reiss, 2001). These rhythmic pulses are also obviously engaged in the musical lives of WS individuals (cf. Bellugi et al., 1999), and also, we hypothesize, play into sociability, underlying the entrainments of the children with social others during interactions (cf. Gill, 2007).

It has been said that WS are slow to develop gestures (Volterra et al. citing Bertrand, Mervis, & Neustat, 1998), and that their gestures, when started, are not frequent (Laing et al., 2002), but other studies at the ISTC in Rome have observed no difference between TD and WS matched for developmental age (Volterra et al., 2005). In their recent work, with 9- to 12-year-old WS children, researchers at the Rome Institute find WS perform gestures in picture-naming and Frog Story narrations at a higher rate than TD children of comparable developmental ages, have more iconic gestures and more pointing gestures, and combine gestures to a greater extent with "social evaluation devices," such as character speech, sound effects, exclamations, and rhetorical questions that function to capture the listener's attention (Bello, Capirci, & Volterra, 2004; Capirci, 2007). More precisely, they found a significant correlation between total spoken social evaluation devices and the use of gestures only for WS children ($p = 0.0078$). A significant correlation was found in particular with iconic gestures ($p = 0.0001$) and beat gestures ($p = 0.004$). Those children with WS who produced more gestures (in particular more iconic gestures and more beat gestures) were also the children who produced more spoken social evaluation devices.

We get a picture of WS children as socially interactive, with gesture a well-established modality for human interaction. Their "enhanced language," we propose, stems from this lively social engagement, as described above. This implicates the GP in the following way. Vygotsky, in his reanalysis of egocentric speech, argued that a child's development is from the outside, the social context, to the inside—the once-social becoming thought. This ontogenetic process has an echo on the much tighter time scale of GP microgenesis, in that the field of oppositions includes, among other information, social interaction variables and the GP itself can be shared interpsychically (cf. McNeill et al., 2010, for descriptions of "mind-merging" in normal adult conversations). We suggest that WS have GPs of this kind. This is not only mimicry; speaking can be self-generated but depend for sustenance on continuing social interactions; closed off is self-directed thought carried by language, including metaphor. Distinctive about WS thinking-for-speaking is its dominant social frame assisted by rhythmic entrainment. Cognitive deficits, including relative inability to access the semantic values of words (Karmiloff-Smith, Brown, Grice, & Paterson, 2003), may deflate the thought circle, but sociability is the key to their language. In this sense, the skill of WS children in language is an aspect of the disability.

However, the facts of actual WS language ability are less than totally clear. In keeping with their sociability and rhythmicity, speech flow is impressively fluent. But the depth of WS language skill is debated. On the one hand are those who argue for near-normal language abilities. Zukowski (2001), for example, compared WS and neurotypical children's language production data on noun-

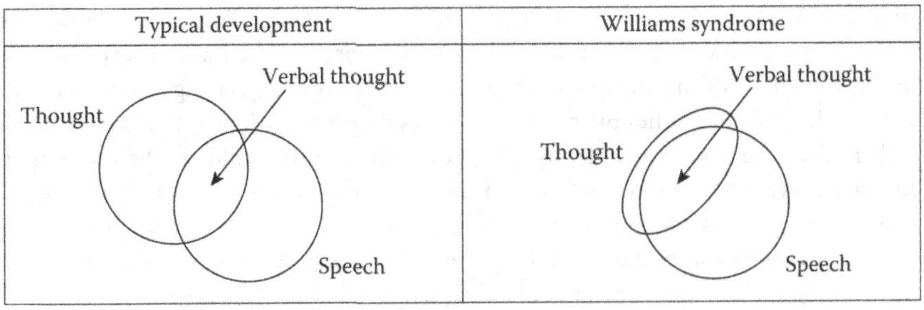

Figure 31.5 Representations in the manner of Vygotsky (1987) of the relationship between thought, speech, and verbal thought, in typically developing and Williams syndrome children.

noun compounds, embedded relative clauses, and yes/no questions; also grammaticality judgments of uses of expressions with "any" and "some." She found performance in the two groups to be similar, concluding, "WS is indeed highly relevant to the modularity debate. The findings also suggest that imperfect levels of language performance in WS may reflect an exaggerated influence of normal processing factors" (from the abstract). On the other hand, Karmiloff-Smith et al. (2003) summarize numerous tests of WS, concluding that "the WS language system is not only delayed but also develops along a different trajectory compared to controls, with individuals with WS placing relatively more weight on phonological information and relatively less weight on semantic information" (p. 230). Karmiloff-Smith et al. (2003) are emphatic in their rejection of innateness linguistic "modularity" claims based on spared WS language skills in the absence of general cognitive ability (cf. Pinker, 1999), citing both the relative inaccessibility of semantic content to WS, and also tests of sentence comprehension, which show "findings inconsistent with the view that WS syntax is intact" (p. 231). In thinking about the modularity issue, it is important to recognize that no general principle relating a given level of cognitive ability or inability to a specific grammatical form presence or absence has ever been defined; so an ability to produce relative clause responses in experiments, for example, may or may not count as evidence of a syntax module, particularly if [as Karmiloff-Smith et al. (2003) propose] WS children reach these abilities over different developmental routes (which may include tracks, not seen in typical development, linked to their hypersociability). And again, in general, sociocentric inputs may create an illusion of structure.

Social framing can also create an appearance of narrative cohesion. Bellugi et al. (1994) observed an abundance of "paralinguistic and linguistic devices for expressive purposes and to maintain audience interest" (p. 16); that is, a cohesion based, not on thematic linkages in discourse, but on the continuation of purposes in social interactions. We can predict that, despite their better than expected language and gesture output, gesture catchments from WS will tend to emphasize this kind of sociocentric cohesion, with few if any catchments built out of recurring gesture references, as we saw created for example by the agrammatic speaker in Figure 31.3. Social but nonreferential catchments may thus be another aspect of the WS syndrome. It is possible that in WS there is an absence of discourse awareness itself (cf. Sullivan, Winner, & Tager-Flushberg, 2003, for WS inability to distinguish lies from irony, where doing so required relating verbal uses to context in comprehension).

To summarize, using Vygotsky's image of overlapping circles, the WS thought-circle is flattened (Figure 31.5).

Childhood autism

Levy (2007, 2008; Levy & Fowler, 2005) has developed a method by which to observe the emergence of spoken discourse cohesion over short intervals—short, but extended enough to permit observation of emergence. A child is shown a classic film, The Red Balloon, and tells the story to a listener. Specific to the method is that the child tells the story repeatedly, over several days (sometimes on the same day), to the same or different listeners. In this way, changes, which typically are consolidations that enhance cohesion, can be tracked as they emerge. The method can be employed with speakers of all sorts and has been used by Levy with autistic children. We concentrate on a case study of a 13-year-old boy (Levy, 2008). While many differences from TD children are found with autistics, we focus, following Levy, on the catchment and its theoretical role in creating fields of oppositions. In his first attempts at retelling the story, speech was fragmented and gestures few, responses were "single utterances or utterance fragments, usually in the absence of focused enactment, and often accompanied by diffuse body motion, for example, shifting position, swaying back and forth, rocking, and fidgeting" (p. 5 ms.).

Levy documents that from this point fully encoded descriptions gradually emerged and—equally striking—also gestures that look typical for such speech; in other words, GPs in what appear to be appropriate fields of oppositions. Coherence increased via catchments: "As D. combined speech with enactment ... he created a sequence that was more temporally coherent than the first: All utterances were accurate descriptions of events, and all occurred in accurate temporal sequence" (p. 11). An example analyzed in detail by Levy involves two catchments at early points in the child's narrative attempts—flying gestures, and holding gestures—that resulted eventually, after several retellings, in a correctly narrated sequence of events (corresponding to the film's sequence). As fields of oppositions, we can see in these catchments how the narrative order was finally straightened out. Initially, the boy first described flying with balloons, then, immediately following, holding onto the balloons (while reversing the film order, the order of D's utterances is the same as by the adults when first prompting the scene). Then the following (Table 31.2, compiled from Levy, p. 23).

Although starting out with an airborne reference, again out of sequence, he had the holding gesture in the correct narrative sequence (holding first). The GP at this point would be something like that suggested in the table: differentiating what could happen while the boy was holding—floating. The child continued with the correct sequence: holding followed by flying. Achieving temporal coherence thus stemmed from catchments and the realization that, eventually, the holding and flying catchments interrelate, one continuing what the other began. This is a kind of imagery-enactment version of the logical relationship of an enabling cause/resultant, which the boy could achieve in this form even if not with a clear vision of the logical connections themselves.

From a GP point of view, as exhibited in this case study, autism seems to involve an imbalance between enactment and speech that was overcome with repeated telling. Like the aphasic in Figure 31.3, a catchment emerged accompanied by coherence (they differ of course in that the autistic child recycles entire descriptions, whereas the aphasic took time to create a single description). In the brain, we speculate, the imbalance focuses on the prefrontal and motor cortexes, with the latter at first flooding the former. Eventually, an awakened prefrontal area is energized and creates something like a normal field of oppositions. In cyclic retelling there is something that activates and/or restores balance across brain regions and leads the autistic speaker toward the realm of the typical. We can imagine that autistic children might seek this kind of cyclic activation on their

Table 31.2 Achieving discourse cohesion by an autistic adolescent

Narrative order	*Speech*	*Gesture*	*Fields of Oppositions (possible):*
1	he floated	start of holding gesture	What Happened While Holding: Floating
2	he hanged on tight	continuation of holding gesture	Still What Happened While Holding: Holding Tight
3	[no speech]	flying gesture	The Thing That Happened: Flying

Source: Based on Levy, 2008.

own—some of the repetitious behavior often remarked upon in the disorder may be an effort to overcome enactment imbalance. At the same time, however, such an effort is a recipe for impaired social communication. What, for an autistic child, may be an effort for eventual enhancement is limited if not actually counterproductive as a kind of social foray. Thus the child would be denied the propulsion from socially engaged cognition that carries WS children so far.

Summary and conclusions: what the GP shows

We began this chapter saying that the four language disorders—agrammatic aphasia, DS, WS, and autism—disrupt different aspects of the GP. We conclude by summarizing the disruptions and what they reveal about human speech and its points of possible breakdown. We suggest that a GP view of language shows the disorders in new light. For this reason, we believe, it is worthy of consideration by clinicians and researchers who deal directly with communication disorders.

Disfluent (agrammatic) aphasia preserves the psychological predicate character of the GP, the point of newsworthy information differentiated from context. Context and catchments are accessible. Broca's aphasia concentrates specifically on the unpacking of GPs via constructions or other syntax. Constructions may also be intact, in part, but are hard to access due to shallow level motor impediments interacting with the vocal articulators. The evidence for this is that, with catchment support and sufficient time, agrammatic aphasics can develop even multiclause unpackings. It is accordingly easy to understand the frustration sometimes shown by agrammatic aphasics, since they experience basically the whole process of thinking-for-speaking but cannot execute it in action. Autism reveals an imbalance of enactment and catchment formation that, with repetition, can be overcome; so the disorder is one of balance, not specifically a breakdown of the GP. In contrast to the aphasic, once balance is reached, speech and discourse appear to function with something like normalcy. Down syndrome speakers, children at least, may not experience thinking-for-speaking in anything like the form it is encountered by normal speakers, the autistic child, or the agrammatic aphasic. The elements opposed semiotically in their GPs are redundant, there is little scope for cognitive movement, and the contexts from which these rigid GPs are differentiated are comparably narrow. The impression one gets of DS speech therefore is of stasis, immobility, and little potential for fueling thinking-for-speaking. Williams speakers unusually seem to have half the normal complement of thinking-for-speaking, missing the other half. Their GPs are socially engaged but do not pass into thought, possibly because their cognitive deficits prevent it. Down and Williams syndrome speakers are mirror images in respect to thinking as well; both are unable to use language as an enriching element of cognition but for opposite reasons—Down cannot break out of limited GPs; Williams cannot translate GPs structured as lively social interactions into cognition.

A further dimension of comparison involves the place of the catchment in the four disorders. Disfluent aphasia retains at least the capability of thematic linkages with spatial, deictically established catchments, as we see in both Figure 31.2 (correct deictic placement of the bowling ball placement) and Figure 31.3 (the overhead locus). Autistics initially cannot form catchments but attain them with appropriate enactments, as in the flying example. This may limit their discourse cohesion to the enactable, just as the aphasic's, with no or little potential in either case to extend imagery metaphorically. Children with DS, because of the near-total redundancy of imagery and speech, possibly cannot form catchments at all. Each image is tied to a specific lexical form. Finally, in Williams, we may find catchments (if sought) based on social interaction, and these catchments could be the richest of all, since interaction can lead the child into complex and enduring forms of cohesive discourse. In respect to catchments, WS and autism differ diametrically. Autistic social catchments may never be reached if recycling is the route, since it is so disruptive to the normal parameters of social interaction, whereas, in WS, where hypersociability is the style, such catchments might be the starting point of almost all of their speech.

Acknowledgments

Preparation supported by research grants from NSF and NIH to the University of Chicago, and award number NIH NIDCD 5R01DC001150–14 to the University of Colorado. We are grateful to Elena Levy and Virginia Volterra for very helpful comments.

Further reading

McNeill, D. (30 August 2012). *How language began: Gesture and speech in human evolution*. New York: Cambridge University Press.

McNeill, D. (7 March 2016). *Why we gesture: The surprising role of hand movements in communication*. New York: Cambridge University Press.

Özer, D., & Göksun, T. (2020). Gesture use and processing: A review on individual differences in cognitive resources. *Frontiers in Psychology, 11*, 573555.

References

Abrahamsen, A., Cavallo, M. M., & McCluer, J. A. (1985). Is the sign advantage a robust phenomenon? From gesture to language in two modalities. *Merrill-Palmer Quarterly, 31*, 177–209.

Bello, A., Capirci, O., & Volterra, V. (2004). Lexical production in children with Williams syndrome: Spontaneous use of gesture in a naming task. *Neuropsychologia, 42*(2), 201–213.

Bellugi, U., Wang, P. P., & Jernigan, T. L. (1994). Williams syndrome: An unusual neuropsychological profile. In S. Broman & J. Grafman (Eds.), *Atypical cognitive deficits in developmental disorders: Implications for brain function* (pp. 23–56). Hillsdale: Lawrence Erlbaum Associates.

Bellugi, U., Lichtenberger, L., Mills, D., Galaburda, A., & Korenberg, J. R. (1999). Bridging cognition, the brain and molecular genetics: Evidence from Williams syndrome. *Trends in Neuroscience, 22*(5), 197–207.

Bertrand, J., Mervis, C. B., & Neustat, I. (1998). Communicative gesture use by preschoolers with Williams syndrome: A longitudinal study. Presentation at the International Conference of Infant Studies, Atlanta, GA.

Butcher, C., & Goldin-Meadow, S. (2000). Gesture and the transition from one- to two-word speech: When hand and mouth come together. In D. McNeill (Ed.), *Language and gesture* (pp. 235–257). Cambridge, UK: Cambridge University Press.

Capirci, O. (2007, December). *Gesture and language in children with Williams syndrome. Presentation at the 2007 ESF exploratory Workshop/ESRC Workshop, sign language vs. gesture: Where is the boundary, and how can we know more?* (pp. 6–7). Rome, Italy: Institute of Cognitive Sciences & Technologies.

Chan, J. B., & Iacono, T. (2001). Gesture and word production in children with Down syndrome. *AAC Augmentative and Attentive Communication, 17*(2), 73–87.

Courchesne, F., Townsend, J., & Saitoh, O. (1994). The brain in infantile autism: Posterior fossa structures are abnormal. *Neurology, 44*(2), 214–223.

De Ruiter, J.-P. (2000). The production of gesture and speech. In D. McNeill (Ed.), *Language and gesture* (pp. 285–311). Cambridge, UK: Cambridge University Press.

Dray, N. L., & McNeill, D. (1990). Gestures during discourse: The contextual structuring of thought. In S. L. Tsohatzidis (Ed.), *Meanings and prototypes: Studies in linguistic categorization* (pp. 465–487). London, UK: Routledge.

Duncan, S. (2006). Co-expressivity of speech and gesture: Manner of motion in Spanish, English, and Chinese. In *Proceedings of the 27th Berkeley linguistic society annual meeting* (pp. 353–370). [Meeting in 2001.] Berkeley, CA: Berkeley Linguistics Society. CA: University of California, Berkeley, Department of Linguistics.

Duncan, S., & Pedelty, L. (2007). Discourse focus, gesture, and disfluent aphasia. In S. D. Duncan, J. Cassell & E. T. Levy (Eds.), *Gesture and the dynamic dimension of language* (pp. 269–283). Amsterdam/Philadelphia: John Benjamins.

Fadiga, L. (2007, December). *Report in OMLL (origin of man, language and languages), ESF EUROCORES program highlights* (p. 13). Retrieved from http://www.esf.org/activities/eurocores/programmes/omll.html

Franklin, A. (2007). Blending in deception: Tracing output back to its source. In S. D. Duncan, J. Cassell & E. T. Levy (Eds.), *Gesture and the dynamic dimension of language* (pp. 99–108). Amsterdam/Philadelphia: John Benjamins.

Furuyama, N., & Sekine, K. (2007). Forgetful or strategic? The mystery of the systematic avoidance of reference in the cartoon story narrative. In S. D. Duncan, J. Cassell & E. T. Levy (Eds.), *Gesture and the dynamic dimension of language* (pp. 75–81). Amsterdam and Philadelphia: Benjamins.

Gill, S. (2007). Entrainment and musicality in the human system interface. *AI and Society, 21*(4), 567–605.

Goldin-Meadow, S., & Butcher, C. (2003). Pointing toward two-word speech in young children. In S. Kita (Ed.), *Pointing: Where language, culture, and cognition meet* (pp. 85–107). Mahwah: Erlbaum Associates.
Goodglass, H. (1993). *Understanding aphasia.* San Diego, CA: Academic Press.
Harris, R. (2003). *Saussure and his interpreters* (2nd ed.). Edinburgh, Scotland: Edinburgh University Press.
Hockett, C. F. (1960). The origin of speech. *Scientific American, 203*(3), 88–96.
Iverson, J. M., Longobardi, E., & Caselli, M. C. (2003). Relationship between gestures and words in children with Down's syndrome and typically developing children in the early stages of communicative development. *International Journal of Language and Communicative Disorders, 38*(2), 179–197.
Johnson, M. (1987). *The body in the mind: The bodily basis of meaning, imagination, and reason.* Chicago, IL: University of Chicago Press.
Karmiloff-Smith, A., Brown, J. H., Grice, S., & Paterson, S. (2003). Dethroning the myth: Cognitive dissociations and innate modularity in Williams syndrome. *Developmental Neuropsychology, 23*(1–2), 227–242.
Kelly, B. F. (2006). The development of constructions through gesture. In E. V. Clark & B. F. Kelly (Eds.), *Constructions in acquisition* (pp. 11–25). Palo Alto: CSLI.
Kimbara, I. (2006). On gestural mimicry. *Gesture, 6*(1), 39–61.
Kimbara, I. (2007). Indexing locations in gesture: Recalled stimulus image and interspeaker coordination as factors influencing gesture form. In S. D. Duncan, J. Cassell & E. T. Levy (Eds.), *Gesture and the dynamic dimension of language* (pp. 213–220). Amsterdam/Philadelphia: John Benjamins.
Kita, S., & Özyürek, A. (2003). What does cross-linguistic variation in semantic coordination of speech and gesture reveal? Evidence for an interface representation of spatial thinking and speaking. *Journal of Memory and Language, 48*(1), 16–32.
Laing, E., Butterworth, G., Ansari, D., Gsodl, M., Longhi, E., Paterson, S., & Karmiloff-Smith, A. (2002). Atypical development of language and social communication in toddlers with Williams syndrome. *Developmental Science, 5*(2), 233–246.
Levelt, W. J. M. (1989). *Speaking: From intention to articulation.* Cambridge, MA: MIT Press/Bradford Books.
Levy, E. (2007). The construction of temporally coherent narrative by an autistic adolescent: Co-construction of speech, enactment and gesture. In S. D. Duncan, J. Cassell & E. T. Levy (Eds.), *Gesture and the dynamic dimension of language* (pp. 285–301). Amsterdam/Philadelphia: Benjamins.
Levy, E. T. (2008). *The mediation of coherent discourse by kinesthetic reenactment: A case study of an autistic adolescent, Part II.* Manuscript. Department of Psychology, University of Connecticut at Stamford.
Levy, E. T., & Fowler, C. A. (2005). How autistic children may use narrative discourse to scaffold coherent interpretations of events: A case study. *Imagination, Cognition and Personality, 24*(3), 207–244.
McNeill, D. (1992). *Hand and mind: What gestures reveal about thought.* Chicago, IL: University of Chicago Press.
McNeill, D. (2000). Catchments and contexts: Non-modular factors in speech and gesture production. In D. McNeill (Ed.), *Language and gesture* (pp. 312–328). Cambridge, UK: Cambridge University Press.
McNeill, D. (2005). *Gesture and thought.* Chicago, IL: University of Chicago Press.
McNeill, D., & Duncan, S. D. (2000). Growth points in thinking for speaking. In D. McNeill (Ed.), *Language and gesture* (pp. 141–161). Cambridge, UK: Cambridge University Press.
McNeill, D., Duncan, S., Cole, J., Gallagher, S., & Bertenthal, B. (2008). Growth points from the very beginning. *Interaction Studies, 9*(1), 117–132.
McNeill, D., Duncan, S., Franklin, A., Goss, J., Kimbara, I., Parrill, F., … Tuttle, R. (2010). Mind-merging. In E. Morsella (Ed.), *Expressing oneself/Expressing one's self: Communication, language, cognition, and identity: A Festschrift in honor of Robert M. Krauss* (pp. 141–164). New York: Taylor & Francis.
Miceli, G., Silveri, M. C., Villa, G., & Caramazza, A. (1984). On the basis of the agrammatic's difficulty in producing main verbs. *Cortex, 20*(2), 207–220.
Pinker, S. (1999). *Words and rules: The ingredients of language.* New York: Basic Books.
Schmitt, J. E., Eliez, S., Warsofsky, I. S., Bellugi, U., & Reiss, A. L. (2001). Enlarged cerebellar vermis in Williams syndrome. *Journal of Psychiatric Research, 35*(4), 225–229.
Slobin, D. I. (1987). Thinking for speaking. In J. Aske, N. Beery, L. Michaelis, & H. Filip (Eds.). *Proceedings of the thirteenth annual meeting of the Berkeley Linguistic Society* (pp. 435–445). Berkeley, CA: Berkeley Linguistic Society.
Stefanini, S., Caselli, M. C., & Volterra, V. (2007). Spoken and gestural production in a naming task by young children with Down's syndrome. *Brain and Language, 101*(3), 208–221.
Sullivan, K., Winner, E., & Tager-Flushberg, H. (2003). Can adolescents with Williams syndrome tell the difference between lies and jokes? *Developmental Neuropsychology, 23*(1–2), 85–103.
Volterra, V., Caselli, M. C., Capirici, O., & Pizzuto, E. (2005). Gesture and the emergence and development of language. In M. Tomasello & D. I. Slobin (Eds.), *Beyond nature-nurture: Essays in honor of Elizabeth Bates* (pp. 3–40). Mahwah, NJ: Lawrence Erlbaum.
Vygotsky, L. S. (1987). *Thought and language. Edited and translated by E. Hanfmann & G. Vakar (revised and edited by A. Kozulin).* Cambridge, MA: MIT Press.

Zinchenko, V. P. (1985). Vygotsky's ideas about units for the analysis of mind. In J. V. Wertsch (Ed.), *Culture communication, and cognition: Vygotskian perspectives* (pp. 94–118). Cambridge, UK: Cambridge University Press.

Zingester, L. B., & Berndt, R. S. (1990). Retrieval of nouns and verbs in agrammatism and anomia. *Brain and Language, 39*(1), 14–32.

Zukowski, A. (2001). *Uncovering grammatical competence in children with Williams syndrome*. PhD dissertation, Boston University.

32
NEURAL ORGANIZATION OF LANGUAGE
Clues from sign language aphasia

Gregory Hickok and Ursula Bellugi

Introduction

A central issue in understanding the neural organization of language is the extent to which this organization is dependent on the sensory and motor modalities through which language is perceived and produced. There are many reasons to think that the neural organization of language should be profoundly influenced by extrinsic factors in development such as sensory and motor experience. The temporal processing demands imposed by the auditory system have been argued to favor left hemisphere systems (Tallal, Miller, & Fitch, 1993), which could, in turn, determine aspects of the lateralization pattern of auditory-mediated language. Superior temporal lobe regions thought to be important for language comprehension are situated in and around auditory cortices—a natural location given auditory sensory input of language. Likewise, Broca's area, which is classically thought to play a role in speech production, is situated just anterior to motor cortex controlling the speech articulators. Thus, it would not be unreasonable to hypothesize that the neural organization of language—including its lateralization and within hemisphere organization—is determined in large part by the particular demands imposed by the sensory and motor interface systems.

By studying the functional neuroanatomy of the signed languages of the deaf, we can test this hypothesis in a straightforward manner. It has been shown that signed languages share much of the formal linguistic structure found in spoken languages, but differ radically in the sensory and motor systems through which language is transmitted (Bellugi, Poizner, & Klima, 1989; Emmorey, 2002; Klima & Bellugi, 1979). In essence, signed language offers a kind of natural experimental manipulation: central linguistic structure and function are held constant, while peripheral sensory and motor experience is varied. Thus, a comparison of the neural organization of signed versus spoken language will provide clues concerning the factors that drive the development of the functional neuroanatomy of language. Here we provide a summary of the findings from studies of the neural organization of the signed languages of the deaf.

Hemispheric asymmetries for sign language processing

Left hemisphere damage (LHD) in hearing/speaking individuals is associated with deficits at sublexical ("phonetic/phonemic"), lexical, and sentence levels, both in production and in comprehension to some degree (Damasio, 1992; Goodglass, 1993; Hillis, 2007). Right hemisphere

DOI: 10.4324/9781003204213-37

damage (RHD), on the other hand, has been associated with supra-sentential (e.g., discourse) deficits (Brownell, Potter, Bihrle, & Gardner, 1986). Given the radical differences in modality of perception and production of sign language, one might expect sign language to differ dramatically in hemispheric asymmetries. But instead, our studies have found very strong evidence of highly similar patterns of hemispheric asymmetries in the deaf signing population compared to hearing/speaking individuals.

Sublexical-, lexical-, and sentence-level processes

A variety of sublexical-, lexical-, and sentence-level deficits has been found in individual LHD deaf signers (Bellugi et al., 1989; Hickok & Bellugi, 2001; Hickok, Kritchevsky, Bellugi, & Klima, 1996b; Poizner, Klima, & Bellugi, 1987). These deficits have been noted both in production, and to varying degrees in comprehension. In production, a range of paraphasic error types have been identified in LHD signers, including "phonemic," morphological, and semantic subtypes, demonstrating the breakdown of these various levels of computation. Some examples of phonemic paraphasias are shown in Figure 32.1. Disorders in sign language sentence formation in LHD signers have emerged both in the form of agrammatism, a tendency to omit grammatical markers, and in the form of paragrammatism, a tendency toward grammatically rich but error prone utterances, showing that sentence-level computations can also be disrupted following LHD in deaf signers (Hickok & Bellugi, 2001; Hickok, Bellugi, & Klima, 1998a). Production errors at all these levels are fairly common in LHD signers, but occur relatively rarely in RHD signers. In our sample of over 50 unilateral brain injured signers, we have found only one RHD signer who was in fact aphasic on standard clinical-type assessment; this individual was left handed and had evidence of a reversed dominance pattern (Pickell et al., 2005). As for comprehension, we have documented deficits at the word (i.e., sign) and sentence level (Hickok, Klima, & Bellugi, 1996a; Hickok, Love-Geffen, &

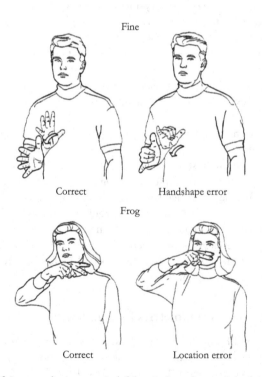

Figure 32.1 Examples of sign paraphasic errors in left hemisphere damaged deaf signers.

Klima, 2002). At the word level, comprehension deficits have been observed only following LHD, not RHD. These deficits are relatively mild and appear to result from breakdowns primarily at the postphonemic level (Hickok, Klima, Kritchevsky, & Bellugi, 1995). At the sentence level, the most severe deficits occur following LHD, but, consistent with findings in the hearing/speaking population, some difficulties in sentence comprehension can be found in RHD signers, particularly as sentence complexity increases (Hickok et al., 2002).

Group studies confirmed the generalizability of these case study observations. In an analysis of 13 LHD and 10 RHD signers, one study (Hickok et al., 1996a) found that LHD signers performed significantly worse than RHD signers on a range of standard language measures, including production, comprehension, naming, and repetition (Figure 32.2). These differences between LHD and RHD signers could not be attributed to variables such as: (a) age at test; (b) onset of deafness; or (c) age of exposure to ASL, as these variables did not correlate with any of the language behaviors tested. Further, reinforcing this finding, it was found that LHD versus RHD group differences showed the same patterns if only native signers were included in the analysis (Figure 32.2; Hickok et al., 2002). This is not to say that these variables have no impact on sign language organization or language ability, because surely they do at some level of detail (Neville et al., 1997; Newport & Meier, 1985), only that the dominant factor that predicts performance on these aphasia assessment measures is whether the left or right hemisphere is damaged.

Supra-sentential (discourse) deficits

One linguistic deficit associated with RHD in hearing/speaking individuals involves discourse-level processes, for example, the ability to appropriately link (in production and comprehension) discourse referents across multiple sentences (Brownell et al., 1986; Wapner et al., 1981). These deficits manifest as failures to integrate information across sentences, including impairments in understanding jokes, in making inferences, and in adhering to the story line when producing a narrative. In contrast, phonological and syntactic processes in these hearing/speaking individuals appear to be intact. Using a story narration task given to two deaf RHD signers, two distinct types of discourse deficits have been documented (Hickok et al., 1999). The first involves a failure to adhere to the story line, evidenced by confabulatory or tangential utterances. The second type of deficit involves errors in the use of the spatialized discourse of ASL. Discourse organization in ASL is unique in that discourse referents are established, referred to, and manipulated in a plane of signing space, and it was the ability to use this spatial mechanism in a discourse that was disrupted in one of the patients studied. These results suggest: (a) the right hemisphere is involved in discourse processing in ASL, as it is in spoken language; and (b) there are dissociable subcomponents of discourse processes in ASL.

Classifier constructions

American Sign Language contains an interesting type of construction, classifier signs, which is not typically assessed on standard aphasia exams in signed or spoken language. Classifier signs are complex forms that can be used to specify a range of spatial information, relative location, movement path, movement manner, object size and shape (see Emmorey, 2002 for a review). These forms are typically comprised of two parts: (1) a handshape configuration, where different handshapes can correspond to different semantic classes of object referents (e.g., people, vehicles, etc.), or to object shape-related properties (e.g., flat, narrow, etc.); and (2) a specification of the location or movement of the referent, denoted by the location/ movement of the hand(s) in signing space. The linguistic status of classifier forms is a matter of debate, but what is clear is that they differ from canonical lexical signs in that they can encode information, for example spatial information, non-categorically. Whereas a lexical sign like DRIVE-TO can indicate that a vehicle was driven from one place

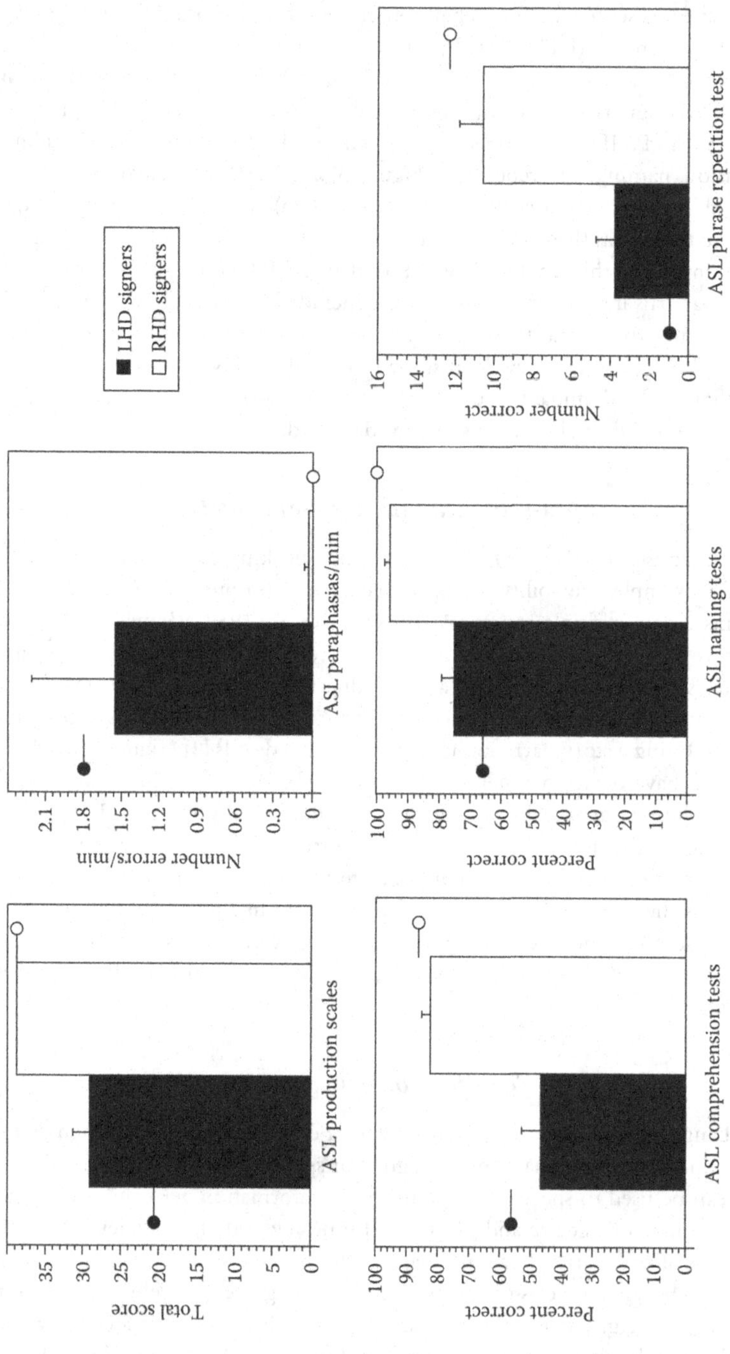

Figure 32.2 Performance of LHD and RHD signers on a range of standard aphasia assessments including production, naming, repetition, and comprehension. Circles indicate average values for the subset of the lesion population that includes only native deaf signers.

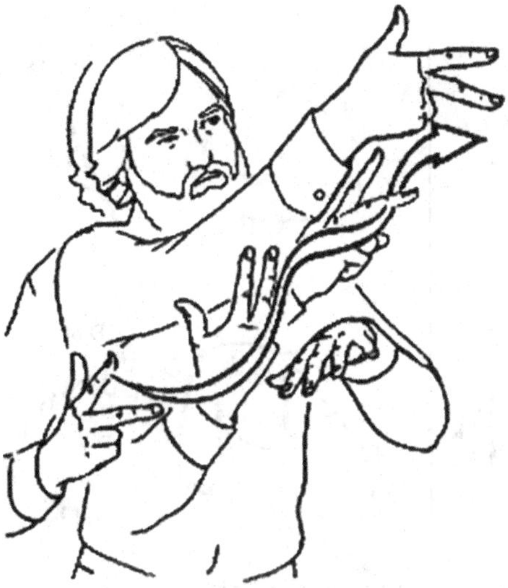

Figure 32.3 An example of classifier form use showing a "vehicle" handshape moving upward along a curvy path. (From Hickok, G., et al., Neuropsychologia, 47, 382–387, 2009. Reprinted with permission.)

to another, a classifier sign can convey more detailed information about the route traversed (e.g., it was curvy and uphill; Figure 32.3).

It has been suggested that the right hemisphere may be more involved in processing classifier signs than in processing canonical lexical signs (Hickok, Bellugi, & Klima, 1998b; Poizner et al., 1987), and a handful of recent functional imaging studies have provided some evidence supporting this idea. For example, a PET study by Emmorey et al. (2002), found that deaf native signers activated parietal regions bilaterally when describing spatial relations using ASL classifier signs (compared to naming objects). See Campbell and Woll (2003), for additional discussion.

A study of ASL production using a narrative task in 21 unilateral brain injured signers (13 LHD) reported that RHD signers made relatively few lexical errors but a substantial number of classifier errors. LHD signers made both lexical and classifier errors in roughly equal proportions. The source of the classifier errors is not clear. For example, it could be that classifier errors in RHD patients are caused by a fundamentally different deficit (e.g., some nonlinguistic spatial deficit) than those in LHD patients (e.g., linguistic form selection). What is clear is that the production of ASL classifier forms is supported to some extent both by the left and right hemispheres, whereas lexical sign production is under the control of predominantly left hemisphere systems.

Hemispheric asymmetries for spatial cognition

It appears that language functions have a similar hemispheric organization in deaf signers compared to hearing/speaking individuals. But what about nonlinguistic spatial functions? Might these abilities be differently organized in the brain of deaf signers? Available evidence suggests that the answer is no, and that the lateralization pattern of nonlinguistic spatial functions is also similar between deaf and hearing people.

Gross visuospatial deficits in RHD signers

RHD in hearing people often leads to substantial visuospatial deficits evidenced, in the most severe cases, by grossly distorted productions in drawing tasks and block arrangement tasks (Kirk & Kertesz, 1994). Deaf RHD signers can have similar kinds of deficits (Figure 32.4). Despite some-

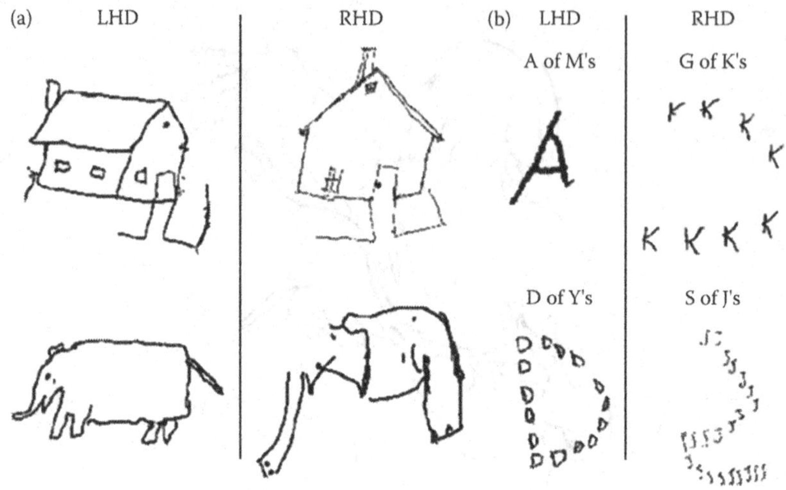

Figure 32.4 Example copy-from-sample drawings by LHD and RHD signers. Note that LHD signers are able to reproduce the basic configuration of the figures but may omit details, whereas the RHD signers often fail to reproduce the configural structure but include many details. Evidence of hemispatial neglect is also apparent in the RHD drawings. (From Hickok, G., et al., Brain and Language, 65, 276–286, 1998. Reprinted with permission.)

times severe nonlinguistic visuospatial impairments, none of the RHD signers had aphasia (Bellugi et al., 1989; Hickok et al., 1998a, 1996a; Poizner et al., 1987).

Local/global differences

While gross visuospatial deficits may more commonly occur with RHD (both in deaf and hearing populations), it has been reported that some visuospatial deficits can be reliably observed in LHD hearing individuals (Delis, Kiefner, & Fridlund, 1988; Kirk & Kertesz, 1994). When LHD individuals have visuospatial deficits, they typically involve difficulties in attending to and/or reproducing the local-level details of a visuospatial stimulus, while global-configuration aspects are correctly identified/reproduced. RHD individuals tend to show the opposite pattern. Thus, it has been suggested that the left hemisphere is important for local-level visuospatial processes, whereas the right hemisphere is important for global-level processes (Delis et al., 1988). Does a similar asymmetry hold for the deaf signing population? To answer this question a group of left or right lesioned deaf signers were asked to reproduce: (1) two line drawings (a house and an elephant); and (2) four hierarchical figures (e.g., the letter "D" composed of small "Y"s). Drawings were scored separately for the presence of local versus global features. Consistent with data from hearing patients, the LHD deaf subjects were significantly better at reproducing global-level features, whereas the RHD deaf subjects were significantly better at reproducing local-level features (Figure 32.4; Hickok, Kirk, & Bellugi, 1998).

Overall, available evidence suggests a similar pattern of hemispheric asymmetries for nonlinguistic spatial cognitive function in the deaf signer population.

Within hemisphere organization

Functional aspects: syndromes and symptoms

To the extent that the types and patterns of deficits found in sign language aphasia are similar to those found in spoken language aphasia, it would suggest a common functional organization for the two forms of language. There are many commonalities in individual language deficits found;

many of the aphasic symptom clusters that have been observed in LHD deaf signers fall within the bounds of classical clinical syndromes defined on the basis of hearing aphasics (Damasio, 1992; Goodglass, 1993; Goodglass & Kaplan, 1983). For example: (a) nonfluent aphasic signers have lesions involving anterior language regions; and (b) fluent aphasic signers have lesions involving posterior language regions. In addition, the range of common deficit types that have been reported in hearing aphasics have been observed regularly in sign language aphasia. Examples of these include the presence of word (i.e., sign) finding problems in most cases of aphasia, paraphasic errors, agrammatism, and the tendency for comprehension deficits to be more closely associated with fluent aphasia than with nonfluent aphasia. In addition, the brain lesions producing these patterns of deficits in LHD signers are roughly consistent with clinical-anatomic correlations in hearing people (Hickok, 1992; Hickok & Bellugi, 2001; Hickok et al., 1998a; Poizner et al., 1987). To a first approximation, the within hemisphere organization of signed and spoken language appear to be remarkably similar.

Role of Broca's area

Broca's area has figured prominently in attempts to determine the anatomy of speech production. We had the opportunity to investigate the role of Broca's area in sign language production through an in-depth case study of LHD-130, a congenitally deaf, native user of ASL, who suffered an ischemic infarct involving the frontal operculum and inferior portion of the primary motor cortex (Figure 32.5, top; Hickok et al., 1996b). Acutely, she presented with sign "mutism," consistent with what one might expect in a hearing/speaking individual. Chronically, she had good comprehension, fluent production with occasional sign finding problems, semantic paraphasias, and what appeared to be a deficit involving the ability to control bimanual movements during sign production. That deficit showed up: (a) in her tendency on one-handed signs, to "shadow," with her nondominant hand, sign-articulatory gestures carried out by her dominant hand; (b) in her tendency on two-handed signs, to assimilate the handshape and/or movement of the nondominant hand with that of the dominant hand; and (c) in her occasional failure to complete the movement of a two-handed sign when the movement's endpoint involved contact between the two hands (Figure 32.5, bottom). We were not able to find any evidence of a bimanual control deficit in nonlinguistic tasks. Blumstein (1995) has suggested that speech production errors in anterior aphasia reflect a breakdown at the phonetic (not phonemic) level caused by a loss of the ability to coordinate independent speech articulators (e.g., larynx, tongue, lips). For a signer, the two hands are independent articulators that are often required to perform independent (i.e., nonsymmetric) movements. The deficit observed in LHD-130 may represent the sign analogue of a phonetic-level breakdown. This case suggests that Broca's area plays an important role in sign production.

A case of sign blindness

"Pure Word Blindness" or "Alexia without Agraphia" has been well-documented in the literature (Friedman & Albert, 1985). Hearing/speaking patients with this disorder are typically blind in the right visual field (right homonymous hemianopia), have normal auditory-verbal language capacity, are able to write, but cannot read. The lesion typically involves left occipito-temporal cortex (explaining the visual field defect) and splenium of the corpus callosum. Language areas are thus preserved, allowing normal production, auditory comprehension, and writing, but according to the classical disconnection analysis of the syndrome (Geschwind, 1965), these areas are isolated from visual input (because of cortical blindness in the right visual field and deafferentation of information coming from the left visual field through the splenium). An alternative possibility is that the occipito-temporal lesion damages a visual word form area that directly affects perceptual reading

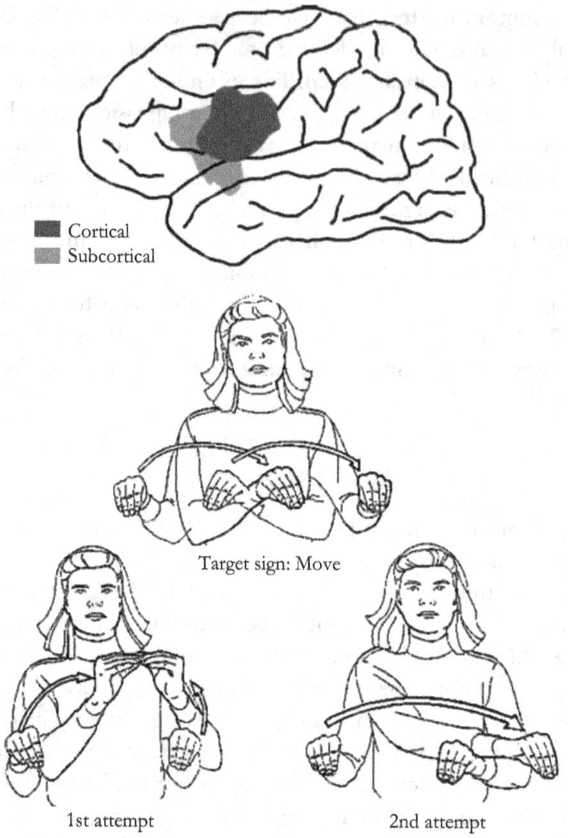

Figure 32.5 Reconstructed brain lesion in a native deaf signer with damage to Broca's region (top), and an example of her bimanual coordination deficit (bottom). (From Hickok, G., et al., Neurocase, 2, 373–380, 1996. Reprinted with permission.)

centers (Beversdorf, Ratcliffe, Rhodes, & Reeves, 1997). Either way, one wonders what effects such a lesion would have on sign language comprehension in a deaf signer.

We had the opportunity to study such a case (Hickok et al., 1995). LHD-111 had a lesion involving all of the left primary visual cortex, most of area 18, with some extension into medial aspects of the temporal lobe (area 37); this lesion also clearly involved white matter fibers lateral to the splenium (Figure 32.6, top). Consistent with the neurological effects of such a lesion in hearing subjects, the deaf patient had a right visual field blindness and was alexic (i.e., she couldn't read written English). Her sign language comprehension was profoundly impaired; she could not follow even simple one-step (ASL) commands such as "point to the floor" (Figure 32.6, bottom). Her single-sign comprehension was also significantly impaired although to a lesser extent than her sentence comprehension, and virtually all of her comprehension errors were semantic in nature. Her visual object recognition, however, was unimpaired: she had no problem naming line-drawings of objects presented to her visually. Her sign production was fluent and grammatical, although she did make occasional paraphasic errors. This case provides strong evidence favoring the view that the left hemisphere is dominant for the comprehension of ASL sentences in deaf individuals because it demonstrates that the right hemisphere by itself is severely constrained in its ability to process signed language. However, the case also suggests a more bilateral organization for early stages of processing in single sign recognition in that her comprehension errors seemed to indicate a semantically underspecified representation rather than a disruption of sign phonological infor-

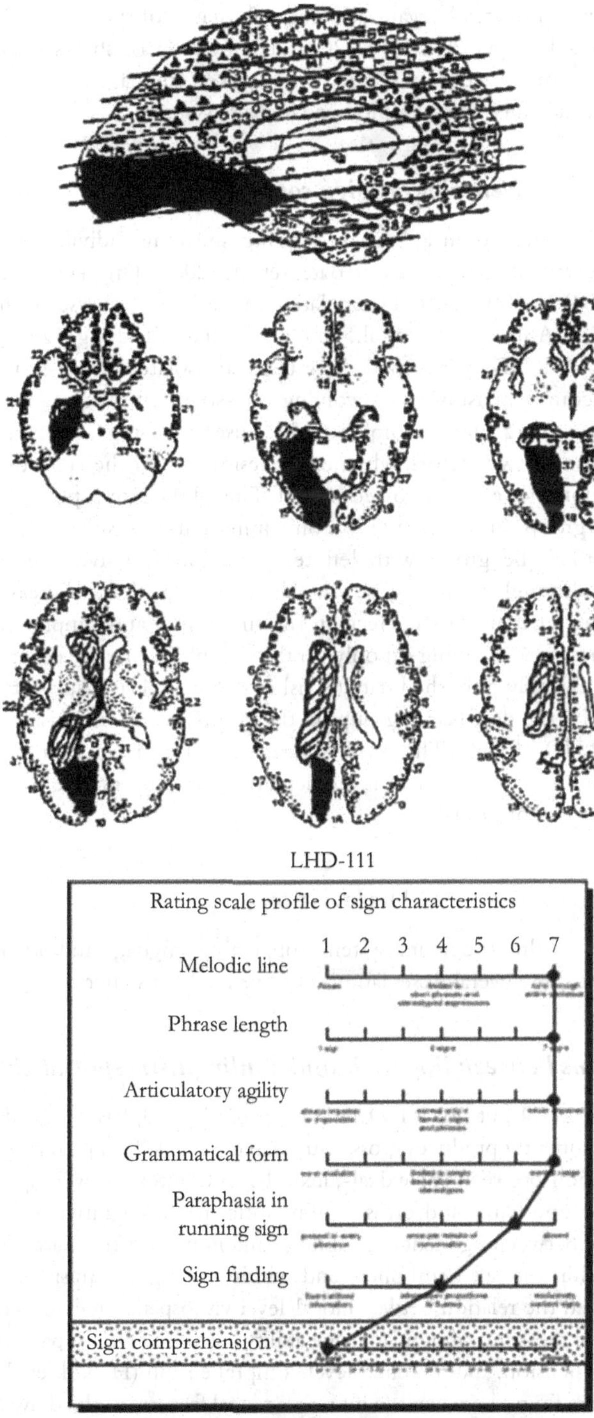

Figure 32.6 A left occipital lesion in a deaf signer (top), and a graph showing her rating profile of sign characteristics. Note the patient's production scales are in the normal or near normal range, whereas her sign comprehension is at floor. (From Hickok, G., et al., Neuropsychologia, 33, 1597–1606, 1995. Reprinted with permission.)

mation. A similar pattern of bilateral organization at early stages of spoken word recognition has been reported (Hickok & Poeppel, 2000, 2004, 2007). Finally, this case shows a dramatic difference in the within hemisphere organization of signed versus spoken language processing resulting from differences in the input modality between the two language systems.

Neurology of sign comprehension

Auditory comprehension deficits in aphasia in hearing/speaking individuals are most closely associated with left temporal lobe damage (Bates et al., 2003; Dronkers, Wilkins, Van Valin, Redfern, & Jaeger, 2004). We investigated the relative role of the left versus right temporal lobe in the comprehension of ASL (Hickok et al., 2002). Nineteen life-long signers with unilateral brain lesions (11 LHD, 8 RHD) performed three tasks, an isolated single-sign comprehension task, a sentence-level comprehension task involving one-step commands, and a sentence-level comprehension task involving more complex multiclause/multistep commands. Performance was examined in relation to two factors: whether the lesion was in the right or left hemisphere and whether the temporal lobe was involved or not. The LHD group performed significantly worse than the RHD group on all three tasks confirming left hemisphere dominance for sign language comprehension. The group with left temporal lobe involvement was significantly impaired on all tasks, although minimally so on the single-sign task, whereas the other three groups performed at better than 95% correct on the single sign and simple sentence comprehension tasks, with performance falling off only on the complex sentence comprehension items. A comparison with previously published data (Swisher & Sarno, 1969) suggests that the degree of difficulty exhibited by the deaf RHD group on the complex sentences is comparable to that observed in hearing RHD subjects. This result suggests that language comprehension, particularly at the lexical-semantic and sentence level, depends primarily on the integrity of the left temporal lobe, independent of modality.

Dissociations

The functional divisions within the neural systems supporting language and other cognitive abilities have been highlighted by several dissociations observed in deaf signers.

Dissociations between linguistic and nonlinguistic spatial abilities

It was noted above that LHD, but not RHD, frequently produces aphasia in deaf signers whereas RHD, but not LHD, frequently produces gross visuospatial deficits. This pattern of deficits constitutes a double dissociation between sublexical-, lexical-, and sentence-level aspects of spatialized linguistic ability on the one hand, and gross nonlinguistic spatial cognitive ability on the other. Additional dissociations between sign language abilities and nonlinguistic spatial abilities have been demonstrated both within the left hemisphere and within the right hemisphere. Within the left hemisphere we examined the relation between local-level visuospatial deficits evident on a drawing copy task and several measures of sign language ability, including rate of paraphasias in running sign, single sign comprehension, and sentence-level comprehension (Hickok et al., 1998). No significant correlations were found between the hit rate for local features in the drawing copy task and any of the sign language performance measures. In fact, cases were identified in which local-level scores were near perfect, yet scores on tests of sign language ability were among the worst in the sample. This suggests that aphasic deficits cannot be reduced to a more general deficit in local-level visuospatial processing. Within the right hemisphere, two case studies have provided evidence that the ability to use the spatialized referential system in ASL discourse does not depend substantially on nonlinguistic visuospatial abilities of the right hemisphere (Hickok et al., 1999). Case RHD-221 had severe visuospatial deficits following a large right perisylvian stroke, yet was not impaired in his ability to set up and utilize spatial loci for referential purposes. Case RHD-207 showed the reverse pattern. Her performance on standard visuospatial tasks was quite good, yet she had difficulty with spatialized aspects of ASL discourse. This finding hints at the possibility that there are nonidentical neural systems within the right hemisphere supporting spatialized discourse functions versus nonlinguistic spatial abilities.

Dissociations between sign and gesture

Evidence supporting the view that deficits in sign language are qualitatively different from deficits in the ability to produce and understand pantomimic gesture comes from a case study of an LHD signer (Corina et al., 1992). Following an ischemic infarct involving both anterior and posterior perisylvian regions, LHD-108 became aphasic for sign language. His comprehension was poor and his sign production was characterized by frequent paraphasias, reduced grammatical structure, and a tendency to substitute pantomime for ASL signs—a tendency not present prior to his stroke. These pantomimic gestures were used even in cases in which the gesture involved similar or more elaborate sequences of movements arguing against a complexity-based explanation of his performance. LHD-108 showed a similar dissociation in his comprehension of signs versus pantomime where he had more trouble matching a sign to a picture than matching a pantomimed gesture to picture. This case makes the point that disruptions in sign language ability are not merely the result of more general disruptions in the ability to communicate through symbolic gesture. Since this initial report, we have seen several additional patients who show a similar tendency to use gesture in place of lexical signs.

Evidence from functional neuroimaging

Lesion evidence has indicated clearly that hemispheric asymmetries for signed and spoken language are similar, and has provided some indication that the within hemisphere organization of signed language is similar in some ways to that of spoken language, but perhaps different in others. But the spatial resolution of the lesion method is relatively poor, particularly in a rare population, limiting the amount of information one can derive from lesion studies alone. Recent functional imaging studies have provided additional insights into the within hemisphere organization of sign language processing and has highlighted both similarities and differences.

Neural systems underlying signed language production

One of the first questions that neuroimaging studies of signed language sought to address was whether Broca's area—a putative speech production region—was involved in signed language production. Lesion evidence has suggested it was (see above) but functional imaging promised to shed additional light on the question and further to assess whether the same degree of left lateralization might be found in sign versus speech production. This was an open question because of the bimanual nature of signed language production. Several studies of signed language production have now been published using PET as well as fMRI methodologies (Corina, San Jose-Robertson, Guillemin, High, & Braun, 2003; Emmorey, Mehta, & Grabowski, 2007; Kassubek, Hickok, & Erhard, 2004; McGuire et al., 1997; Pa, Wilson, Pickell, Bellugi, & Hickok, 2008; Petitto et al., 2000). A consistent finding is that indeed Broca's area is involved in signed language production, and this activity is strongly left dominant; this is true even when the sign articulation involved one-handed signs produced with the nondominant hand (Corina et al., 2003). Such a result could be interpreted in one of two ways. Either a canonical "speech area," Broca's region, has been recruited to support manual language production in deaf signers, or Broca's area is not a speech-dedicated region. Given that Broca's area has been implicated in a range of nonspeech, even nonlanguage functions in the last several years (Fink et al., 2006; Schubotz & von Cramon, 2004), the latter possibility seems likely. More research is needed to sort out the functional organization of this brain region.

Language production is not merely a function of the frontal lobe. Regions of the posterior temporal lobe also play an important role in speech production (Hickok & Poeppel, 2007; Indefrey & Levelt, 2004). Signed language production also involves nonfrontal structures including some areas in the posterior inferior temporal lobe that appear to be shared with spoken language production (Emmorey et al., 2007). Signed language production also seems to recruit structures in the posterior parietal lobe that are unique to sign (Buchsbaum et al., 2005; Corina et al., 2003; Emmorey et al., 2007). The involvement of these regions may reflect sensory–motor functions that are specific to manual gestures (Buchsbaum et al., 2005; Emmorey et al., 2007).

Neural systems underlying sign language perception/comprehension

A number of studies of signed language perception have found activation of superior temporal regions; that is, regions that are also typically implicated in spoken language perception (Binder et al., 2000; Hickok & Poeppel, 2007). One of the early fMRI studies hinted that sign perception may involve a more bilateral network than processing spoken language (studied via written presentation; Neville et al., 1998), but subsequent work has shown similar lateralization patterns when sign perception is compared to audio-visually presented speech (MacSweeney et al., 2002). There are differences, however, in the within hemisphere activation pattern for the perception of signed and spoken language. Pa et al. (2008) presented ASL nonsigns and English nonwords (forms that are phonotactically permissible in their respective languages but do not correspond to a word) to bilingual hearing signers who had native-level proficiency in both languages (they were hearing offspring of deaf signing adults). This allowed the direct comparison of activation patterns for sign and speech perception within the same individual's brain. Sign perception activated large regions of occipito-temporal cortex, portions of the posterior superior temporal lobe bilaterally, posterior parietal cortex, and posterior frontal regions. Speech perception activated most of the superior temporal lobe and posterior frontal regions. Overlap between the two language forms was found in the posterior superior temporal cortex and in the posterior frontal lobe (Figure 32.7). Thus, speech activated auditory-related areas in the superior middle and anterior temporal lobe greater than sign (consistent with the input modality for speech), and sign activated visual-related areas in the ventral occipito-temporal lobe greater than speech (consistent with the input modality for speech). Sign also activated posterior parietal areas whereas speech did not, possibly reflecting visual-manual sensory–motor mechanisms.

One fMRI study attempted to identify regions that are specifically activated during sign perception above and beyond perception of nonlinguistic gestures (MacSweeney et al., 2004). These investigators showed videos of British Sign Language (BSL) or videos of a non–BSL gestural communication system ("TicTac," a gestural code used by racetrack bookmakers) to hearing nonsigners and deaf native signers of BSL. Deaf BSL signers showed greater activation in the left posterior superior temporal sulcus and temporal-parietal boundary during the perception of BSL compared to TicTac. Hearing nonsigners showed no differences in their brain response within this region (although there were differences elsewhere). It is unclear from these findings exactly what this brain region is doing with respect to sign language processing, however, it is interesting that in the study described above a very similar region showed responsivity to both speech and sign in hearing bilingual (English and ASL) signers. This hints that the region supports some type of linguistic specific function.

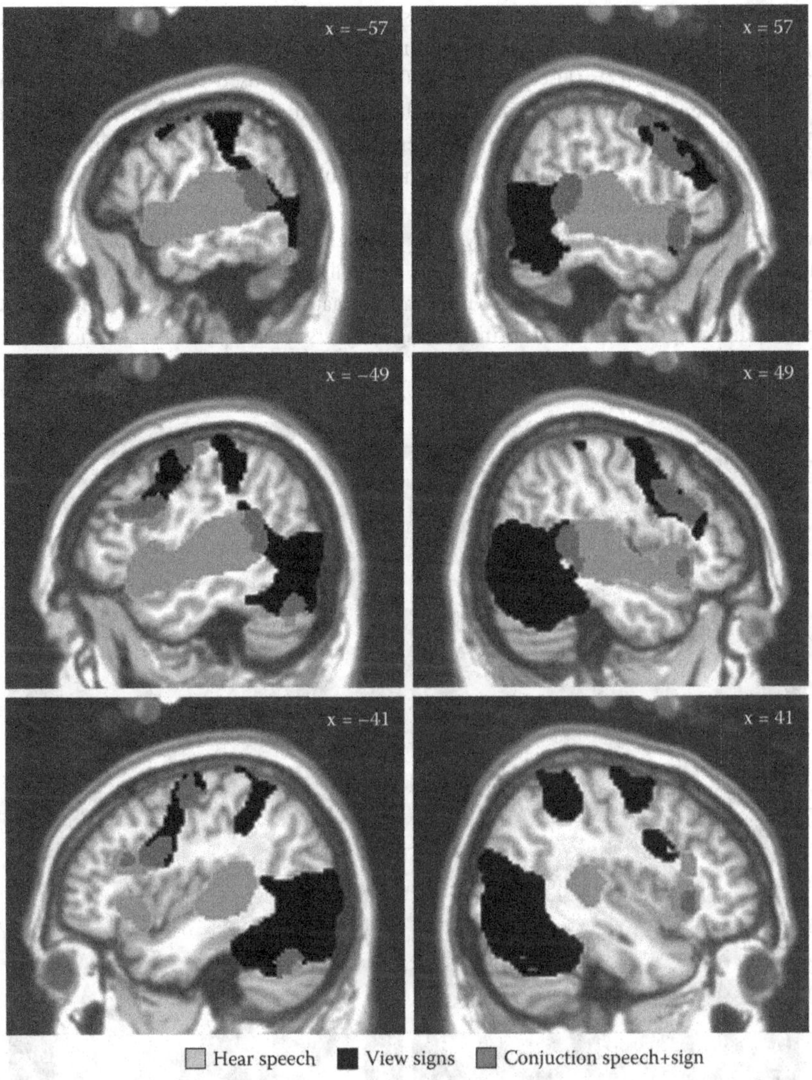

Figure 32.7 fMRI activations during the perception of speech versus sign in hearing bilingual (English and ASL) participants. (From Pa, J., et al., Journal of Cognitive Neuroscience, 20, 2198–2210, 2008. Reprinted with permission.)

Neural substrate for working memory for signs

The neural basis of sign language working memory is an area that has not received extensive attention, but one that has the potential for shedding light on some fundamental questions regarding short-term memory generally. For example, the nature of the representations maintained in verbal working memory is still open to debate. Some authors argue for sensory–motor based codes (modality-dependant; Buchsbaum & D'Esposito, 2008; Hickok, Buchsbaum, Humphries, & Muftuler, 2003; Wilson, 2001) while others promote a modality-independent model (Baddeley, 1992; Jones & Macken, 1996). Sign language provides a unique perspective on this issue because it is possible to manipulate the sensory–motor modality, while keeping the linguistic nature of the stimuli effectively constant. One can then ask, is the neural organization of working memory for an acoustic-vocal language different from that for a visual-manual language?

One study examined working memory for sign language in deaf native signers using fMRI (Buchsbaum et al., 2005) and compared its findings to a similar published study involving speech and hearing nonsigner subjects (Hickok et al., 2003). This study used a design with a several second delay period between encoding and recall, which allowed for the measurement of storage-related activity. The pattern of activation during the retention phase was substantially different from what had been found in hearing participants performing a similar task with speech. Short-term maintenance of sign language stimuli produced prominent activations in the posterior parietal lobe, which were not found in the speech study. This parietal activation was interpreted as a reflection of visual–motor integration processes. Posterior parietal regions have been implicated in visual–motor integration in both human and nonhuman primates (Andersen, 1997; Milner & Goodale, 1995), and studies of gesture-imitation in hearing subjects report parietal activation (Chaminade,

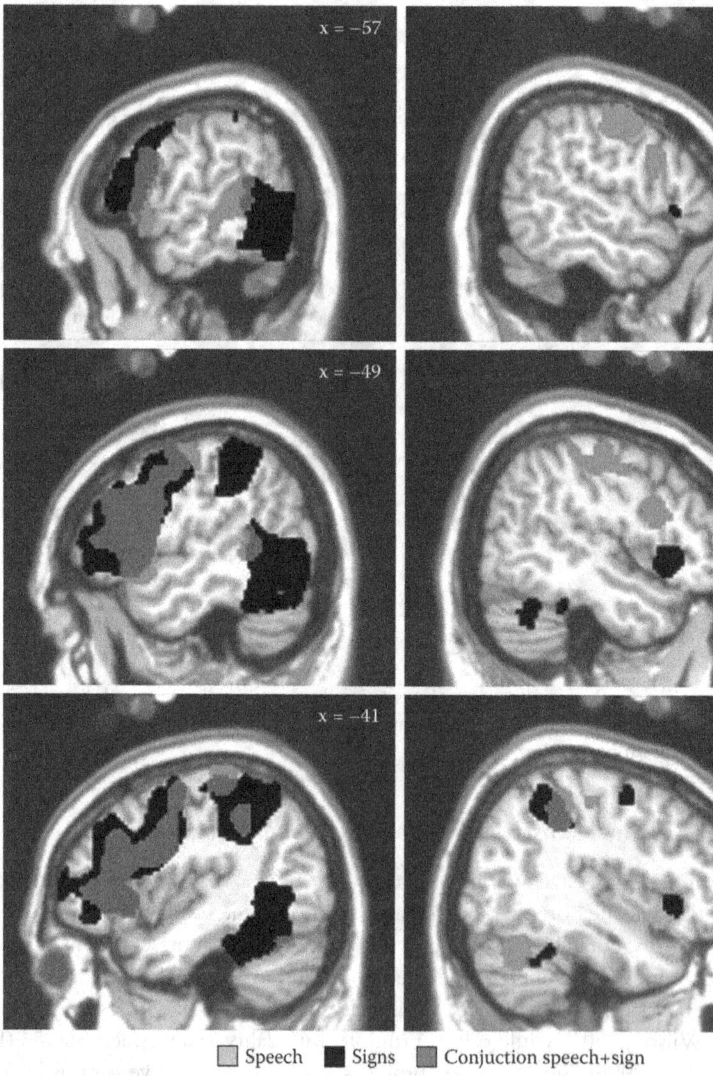

Figure 32.8 fMRI activations during the short-term maintenance of speech versus sign in hearing bilingual (English and ASL) participants. (From Pa, J., et al., Journal of Cognitive Neuroscience, 20, 2198–2210, 2008. Reprinted with permission.)

Meltzoff, & Decety, 2005). It seems likely, therefore, that parietal activation in an STM task for sign language does not reflect activity of a sensory store, but instead results from sensory–motor processes underlying the interaction of storage and manual articulatory rehearsal. Additional maintenance activity was found in the posterior superior temporal lobe, as well as in posterior frontal regions, both of which have been shown to activate during maintenance of speech information, suggestive of some form of common process. However, because cross-modality comparisons could only be made between subjects and studies, it is difficult to make solid inferences about patterns of overlap and dissociation. No maintenance activity was found in visual-related areas in that study, such as the ventral temporal–occipital regions that are so strongly activated during sign perception. Activation in these regions would provide more convincing support for sensory-dependent working memory storage systems.

A follow-up study directly compared working memory for signed and spoken language using hearing bilinguals (native in English and ASL; Pa et al., 2008). This study clearly demonstrated sensory modality-specific activity in working memory. Delay activity was found in left ventral occipito-temporal (i.e., visual) areas during sign maintenance but not for speech maintenance, whereas delay activity was found in left superior temporal (i.e., auditory) areas for speech maintenance but not sign maintenance. However, regions of overlap were also noted in both lateral frontal lobe regions as well as a small focus in the posterior superior temporal lobe (Figure 32.8). These findings indicate there may be both modality dependent and modality independent components to working memory for linguistic stimuli.

Summary

The lateralization pattern of neural systems supporting sign language processing is remarkably similar to that found for spoken language. Likewise, the patterns of aphasic deficits found among brain injured deaf signers are quite recognizable in the context of aphasiological research on hearing individuals with acquired language disorders. However, differences in the neural organization of signed and spoken language processing have emerged in recent years. These differences appear to be tied to the unique sensory–motor demands of the two language forms.

Further reading

Caselli, N. K., & Pyers, J. E. (2020). Degree and not type of iconicity affects sign language vocabulary acquisition. *Journal of Experimental Psychology: Learning, Memory, and Cognition, 46*(1), 127.

Krebs, J., Malaia, E., Wilbur, R. B., & Roehm, D. (2021). Psycholinguistic mechanisms of classifier processing in sign language. *Journal of Experimental Psychology: Learning, Memory, and Cognition, 47*(6), 998.

References

Andersen, R. (1997). Multimodal integration for the representation of space in the posterior parietal cortex. *Philosophical Transactions of the Royal Society of London B: Biological Sciences, 352*(1360), 1421–1428.

Baddeley, A. D. (1992). Working memory. *Science, 255*(5044), 556–559.

Bates, E., Wilson, S. M., Saygin, A. P., Dick, F., Sereno, M. I., Knight, R. T., & Dronkers, N. F. (2003). Voxel-based lesion-symptom mapping. *Nature Neuroscience, 6*(5), 448–450.

Bellugi, U., Poizner, H., & Klima, E. (1989). Language, modality, and the brain. *Trends in Neurosciences, 10*, 380–388.

Beversdorf, D. Q., Ratcliffe, N. R., Rhodes, C. H., & Reeves, A. G. (1997). Pure alexia: Clinical-pathologic evidence for a lateralized visual language association cortex. *Clinical Neuropathology, 16*(6), 328–331.

Binder, J. R., Frost, J. A., Hammeke, T. A., Bellgowan, P. S., Springer, J. A., Kaufman, J. N., & Possing, E. T. (2000). Human temporal lobe activation by speech and non-speech sounds. *Cerebral Cortex, 10*(5), 512–528.

Blumstein, S. (1995). The neurobiology of the sound structure of language. In M. S. Gazzaniga (Ed.), *The cognitive neurosciences* (pp. 913–929). Cambridge, MA: MIT Press.

Brownell, H. H., Potter, H. H., Bihrle, A. M., & Gardner, H. (1986). Inference deficits in right brain-damaged patients. *Brain and Language, 27*(2), 310–321.
Buchsbaum, B. R., & D'Esposito, M. (2008). The search for the phonological store: From loop to convolution. *Journal of Cognitive Neuroscience, 20*(5), 762–778.
Buchsbaum, B. R., Pickell, B., Love, T., Hatrak, M., Bellugi, U., & Hickok, G. (2005). Neural substrates for verbal working memory in deaf signers: fMRI study and lesion case report. *Brain and Language, 95*(2), 265–272.
Campbell, R., & Woll, B. (2003). Space is special in sign. *Trends in Cognitive Sciences,* 7(1), 5–7.
Chaminade, T., Meltzoff, A. N., & Decety, J. (2005). An fMRI study of imitation: Action representation and body schema. *Neuropsychologia, 43*(1), 115–127.
Corina, D. P., Poizner, H., Bellugi, U., Feinberg, T., Dowd, D., & O'Grady-Batch, L. (1992). Dissociation between linguistic and non-linguistic gestural systems: A case for compositionality. *Brain and Language, 43*(3), 414–447.
Corina, D. P., San Jose-Robertson, L., Guillemin, A., High, J., & Braun, A. R. (2003). Language lateralization in a bimanual language. *Journal of Cognitive Neuroscience, 15*(5), 718–730.
Damasio, A. R. (1992). Aphasia. *New England Journal of Medicine, 326*(8), 531–539.
Delis, D. C., Kiefner, M. G., & Fridlund, A. J. (1988). Visuospatial dysfunction following unilateral brain damage: Dissociations in hierarchical and hemispatial analysis. *Journal of Clinical and Experimental Neuropsychology, 10*(4), 421–431.
Dronkers, N. F., Wilkins, D. P., Van Valin Jr., R. D., Redfern, B. B., & Jaeger, J. J. (2004). Lesion analysis of brain regions involved in language comprehension. *Cognition, 92*(1–2), 145–177. (special issue entitled, "The New Functional Anatomy of Language", eds., G. Hickok & D. Poeppel).
Emmorey, K. (2002). *Language, cognition, and the brain: Insights from sign language research.* Mahwah: Lawrence Erlbaum and Associates.
Emmorey, K., Damasio, H., McCullough, S., Grabowski, T., Ponto, L. L., Hichwa, R. D., & Bellugi, U. (2002). Neural systems underlying spatial language in American sign language. *Neuroimage, 17*(2), 812–824.
Emmorey, K., Mehta, S., & Grabowski, T. J. (2007). The neural correlates of sign versus word production. *Neuroimage, 36*(1), 202–208.
Fink, G. R., Manjaly, Z. M., Stephan, K. E., Gurd, J. M., Zilles, K., Amunts, K., & Marshal, J. C. (2006). A role for Broca's area beyond language processing: Evidence from neuropsychology and fMRI. In Y. Grodzinsky & K. Amunts (Eds.), *Broca's region* (pp. 254–268). Oxford, UK: Oxford University Press.
Friedman, R. B., & Albert, M. L. (1985). Alexia. In K. M. Heilman & E. Valenstein (Eds.), *Clinical neuropsychology.* New York: Oxford University Press.
Geschwind, N. (1965). Disconnexion syndromes in animals and man. *Brain, 88,* 237–294, 585–644.
Goodglass, H. (1993). *Understanding aphasia.* San Diego, CA: Academic Press.
Goodglass, H., & Kaplan, E. (1983). *The assessment of aphasia and related disorders* (2nd ed.). Philadelphia: Lea & Febiger.
Hickok, G. (1992). *Agrammatic comprehension and the trace-deletion hypothesis (Occasional Paper 45).* Cambridge, MA: MIT Center for Cognitive Science.
Hickok, G., & Bellugi, U. (2001). The signs of aphasia. In R. S. Berndt (Ed.), *Handbook of neuropsychology,* (2nd ed., Vol. 3, pp. 31–50). New York: Elsevier.
Hickok, G., & Poeppel, D. (2000). Towards a functional neuroanatomy of speech perception. *Trends in Cognitive Sciences, 4*(4), 131–138.
Hickok, G., & Poeppel, D. (2004). Dorsal and ventral streams: A framework for understanding aspects of the functional anatomy of language. *Cognition, 92*(1–2), 67–99.
Hickok, G., & Poeppel, D. (2007). The cortical organization of speech processing. *Nature Reviews. Neuroscience, 8*(5), 393–402.
Hickok, G., Klima, E., Kritchevsky, M., & Bellugi, U. (1995). A case of "sign blindness" following left occipital damage in a deaf signer. *Neuropsychologia, 33*(12), 1597–1606.
Hickok, G., Klima, E. S., & Bellugi, U. (1996a). The neurobiology of signed language and its implications for the neural basis of language. *Nature, 381,* 699–702.
Hickok, G., Kritchevsky, M., Bellugi, U., & Klima, E. S. (1996b). The role of the left frontal operculum in sign language aphasia. *Neurocase, 2*(5), 373–380.
Hickok, G., Bellugi, U., & Klima, E. S. (1998a). The neural organization of language: Evidence from sign language aphasia. *Trends in Cognitive Sciences, 2*(4), 129–136.
Hickok, G., Bellugi, U., & Klima, E. S. (1998b). What's right about the neural organization of sign language? A perspective on recent neuroimaging results. *Trends in Cognitive Science, 2*(12), 465–468.
Hickok, G., Kirk, K., & Bellugi, U. (1998c). Hemispheric organization of local- and global-level visuospatial processes in deaf signers and its relation to sign language aphasia. *Brain and Language, 65*(2), 276–286.

Hickok, G., Wilson, M., Clark, K., Klima, E. S., Kritchevsky, M., & Bellugi, U. (1999). Discourse deficits following right hemisphere damage in deaf signers. *Brain and Language*, *66*(2), 233–248.

Hickok, G., Love-Geffen, T., & Klima, E. S. (2002). Role of the left hemisphere in sign language comprehension. *Brain and Language*, *82*(2), 167–178.

Hickok, G., Buchsbaum, B., Humphries, C., & Muftuler, T. (2003). Auditory-motor interaction revealed by fMRI: Speech, music, and working memory in area Spt. *Journal of Cognitive Neuroscience*, *15*(5), 673–682.

Hickok, G., Pickell, H., Klima, E. S., & Bellugi, U. (2009). Neural dissociation in the production of lexical versus classifiers signs in ASL: Distinct patterns of hemispheric asymmetry. *Neuropsychologia*, *47*(2), 382–387.

Hillis, A. E. (2007). Aphasia: Progress in the last quarter of a century. *Neurology*, *69*(2), 200–213.

Indefrey, P., & Levelt, W. J. (2004). The spatial and temporal signatures of word production components. *Cognition*, *92*(1–2), 101–144.

Jones, D. M., & Macken, W. J. (1996). Irrelevant tones produce an irrelevant speech effect: Implications for phonological coding in working memory. *Journal of Experimental Psychology: Learning, Memory, and Cognition*, *19*(2), 369–381.

Kassubek, J., Hickok, G., & Erhard, P. (2004). Involvement of classical anterior and posterior language areas in sign language production, as investigated by 4 T functional magnetic resonance imaging. *Neuroscience Letters*, *364*(3), 168–172.

Kirk, A., & Kertesz, A. (1994). Localization of lesions in constructional impairment. In A. Kertesz (Ed.), *Localization and neuroimaging in neuropsychology* (pp. 525–544). San Diego: Academic Press.

Klima, E., & Bellugi, U. (1979). *The signs of language*. Cambridge, MA: Harvard University Press.

MacSweeney, M., Woll, B., Campbell, R., McGuire, P. K., David, A. S., Williams, S. C., ... Brammer, M. J. (2002). Neural systems underlying British Sign Language and audio-visual English processing in native users. *Brain*, *125*(7), 1583–1593.

MacSweeney, M., Campbell, R., Woll, B., Giampietro, V., David, A. S., McGuire, P. K., ... & Brammer, M. J. (2004). Dissociating linguistic and nonlinguistic gestural communication in the brain. *Neuroimage*, *22*(4), 1605–1618.

McGuire, P. K., Robertson, D., Thacker, A., David, A. S., Kitson, N., Frackowiak, R. S., & Frith, C. D. (1997). Neural correlates of thinking in sign language. *NeuroReport*, *8*(3), 695–698.

Milner, A. D., & Goodale, M. A. (1995). *The visual brain in action*. Oxford, UK: Oxford University Press.

Neville, H. J., Coffey, S. A., Lawson, D. S., Fischer, A., Emmorey, K., & Bellugi, U. (1997). Neural systems mediating American sign language: Effects of sensory experience and age of acquisition. *Brain and Language*, *57*(3), 285–308.

Neville, H. J., Bavelier, D., Corina, D., Rauschecker, J., Karni, A., Lalwani, A., ... Turner, R. (1998). Cerebral organization for language in deaf and hearing subjects: Biological constraints and effects of experience. *Proceedings of the National Academy of Sciences*, *95*(3), 922–929.

Newport, E., & Meier, R. (1985). The acquisition of American sign language. In D. I. Slobin (Ed.), *The crosslinguistic study of language acquisition: Volume 1: The data* (pp. 881–938). Hillsdale: LEA.

Pa, J., Wilson, S. M., Pickell, B., Bellugi, U., & Hickok, G. (2008). Neural organization of linguistic short-term memory is sensory modality-dependent: Evidence from signed and spoken language. *Journal of Cognitive Neuroscience*, *20*(12), 2198–2210.

Petitto, L. A., Zatorre, R. J., Gauna, K., Nikelski, E. J., Dostie, D., & Evans, A. C. (2000). Speech-like cerebral activity in profoundly deaf people processing signed languages: Implications for the neural basis of human language. *Proceedings of the National Academy of Sciences*, *97*(25), 13961–13966.

Pickell, H., Klima, E., Love, T., Kritchevsky, M., Bellugi, U., & Hickok, G. (2005). Sign language aphasia following right hemisphere damage in a left-hander: A case of reversed cerebral dominance in a deaf signer? *Neurocase*, *11*(3), 194–203.

Poizner, H., Klima, E. S., & Bellugi, U. (1987). *What the hands reveal about the brain*. Cambridge, MA: MIT Press.

Schubotz, R. I., & von Cramon, D. Y. (2004). Sequences of abstract nonbiological stimuli share ventral premotor cortex with action observation and imagery. *Journal of Neuroscience*, *24*(24), 5467–5474.

Swisher, L. P., & Sarno, M. T. (1969). Token Test scores of three matched patient groups: Left brain-damaged with aphasia, right brain-damaged without aphasia, non-brain damaged. *Cortex*, *5*(3), 264–273.

Tallal, P., Miller, S., & Fitch, R. H. (1993). Neurobiological basis of speech: A case for the preeminence of temporal processing. *Annals of the New York Academy of Sciences*, *682*, 27–47.

Wapner, W., Hamby, S., & Gardner, H. (1981). The role of the right hemisphere in the apprehension of complex linguistic materials. *Brain and Language*, *14*(1), 15–33.

Wilson, M. (2001). The case for sensorimotor coding in working memory. *Psychonomic Bulletin and Review*, *8*(1), 44–57.

33

SIGN LANGUAGE AND SIGN LANGUAGE RESEARCH

Myriam Vermeerbergen and Mieke Van Herreweghe

Introduction

The first version of this chapter was written in 2008, almost 15 years ago. Although during this period, the domain of sign language linguistics has seen several important developments, sign languages themselves obviously haven't changed all that much and our approach to and understanding of these visual-gestural languages have also largely remained the same. Therefore, we have chosen to maintain most of our chapter from the 2010 edition of this book with only minimal changes. This concerns the sections titled "The linguistic status of sign languages," "Some salient characteristics of sign languages," and "Two important developments in sign linguistics." The last part of the chapter, originally titled "Sign language research today" is obviously very dated and needed revision. Hence, the title of the new section is "Sign language research – from 2010 to today."

The linguistic status of sign language

In the past, sign languages were generally ignored, not only in mainstream society, but also in linguistic research. The main reason for this indifference was that sign languages were not considered to be genuine natural languages. Before the start of modern sign linguistics, it was often assumed that all deaf people across the world used a kind of universal, primitive system of gestures and pantomime. At the same time, many people seemed (and some still seem) to believe that *sign language* is nothing but a word for word transliteration of the local spoken language in which the signs are produced simultaneously with the spoken (content) words. Neither assumption is correct and these false beliefs only gradually started to change after the publication of the book *Sign Language Structure* by the American linguist Stokoe in 1960. One of the effects of the publication was that interest into sign linguistics was steadily aroused, and today, even though still not all linguists and non-linguists are equally convinced of the linguistic status of sign languages, linguistic research into sign languages has conquered a solid position in various linguistic subdisciplines. Among other things, Stokoe maintained in this book that the signs used in American Sign Language (or ASL) should not be considered unanalyzable wholes but should be regarded as consisting of various smaller meaning-distinguishing component parts. As such he was the first to show that a sign language exhibits *duality of patterning*, exactly as is the case for spoken languages.[1] ASL could be considered a genuine human language as in mainstream linguistics duality of patterning is considered to be a:

DOI: 10.4324/9781003204213-38

> defining property of human language, which sees language as structurally organized into two abstract levels; also called double articulation. At one level, language is analysed into combinations of meaningful units (such as words and sentences); at the other level, it is analysed as a sequence of phonological segments which lack meaning.
>
> *(Crystal, 1999, p. 94)*

Stokoe's (1960) first modern linguistic analysis of a sign language[2] received a great deal of attention and particularly during the 1970s other researchers began to express an interest in the linguistic structure of signs and sign languages, first mainly in the USA, and from the 1980s onwards also in other countries. This has led to detailed analyses of ASL and other sign languages in various linguistic domains. Providing a survey of all of this research lies outside the scope of this paper, but to give some idea, attention has been paid to various aspects in phonetics/phonology (Loncke, 1983 and Demey, 2005 for Flemish Sign Language; Van der Kooij, 2002 and Crasborn, 2001 for Sign Language of the Netherlands), morphology (Bergman, 1983 for Swedish Sign Language; Pizzuto, 1986 for Italian Sign Language; Engberg-Pedersen, 1993 for Danish Sign Language; Brennan, 1990 for British Sign Language), syntax (Deuchar, 1984 for British Sign Language; Vermeerbergen, 1996 and 1997 for Flemish Sign Language; Rissanen, 1986 for Finnish Sign Language), lexicography/lexicology (Johnston, 1989 for Australian Sign Language; De Weerdt, Vanhecke, Van Herreweghe, & Vermeerbergen, 2003 for Flemish Sign Language), and so on.[3]

Early modern sign linguistics often emphasized the differences between sign languages. Publications from the 1970s and 1980s regularly begin by stating that there is not one universal sign language but instead many different, mutually unintelligible sign languages.[4] At that time, cross-linguistic sign language studies were rare, and the limited amount of comparative research mainly concentrated on the lexicon, more specifically on signs belonging to the established lexicon. Towards and in the 1990s, there was an increase in the number of sign languages being studied (although this evolution remained mostly limited to North America, Australia, and Western Europe). Johnston (1989, p. 208) noted in his doctoral dissertation on Auslan or Australian Sign Language:

> Overall, fragmentary studies of parts of the grammar of a number of natural sign languages do nonetheless contribute to an impression of shared syntactic patterning across sign languages. The lexical diversity among sign languages – long established and recognised – remains a valid observation. Only now, as studies such as the present are being made of other sign languages, is the degree of commonality among sign languages on the grammatical level coming to light.

Apart from such *explicit* references to the similarities between the grammars of different sign languages, it seemed to be common practice for researchers to compare their own interpretation of a specific grammatical mechanism in sign language A to the interpretation of another researcher studying the same mechanism in sign language B as if both researchers were dealing with one and the same language – or at least with one and the same mechanism across the sign languages (e.g., Van Herreweghe, 1995). From this, it seemed that a high degree of similarity was at least implicitly assumed. And indeed, the overall picture one got from the body of sign language literature available at that time was that sign languages are typologically more similar than spoken languages.

However, with the increasing number of cross-linguistic analyses and typological studies and the addition of previously unstudied or understudied languages the field moved on again. Some of the cross-linguistic studies seemed to confirm the high degree of similarity between sign languages (which may lead scholars to comment on this issue, e.g., Liddell, Vogt-Svendsen, & Bergman, 2007) whereas other studies, often involving more "exotic" sign languages (e.g., Nyst, 2007), seemed to point at more variation than previously assumed. There is clearly a need for much more comparative work – and for yet more sign languages to be documented – before more conclusive answers can be given. Nevertheless, the similarities that were found between different sign languages have been attributed to a number of different reasons, both internally linguistic and sociolinguistic. Johnston (1989, p. 211) discusses

> four major constraints on grammatical organization to show how they variously contribute to produce particular characteristics of Auslan and other sign languages. The four constraints are: 1) the visual-gestural nature of sign languages, 2) the absence of a written form for sign languages, 3) the unique contact features of sign languages and their host languages, and 4) the patterns of acquisition of sign languages by their speakers.

Woll (2003, p. 25) adds a number of mutually compatible and to some extent overlapping reasons of which (a) iconicity and (b) a link between sign languages and gesture are the most relevant here.

Since these characteristics seem to be defining factors for many (or maybe even all?) sign languages, we shall briefly discuss them in the following section.

Some salient characteristics of sign language

A visual-gestural modality

Sign languages make use of the visual-gestural modality and this opens up structural possibilities that are not – or to a (much) lesser extent – available for spoken languages, which are oral-aural languages. These possibilities are: (1) the use of three dimensional space for linguistic expression; and (2) the availability of a range of articulators, including both hands and arms, the torso, the mouth and the eyes, as well as other parts of the face. As a result, rather than showing a primarily linear patterning similar to that of spoken languages, sign languages exhibit a highly simultaneous organization .[5]

In the VGT-utterance the construction illustrated in Figure 33.1 has been taken from, the signer expresses the actions of a cat sitting on a fence looking tight from left to right. The dominant hand refers to the figure (the cat) while the non-dominant hand represents the ground (the fence). The way these manual articulators are positioned in signing space is meaningful; the spatial arrangement not only reflects the locative relation between figure and ground but also expresses the position

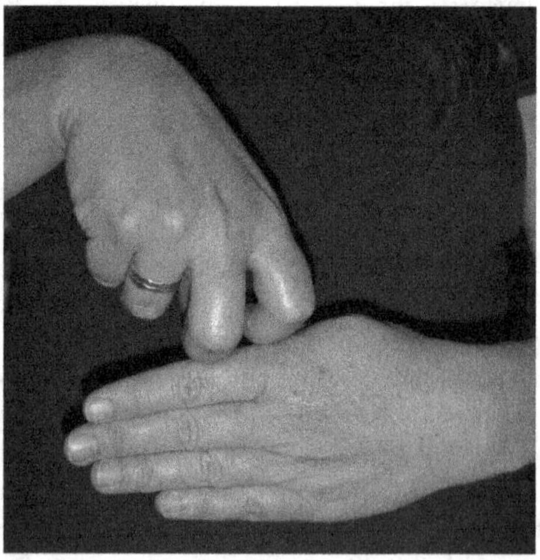

FIGURE 33.1 "Classifier construction" in VGT referring to a cat sitting on a fence.

of the fence relative to other parts of the scene (for example, the house from which the narrator witnesses the event).[6] In order to further refer to the cat's activities and emotional state the signer moves her head and uses her eye-gaze and facial expressions, which results in an even higher level of simultaneous organization.

The utterance discussed here is an example of *multichannel simultaneity involving non-manual articulators other than the mouth.* This type of simultaneity is often related to the simultaneous expression of different elements of a multifaceted event or to the simultaneous expression of different points of view (Leeson & Saeed, 2007; Perniss, 2007; Sallandre, 2007). It can also occur with non-manual sentence type marking; in order to "transfer" a positive declarative sentence into a negative one, users of a wide range of sign languages may simply combine the manual part of the sentence (in the same word – or sign – order) with a headshake. Furthermore, the same utterance can become a (negative) polar question by adding a nonmanual marker to the same sequence of signs. The non-manual marker typically consists of "a combination of several features, including raised eyebrows, wide open eyes, eye contact with the addressee, and a forward head and/or body position" (Zeshan, 2006b, p. 40).

Many examples of simultaneity described in the literature involve *manual simultaneity* where each hand is used to convey different information. This may take the form of one hand holding a sign in a stationary configuration while the other hand produces one or more other signs. In an example from Flemish Sign Language, the signer narrates a scene from an animated movie. The signer first explains that the two main characters are driving in a car and are being followed by two men in a second car. The final sign in this utterance is FOLLOW, which is produced with two "fist-with-thumb-up" hand configurations, each representing one car. After the production of this sign, one hand remains in place, still showing the "fist-with-thumb-up" configuration, while the dominant hand produces the following signs:[7]

Example 33.1

Right hand: FOLLOW // Ps KNOW NOTHING BEHIND FOLLOW // Ps STOP

Left hand: FOLLOW --

"They (*i.e., the men in the first car*) don't know they are being followed. They stop."

Thus, the sign FOLLOW is "held" by the left hand, while the other hand continues to sign the rest of the story (Vermeerbergen & Demey, 2007, p. 269).

Examples such as the one above contrast with cases of *full manual simultaneity*; that is, the simultaneous production of two different full lexical items. With full manual simultaneity, one of the two signs that are simultaneously produced often shows a relatively simple form, for example, a pointing sign (Ps) or a numeral (handshape). In the following example, again taken from Flemish Sign Language, the sign simultaneously produced by the nondominant hand is a Ps directed towards a locus previously associated with a specific boy (Vermeerbergen & Demey, 2007, p. 270):

Example 33.2

Right hand: GRAND^PARENTS DEAF GRAND^PARENTS

Left hand: Ps --------------------------

"His grandparents are deaf." or "He has deaf grandparents."

Finally, *manual-oral simultaneity* occurs when the oral and manual channels are used at the same time, for example, when a manual sign is combined with the (silent) production of a spoken word (so-called *mouthings*, see also further down). Often the meaning of the mouthing and the manual sign is related, for example, when a signer signs SIT and produces the mouthing "sit," but in some cases the mouthing is combined with a sign that is morphologically and/or lexically unrelated, for example, when a Flemish signer produces SIT and simultaneously (silently) articulates the Dutch word "op" (on) resulting in the meaning "sit on." Other examples of manual-oral simultaneity involve *mouth gestures*: activities of the mouth that are unrelated to spoken languages, such as the use of a fff-sound when manually signing the meaning "fill-with-water-from-tap" (Vermeerbergen & Demey, 2007, p. 261).[8]

With regard to the use of space in sign languages, it should be noted that space is not only used to convey spatial information, for example, to express the locative relationship between different referents as in Figure 33.1, but also to encode grammatical information. In most – if not all – of the sign languages described so far, space is used as a medium to express agreement with a certain group of verbs. In order to indicate the relationship between the verb and its argument(s), the signer may alter the movement, orientation or place of articulation of the verb with respect to the location of the argument(s). An example of a spatially modified verb in Flemish Sign Language is the verb sign INVITE. The production of this sign always involves a linear horizontal movement of the hand, but the signer can relocate the beginning and end points of the movement. If the arguments of the verb are actually present, the movement begins close to (or in the direction of) the body of the "invited referent" and the end point relates to the actual location of the "inviting referent." If a referent is not present, the signer may decide to establish a *locus*, that is, s/he may relate the non-present referent to a certain area in space. In order to talk about her non-present colleague, for example, a signer can produce the signs MY and COLLEAGUE and consequently point at a certain area or locus in signing space. This area now "represents" the colleague. The choice of a locus is often motivated, for example, when that particular colleague was in the room before, the signer will most probably choose a locus in relation to the place where s/he was actually standing, sitting, … while s/he was present. Or the locus is related to his/her now empty chair/desk/office. After having established the loci for two referents, for example, "colleague" and "son," INVITE can be produced with a movement away from the locus for "son" and towards the locus for "colleague", meaning "the/my colleague invited his/her son" (or: "the son was invited by my colleague"). Loci can also be pointed at, for example for the purpose of anaphoric reference, another example of nonlocative use of signing space.

The example shown in Figure 33.2 from Flemish Sign Language illustrates both the use of space and the simultaneous use of a range of manual and nonmanual articulators. The sentence contains only one single manual sign: the verb sign INVITE, but its spatial configuration results in the

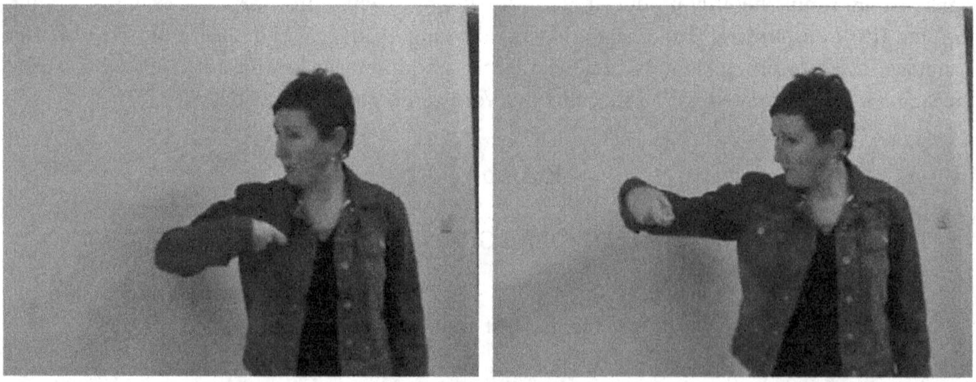

FIGURE 33.2 VGT-sentence meaning "Don't/Didn't you invite me?"

"incorporation" of the patient "I/me" and the agent "You": "you invite me" (or: "I am invited by you"). The manual production is combined with a headshake to add a negative reading and there is also nonmanual polar question marking (see Figure 33.2). This whole combination results in the expression of the utterance "Don't/Didn't you invite me?".

An atypical acquisition process

In most western countries it is maintained that 90 to 95% of deaf children have hearing parents (Schein, 1989), so that only 5 to 10% of deaf children have deaf parents and are as such potential "native signers". The majority of deaf children are born to hearing parents who are not likely to know any sign language. Most of these children start acquiring the local sign language only when beginning (pre)school. This can be quite early in life, e.g., in Belgium preschool starts at the age of two years and six months, but the first contact with (a form of) the local sign language may sometimes be much later, for example, in a recent past in South Africa some children occasionally only started attending school at age 11 or 12 (Van Herreweghe & Vermeerbergen, 2010, p. 129), either because their deafness was only detected later and/or because schooling is not deemed important by or simply not possible for the parents. Sometimes such children develop a form of what is called "home signing" in the literature, which is a form of gestural communication "invented" by deaf children, together with one or more of their hearing relatives, when these children are not able to spontaneously acquire a spoken language and at the same time are not exposed to a conventional sign language (Goldin-Meadow, 2003; Mylander & Goldin-Meadow, 1991).[9] It is possible that these early home sign systems have a certain influence on an individual's later sign language acquisition and usage, and also on the language itself. Especially in deaf communities where a good number of the signers have gone through a similar pattern of development and where many of them did not come into contact with the conventional sign language until later in life, the impact of home sign systems on the community sign language may be far-reaching. Following Labov's "Uniformitarian Principle" (Labov, 1972), what happens now may have happened in the past as well. It may well be that for sign languages such as Flemish Sign Language or American Sign Language, which are used in a community in which today (most) deaf children have access to an adequate language model relatively early in life (so that the use of home sign systems may be more limited, at least in length of time), there once was a time when there was more homesigning and possibly also more contact between home sign systems and the community sign language. Hence the structure of the sign language as we know it today, may have been influenced by home sign systems in the past. It will be clear to the reader that many questions regarding the impact of home sign systems on the structure of sign languages remain to be explored, including questions related to the significance of home signing in communities where usable language models are available relatively early in the lives of deaf children.

Moreover, because of the atypical acquisition process, schools for the deaf, especially if they are residential schools, play an important role in the development of sign languages. In many countries sign languages are not widely used as medium of instruction in deaf education. The language of instruction in the deaf classroom is not a signed language but a spoken language (possibly in its written form) and/or a "signed spoken language"; that is, a (simplified form of the) spoken language combined with signs (Loncke, 1990), also known as "sign supported speech" or "simultaneous communication". Consequently, in the (residential) deaf schools significant deaf peers function as linguistic role models, rather than significant hearing adults. Nevertheless, in the last decades there have been important changes in this respect. On the one hand, in some (residential) deaf schools there has been a movement towards bilingual–bicultural education with more and more deaf adults being active in deaf education and as such also functioning as linguistic role models. At the same time, especially in Western countries, there has been a movement towards mainstream education, so that deaf adults/peers are not or no longer present as linguistic role models in the lives of many young deaf mainstreamed pupils, especially in those countries where the degree of cochlear implantation is high. In the latter countries in particular, many deaf adults are concerned about the survival of their Deaf communities (Johnston, 2004; Meurant, Sinte, Van Herreweghe, & Vermeerbergen, 2013).

The unique contact features with the surrounding spoken language

One of the factors by which all sign languages seem to be influenced is/are the surrounding spoken language(s), especially in their written form. Since sign languages have only recently begun to be written down, there is no tradition of literacy in any sign language to date. That means that

> literacy in any signing community is, strictly speaking, always literacy of another language (usually the host spoken language) rather than knowledge of a written form of sign. It is possible for this knowledge of the host spoken language to interfere with and influence the sign language of the community lexically and grammatically.
>
> *(Johnston, 1989, p. 234)*

This also means that sign languages and spoken languages have a different function: the sign language will be the preferred language for face-to-face communication with other signers, whereas the spoken language will mostly be used in written forms of communication and in interactions with hearing people, since most hearing people don't sign and interpreters are not always available. Moreover, sign languages are not as prestigious as spoken languages. In some countries many people – both deaf and hearing – do not consider sign languages as bona fide languages to be used in society, but as a form of in-crowd code (see, e.g., Raičević Bajić, Gordana, Gordić, Mouvet, & Van Herreweghe, 2021 for a recent study). Signers' knowledge and use of (the written form of) a spoken language may leave its mark on their sign language:

> For example, in Flanders, the northern part of Belgium, the influence from spoken Dutch can be seen in the lexicon and possibly also the grammar of VGT (Vlaamse Gebarentaal or Flemish Sign Language) (cf. Van Herreweghe and Vermeerbergen 2004, Vermeerbergen 2006). One example from the lexicon is the parallelism between Dutch compounds and VGT compounds; often Dutch compounds such as *schoonbroer* (meaning *brother-in-law* but in fact a compound consisting of *beautiful* and *brother*) are also compounds in VGT consisting of the same component parts (SCHOON^BROER). [...] It should be noted here that the influence from a spoken language on a signed language may be the result of "direct import" from the oral language (i.e. the language in its spoken/written form), or may be related to the knowledge and use of a signed spoken language (i.e. the "signed version" of the spoken language).
>
> *(Akach, Demey, Matabane, Van Herreweghe & Vermeerbergen, 2009, p. 337)*

Other direct influences from the surrounding spoken language can be seen in finger spelling (which constitutes direct borrowing from the spoken language into the sign language) and the fact that a sign, especially a sign from the established or *frozen* lexicon, can be accompanied by a *mouthing* that refers to a mouth pattern derived from the equivalent word in the surrounding spoken language (Boyes, Braem, & Sutton-Spence, 2001). As already mentioned, mouthing leads to manual-oral simultaneity. However, mouthing can sometimes be misleading, in that people seem to think that the lexical properties of the spoken word are automatically transferred to the lexical properties of the sign. Needless to say, that this is not necessarily the case.

Sign languages as oral or face-to-face languages

Sign languages are in essence *oral* or *face-to-face* languages and as such they are better comparable to spoken languages in nonliterate communities than to spoken languages with a long tradition of literacy. One of the characteristics that sign language communities have in common with nonliterate spoken language communities is that "they have a much wider and tolerant concept of acceptability that takes into account innovation and improvisation with no clear idea of 'right' or 'wrong' or even of what is 'grammatical' in sign language" (Johnston, 1989, p. 232). This lack of codification and the fact that these oral tradition languages are not used in education seems to have led to more variation and a greater instability in the lexicon and maybe also in the grammar "and there is no reason why the characteristics known to result from the lack of a written form in spoken languages should not be there for sign languages" (Vermeerbergen, 2006, p. 179). The influence of a "strictly oral tradition" on language structure has been well documented (Ong, 1982; Givón, 1979). Johnston (1989, p. 233) gives the following example:

> In particular, both parataxis and topicalization seem to be strongly encouraged by the face to face, unplanned nature of communications in sign language which are always rooted in a shared communicative context between signer and addressee (e.g., Ochs, 1979). Topic-prominence can thus be seen to stem from both (a) conversational face to face discourse patterning of oral cultures and (b) the need to locate in space the agreement point.

Iconicity

Another intrinsically linguistic characteristic that all sign languages have in common is iconicity that can be found at different levels of linguistic organization. Taub defines "pure iconicity" as follows:

> Let me give a strict definition of those items which I consider purely iconic. In iconic items, some aspect of the item's physical form (shape, sound, temporal structure, etc.) resembles a concrete sensory image. That is, a linguistic item that involves only iconicity can represent only a concrete, physical referent (...). Thus, ASL TREE (...), whose form resembles the shape of a prototypical tree, is purely iconic: Its form directly resembles its meaning.
>
> *(Taub, 2001, pp. 20–21)*

In sign languages iconicity is far more pervasive than in spoken languages since "objects in the external world tend to have more visual than auditory associations. Many entities and actions have salient visual characteristics. It is difficult (...) to imagine any characteristic sounds which might be associated with any of these meanings" (Deuchar, 1984, p. 12). Still, iconicity does not lead to complete transparency and thus to complete similarity between sign languages in the world, since also culture, conventionalization, and conceptualization need to be taken into account. In certain sign languages, WATER is signed by means of a sign referring to the sea, in other sign languages the sign refers to a tap, in yet other sign languages, the sign mirrors a drinking action. All these signs can be considered iconic, yet they are clearly different from each other:

> Iconicity is not an objective relationship between image and referent; rather, it is a relationship between our mental models of image and referent. These models are partially motivated by our embodied experiences common to all humans and partially by our experiences in particular cultures and societies.
>
> *(Taub, 2001, pp. 19–20)*

For some time, one of the central questions in sign phonology was whether iconicity plays a part in the linguistic structure of sign languages. Put more simply: Do sublexical elements carry meaning? This is an important question with respect to the phonological or morphological status of sublexical elements (i.e., the elements signs are composed of). Traditionally sub-lexical elements have been characterized in terms of place of articulation, movement, handshape and orientation and as such they have been characterized as phonemes (i.e., meaningless elements). However, take for instance the handshape featuring an extended index-finger (the handshape often used to point at things), with the finger pointing upwards. In some signs, for example, MEET in Flemish Sign Language and a number of other sign languages, the form of this handshape can be associated with an upright person and as such it can be said to carry meaning. A second, related, question is: When signers use the handshape just mentioned as part of a sign (e.g., MEET in Flemish Sign Language), are they aware of the form-meaning association? Do they only use this handshape to refer to one upright person and not a bent one for instance, or to two people meeting two other people, or is this irrelevant? If sublexical elements carry meaning, that conflicts with the idea that signs – like words – are composed of phonemes (i.e., meaningless but meaning-distinguishing sub-lexical elements) and as such with duality of patterning (see the first section of this chapter). Demey (2005) tries to resolve this enigma by proposing the idea that the sublexical form elements have potential meaningfulness, but this meaningfulness need not be accessed. The sign language user has the possibility to step into

> an iconic superstructure that can remotivate the sublexical form-meaning relations. This superstructure offers the language user the possibility – either productively or receptively – to relate a phonetic form element directly with a meaning. Nevertheless, as stated before, the *potential* meaningfulness of sublexical form elements does not indicate a modality difference between sign languages and spoken languages. Iconic – or otherwise motivated – relations between form and meaning can be found in both signed and spoken languages. However, the enormous potentiality of the visual-gestural signal for iconic motivation, and specifically for image iconicity, is a modality consequence.
>
> *(Demey, Van Herreweghe, & Vermeerbergen, 2008, p. 212)*

Iconicity is an undeniable characteristic of sign languages, present at all levels of organization. However, iconicity also exists in spoken languages. It cannot only be found in onomatopoeia, but also in intonation, in sound symbolism, and so on. The two modalities (sign and speech) "do not produce differences in kind, but only in degree"

(Demey, Van Herreweghe, & Vermeerbergen, 2008, p. 212).

A link between sign languages and gesture?

Because in the early stages of sign linguistics the linguistic status of sign languages was emphasized, attention for the presence of gesture in sign language usage was obscured. However, that has clearly changed. Some of the more recent analyses seem to provide support for a model of sign language structure that incorporates both linguistic and gestural elements (e.g., Liddell, 2003a; Schembri, 2001; Schembri, Jones, & Burnham, 2005; Vermeerbergen & Demey, 2007, among others). From our own cross-linguistic study of aspects of the grammars of Flemish Sign Language and South African Sign Language (Vermeerbergen, Van Herreweghe, Akach, & Matabane, 2007; Van Herreweghe & Vermeerbergen, 2008) it has become clear that a different choice of data can lead to very different answers to the question of whether or not gesture is a part of sign language production. Narratives resulting from a description of picture stories are a completely different set of data when compared to elicited sentences produced in isolation. *Visual imagery* for instance, is much more prominent in the narratives than in the isolated sentences and it is exactly in the domain of visual imagery that there is overlap with gesture. A very clear example is *constructed action*; that is, the narrator's construction of another person's actions (Metzger, 1995), which seems to be very similar in sign languages and in gesture (Liddell & Metzger, 1998). As part of the study just mentioned both a Flemish signer and a South African signer used constructed action to personify a pigeon which comfortably sits down on a nest with three eggs to start brooding. This is very similar in both signed stories. The relation between gesture and sign language will be further discussed in the final part of this chapter.

Two important developments in sign linguistics

Moving away from a description of sign languages as essentially analogous to spoken languages

The early days of modern sign linguistics showed the desire to emphasize the equivalence of the linguistic status of sign languages and spoken languages. Characteristics that seem to be more typical of sign languages were often ignored, minimized, or interpreted as being comparable to certain spoken language mechanisms (see e.g., Johnston, 1989, for a discussion of the minimization of the importance of iconicity). Moreover, the theories, categories, terminology, and so on, developed and used for spoken language research were considered appropriate for the analysis and description of sign languages as well.[10] Since the 1990s, in part because the status of sign languages has become established, there is a growing interest in the properties typical of (although not always unique to) sign languages. It is also less taken for granted that spoken language research tools automatically "fit" sign language research. This evolution will be briefly illustrated here with regard to: (1) the use of space in verb agreement; and (2) the analysis of classifiers and classifier constructions (see also Vermeerbergen, 2006).

The use of space in verb agreement

As already explained, in many sign languages the form of certain verb signs may be adapted in order to spatially refer to one or more of the arguments of the verb, whether they are present or non-present referents. For non-present referents, signers may establish loci, which can also be used for pronominal reference.

In the (earlier) literature (especially on ASL, e.g., Padden, 1988a; Poizner, Klima, & Bellugi, 1987), the use of space in such spatialized grammatical mechanisms is differentiated from "spatial mapping techniques." The latter are said to occur in "topographical space," in which very detailed representations of locative relations can be visualized. The "syntactic space" on the other hand is used to express syntactic or semantic non-locative information mostly through the use of loci. A locus in this type of space is described as an "arbitrary, abstract point" in space "referring" to a certain referent, but its actual location in signing space is considered to be irrelevant. In the 1970s and 1980s we generally see similar interpretations of the use of syntactic space for agreement verbs (also called "inflecting verbs") and – in connection with this – the use of loci. These interpretations are expressed in grammatical terminology which is regarded as analogous to "agreement" in spoken language, for example, morpheme, cliticization, pronoun, agreement in person and number, and so forth.

In the 1990s the clear-cut distinction between "spatial mapping" and "spatialized syntax" was being questioned (e.g., Bos (1990) for Sign Language of the Netherlands, Johnston (1991) for Australian Sign Language, Engberg-Pedersen (1993) for Danish Sign Language and Vermeerbergen (1998) for Flemish Sign Language):

> It is argued that the spatialised representation is, for at least part of the syntactical mechanisms, not based on "abstract linguistic properties" (Poizner et al., 1987, p. 211) but on the inherent locative relationships among real world people, objects and places. At the same

> time Engberg-Pedersen (1993) and Liddell (1990) challenge the interpretation of a locus as an arbitrary, abstract
>
> point in space. They argue that instead a locus should be seen as a "referent projection" (Engberg-Pedersen, 1993, p. 18) or as being based on the real-world location and extension of imagined referents (Liddell, 1990).
>
> *(Vermeerbergen 2006, p. 176)*

Liddell (2003a) moves even further on this path and considers the directionality in ASL verb signs such as GIVE[11] to be gestural in nature. He analyses these spatially modified signs as being composed of a linguistic part expressed by the handshape, type of movement and certain aspects of the hand's orientation, and a gestural part relating the sign to a locus. (Vermeerbergen 2006, pp. 176–177). Agreement verbs (or *indicating verbs* as Liddell calls them) are thus considered to be heterogeneous elements, partly linguistic and partly gestural.

The analysis of classifiers and classifier constructions

In many sign languages, signers may "represent" referents by means of a handshape or a combination of a handshape and a specific orientation of the hand. This is illustrated in Figure 33.1 in this chapter, where one hand refers to a (sitting) cat and the other hand to a fence. Such handshapes are generally called "classifiers," a notion introduced in the sign language literature by Frishberg (1975) in a paper on historical change in American Sign Language. As can be seen from the example in this chapter, aspects of the form or dimensions of the referent (usually) play an important part in the choice of a certain (classifier) handshape. In some earlier descriptions (e.g., McDonald, 1982; Supalla, 1978), sign languages are compared to predicate classifier languages, such as the Athapaskan languages, which represent one of the four types in Allan's (1977) typology of spoken classifier languages (Engberg-Pedersen, 1993). This parallel between classifiers and classifier constructions in sign languages on the one hand and classificatory verbs in Athapaskan languages, especially in Navaho, on the other hand, often quoted in (earlier) sign language publications, was (later) shown to be problematic (Engberg-Pedersen, 1993; Schembri, 2003). This, among other reasons, has led a number of sign linguists to argue against an analysis of the handshape in these so-called "classifier constructions" as classifiers (see Schembri, 2003, for an elaborate discussion of this issue). The idea that all component parts of these constructions are discrete, listable and specified in the grammar of individual sign languages, each having morphemic status (e.g., Supalla, 1982) has also been questioned.[12] Some sign linguists consider the possibility of dealing with mixed forms; that is, structures involving both linguistic and "nonlinguistic components"[13] (e.g., Liddell, 2003a; Schembri, Jones, & Burnham, 2005), which is closer to the view of Cogill-Koez (2000), who argues that a "classifier construction" may be a visual representation of an action, event, or spatial relationship rather than a lexical or a productive sign.

A growing number of sign languages studied

A second important development in the field of sign linguistics relates to the number of sign languages studied. In the early stages of sign linguistics most of the research concerned ASL and there was very little cross-linguistic research. According to Perniss, Pfau, and Steinbach (2007) this last issue remained unchanged in the "postmodern area starting in the 1980s" when sign language researchers continued to focus on a comparison of sign languages to spoken languages. Since the turn of century, however, there has been a growing interest in the cross-linguistic comparison of sign languages. Whereas most cross-linguistic analyses involve a limited number of sign languages (often two or three), there are also some larger scale typological projects (Zeshan & Perniss, 2008; Zeshan, 2006a). At the same time, the number of sign languages being studied is increasing and now also includes (more) non-Western sign languages as well as previously un(der)studied

(Eastern) European sign languages (e.g., Indo-Pakistan Sign Language, Adamorobe Sign Language, Jordanian Sign Language, Croatian Sign Language).

Sign language research – from 2010 to today

As announced in the preface, this section of the chapter is not, like the previous sections, taken from the 2010 edition, but it rather is almost completely new. In the last 15 years, the field of sign language research has greatly expanded and evolved. Therefore, we have to limit ourselves to some of the most important developments: the continued increase in the number of sign languages studied and the diversity within them; the relationship between gesture and sign; the creation of sign language corpora; and recent research on automatic sign language recognition and translation.

More and other sign languages

The evolution outlined above with respect to the increasing number of sign languages being studied has continued over the past 15 years. Not only the number of (non-) institutionalized macro-community sign languages being studied has increased, research into micro-community sign languages, i.e., sign languages used in small and sometimes very isolated language communities, has expanded too (de Vos, 2012; Schuit, 2014; Safar, 2020, among others). Often these are indigenous signed languages used in areas with high incidences of congenital deafness (Zeshan & de Vos, 2012). Research on *homesign* is increasingly focusing on adult homesigners (e.g., Richie, Yang, & Coppola, 2014; Safar & de Vos, 2022) rather than children. Also worth mentioning is the study of International Sign. *International Sign* (IS) is not a specific signed language but rather refers to a set of variable communicative practices used for the interaction between signers who do not share a common sign language (Rosenstock & Napier, 2016). It is a translanguaging practice. Different forms of IS vary depending on the signers involved and on the setting. IS may be created ad hoc when two signers with different sign languages meet for the first time, but it is also used in formal international contexts, such as meetings and congresses of the World Federation of the Deaf, Deaflympics and other international sports events and academic conferences. International institutions and organisations increasingly offer IS interpreting services and there now also is an accreditation system for International Sign interpreters.

The communicative success of IS is linked to various factors, including shared contextual knowledge and shared knowledge of a spoken language (Hiddinga & Crasborn, 2011).

Gesture and/in sign languages

Another evolution that had started earlier but has gained in importance in recent years is the attention paid to the relationship between sign languages and gesture. Certain structures and mechanisms appear to be used by both signers and speakers in a surprisingly similar way (Vermeerbergen & Demey, 2007). Examples here include pointing gestures/signs and *list buoys*. When using a list buoy, the extended fingers of the non-dominant hand are used to refer (back) to the elements of an ordered list, for example, children within a family or the different dishes from a menu (Liddell, 2003a). The use of list buoys has been described for several sign languages and also occurs in the co-speech gesture of speakers of several spoken languages. Moreover, in the last decade considerable attention has been paid to enactment in sign languages (Ferrara, 2012; Ferrara & Hodge, 2018; Beukeleers, 2020; see Beukeleers & Vermeerbergen, 2022 for an overview). The terms *enactment* or *enacting gestures* are often used interchangeably with the slightly older notion of *constructed action* (cf. the section on "A link between sign languages and gesture?") to refer to the use of the signer's body (the head, face, arms and torso) to represent the thoughts, feelings or actions of a referent using the surrounding space on a real-world scale. The practice of demonstrating the thoughts, words or actions of referents is also available in the multi-modal communicative repertoire of speakers. The study of enactment by signers and speakers further illustrates that when the communication of signers and speakers is being compared, it is speech in combination with (co-speech) gesture – and not speech by itself – that constitutes the appropriate level for cross-linguistic analysis (Vermeerbergen & Demey, 2007).

This premise, along with the increasing interest in multi-modal approaches to spoken languages, including the role of prosody, eye-gaze, and manual and non-manual gesture, helps ensure that the division between the fields of gesture research, sign language research, and spoken language research gradually diminishes.

Sign languages corpora

In the early days of sign language research, sign language data were recorded on video-tapes and transcription was done by means of pencil and paper while viewing the data with a video player that would, at best, allow the researcher to view the recording in slow motion. This obviously had an impact on the size of the corpus that could be studied: a corpus consisting of ten hours of data was considered to be a very large corpus (Vermeerbergen & Nilsson, 2018).

Today, for a growing number of sign languages, a comprehensive corpus, maximally representative of the language and its users, has been or is being created (Van Herreweghe & Vermeerbergen, 2012). One of the first (if not *the* first) large-scale sign language corpus projects was the corpus of American Sign Language (ASL) collected by Ceil Lucas, Robert Bayley, and their team. In the course of 1995, they collected data in seven cities in the United States that were considered to be representative of the major areas of the country (see, for instance, Lucas, Bayley, & Valli, 2001). However, their corpus is not machine-readable. Sign language corpora are only machine-readable when transcriptions and/or annotations are included. According to Johnston (2010) two types of annotation are essential: ID glossing and a translation into a written language. The first projects to build a machine-readable sign language corpus began in 2004 in Australia and in Ireland, soon followed by a number of similar projects for other European signed languages, including Flemish Sign Language. The Flemish Sign Language Corpus contains approximately 140 hours of digital video recordings of naturalistic and elicited signing, by 119 native or near-native deaf men and women from the five regions in Flanders, aged between 12 and 90 (Van Herreweghe, Vermeerbergen, Demey, De Durpel, Nyffels, & Verstraete, 2015; www.corpusvgt.be).

Sign language corpora obviously make it possible to verify and, where necessary, revise the results of earlier research, which was often based on the sign language production of a limited number of signers. Furthermore, modern corpora also make it possible to ask research questions that are impossible to answer without a comprehensive, machine-readable corpus, questions about frequency, for example, or about stylistic or sociolinguistic variation. However, a major problem with respect to corpora is the time required for annotation of the data. This turns out to be so labor intensive and time consuming that for almost all existing sign language corpora only a minority of the data has been annotated.

Automatic sign (languages) recognition and translation

It is hoped that the annotation of sign language data can be facilitated in the future through automatic sign language recognition and/or translation. Research into automatic sign language recognition, automatic sign language translation, and Avatar technology is not really new, but until fairly recently the research projects were, as it were, outside the domain of sign language linguistics. Cormier, Fox, Woll, Zisserman, Camgöz, & Bowden (2019) state that "part of the problem is that most computer scientists in this research area do not have the required in-depth knowledge of sign language, and often have no connection with the Deaf community or sign linguists. For example, one project described as translation into sign language aimed to take subtitles and turn them into fingerspelling. This is one of many reasons why much of this technology, including sign-language gloves, simply doesn't address the challenges." Fortunately, this has changed in recent years. There are currently at least four large-scale multidisciplinary projects working on automatic sign language recognition/translation and involving sign language researchers: the English ExTOL project (https://cvssp.org/projects/extol), the German GIGA- Gebärdensprache project (https://www.wi.uni-muenster.de/news/4131-nrw-funding-project-giga-gebardensprache), and two European funded Horizon 2020 projects, i.e., the SignON project (https://signon-project.eu) and the EASIER project (https://www.project-easier.eu).

Important in such projects is not only the interdisciplinary collaboration between sign language researchers, computer scientists, and experts in AI, but also the involvement of the Deaf community (Krausneker & Schügerl, 2022). This is particularly important in view of the existing suspicion towards avatar technology and the fear that this technology will be seen by policy makers as an alternative for sign language interpreters (World Federation of the Deaf, 2018), but it is also important with respect to "expectation management." It is unlikely that in the near future these research projects will lead to machine translation programs for sign languages comparable to the current capabilities and quality of, e.g., Deep-L and Google Translate (McDonnald et al., 2021).

In conclusion

In the preface to the revised version of this chapter, we wrote that sign languages haven't changed all that much, but that is not quite correct. For at least some sign languages, it may be the case that they are currently undergoing significant changes. For example, greater access to tertiary education for deaf signers, often involving educational sign language interpreting, may lead to an exponential growth of the lexicon and most probably also to the development of a formal/informal register (Meurant, Sinte, Van Herreweghe, & Vermeerbergen, 2013). Recent technological developments, in turn, make it possible to use sign languages for remote communication, both for real-time (online) communication, and for recording video messages that will only be viewed at a later time. This means that sign languages are no longer used exclusively for communication between interlocutors who are in the same place at the same time. Research into the potential impact of this on the linguistic structure of sign languages has only very recently begun.

Whereas only 50 years ago sign language researchers often felt they needed to explain and prove that studying a sign language is indeed genuine linguistics, today it is clear – and accepted – that a better understanding of various aspects of the structure and use of sign languages constitutes an important contribution to a better understanding of human multi-modal communication. Also, thanks to some more recent developments within the research on spoken languages, as briefly outlined above, and an increasing specialization among sign language researchers (Vermeerbergen & Nilsson, 2018), sign language research no longer is a highly specific, segregated, research domain.

Notes

1 However, the focus on duality of patterning in sign languages only started later (Padden, 1988b; Siple, 1982).

2 In fact, Stokoe was not the first to study a sign language. In 1953, the Dutch linguist Tervoort had presented a doctoral dissertation on the use of signs by deaf children, but his work remained largely unknown for quite some time, and what's more, he didn't present his work as research on a "sign language" but talked about an "esoteric language" of deaf children.

3 For a fuller bibliography we would like to refer the reader to the International Bibliography of Sign Language compiled by Joachim and Prillwitz (1993) and the more recent bibliography focusing on 2008–2017 published by Brill (https://www.jstor.org/stable/10.1163/j.ctv2gjwnkg).

4 Woll (2003, p. 20) mentions the following studies: Baker and Cokely, 1980; Fischer, 1974; Klima and Bellugi, 1979; Kyle and Woll, 1985; Lane, 1977; Stokoe, 1972.

5 We want to point out here that with regard to the linear/sequential versus simultaneous organization the difference between sign languages and spoken languages is one of degree: spoken languages too show simultaneous patterning, for example, tones in tone languages and intonation in other languages. More recently co-speech gesture is also increasingly considered to be an integrated part of spoken language communication. And of course, not all elements of a signed utterance are produced at the same time.

6 The locative relation between the cat and the fence is expressed by the position of the hands with respect to each other, while the relation between the fence and the house is expressed by the position of the hands with respect to the body of the signer (and this is not clearly visible in the picture: the hands are in a horizontal plane on the left side of the signer).

7 Manual signs are represented here as English *glosses*: words (more or less closely) representing the meaning of the sign. Pointing signs are glossed "Ps". The lengthened production of a sign is indicated by a line following its gloss. // indicates a clause boundary.

8 We would like to refer the reader to Vermeerbergen, Leeson, & Crasborn (2007) for a collection of papers dealing with different aspects of simultaneity across a wide range of sign languages.

9 When at a later age there is still no or insufficiently accessible linguistic input these home sign systems continue to develop and become "emerging sign languages" (Fusellier-Souza, 2004, 2006).

10 It may be pointed out, however, that in his 1960 book on ASL, Stokoe did propose some sign language specific terminology such as chereme and cherology instead of phoneme and phonology. However, his attempt did not meet with much approval.

11 As is the case for INVITE in Flemish Sign Language (as well as for GIVE in Flemish Sign Language), ASL GIVE includes a linear movement which may be altered to relate the verb to one or more of its arguments.

12 Already in 1977, DeMatteo argued in favor of an analysis of classifier constructions as visual analog reconstructions of an actual scene. However, as noted by Liddell (2003b, pp. 202–203):
DeMatteo's (1977) analysis appeared at a time when linguists were demonstrating remarkable parallels between signed and spoken language grammars. By doing so, they were amassing evidence that ASL should be treated as a real human language. Given this progress in finding linguistic structure underlying ASL utterances, DeMatteo's proposal did not receive a welcome reception. After all, his claim was that the underlying representation of a classifier predicate cannot be analyzed as one would analyze a spoken language utterance (i.e., as combinations of morphemes). It would follow, then, that ASL was different in an important way from spoken languages.

13 "Nonlinguistic" meaning "traditionally regarded as not being linguistic in nature."

Further reading

Anible, B. (2020). Iconicity in American sign language–English translation recognition. *Language and Cognition, 12*(1), 138–163.

Quer, J., & Steinbach, M. (2019). Handling sign language data: The impact of modality. *Frontiers in Psychology, 10*, 483.

Slonimska, A., Özyürek, A., & Capirci, O. (2020). The role of iconicity and simultaneity for efficient communication: The case of Italian Sign Language (LIS). *Cognition, 200*, 104246.

References

Akach, P., Demey, E., Matabane, E., Van Herreweghe, M., & Vermeerbergen, M. (2009). What is South African sign language? What is the South African Deaf community? In B. Brock-Utne & I. Skattum (Eds.), *Languages and education in Africa. A comparative and transdisciplinary analysis* (pp. 333–347). Oxford, UK: Symposium Books.

Allan, K. (1977). Classifiers. *Language, 53*(2), 285–311.

Baker, C., & Cokely, D. (1980). *American Sign Language: A teacher's resource text on grammar and culture.* Silver Spring, MD: T.J. Publishers.

Bergman, B. (1983). Verbs and adjectives: Morphological processes in Swedish Sign Language. In J. Kyle & B. Woll (Eds.), *Language in sign: An international perspective on sign language* (pp. 3–9). London, UK: Croom Helm.

Beukeleers, I. (2020). *On the role of eye gaze in Flemish Sign Language: A multifocal eye-tracking study on the phenomena of online turn processing and depicting.* Doctoral Dissertation. KU Leuven, Leuven.

Beukeleers, I., & Vermeerbergen, M. (2022). Show me what you've b/seen: A brief history of depiction. *Frontiers in Psychology, 13*, 808814. https://doi.org/10.3389/fpsyg.2022.808814

Bos, H. (1990). Person and location marking in SLN: Some implications of a spatially expressed syntactic system. In S. Prillwitz, & T.Vollhaber (Eds.), *Current trends in European sign language research. Proceedings of the third European congress on sign language research* (pp. 231–248). Hamburg, Germany: Signum Press.
Boyes Braem, P.,& Sutton-Spence, R. (Eds.) (2001). *The hands are the head of the mouth: The mouth as articulator in sign languages*. Hamburg, Germany: Signum Press.
Brennan, M. (1990). *Word formation in British Sign Language*. Stockholm, Sweden: University of Stockholm.
Cogill-Koez, D. (2000). Signed language classifier predicates: Linguistic structures or schematic visual representation? *Sign Language and Linguistics, 3*(2), 153–207.
Cormier, K., Fox, N., Woll, B., Zisserman, A., Camgöz, N. C., & Bowden, R. (2019). ExTOL: Automatic recognition of British Sign Language using the BSL corpus. Paper presented at the 6th Workshop on Sign Language Translation and Avatar Technology (SLTAT 2019).
Crasborn, O. (2001). *Phonetic implementation of phonological categories in Sign Language of the Netherlands*. Utrecht, The Netherlands: LOT.
Crystal, D. (1999). *The penguin dictionary of language*. London, UK: Penguin.
de Vos, C. (2012). *Sign-spatiality in Kata Kolok: How a village sign language of Bali inscribes its signing space*. Doctoral Dissertation, Radboud University Nijmegen.
De Weerdt, K., Vanhecke, E., Van Herreweghe, M., & Vermeerbergen, M. (2003). *Op (onder)zoek naar de Vlaamse gebaren-schat. [In search of the Flemish sign lexicon]*. Gent, Belgium: Cultuur voor Doven.
DeMatteo, A. (1977). Visual imagery and visual analogues. In L. Friedman (Ed.), *On the other hand: Recent perspectives on American Sign Language* (pp. 109–136). New York: Academic Press,.
Demey, E. (2005). *Fonologie van de Vlaamse Gebarentaal: Distinctiviteit en iconiciteit* [*Phonology of Flemish Sign Language: Distinctivity and iconicity*] Doctoral dissertation, Ghent University, Ghent.
Demey, E., Van Herreweghe, M., & Vermeerbergen, M. (2008). Iconicity in sign languages. In K. Willems, & L. De Cuypere (Eds.), *Naturalness and iconicity in linguistics* (pp. 189–214) (Iconicity in Language and Literature Series, Vol. 7). Amsterdam, The Netherlands: Benjamins.
Deuchar, M. (1984). *British Sign Language*. London: Routledge & Kegan Paul.
Engberg-Pedersen, E. (1993). *Space in Danish Sign Language*. Hamburg, Germany: Signum-Verlag.
Ferrara, L. (2012). *A grammar of depiction: Exploring gesture and language in Australian Sign Language* (Auslan). Doctoral Dissertation, Macquarie University, Sydney.
Ferrara, L., & Hodge, G. (2018). Language as description, indication and depiction. *Frontiers in Psychology, 9*, 716. https://doi.org/10.3389/fpsyg.2018.00716
Fischer, S. (1974). Sign language and linguistic universals. In *Actes du colloque Franco-Allemand de grammaire transformationelle* (pp. 187–204). Tubingen, Germany: Niemeyer.
Frishberg, N. (1975). Arbitrariness and iconicity: Historical change in American Sign Language. *Language, 51*(3), 676–710.
Fusellier-Souza, I. (2004). *Sémiogenèse des langues des signes : Étude de langues des signes primaires (LSP) pratiquées par des sourds brésiliens. [Semiogenesis of sign languages: Study of primary sign languages used by Brazilian deaf people]*. Doctoral dissertation, Université Paris 8, Saint-Denis.
Fusellier-Souza, I. (2006). Emergence and development of signed languages: From diachronic ontogenesis to diachronic phylogenesis. *Sign Language Studies*, 7(1), 30–56.
Givón, T. (1979). From discourse to syntax: Grammar as a processing strategy. In T. Givón (Ed.), *Syntax and semantics, 12 Discourse and syntax* (pp. 81–109). New York: Academic Press.
Goldin-Meadow, S. (2003). *The resilience of language. What gesture creation in deaf children can tell us about how all children learn language*. New York: Psychology Press.
Hiddinga, A., & Crasborn, O. (2011). Signed languages and globalization. *Language in Society, 40*(4), 483–505.
Joachim, G. & Prillwitz, S. (Eds) (1993). *International Bibliography of Sign Language*. Hamburg: Signum Verlag Books.
Johnston, T. (1989). Auslan. *The sign language of the Australian deaf community*. Doctoral dissertation, University of Sydney, Sydney.
Johnston, T. (1991). Spatial syntax and spatial semantics in the inflection of signs for the marking of person and location in Auslan. *International Journal of Sign Linguistics, 2*(1), 29–62.
Johnston, T. (2004). W(h)ither the deaf community? Population, genetics, and the future of Australian Sign Language. *American Annals of the Deaf, 148*(5), 358–375.
Johnston, T. (2010). From archive to corpus: Transcription and annotation in the creation of signed language corpora. *International Journal of Corpus Linguistics, 15*(1), 106–131.
Klima, E. S., & Bellugi, U. (1979). *The signs of language*. Cambridge, MA: Harvard University Press.
Krausneker, V., & Schügerl, S. (2022). Avatars for sign languages: Best practice from the perspective of deaf users. In A. Petz, E.-J. Hoogerwerf & K. Mavrou (Eds.), *ICCHP-AAATE 2022. Open access compendium "assistive technology, accessibility and (e)inclusion* (pp. 156–164). Linz: Association ICCHP.

Kyle, J. G., & Woll, B. (1985). *Sign language. The study of deaf people and their language*. Cambridge, UK: Cambridge University Press.
Labov, W. (1972). *Sociolinguistic patterns*. Philadelphia: University of Pennsylvania Press.
Lane, H. (1977). *The wild boy of Aveyron*. London, UK: Allen & Unwin.
Leeson, L., & Saeed, J. I. (2007). Conceptual blending and the windowing of attention in simultaneous constructions in Irish Sign Language. In M. Vermeerbergen, L. Leeson & O. Crasborn (Eds.), *Simultaneity in signed languages: Form and function* (pp. 55–72). Amsterdam, The Netherlands: John Benjamins.
Liddell, S. K. (1990). Four functions of a locus: Reexamining the structure of space in ASL. In C. Lucas (Ed.), *Sign language research: Theoretical issues* (pp. 176–198). Washington DC: Gallaudet University Press.
Liddell, S. K. (2003a). *Grammar, gesture, and meaning in American sign language*. Cambridge, UK: Cambridge University Press.
Liddell, S. K. (2003b). Sources of meaning in ASL classifier predicates. In K. Emmorey (Ed.), *Perspectives on classifier constructions in sign languages* (pp. 199–220). Mahwah, NJ: Lawrence Erlbaum Associates.
Liddell, S. K., & Metzger, M. (1998). Gesture in sign language discourse. *Journal of Pragmatics, 30*(6), 657–697.
Liddell, S. K., Vogt-Svendsen, M., & Bergman, B. (2007). A crosslinguistic comparison of buoys. Evidence from American, Norwegian, and Swedish sign language. In M. Vermeerbergen, L. Leeson & O. Crasborn (Eds.), *Simultaneity in signed languages: Form and function* (pp. 187–216). Amsterdam, The Netherlands: John Benjamins.
Loncke, F. (1983). Fonologische aspecten van gebaren [Phonological aspects of signs]. In B. T. Tervoort (Ed.), *Hand over hand: Nieuwe inzichten in de communicatie van de doven*. [Hand over hand: New insights in the communication of deaf people] (pp. 105–119). Muiderberg, The Netherlands: Coutinho.
Loncke, F. (1990). *Modaliteitsinvloed op taalstructuur en taalverwerving in gebarencommunicatie. [Modality influence on language structure and language acquisition]*. Unpublished doctoral dissertation. Vrije Universiteit Brussel.
Lucas, C., Bayley, R., & Valli, C. (2001). *Sociolinguistic variation in American sign language*. Washington, DC: Gallaudet University Press.
McDonald, B. (1982). *Aspects of the American Sign Language predicate system*. Unpublished doctoral dissertation. University of Buffalo.
McDonald, J. C., Wolfe, R., Efthimiou, E., Fontinea, E., Picron, F., Van Landuyt, D., … Krausneker, V. (2021). The myth of signing avatars. In Proceedings of the 18th Biennial Machine Translation Summit, Virtual, August 16–20, 2021 (pp. 33–42).
Metzger, M. (1995). Constructed dialogue and constructed action in American sign language. In C. Lucas (Ed.), *Sociolinguistics in deaf communities* (pp. 255–271). Washington DC: Gallaudet University Press,.
Meurant, L., Sinte, A., Van Herreweghe, M., & Vermeerbergen, M. (2013). Sign language research, uses and practices: A Belgian perspective. In L. Meurant, A. Sinte, M. Van Herreweghe & M. Vermeerbergen (Eds.). *Sign language research, uses and practices: Crossing views on theoretical and applied sign language linguistics* (pp. 1–14). Boston/Berlin: De Gruyter Mouton & Nijmegen: Ishara Press.
Mylander, C., & Goldin-Meadow, S. (1991). Home sign systems in deaf children: The development of morphology without a conventional language model. In P. Siple & S. D. Fischer (Eds.), *Theoretical issues in sign language research, Vol. 2: Psychology* (pp. 41–63). Chicago: University of Chicago Press.
Nyst, V. (2007). Simultaneous constructions in Adamorobe Sign Language (Ghana). In M. Vermeerbergen, L. Leeson, & O. Crasborn (Eds.), *Simultaneity in signed languages: Form and function* (pp. 127–145). Amsterdam, The Netherlands: John Benjamins.
Ochs, E. (1979). Planned and unplanned discourse. In T. Givón (Ed.), *Syntax and semantics. Vol 12 Discourse and syntax* (pp. 51–80). New York: Academic Press.
Ong, W. (1982). *Orality and literacy: The technologizing of the word*. London, UK: Methuen.
Padden, C. (1988a). *Interaction of morphology and syntax in American Sign Language*. New York, NY: Garland Publishing.
Padden, C. (1988b). Grammatical theory and signed languages. In F. Newmeyer (Ed.), *Linguistics: The Cambridge survey, 2* (pp. 250 –266). Cambridge, UK: Cambridge University Press,.
Perniss, P., Pfau, R., & Steinbach, M. (2007). Can't you see the difference? Sources of variation in sign language structure. In P. Perniss, R. Pfau & M. Steinbach (Eds.), *Visible variation. Comparative studies on sign language structure* (pp. 1–34). Berlin, Germany: Mouton de Gruyter.
Perniss, P. (2007). Locative functions of simultaneous perspective constructions. In M. Vermeerbergen & L. Leeson (Eds.), & 0. Crasborn (Eds.). *Simultaneity in signed languages: Form and function* (pp. 27–54). Amsterdam, The Netherlands: John Benjamins.
Pizzuto, E. (1986). The verb system of Italian Sign Language. In B. Tervoort (Ed.), *Signs of life. Proceedings of the second European congress on sign language research*. Amsterdam: The Netherlands Foundation for the deaf and Hearing-Impaired Child and the Insitute for General Linguistics of the University of Amsterdam.
Poizner, H., Klima, E., & Bellugi, U. (1987). *What the hands reveal about the brain*. Cambridge, MA: MIT Press.

Raičević Bajić, D., Nikolić, G., Gordić, M., Mouvet, K., & Van Herreweghe, M. (2021). Language attitudes towards Serbian Sign Language and experiences with deaf education in Serbia. *DiGeSt: Journal of Diversity and Gender Studies, 8*(1), 76–90.

Richie, R., Yang, C., & Coppola, M. (2014). Modeling the emergence of lexicons in homesign systems. *Topics in Cognitive Science, 6*(1), 183–195.

Rissanen, T. (1986). The basic structure of Finnish Sign Language. In B. Tervoort (Ed.), *Signs of life: Proceedings of the second European congress on sign language research*. Amsterdam: The Netherlands Foundation for the deaf and Hearing-Impaired Child and the Institute for General Linguistics of the University of Amsterdam.

Rosenstock, R., & Napier, J. (Eds.) (2016). *International Sign. Linguistic, usage, and status issues*. Washington, DC:: Gallaudet University Press.

Safar, J. (2020). *A comparative study ofYucatec Maya Sign Languages*. Doctoral Dissertation, Stockholm University, Stockholm.

Safar, J., & de Vos, C. (2022). The role of common ground in repair sequences in Balinese homesign. Paper presented at ISGS 2022, Chicago, IL.

Sallandre, M.-A. (2007). Simultaneity in French Sign Language discourse. In M. Vermeerbergen & L. Leeson (Eds.), & 0. Crasborn (Eds.). *Simultaneity in signed languages: Form and function* (pp. 187–216). Amsterdam, The Netherlands: John Benjamins.

Schein, J. (1989). *At home among strangers. Exploring the deaf community in the United States*. Washington, DC: Gallaudet University Press.

Schembri, A. (2001). *Issues in the analysis of polycomponential verbs in Australian Sign Language* (Auslan) [Doctoral Dissertation]. Sydney: University of Sydney.

Schembri, A. (2003). Rethinking "classifiers" in signed languages. In K. Emmorey (Ed.), *Perspectives on classifier constructions in sign languages* (pp. 3–34). Mahwah, NJ: Lawrence Erlbaum Associates.

Schembri, A., Jones, C., & Burnham, D. (2005). Comparing action gestures and classifier verbs of motion: Evidence from Australian Sign Language, Taiwan Sign Language, and non-signers' gestures without speech. *Journal of Deaf Studies and Deaf Education, 10*(3), 272–290.

Schuit, J. (2014). *Sign of the arctic. Typological aspects of Inuit Sign Language*. Doctoral Dissertation, University of Amsterdam, Amsterdam.

Siple, P. (1982). Signed language and linguistic theory. In L. Obler & L. Menn (Eds.), *Exceptional language & linguistics* (pp. 313–333). New York: Academic Press.

Stokoe, W. (1960). *Sign language structure. An outline of the visual communication system of the American Deaf.* Silver Spring, MD: Linstok Press.

Stokoe, W. (1972). *Semiotics and human sign languages*. The Hague, The Netherlands: Mouton.

Supalla, T. (1978). Morphology of verbs of motion and location in American Sign Language. In F. Caccamise & D. Hicks (Eds.), *American sign language in a bilingual, bicultural context. Proceedings of the second national symposium on sign language research and teaching* (pp. 27–46). Coronado, CA: National Association of the Deaf.

Supalla, T. (1982). *Structure and acquisition of verbs of motion and location in American Sign Language*. Doctoral dissertation, University of California, San Diego.

Taub, S. (2001). *Language from the body. Iconicity and metaphor in American Sign Language*. Cambridge, UK: Cambridge University Press.

Tervoort, B. (1953). *Structurele analyse van visueel taalgebruik binnen een groep dove kinderen. [Structural analysis of visual language use within a group of deaf children]*. Amsterdam, The Netherlands: Noord-Hollandse uitgevers maatschappij.

Van der Kooij, Els (2002). *Phonological categories in Sign Language of the Netherlands. The role of phonetic implementation and iconicity*. Utrecht, The Netherlands: LOT.

Van Herreweghe, M. (1995). *De Vlaams-Belgische Gebarentaal: Een eerste verkenning, [Flemish-Belgian Sign Language. An initial exploration]*. Gent, Belgium: Academia Press.

Van Herreweghe, M., & Vermeerbergen, M. (2004). Flemish Sign Language: Some risks of codification. In M. Van Herreweghe & M. Vermeerbergen (Eds.), *To the lexicon and beyond: Sociolinguistics in European deaf communities* (pp. 111–137). Washington, DC: Gallaudet University Press.

Van Herreweghe, M., & Vermeerbergen, M. (2008). Referent tracking in two unrelated sign languages and in home sign systems. Paper presented at the 30th Annual Meeting of the German Linguistics Society DGfS, Bamberg.

Van Herreweghe, M., & Vermeerbergen, M. (2010). Deaf perspectives on communicative practices in South Africa: Institutional language policies in educational settings. *Text and Talk, 30*(2), 125–144.

Van Herreweghe, M., & Vermeerbergen, M. (2012). Data collection. In R. Pfau, M. Steinbach & B. Woll (Eds.), *Sign language: An international handbook* (vol. 37, pp. 1023–1045). Berlin: De Gruyter.

Van Herreweghe, M., Vermeerbergen, M., Demey, E., De Durpel, H., Nyffels, H., & Verstraete, S. (2015). *Het corpus VGT. Een digitaal open access corpus van video's en annotaties van Vlaamse Gebarentaal, ontwikkeld aan de Universiteit Gent ism KU Leuven*. https://corpusvgt.be

Vermeerbergen, M. (1996). ROOD KOOL TIEN PERSOON IN. *Morfo-syntactische aspecten van gebarentaal. [RED CABBAGE TEN PERSON IN. Morphosyntactic aspects of sign language]* Doctoral dissertation. Vrije Universiteit Brussel.

Vermeerbergen, M. (1997). Grammaticale aspecten van de Vlaams-Belgische Gebarentaal. [Grammatical aspects of Flemish-Belgian Sign Language]. *Gentbrugge, Belgium: Cultuur voor doven.*

Vermeerbergen, M. (1998). The use of space in Flemish Sign Language. In S. Santi, I. Guaïtella, C. Cavé, & G. Konopczynski (Eds.), *Oralité et Gestualité [Orality and gestuality]* (pp. 131–136). Paris, France: L'Harmattan.

Vermeerbergen, M. (2006). Past and current trends in sign language research. *Language and Communication, 26*(2), 168–192.

Vermeerbergen, M., & Demey, E. (2007). Sign + gesture = speech + gesture? Comparing aspects of simultaneity in Flemish Sign Language to instances of concurrent speech and gesture. In M. Vermeerbergen, L. Leeson, & 0. Crasborn (Eds.). *Simultaneity in signed languages: Form and function* (pp. 257–282). Amsterdam, The Netherlands: John Benjamins.

Vermeerbergen, M., & Nilsson, A.-L. (2018). Introduction. In A. Aarssen, R. Genis & E. Van der Veken (Eds.). *A bibliography of sign languages, 2008-2017* (pp. 9–31). Leiden: Brill.

Vermeerbergen, M., Leeson, L., & Crasborn, O. (Eds.) (2007). *Simultaneity in signed languages: Form and function.* Amsterdam, The Netherlands: John Benjamins

Vermeerbergen, M., Van Herreweghe, M., Akach, P., & Matabane, E. (2007). Constituent order in Flemish Sign Language and South African Sign Language. A cross-linguistic study. In *Sign Language and Linguistics, 10*(1), 25–54.

Woll, B. (2003). Modality, universality, and the similarities among sign languages: An historical perspective. In A. Baker, B. van den Bogaerde & O. Crasborn (Eds.), *Cross-linguistic perspectives in sign language research* (pp. 17–27). Hamburg, Germany: Signum.

World Federation of the Deaf (2018). WFD and WASLI statement of use of signing avatars. Retrieved from https://wfdeaf.org/news/resources/wfd-wasli-statement-use-signing-avatars/

Zeshan, U. (Ed.) (2006a). *Negatives and interrogatives across signed languages.* Nijmegen, The Netherlands: Ishara Press.

Zeshan, U. (2006b). Negative and interrogative constructions in sign languages: A case study in sign language typology. In U. Zeshan (Ed.), *Negatives and interrogatives across signed languages* (pp. 28–68). Nijmegen, The Netherlands: Ishara Press.

Zeshan, U., & de Vos, C. (2012). *Sign languages in village communities: Anthropological and linguistic insights.* Berlin, Boston: De Gruyter Mouton.

Zeshan, U., & Perniss, P. (Eds.) (2008). *Possessive and existential constructions in sign languages.* Nijmegen, The Netherlands: Ishara Press.

34
PSYCHOLINGUISTICS AND AUGMENTATIVE AND ALTERNATIVE COMMUNICATION

Filip Loncke and Emma Willis

Introduction

The psycholinguistic relevance of augmentative and alternative communication

The term *Augmentative and Alternative Communication* (AAC) refers to the methods, tools, and theories of the use of non-standard linguistic and non-linguistic forms of communication by and with individuals without or with limited functional speech. Standard linguistic forms of communication are speech/listening and writing/reading. We call them standard forms because they appear to be the most effective linguistic forms for typical language users.

Non-linguistic forms of communication can include natural gestures and pictographic representation. AAC also includes the use of object communication, manual signs, pictographic symbols, and speech generating devices with varying degrees of technological complexity. AAC is meant to compensate and/or replace communication forms that are less accessible for individuals with limitations that can be of a neuromotor, cognitive, and/or developmental nature.

AAC is an applied discipline. This means that it uses information from other fields and sciences. Disciplines that inform our understanding of AAC (i.e., how AAC should be practiced) include developmental psychology, psycholinguistics, educational sciences, rehabilitation science, sociology, neuropsychology, computer sciences, and perception psychology. One could also consider AAC to be a translational discipline as it tries to find ways how developments and discoveries in other fields find their way to improvements in the communication and interaction by individuals with limited functional speech. While AAC has emerged primarily as an applied educational and therapeutic field, it offers a unique opportunity to observe the effect of non-typical conditions on linguistic production and reception. For example, the rate of message generating is significantly usually significantly slower than is the case in typical speech communication. This basic fact may influence internal planning of an utterance by the sender as well as processing strategies by the receiver.

Historical backgrounds of the psycholinguistics of augmentative and alternative communication

It is probably no co-incidence that AAC started to develop in the 1970s. In that period psycholinguistic research had developed an interest in the flexibility of the human language capacity. The discovery that sign languages of deaf communities are linguistically full-fledged languages (Klima & Bellugi, 1979) stands as an example of this renewed and refreshed look at communication and

DOI: 10.4324/9781003204213-39

language (Vermeerbergen & Van Herreweghen, this volume). Although speech is clearly and without doubt the preferred modality for direct linguistic communication, other modalities function as alternatives.

The discovery of language in the gestural modality also led to exploring the transitions and the dividing lines between non-linguistic communication and linguistic communication. This is exemplified in the description of gestures versus manual signs: gesturing is typically a phenomenon that is co-occurring with speech (McNeill & Duncan, this volume) with which it has a dynamic relation. In many instances, gestures do not have any meaning as such but serve as a psychomotor underpinning – or reinforcement – of the speech process. Gesturing can move to the foreground by assuming meaning through the use of conventionalized or semi-conventionalized forms. Deaf children of hearing parents with limited contact to sign language users have been described to develop "home signs," gestures that have taken on a meaning that is understood by a limited number of individuals with whom the person interacts. For example, pointing to the chin may be sign that refers to a specific person (e.g., a neighbor) who has a small beard (Vermeerbergen & Van Herreweghen, this volume). Gestures can also become more prevalent in situations of processing difficulties in speech. One example is lexical access. An increasing number of studies shows that gesturing facilitates in cases of word finding (Ravizza, 2003), possibly as a result of both iconic facilitation and neurological activation.

As linguistic processing in the spoken modality becomes less available, gesturing tends to overtake language role. Goldin-Meadow's (1998) research has shown how gesture assumes linguistic value in instances where a developing person does not have sufficient exposure to spoken language. Gestural applications within AAC capitalize on this principle. Gesturing and manual signing have been forms of AAC since the earliest days and remain in use until today. Since the 1970s sign language has regained recognition as full-fledged languages and manual signs are consider being powerful linguistic elements that will foster communication. In the past, educators often feared that signing would impede the development of natural speech. Although some of these fears still subsist, manual signing is now often used as a complement, a replacement, or as a trigger for speech. The (in)compatibility hypothesis will be discussed later in this chapter.

This early development coincided with an increased interest in presymbolic and pre-linguistic communication. What are the mechanisms and dynamics between birth and the first expressed word that move a child into the use of a symbolic system? Several indications point to the fact that gestures provide a bridge between primarily sensorimotor functioning in the first months of life toward symbolic conceptualization and language use. A major part of AAC-practice is focused on facilitating communication through the systematic use of external symbols or referents, as well as attempts to help transition a person to symbolic and/or linguistic communication. For example, low functioning children with autism may be taught to use an object (e.g., a cereal box) as a tangible referent for breakfast. The object becomes part of a ritualized routine sequence in which it assumes the function of a signal or a pre-symbol. Systematic use of pre-symbols is reinforced and shaped toward genuine symbolic and linguistic functioning. This type of intervention usually is part of a concept of trainability through stages toward internalized symbol use (Taylor & Iacono, 2003).

In short, the breakthrough of AAC practice has been facilitated by the recognition that non-speech modalities can be communicative and linguistic. The potential of modalities other than speech was also explored through the use of graphic symbols or pictures that were used on a communication board (Archer, 1977) to function as lexical elements, replacing spoken words or spoken messages. The development of synthetic and computer-generated speech in the past thirty years made it clear the natural articulation can be substituted by machine-generated speech.

It is impossible to draw a strict distinction between AAC and standard forms of communication. As electronic forms of communication have become common, the distinction between standard communication and AAC tends to become less clear. For example, cell phone technology and email communication are increasingly used as assistive devices or techniques. Applied applications are reflected in identifying the aids that will help a person and his/her communication environment to interact.

Compatibility or incompatibility of modalities

This discussion that started from the beginning of public education for deaf children would continue through the 20th century and into the present day. Few debates throughout the history of special education have stirred up as many emotions and divided individuals into vehemently opposing camps as this dispute. Why is that? One explanation is that this issue is much more than a mere continuum of opinion about what would be the better method to teach deaf children. It touches on a deeper, underlying difference of opinion about how the human mind works. It essentially comes down to assuming or rejecting the compatibility (or incompatibility) between modalities. Does manual signing prevent the development of speech—or, on the contrary, could it be beneficial for speech articulation? In other words, the question is whether the human mind tends to limit primary language expression to one single modality (speech or language), one sensory mode (visual or auditory), and one linguistic structure (spoken language grammar or sign language grammar), or whether no such limitations exist.

These opposing visions about the compatibility between natural speech and an alternative mode of communication have not remained limited to educational decisions in deaf education. A similar concern has risen in the field of augmentative and alternative communication. Educators and parents often fear that the introduction of a non-speech form of communication will be detrimental for the acquisition of the spoken language and especially of natural speech. In their 2005 article, Romski and Sevcik characterized this fear as one of the five persistent myths about AAC.

The incompatibility hypothesis

What exactly are the concerns of those who believe the use of AAC might have a negative impact on natural speech and language use? The following underlying issues and assumptions are the main concerns:

(1) The use of AAC could lead to less overall effort by the user as he or she may lose the drive and the motivation to communicate through natural speech.
(2) The use of AAC will lead to the use of messages that structurally deviate from English (or whichever the spoken language is that is used in the environment of the person).

What are the underlying assumptions in this AAC debate? It is related to

(a) A view on the compatibility between natural speech and the non-speech modalities: is there a mutual inhibitory effect, a facilitation effect, or none of the above?
(b) A view on trans-modal interference: will the syntactical structure of one modality (e.g., manual signing) be transposed to the syntactical structure of English (or the spoken language of the user)?
(c) A view on total mental lexical storage capacity across modalities (will symbolic capacity have to be distributed over modalities?).
(d) A view on the motivational effects of the use of one modality toward the other: will effective communication in one modality encourage or discourage the user to make efforts in the speech modality?

Some clues may come from the existing knowledge on bilingualism, multimodality, and motivation toward the use of communication modalities.

The microgenesis of an AAC utterance

Levelt's blueprint of the speaker and its variants has been the most prevalent model of the microgenesis of speech, a description of components and processes that are active in running speech. It shows that speakers fluently and speedily perform the following mental operations in a coordinated (partially sequential, partially parallel) way: lexical selection, syntactic planning, and phonological encoding, while monitoring their own speech. The questions now are: can the same fluency, speed, and effortlessness be achieved in AAC?

Can the AAC user be as fast, or is the nature of the use of AAC such that nobody can achieve the same speed? One of the key processes in speech is lexical access: the ability of speakers to find a word in their internal lexicon and activate it. Is word finding in AAC as easy or is it more burdensome. If it is inherently more difficult, then AAC users are at a disadvantage in their conversations. Is lexical access in AAC still an exclusively internal process?

How are lexical elements stored in the head of the AAC user? Lexical search in AAC is often partially an external process: the AAC user needs to decide which words they want to express (i.e., they need to find them in their brain) and then find the symbol on their device. Chris Klein, an AAC user, describes how he feels he must manage two lexicons, an internal lexicon (in his head) and an external lexicon (in the device) (personal communication).

Lexicon size, lexical development, lexical search, and AAC

Lexical development is an important topic in AAC as this is amongst the central features of language acquisition. Building a vocabulary, or a lexicon, is important to our increasing abilities to express the variety of wants, needs, and thoughts we have in our daily lives. There are continuing discussions in how best to support lexical development for individuals who use AAC. The only vocabulary the user has access to are those words that are included on their device in that moment – there is less flexibility in being able to use new words on the fly.

So why exactly is there decreased flexibility when it comes to the lexicon on AAC devices for individuals acquiring language? In typical language development, the lexicon can grow much more sporadically through life experiences and exposure. When a word has been added to the internal lexicon, an individual who communicates through a verbal modality is much more readily able to use that word at any point in the future. However, for an individual who uses AAC, whose communicative lexicon exists externally from themselves, is not as readily able to use a spontaneously learned word to communicate with communicative partner.

It is difficult to perfectly mirror natural lexical development because of the external nature of the lexicon on AAC. Because of this, lexical development currently relies more on *teaching* to expand the lexicon. Many AAC-systems could add new vocabulary on the fly; however, the user will still have to learn the location of this icon to be able to use it in the future.

Lexicon size

Selecting a word in the lexicon implies activation of the lexical item, but at the same time one must reject competitors. Despite an enormous lexicon, most typical language users experience only problems sporadically because of one competitor blocking the real word to "come out" (this is one of the explanations of the "tip of the tongue" phenomenon).

But AAC users may be in a different situation. Could it be that processing will be facilitated if fewer choices are available? Some educators believe that for some (certainly not all) AAC users, "less can be more." A well-selected small lexicon might be a help.

The sender's lexical selection (i.e., the decision which symbols to use) can be facilitated in a few ways. Within AAC, this is often done by presenting the person with a pre-selected and limited number of choices, such as the graphic symbols on communication boards. Symbols also need to be made mentally accessible, i.e., the user needs to be able to retain them and decode them. Often this is done by simply offering visual (rather than auditory). Symbols are easier to access when they are easier to be decoded, e.g., when the user can recognize which parts they are made of. Lexical searches can also be made easier. The better symbols are organized, the easier and faster their retrieval will be. This is obviously the case for any typical lexical access (Levelt, Roelofs, & Meyer, 1999). It is certainly also true for access in AAC. This can be done by spatially organizing symbols in a meaningful way on a communication board. For example, nouns and verbs can be assigned specific areas on the display, which would be a linguistic-categorical organization. Often, communication displays are organized in a semantic way (e.g., food items are placed together). If the person is literate, a keyboard (or letter board) is the best possible lay out: as in typing, the person constructs the words with the letters, sometimes aided by word prediction.

Limiting the lexical selection – the core words approach

The rationale for the use of core words is partially based on the observation that users need to have easy access to words – communication needs to go fast, and a limitation of the number of words may make it easier to "find" the words that you are looking for. This leads to the question how many words you should have in a device (or in a lexicon) to keep working with them manageable. Instead of having to choose between enormous multitudes of symbols that are unmanageable or a limited number that will cause frustration, some educators suggest that the solution lies in the *combinatoriality principle*: to create words and phrases by combining elements of the selection set. One clear example is the use of the alphabetic principle. Literate AAC-users often employ letter boards or devices, which have a typical computer keyboard. By pointing to the letters of the alphabet, the user can form words. When you type the message on a device, it appears on a screen and it can be activated into speech output. This is one reason why literacy needs to be a prime objective in intervention and education of AAC-users. Literacy will empower and increase the possibilities for expression. However, some AAC-users may not be able to become literate. Baker (2012), a linguist, developed an icon-based combinatorial system, called Minspeak. Though the system was originally intended for literate users for rate enhancement, it can be a significant help for non-reading people. Minspeak, installed on communication devices from Prentke Romich Company, is a system that allows users to combine a limited number of graphic symbols to generate a range of meanings. The user does not have to remember the location of hundreds of graphic symbols. Instead, the user simply needs to know the combination code to create the words or phrases.

The Minspeak® code has been developed by Baker (2012). Minspeak is a combination of symbols (called icons) that, for the most part, do not represent direct meanings. Using a combination code generates meanings. For example, for "I love coffee" you will need to hit the "I" icon twice, then the LOVE icon (illustrating a mother holding a baby), followed by the MR. ACTION MAN, verb icon (illustrating worker with bucket and hammer), and finally the DRINK button, followed by the COFFEE button in the activity row. This system may be less intuitive at first sight, but it allows the user to stay away from navigation and proceed faster.

From a cognitive processing point of view, navigation requires time and memory (knowing where the message is stored). Icon sequencing (such as Minspeak®) requires the person initially to remember the "code." Proponents of the Minspeak system believe that this is mainly a process of motor learning and motor memory – comparable to what individuals "know" about a computer keyboard. Many keyboard users may not be able to answer if you ask them where is the "g" on the keyboard, but they may be fast and flawless when they have to type a word that contains a "g."

Motor planning

A number of authors (Center for AAC and Autism, 2009) have suggested that "language acquisition through motor planning" (or LAMP) is what is needed. Producing symbol sequences could be compared with the complex motor patterns of natural speech (Browman & Goldstein, 1990), except that augmented communicators are using symbols to construct messages. Fluent communication on an AAC device is facilitated by learned and repetitive patterns that have become automatized. Constructing messages using the LAMP approach is also an assembly process that requires the communicator to sequence a series of choices and actions. In many ways, this is similar to the morphological and syntactical planning and execution in typical speech, although it can have its specific characteristics in AAC. For example, the use of Minspeak® requires a unique serial combination of icons (icon sequencing), an operation that does not have a direct equivalent in typical speech production. The production of syntactic sequences is a different process in AAC because the assembly and production process typically take more time, which can lead to a discrepancy between planning time (thinking of the utterance to express) and execution time. One challenge and a matter of debate of the system is its learnability by young children (Drager & Light, 2010). In order to study how the system is best acquired by young children, a methodology will be needed that focuses on the acquisition of coding rules, not single words and meanings.

It is clear that memory and automaticity play a role in fast accessing symbols, words, and phrases and in executing their production. What kind of memory? Thistle and Wilkinson (2013) analyzed the cognitive operations involved in typical AAC device use and reasoned that seemingly fluent use of an AAC system must rely on short working-memory processes. They identify a number of special challenges or heightened memory risks for AAC users such as (1) locating symbols in the device or board, (2) coordinating attention across AAC display, partner, and topic, (3) inconsistent carry-over to new device, (4) loss of track of message during production.

Effects of the rate of communication

Baker (in Musselwhite, 1987) suggested that the actual production of a communication utterance is dependent on a number of factors. His so-called *ergonomic principle* states

$$\frac{\textit{Motivation to say something}\left(\textit{use a method or device}\right)}{\left(\textit{Cognitive, linguistic and Physical Effort}\right)\left(\textit{Needed time}\right)}$$

This equation needs to equal 1 or be larger than 1. It is an attempt to grasp the psychological "worthwhileness" of the effort to speak. Baker (personal communication, 2019) meant this to be a universal statement, that is, in fact, not specific or limited to AAC. If a typical speaker is asked a question but feels too tired to answer it, they may say "do you mind if I tell you about that later?" This general principle, that one (1) needs to be in the mood, (2) have the time, (3) find it worth the effort, is formalized in the equation. It has the advantage that it provides an explanation for a number of observations and issues in AAC, including why AAC users often do not seem to take initiative to communicate, or why there is often so much device or method abandonment. One of the challenges for AAC developers and professionals is to find way to minimize the effort it takes to produce an utterance.

The rate of typical speech (up to 200 words a minute) is generally assumed to be commensurate with comfortable information expression and reception. As discussed in the previous chapter, the use of channels other than natural speech, as happens in AAC, holds the risk to slow down the speed of conveying strings of words. The slowdown of the utterance speed is a major issue of concern regarding AAC. The lack of speed can have an impact on:

1) The interaction of cognitive planning and communicative expression. If communication production slows down the communication partners could start to struggle with short-term memory problems. During speech production of an utterance, speakers know and remember how they start a sentence until the end of the utterance. In typical speech, fragments of the utterance are prepared in the head of the speaker and kept in a "syntactic buffer" waiting to be processed by the phonological encoder, i.e., the part of the message generator that plans the actual speech articulation. In the case of AAC, the waiting time of the planned utterance parts is likely to be increased. The speed of speaking needs to keep pace with the speaker's unfolding of thought. The frustration that this causes may be one of the reasons (not the only one) why there is AAC-device and AAC-system abandonment, i.e. the phenomenon that AAC-users and their partners cease to use the system.
2) The trade-off between invested effort (cognitively, linguistically, and physically) and result: because augmented speech requires more effort, speakers may tend to simplify and economize linguistic structure, e.g., dropping morphological endings, limiting the message to key words and symbols.
3) The willingness and ability of communication partners to participate in the communication exchange: a decreased rate of communication affects all communication partners. Listening to a person who uses AAC may require more attention, patience, and interaction discipline (e.g., waiting your turn) than is needed in communication with a typical speaker.

Another psycholinguistic issue: iconicity

Iconicity is the term used to indicate that a symbol bears a physical resemblance to its referent. Klima and Bellugi (1979) propose two degrees of iconicity: transparency and translucency. A symbol is transparent if the meaning is readily available to the observer. Translucency refers to situations where the observer can understand the link with the referent once this connection is made explicit. For example, the meaning of the American Sign Language (ASL) sign BALL (curving the hands around an imaginary ball) is likely to be understood, while the sign GIRL (tip of extended thumb slides down the cheek) can only be grasped after one explains that it refers to the string of the bonnet that girls and women used to wear in the late 18th century in France (the time of heightened interest in signing, and a time that signs were recorded onto books).

There are a few considerations for creating iconicity in symbols. One of the first considerations is the age of the target-user. Are these symbols intended for use by a child gaining language? Or are these symbols intended for use by an adult who has already acquired language? How to achieve iconicity in a symbol is different if the target is a child or an adult. The key reason behind this is the type of memory that each population uses to gain meaning from the symbol. Children rely on their episodic memory to gain meaning.

This means that children rely heavily on drawing from their memory of situations and events that they have experienced before. This is a distinct difference from adults, who rely significantly more on semantic memory to apply meaning to symbols. Semantic memory is recalling the meaning associated with different words, concepts, etc. It does not require recalling a specific event to derive meaning.

A second consideration is the disorder area of the target user. Is it intended for an adult without language impairment, but loss of verbal speech? Or perhaps an adult with either a sudden or gradual loss of language skill? How to best design an icon for adults with varying acquired language disorders is an important future direction for AAC research.

Conclusion

Besides the clinical and educational possibilities of AAC, it also provides us with an exciting intellectual and scientific perspective. AAC explores the flexibility and the resilience that humans have with their communication. When the standard forms of communication are not available, humans can elevate other modalities and re-configure them to establish valuable communication and to realize their human potential.

Further reading

Dukhovny, E., & Gahl, S. (2014). Manual motor-plan similarity affects lexical recall on a speech-generating device: Implications for AAC users. *Journal of Communication Disorders*, *48*, 52–60.

Dukhovny, E., & Thistle, J. (2017). An exploration of motor learning concepts relevant to use of speech-generating devices. *Assistive Technology*, *13*, 1–7.

Icht, M., Levine-Sternberg, Y., & Mama, Y. (2020). Visual and auditory verbal long-term memory in individuals who rely on augmentative and alternative communication. *AAC: Augmentative and Alternative Communication*, *36*(4), 238–248. https://doi.org/10.1080/07434618.2020.1852443

Loncke, F. (2021). *Augmentative and alternative communication. Models and applications* (2nd ed.). San Diego: Plural Publishing. ISBN13: 978-1-63550-122-3

Wagner, B. T., Shaffer, L. A., Ivanson, O. A., & Jones, J. A. (2021). Assessing working memory capacity through picture span and feature binding with visual-graphic symbols during a visual search task with typical children and adults. *AAC: Augmentative and Alternative Communication*, *37*(1), 39–51. https://doi.org/10.1080/07434618.2021.1879932

References

Archer, L. A. (1977). Blissymbolics: A nonverbal communication system. *Journal of Speech and Hearing Disorders*, *42*(4), 568–579.

Baker, B. (2012). *How Minspeak® allows for independent communication by giving anyone access to core vocabulary. Message posted to* http://www.minspeak.com/CoreVocabulary.php

Browman, C. P., & Goldstein, L. (1990). Gestural specification using dynamically-defined articulatory structures. *Journal of Phonetics*, *18*(3), 299–320.

Center for AAC and Autism (2009). What is LAMP? (language acquisition through motor planning). Retrieved from http://www.aacandautism.com/lamp

Drager, K. D. R., & Light, J. C. (2010). A comparison of the performance of 5-year-old children with typical development using iconic encoding in AAC systems with and without icon prediction on a fixed display. *Augmentative and Alternative Communication*, *26*(1), 12–20. https://doi.org/10.3109/07434610903561464

Goldin-Meadow, S. (1998). The development of gesture and speech as an integrated system. In J. M. Iverson, S. Goldin-Meadow, J. M. Iverson & S. Goldin-Meadow (Eds.), *The nature and functions of gesture in children's communication* (pp. 29–42). San Francisco: Jossey-Bass.

Klima, E. S., & Bellugi, U. (1979). *The signs of language*. Cambridge, MA: Harvard University Press.

Levelt, W. J. M., Roelofs, A., & Meyer, A. S. (1999). A theory of lexical access in speech production. *Behavioral and Brain Sciences*, *22*(1), 1–38.

Musselwhite, C. (1987). *What is Minspeak?* Pittsburgh: Semantic Compaction Systems.

Ravizza, S. (2003). Movement and lexical access: Do noniconic gestures aid in retrieval? *Psychonomic Bulletin and Review*, *10*(3), 610–615.

Romski, M., & Sevcik, R. A. (2005). Augmentative communication and early intervention: Myths and realities. *Infants and Young Children*, *18*(3), 174–185.

Taylor, R., & Iacono, T. (2003). AAC and scripting activities to facilitate communication and play. *Advances in Speech-Language Pathology*, *5*(2), 79–93.

Thistle, J., & Wilkinson, K. M. (2013). Working memory demands of aided augmentative and alternative communication for individuals with developmental disabilities. *Augmentative and Alternative Communication*, *29*(3), 235-245. doi:10.3109/07434618.2013.815800

35
EPILOGUE
Applying psycholinguistic theories to conversation data in the context of dementia

Jackie Guendouzi

Introduction

Since the publication of the first edition of this collection, students have frequently asked how the theories presented in this book apply to everyday communication or clinical practice. In addition to the questions from my students, caregivers frequently ask me to explain why their family member is so confused when they speak to them, and ask why the person with dementia does not understand simple requests or instructions. There is often an assumption, on the part of the neurotypical caregiver, that the person with dementia's responses are random errors; a result of psychosis caused by the disease. However, if we carefully review transcripts of conversations with people with dementia in relation to theories of cognition and language processing we can explain many of the communication patterns that arise in the interactions.

Psycholinguistic theories are more commonly associated with experimental research or model building (see Chapter 8). With some exceptions (e.g., Guendouzi, 2013; Guendouzi & Pate, 2014; Wray, 2002) psycholinguistic approaches are less likely to be used when discussing analysis of conversational data. Traditionally, qualitative researchers have relied on socio-pragmatic approaches and analytical methods associated with discourse analysis (e.g., Brown & Levinson, 1987; Goffman, 1987; Goodwin, 1981, 2017; Sacks, Schegloff, & Jefferson, 1974; Schiffrin, 1994). Without doubt, such research extended our understanding of the features and patterns of talk that arise in the context of dementia (e.g., Davis, 2005; Guendouzi & Davis, 2013; Guendouzi & Muller, 2006; Hamilton, 1994; Orange, Lubinski, & Higginbottom, 1996; Ramanathan, 1997). It has also assisted in the development of clinical approaches that support person-centered care strategies (Burshnic & Bourgeois, 2020; Coelho, Cherney & Shadden, 2023). This chapter will draw on ideas associated with relevance theory (Sperber & Wilson, 2002), cognitive schemas (Evans, 2019), and formulaic or familiar language (see Chapter 12; Van Lancker-Sidtis, 2011; Sidtis, 2022) to discuss conversations involving people with dementia, within a connectionist paradigm (Dell & Kittredge, 2011; see also Chapter 8). The goal is to illustrate how psycholinguistic theories can add to our understanding of everyday communication in the context of acquired communication disorders.

Language processing, social interaction, and cognition

The brain stores a vast amount of information, which logically suggests the need to develop a language processing system (LPS) that allows us to reduce or bypass the need for item-by-item linear processing. The cognitive mechanisms that store and organize information are created from stimuli

DOI: 10.4324/9781003204213-40

and inputs experienced over our lifespan. When interacting with others we draw on both acquired social knowledge and underlying bio-cognitive mechanisms to support our LPS. For example, when engaged in a conversation we need to pay attention to the context of the speech event, focus on the incoming information (both verbal and non-verbal), hold this information in our working memory, and then match or assimilate it to information already stored in our long-term memories. However, memory is not like a filing cabinet that stores things in folders side by side, nor is the information necessarily stored in close physical proximity within the brain. It is more likely, as connectionist models (see also Chapter 8) suggest, that information with semantic connections (e.g., "birthday" and "cake") or words that are frequently utilized together (e.g., the words "good" and "morning") become strongly linked in our neural networks. Walker (Chapter 8) notes that the activation of feature units across semantic networks requires activation at several layers and is bidirectional. It is likely that, over our lifetime, the LPS develops the equivalent of procedural algorithms (through strongly linked neural connections) that allow us to process information more efficiently.

Accordingly, we rely on a range of bio-cognitive resources including focus, attention, inhibition, working memory, and declarative memory to support the use of information in our daily interactions. Disruption or damage to any part of the system can result in a communication breakdown: for example, if we fail to pay attention to an interlocutor's tone of voice, we may not recognize they were being sarcastic and interpret their remark literally. Alternatively, if we cannot hold the components of a grammatically complex utterance in our working memory before the memory trace fades or decays (Cowan, 2011) we may not be able to understand the propositional content of the remark. By processing the various stimuli around us (e.g., verbal message, other people, background noises, visual distracters, etc.) the LPS identifies which specific indices in the situation are relevant to the intended message of our interlocutor. In the case of neuro-typical people, we can generally assume that their cognitive resources are functioning at a near optimal level; therefore, conversations typically flow smoothly and communication breakdowns are less frequent. In the case of neuro diverse people, disruption to the LPS results in interactions that often breakdown or become confused.

Cognitive schemas: contextualizing interactions

Early psycholinguistic researchers (e.g., Bartlett, 1932; Minsky, 1975) suggested that we organize and store knowledge in cognitive/semantic schemas. Guendouzi (2022) suggested that a schema is a cognitive mechanism that allows us to frame an interaction within a recognizable context. It is generated when a sufficient number of semantically associated nodes in the LPS network are activated in response to particular interactional inputs/stimuli. Semantic associations can be shared across social groups that is, we may all have a similar schema for a visit to the grocery store. However, over time we create semantic associations that are more individual to our specific life experiences, thus our schemas may not always match. For an excellent and thorough discussion of frame and schema semantics, see Evans's work on cognitive linguistics (2019). Schema for the purpose of this discussion is a term that refers to a cognitive mechanism that functions within the LPS to frame interactions, or to put it another way schemas help us to recognize the context of our interactions and thus help us draw the appropriate inferences from our conversations. For example, if I am in an environment where I see shopping carts, shelves with boxes, cans, and checkout registrars, the items and their semantic associations activate a generic schema related to a grocery store. From a cognitive perspective, this can be considered lower level processing; a process that needs to happen reflexively at rapid speeds so is likely more of a procedural task. Once the incoming information has been integrated and an appropriate schema activated, the LPS then establishes the reason, or *relevance* for why we might be in this situation. That is, the LPS needs to focus on organizing and assembling information that will help to produce the appropriate behaviors (verbal and non-verbal) that we should now engage in to achieve our interactional goals.

Relevance theory

Relevance theory (RT) is an "inferential approach to pragmatics which situates itself within cognitive science" (Jagoe, 2015, p. 55). Sperber and Wilson (2002) conceptualized RT as a cognitive processing mechanism that acted to filter the multiple stimuli we encounter when engaged in an interaction. RT posits a processing mechanism that operates to narrow our focus of attention on what is meaningful or important in a particular situation, inhibiting information that is irrelevant in order to reduce the interactional demands on our cognitive resources. As noted elsewhere (Guendouzi, 2013; Guendouzi & Savage, 2017) RT suggests that relevance is determined by predictability and/or a "best fit" scenario. Sperber and Wilson (2002) argued RT represents a "hard-wired" behavior that develops over time. Piaget (1977) suggested when we encounter new information, our cognitive processing systems attempt to assimilate or match the incoming information into existing schemas, particularly if the information shares semantic, linguistic, experiential or functional associations. From a connectionist perspective, relevance is achieved at the point, at which a sufficient number of units in a network are activated (at all levels) to create a condition of relevance that will allow us to correctly interpret the situation.

However, it is important to be aware that even in the case of neuro-typical people, this process may misfire and miscommunications can arise. The incoming stimuli/inputs may activate semantic schemas that are idiosyncratic; the inputs may trigger highly individual associations resulting in very different interpretations of meaning. For example, on passing a sign on building advertising that you could "Book Parties Here" a friend of the author commented, "I didn't know they held book parties." The company organized corporate parties and most of us would have interpreted this sign the way it was intended, as an advertisement to encourage potential customers to book their parties at this location. However, the friend was an avid reader, and spent most of their time in bookstores or reading. She most frequently came across or used the word "book" in its' role as a noun. Therefore, her LPS activated units associated with the word "book" that had developed strong links based on her own life experience. This example of an inference error is something we have probably all experienced at some time, but it demonstrates how the interpretation of a simple sentence can become ambiguous. Additionally, it serves to remind us that standardized clinical assessments using picture or word card stimuli may activate information in an individual's LPS resulting in an unusual response that seems incorrect but overlaps with an associated schema relevant to the client's own life.

Sperber and Wilson suggested that contextual details are "the set of premises used in interpreting an utterance" and represent a "subset of the hearer's assumptions about the world" (1986/1995, p. 15). Additionally, communication routines or "scripts" (Schank & Abelson, 1977) associated with particular situations become strongly linked to a schema. I have used the example of a hospital schema elsewhere (Guendouzi, 2022); however, it is a useful example to illustrate the story a caregiver recalled when talking about the behaviors of her mother, a person with dementia. A generic hospital schema might include representations of the concepts and words for people and things associated with a healthcare institution (e.g., nurses, doctors, medical equipment, medical procedures, medications, etc.). Communication routines (scripts) associated with a hospital schema might include questions such as "how are you feeling today" or "I just need to examine your chest." When faced with a visual cue (e.g., person with scrubs and a stethoscope) the LPS activates other stored items associated with a hospital visit and we then recognize the request "I need to listen to your chest, can you lift your shirt" as both relevant and appropriate.

However, a person with dementia's assumptions about a situation may be based on fragmented or mismatched schemas that is, schemas where higher-level information is not fully activated so they misinterpret a situation. During interviews with caregivers of people with dementia, a daughter described an incident involving her mother who had recently moved to a nursing home. The mother did not recognize a new male care assistant who had come to help her get dressed; all she saw was an unknown man who appeared to be taking off her nightclothes. The woman perceived the care assistant as an intruder to her bedroom and she became very agitated and combative. Staff informed the daughter that her mother's aggressive behavior was a general symptom of her dementia. However, the woman's reaction was not random or psychotic behavior but rather the result of a misinterpretation caused by weakened cognitive resources and a degraded LPS. The woman's LPS appeared to stall at a lower level therefore the information available to create an appropriate cognitive schema was not fully activated (or connected) to higher processing levels needed to complete her interpretation of the situation (Guendouzi & Savage, 2017). It is likely that the cognitive processing effort required to create a schema that provided the correct interpretation of the event was too great. A processing task that would require the woman recalling the following, who the care assistant was, the duties of his professional role, his relationship to her, and why she might need assistance dressing.

Familiar language: formulaic expressions

Formulaic expressions are another feature of language that may play a role in the LPS to reduce or minimize the cognitive processing load. Familiar language (Sidtis, 2022) has become an active area of linguistic study. Familiar language was neglected for a long period due to a "myopic perspective that … formulas, idioms and conventional expressions…take the form of a mundane look-up list" (Van Lancker Sidtis, 2011, p. 247) and were of little interest to researchers examining grammar. One of the problems with the study of familiar language is that, at times, it is hard to pin down what exactly constitute formulaic expressions. There is a general consensus that familiar language is comprised of formulaic expressions that carry meaning as a whole unit such as idioms or proverbs, but there has been some discussion over non-propositional expressions such as *how are you today.* Van Lancker Sidtis suggests the "best operational definition … is an exclusionary one" that applies "non-novel as the selection criteria" (2011, p. 248). The feature formulaic expressions have in common is that the words contained in the string do not require online processing from a set of grammatical rules. Formulaic expressions are likely stored as whole units; their canonical form reflects "conventionalized meaning and conditions of use" and contains specific words, word order and a "set intonation contour" (Van Lancker Sidtis, 2011, p. 248).

Formulaic expressions often carry a meaning that is much greater than the sum of the literal words. Sidtis (2022) has recently extended her work to include formulaic expressions, lexical bundles, and collocations as examples that fall under the umbrella term familiar language. It is also possible to include several types of language used in everyday conversations as formulaic expressions, the most obvious being proverbs and idioms (e.g., *don't look a gift horse in the mouth*) and metaphor (e.g., *all the world's a stage*). We would also include frequently used formulaic expressions such as "how are you doing?" or "lovely day today," and idiosyncratic formulaic expressions, that is, word strings used frequently by individual speakers but not necessarily used by the speech community in general. In addition, adverbial tags that act as politeness markers in requests or commands (e.g., "could you possibly," "if you don't mind") are also examples of familiar language. Thus, as is the case with semantic schemas, formulaic expressions can be either generic (e.g., phrases we all use such as "good morning") or more specific to a sub-culture or speech community. As will be discussed in example three, individuals may also use a particular statement so frequently it comes to function as an idiosyncratic formulaic expression.

The data: conversations in the context of dementia

The examples discussed below are from a database of interactions that involved conversations between the researcher and people with dementia of the Alzheimer's type. The first two conversations took place in a nursing home in the United Kingdom and were audio-recorded. The third conversation took place in the community speech-hearing clinic located at Southeastern Louisiana University and was video-recorded. IRB permissions were obtained before recordings commenced. The author, who carried out the interactions, transcribed all recordings. A colleague of JG and two graduate assistants reviewed copies of transcripts and recordings for accuracy and consensus of interpretation.

Example one: conversation with a neuro-typical person

The LPS of a person with dementia reflects a system that is not functioning at an optimal performance level and therefore, errors and miscommunication frequently arise. Identifying linguistic production errors (e.g., misuse of vocabulary, unfinished sentences etc.) in people with acquired neurogenic disorders is somewhat easier than recognizing misaligned cognitive schemas. Consider the conversation in extract one below where the author (JG), visited an elderly woman, named Ann, who had no cognitive impairment. Ann was in the hospital following a minor routine surgery. The previous week JG had been introduced to Ann as a researcher from the nearby university who was investigating lifespan issues. In this interaction, the conversational moves follow a predictable pattern of routine speech acts that would be expected in the context of a hospital visit. Comments in *italics* refer to the speech acts present in each turn.

Extract 1

1. JG: Hi remember me? I came last week (*politeness token – greeting*)
2. Ann: Oh yes hi, it's J the researcher from the university, isn't it? (*appropriate response – greeting with acknowledgement of JG's identity*)
3. JG: So how is it going today? How are you feeling? (*appropriate request for information/politeness token*)
4. Ann: Well it's a bit sore but not too bad I can manage (*appropriate response/ politeness token*)
5. JG: So what did you have for lunch then? (*request for information triggered by B's empty plate*)
6. Ann: Oh they gave us steak and salad not too bad (*appropriate response with comment*)

Example two: conversation with a person with dementia

However, when we compare the conversation in extract one to a similar speech event involving JG and Flo, a woman with dementia in a nursing home, there is a noticeable difference. Comments in square brackets indicate the potential interpretation of Flo's responses if associated with generic schema relating to education.

Extract 2

1. JG: Hi remember me? I came last week (*politeness token – greeting*)
2. Flo: Oh the book? (*Inappropriate response*) [Educational schema: acknowledging researcher's identity, *attempt at greeting?*]
3. JG: So how is it going today? How are you feeling? (*Appropriate request for information, politeness token, trying to remain on topic*)
4. Flo: But I didn't, it was yesterday (looks closely at JG) (*inappropriate response*) [*potential acknowledgement* of meeting a week previously]
5. JG: So what did you have for lunch then? (*Topic redirection the topic to daily events*)
6. Flo: It wasn't good (*Potentially appropriate reply*) [Acknowledgment of educational schema reference to JG's work and the book]
7. JG: The lunch wasn't good? (*Request for clarification – a assumes Flo is referring to the topic of lunch*)

8. Flo: The points I didn't get the points with the writing? (*Inappropriate response to lunch topic*) [Educational schema, appears to be implying she didn't get the points for her work, or contribution to book]
9. JG: Well you did OK with your writing (*A has decided to go with B's conversational topic line*)

When compared to extract one, the conversation in extract two might appear confused until we consider it in relation to the notion of an incomplete pattern for a cognitive schema that represents JG specifically. Flo had been told during their first meeting that JG was a college professor writing a book about retired people living in assisted care. Flo's responses suggest that she has retained some of this information. JG's appearance in the room appears to activate some words associated with a more generic schema of education rather than remembering her actual name and identity. Although JG did not make the connection during the first interaction, as references to words and items related to teaching, education, or the process of writing began to occur more frequently it became clear these were not random utterances, Flo's LPS was attempting to create a condition of relevance for their conversation. Flo's declarative memory and partially activated schemas provided words and ideas from her past childhood experiences of education that included completing homework and references to items associated with school or writing. See Guendouzi (2022) for a further example of Flo's use of an educational schema in conversations with JG.

Although it is difficult to confirm the meaning of Flo's contributions definitively, it is notable that they were associated to JG's profession as an academic, and the actual purpose of JG's visit to Flo (researcher investigating language in the elderly). Once an incomplete schema is activated, it may provide information that has enough connections to the current situation that the search for the "best fit" match shuts down, thus requiring less processing effort. Although in Flo's case she could not actually specify JG's name or professional role there was a close enough association in her LPS to switch off the search for further information. This suggests that the LPS of people with dementia is still attempting to function and create a state in the system where conditions needed for relevance occur. On this occasion the condition of relevance was satisfied because there was "a great enough *positive effect* to offset" any further "*cognitive processing effort*" (Guendouzi, 2013, p. 42). That is, JG began to acknowledge and validate any of Flo's remarks that related to education. For example, on another occasion when Flo mentioned poetry and asked if "the poem was finished," JG, replied with "yes it was good" and this appeared to lift Flo's spirits and she became more engaged in the ensuing conversation.

It is probable that the LPS activates generic features of incoming stimuli first. Once all the necessary information is activated the LPS produces the most likely interpretation. In the case of Flo, it appeared that her LPS was not able to activate and process information beyond the level needed to create a generic schema related to education. Higher-level activation processes, that would normally help retrieve information necessary to identify JG, by her name, job title, or place of work, do not appear to be functioning or connecting. A question that is less clear is whether there enough evidence to suggest that, at some level, Flo understood whom she was talking to, and simply could not access or connect all the information units in her LPS needed to complete the pattern. Thus, were her responses a compensatory strategy or simply an artifact of automatic processing hardwired into the LPS? What the data does suggest, is that the LPS continues to try and create relevance and will stop this process if there are sufficient units activated to make a connection, albeit a tenuous association.

Formulaic expressions in the case of dementia

In Sidtis's (2022) investigation of familiar language in the context of neurological disorders, she notes the case of a man with dementia who was able to remember and articulate lengthy portions of poetry. When asked how he did this, he responded that he "hadn't really tried" to memorize poetry but "the lines stuck like burrs, inscribing themselves in his memory" (2022, p. 234). Sidtis suggests that because "subcortical structures remain functional … implying implicit memory" (2022, p. 234) people with dementia are able to better remember formulaic expressions. Bridges and Sidtis (2013) found that individuals with dementia "used significantly more formulaic expressions than healthy controls" (Sidtis, 2022, p. 236). Researchers have also noted that social phrases remain intact even in the later stages of Alzheimer's disease (Bayles et al., 2004; Kempler et al., 1995). In contrast, under experimental conditions it has been shown that people with dementia perform poorly on tasks involving formulaic language such as idioms, metaphors, and proverbs (Amanzio, Geminiani, Leotta, & Cappa, 2008; Papagno, Lucchelli, Muggia, and Rizzo, 2003).

Based on findings in empirical studies, some researchers have advised caregivers to avoid the use of figurative language because it requires "pragmatic decoding and abstract thinking" (Wray, 2011, p. 605). For example, Papagno et al. (2003) suggested that inadequate suppression of literal meanings and/or extraneous extra linguistic factors might play a role in people with dementia's performance during proverb-based tasks. Similarly, Lindholm and Wray found that people with dementia's performance on proverbs in an interactional setting in Finland was below what was expected given that proverbs represent a subset of formulaic language (Lindholm & Wray, 2011). On the other hand, the ability to produce some forms of formulaic politeness tokens in conversational contexts may act as a compensatory strategy for people with dementia (Guendouzi & Müller, 2001). In some studies, researchers suggested that formulaic language might be of use in rehabilitation programs (e.g., Arkin & Mahendra, 2001; Chapman, Ulatowska, Franklin, Shobe, & Thompson, 1997). The occurrence of formulaic language in the talk of people with dementia has been well-documented (Davis, 2005; Davis & Bernstein, 2005; Davis & Maclagan, 2010; Guendouzi & Müller, 2006; Hamilton, 1994; Orange & Purves, 1996; Sidtis, 2022).

Citing the work of Nicholas, Obler, Albert, and Helm-Estabrooks (1985), Sidtis notes that the "speech of persons with Alzheimer's disease is generally described as plentiful in high frequency words and empty of propositional information" (2022, p. 233). She suggests that formulaic expressions may be preserved because they are "routinized verbal motor gestures based in social contexts" (2022, p. 2333) and thus rely on cognitive mechanisms associated with procedural memory. Procedural memory tasks are associated with the sub-cortical levels of the brain therefore, as there is less damage to basal ganglia in Alzheimer's dementia, formulaic expressions may be less affected than language with more complex propositional content. However, this raises an interesting question – do people with dementia in the early stages overtly use formulaic expressions to help them convey propositions that are more complex? Example three below considers this question in relation to a man with dementia who repeatedly used the formulaic expression "my wife's a driver."

Example three: the propositional flexibility of formulaic expressions

Ed, a man with dementia, had developed the use of a formulaic expression "my wife's a driver" that he frequently used within his conversations. His wife confirmed that he had used the expression before he had developed dementia but it had started to occur far more frequently as the dementia progressed. Typically, Ed used this formulaic expression when he was unable to respond to a question or when he appeared to be having word finding difficulties (Guendouzi & Müller, 2006). In this particular conversation, the formulaic expression appears to stand in for at least five separate propositional statements [PS].

Extract 3

1. Clinician: Are you going anywhere today?
2. Ed: My wife's a driver [PS1: I can't go out, my wife is at work and she has the car]

Extract 4

1. Clinician: What about this weekend what are you doing?
2. Ed: My wife's a driver [PS2: I don't know, my wife will make that decision]

Extract 5

1. Clinician: Are you going to see if you can get more of that medication?
2. Ed: My wife's a driver [PS3: my wife will take care of that]

Extract 6

1. Clinician: It's Friday so where are you going for lunch?
2. Ed: My wife's a driver [PS4: My wife will decide where we go]

Extract 5

1. Clinician: What did you watch on TV yesterday?
2. Ed: My wife's a driver [PS5: My wife chooses what we watch on TV]

Ed had worked at an engineering plant until he developed dementia; he had made most of the decisions in the couple's lives – now his wife was the person who made financial decisions, drove them around, and went to work. In the above interactions, Ed appeared to use this particular formulaic expression when asked questions about his well-being or what he was going to do or had been doing. His response may have been a literal reference to the fact that his wife was now the only person who could drive their car (Ed's license had been revoked). However, taken in conjunction with Ed's non-verbal behaviors, whether intentional or not, this formulaic expression served as a means to respond to JG's questions. Based on the number of times used, it appeared easy for Ed (or his LPS) to retrieve and produce this formulaic expression in conversations. Thus, it allowed Ed to express several different propositions without the LPS expending a great deal of cognitive energy. Although whether Ed was using this particular formulaic expression, as a compensatory strategy is more difficult to say, it may have been a predictable outcome of a disrupted LPS. At that point, in his life, an appropriate response to the researcher's questions would have involved some reference to Ed's wife due to his inability to drive, go the pharmacy, or use the TV control system, highlighting her role as a caregiver. His LPS did produce information that was related to the researcher's questions; it did not, however, give an explicit or detailed response nor one that allowed for the development of the topic.

Conclusions: why psycholinguistic approaches

This chapter focused on highlighting how psycholinguistic theories may help to explain some of the effects of disruption to the LPS in the context of dementia. To summarize, the LPS including cognitive systems such as memory, attention, and focus, helps us recognize and interpret the linguistic messages we encounter in our daily interactions. Through reference to schemas that frame the context, and the establishment of relevance, neuro-typical interlocutors will generally infer the correct meaning of an utterance and produce an appropriate response. The LPS integrates incoming information/stimuli by activating and linking associated information nodes across our semantic networks, this information is stored through the strength of connections created by frequent co-occurrence. Disruption to any part of the LPS results in less than optimal processing capacity, making it difficult to access, retrieve, or combine the necessary information units required to produce coherent propositional language. Examination of naturally occurring interactions involving people with dementia suggests that some of the communication issues associated with this disease result from LPS mechanisms that although disrupted, are attempting to function in a predictable manner and do their job. As the disease progresses and the brain loses grey and white matter (and therefore neurons) activation levels and the ability to transmit information across networks is greatly impeded.

In my own research, there is evidence that supports ideas that have emerged from work on relevance theory, cognitive schemas, and theories of familiar and formulaic language. When my students ask, why do we need to learn these theories? What relevance do they have to clinical practice? I typically respond by saying, that without reference to these theories, it would be very difficult to explain to a caregiver why Flo randomly inserted words related to education into our conversations, or why Ed continually answered questions with the formulaic expression "my wife's a driver." Once we had identified this linguistic pattern in Ed's conversations, we could predict this utterance as being his likely response to particular types of questions. Similarly, when talking to Flo I began to pay attention to particular words or references that occurred during our conversations and look for associations or collocations that might suggest schemas that gave clues as to how she was contextualizing our interactions. In the case of both Ed and Flo, discerning the irregular patterns in their communication assisted with developing strategies for interacting with them on a regular basis.

Examining conversational data from the perspective of psycholinguistic theories also raises important questions about how we clinically assess the language abilities of people with acquired neurogenic disorders. People with dementia may perform very poorly on a cognitive screener or picture naming task yet in the early stages manage their daily conversations relatively well. In interviews with the author, caregivers often reported that a family member was able to "hide" their dementia for some time by adjusting their ways of talking (e.g., greater use of formulaic expressions or politeness tokens).

Future directions

Psycholinguistic theories that attempt to model how the LPS functions could also help us predict what is likely to happen if the LPS breaks down. Constructing language-processing models was a major part of early computational linguistic research. For example, computerized models attempted to calculate and predict the probability of which particular language strings a computer would generate when different sequences of words or other information was entered into the system. This type of research played a role in the later development of automated chat and phone helplines and eventually led to computerized assistants such as Alexa or Siri. If we take this approach with conversational data in the context of dementia, it is more likely, that we will be able achieve translatable outcomes. Research that attempts to predict what will happen in the context of specific interactional routines should be carried out. In the first instance, we can use 'naturally' occurring conversational databases and then compare the patterns that emerge in the interactions to models of language processing. For example, one potential finding that emerged from the data discussed here, is that the LPS relies on multiple connections and higher level processing to activate the schemas that allow us to contextualize our interactions and adjust our communication behaviors accordingly. However, if as in the case of Flo, a person with dementia is unable to completely process all the pieces, the contributions they make are not necessarily random errors rather, their LPS produces fragments of a schema that are related in some way to the conversation at hand.

There is less need to collect data to identify the errors people with dementia are making; the features of language in dementia have been well documented. Rather we need to think in terms of whether we can train care-partners (professional and familial) to become more aware of the effects of a disrupted LPS. Researchers such as the contributors to this collection, play a valuable role in giving us the tools to explore the functional dynamics of conversations involving people with dementia. However, there is also a need for more translatable research that helps to develop better management plans and reassess how we measure communication abilities in people with dementia. In order to create person-centered care for people with dementia (Sabat, 2001), we need to work continually towards improving and extending communication-training programs for care-partners. In order, to succeed in doing this, we need to do more than just describe the features of conversations, we also need to use theories and models to hypothesize and predict situations in which communication is most likely to break down. This will enable us to develop communication programs that not only use augmentative technology, social technology (e.g., social robots), and importantly linguistic strategies but also programs based on what we have learned from psycholinguistic and cognitive theories.

Further reading

Guendouzi, J. (2014). Who am I talking to anyway?: Relevance theory in the case of dementia. In B. Davis & J. Guendouzi (Eds.), *Pragmatics in dementia discourse: Applications and issues* (pp. 29–54). Cambridge: Cambridge Scholars Publishing.

Guendouzi, J., & Pate (2014). Interactional resources and cognitive resources in dementia: A perspective from Politeness Theory. In R. Schrauf & N. Mueller (Eds.), *Dialogue and dementia: Cognitive and communicative resources for engagement*. London: Blackwell.

References

Amanzio, M., Geminiani, G., Leotta, D., & Cappa, S. (2008). Metaphor comprehension in Alzheimer's disease: Novelty matters. *Brain and Language, 2107*(1), 1–10. https://doi.org/10.1016/j.bandl.2007.08.003

Arkin, S., & Mahendra, N. (2001). Discourse analysis of Alzheimer's patients before and after intervention: Methodology and outcomes. *Aphasiology, 15*(6), 533–569.

Bartlett, F. C. (1932). *Remembering: A study in experimental and social psychology*. Cambridge, UK: Cambridge University Press.

Bayles, K. A., Tomoeda, C. K., McKnight, P. E., Estabrooks, N. H., & Hawley, J. H. (2004). *Seminars in Speech and Language, 25*(4), 335–347.

Bridges, A. & Van Lancker Sidtis, D. (2013). Formulaic language in Alzheimer's Disease. *Aphasiology*, 27(7), 799–810.

Brown, P., & Levinson, S. C. (1987). *Politeness: Some universals in language usage*. Cambridge University Press.

Burshnic, V., & Bourgeois, M. (2020). A seat at the table: Supporting persons with severe dementia in cmmunicating their preferences, *Clinical Gerontologist*, 1–14.

Chapman, S. B., Ulatowska, H. K., Franklin, L. R., Shobe, A. E., Thompson, J. L., & McIntire, D. D. (1997) Proverb interpretation in fluent aphasia and Alzheimer's disease: Implications beyond abstract thinking. *Aphasiology, 11*, 337–350.

Coelho, C. A., Chereny, L. R., & Shadden, B. (2022). *Discourse Analysis in Adults with and without Communication Disorders: A Resource for Clinicians and Researchers*. San Diego, CA: Plural Publishers.

Cowan, N. (2011). Working memory and attention in language use. In J. Guendouzi, F. Loncke & M. Williams (Eds.), *Handbook of psycholinguistics & cognitive processes: Perspectives in communication disorders*. New York: Psychology Press.

Davis, B. H. (2005). *Alzheimer talk, text, and context*. New York: Palgrave MacMillan.

Davis, B. H., & Maclagan, M. (2018). Narrative and ageing: Exploring the range of narrative types in dementia conversation. *European Journal of English Studies, 22*(1), 76–90.

Davis, B. H., & Maclagan, M. (2013). Talking with Maureen: Pauses, extenders, and formulaic language in small stories and canonical narratives by a woman with dementia. In R. Schrauf & N. Müller (Eds.), *Dialogue and dementia: Cognitive and communicative engagement* (pp. 87–121). New York: Psychology Press.

Davis, B. H., & Maclagan, M. (2010). Pauses, placeholders and fillers in Alzheimer's discourse: Glueing relationships as impairment increases. In N. Amiridze, B. Davis & M. Maclagan (Eds.), *Fillers, pauses and placeholders in discourse and grammar* (pp. 189–215). Amsterdam: John Benjamins.

Dell, G., & Kittredge (2011). Connectionist models of aphasia and other language impairments. In J. Guendouzi, F. Loncke & M. Williams (Eds.), *Handbook of psycholinguistics & cognitive processes: Perspectives in communication disorders*. New York: Psychology Press.

Evans, V. (2019). *Cognitive linguistics: A complete guide*. Edinburgh: Edinburgh University Press.

Goodwin, C. (2017). *Co-Operative action*. Cambridge: Cambridge University Press.

Goodwin, C. (1981). *Conversational organization: Interaction between speakers and hearers*. London: Academic Press.

Guendouzi, J. (2022). What discourse analysis reveals about conversation & language processing in the context of dementia of the Alzheimer's type. In Cherney, Shadden & Coelho (Eds.), *Discourse analysis in adults with and without communication disorders: A resource for clinicians and researchers*. San Deigo, CA: Plural Publishers.

Guendouzi, J. (2013). 'So what's your name?': Relevance in dementia. In B. Davis & J. Guendouzi (Eds.), *Pragmatics in dementia discourse* (pp. 29–54). Newcastle upon Tyne: Cambridge Scholars Publishing.

Guendouzi, J., & Davis, B. (2013). Dementia discourse and pragmatics. In B. Davis & J. Guendouzi (Eds.), *Pragmatics in dementia discourse: Applications and issues*. Cambridge Scholars Publishing.

Guendouzi, J., & Müller, N. (2006). *Approaches to discourse in dementia*. Mahwah: Lawrence Erlbaum Associates.

Guendouzi, J., & Pate, A. (2014). Interactional and cognitive resources in dementia: Aperspective from politeness theory. In R. Schrauf & N. Müller (Eds.), *Dialogue and dementia: Cognitive and communicative resources for engagement* (pp. 121–146). London: Blackwell.

Guendouzi, J., & Savage, M. (2017). Alzheimer's disease. In L. Cummings (Ed.), *Research in clinical pragmatics*. New York: Springer.

Guendouzi, J., Davis, B., & Maclagan, M. (2015). Listening to narratives from people recently diagnosed with dementia. *Topics in Language Disorders. 35*(3), 237–257

Hamilton, H. E. (1994). *Conversations with an Alzheimer's patient: An interactional sociolinguistic study*. Cambridge: Cambridge University Press.

Jagoe, C. (2015). Collaborative meaning-making in delusional talk as a search for mutual manifestness: A relevance theory approach. *Journal of Interactional Research in Communication Disorders, 6*(1), 53–70.

Kempler, D., Andersen, E. S., & Henderson, V. W. (1995). Linguistic and attentional contributions to anomia in Alzheimer's disease. *Neuropsychiatry, Neuropsychology, and Behavioral Neurology, 8*(1), 33–37.

Lindholm, C., & Wray, A. 2011. Proverbs and formulaic sequences in the language of elderly people with dementia. *Dementia, 10*(4), 603–623.

Minsky, M. (1975). A framework for representing knowledge. In P. H. Winston (Ed.), *The psychology of computer vision* (pp. 211–277). New York: McGraw-Hill.

Nicholas, M., Obler, L. K., Albert, M. L., & Helm-Estabrooks, N. (1985) Empty speech in Alzheimer's disease and fluent aphasia. Journal of Speech Hearing Research(3), 405-410.

Orange, J. B., Lubinski, R. B., & Higginbotham, J. (1996). Conversational repair by individuals with dementia of the Alzheimer's type. *Journal of Speech and Hearing Research, 39*(4), 881–895.

Papagno, C., Lucchelli, F., Muggia, S., & Rizzo, S. (2003 November). Idiom comprehension in Alzheimer's disease: The role of the central executive. *Brain, 126*(11), 2419–2430. https://doi.org/10.1093/brain/awg243.

Piaget, J. (1977). The role of action in the development of thinking. In *Knowledge and development* (pp. 17–42). New York: Springer.

Ramanathan, V. (1997). *Alzheimer's discourse: Some sociolinguistic dimensions*. Mahwah, NJ: Lawrence Erlbaum.

Sabat, S.R. (2001). *The experience of Alzheimer's Disease: Life through a tangled veil*. Oxford, U.K.: Blackwell Publishers.

Sacks, H., Schegloff, E., & Jefferson, G. (1974). A simplest systematic for the organization of turn taking for conversation. *Language, 50*(4), 696–735.

Schank, R. C., & Abelson, R. (1977). *Scripts, plans, goals, and understanding*. Hillsdale: Erlbaum Associates.

Schiffrin, D. (1994). *Approaches to discourse: Language as social interaction*. Oxford: Blackwell.

Sperber, D., & Wilson, D. (2002). Pragmatics, modularity and mind-reading. *Mind and Language, 17*(1–2), 3–23.

Sidtis, D. (2022). *Foundations of Familiar Language: Formulaic expressions, Lexical Bundles, & Collocations at Work and Play*. Oxford: Wiley Blackwell.

Van Lancker-Sidtis, D. (2011). Formulaic expressions in mind and brain: Empirical studies and a dual-process model of language competence. In J. Guendouzi, F. Loncke & M. Williams (Eds.), *Handbook of psycholinguistics & cognitive processes: Perspectives in communication disorders*. New York: Taylor & Francis.

Wray, A. (2002). *Formulaic language and the lexicon*. Cambridge: Cambridge University Press. https://doi.org/10.1017/CBO9780511519772

INDEX

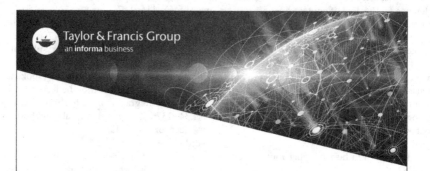